Global Perspectives in Cancer Care

T0177538

Global Perspectives in Cancer Care

Religion, Spirituality, and Cultural Diversity in Health and Healing

Edited by

MICHAEL SILBERMANN AND ANN BERGER

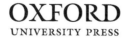

OXFORD
UNIVERSITY PRESS

OXFORD
UNIVERSITY PRESS

Oxford University Press is a department of the University of Oxford. It furthers
the University's objective of excellence in research, scholarship, and education
by publishing worldwide. Oxford is a registered trade mark of Oxford University
Press in the UK and certain other countries.

Published in the United States of America by Oxford University Press
198 Madison Avenue, New York, NY 10016, United States of America.

Library of Congress Cataloging-in-Publication Data
Names: Silbermann, Michael, 1935– editor. | Berger, Ann (Ann M.), editor.
Title: Global perspectives in cancer care : religion, spirituality,
and cultural diversity in health and healing / [edited by] Michael Silbermann and Ann Berger.
Description: New York, NY : Oxford University Press, [2022] |
Includes bibliographical references and index.
Identifiers: LCCN 2021033959 (print) | LCCN 2021033960 (ebook) |
ISBN 9780197551349 (paperback) | ISBN 9780197551363 (epub) |
ISBN 9780197551370 (online)
Subjects: MESH: Neoplasms—therapy | Neoplasms—psychology | Spiritual Therapies |
Spirituality | Cultural Diversity | Religion and Medicine
Classification: LCC RC263 (print) | LCC RC263 (ebook) | NLM QZ 266 |
DDC 362.19699/4—dc23
LC record available at https://lccn.loc.gov/2021033959
LC ebook record available at https://lccn.loc.gov/2021033960

DOI: 10.1093/med/9780197551349.001.0001

This material is not intended to be, and should not be considered, a substitute for medical or other professional
advice. Treatment for the conditions described in this material is highly dependent on the individual
circumstances. And, while this material is designed to offer accurate information with respect to the subject
matter covered and to be current as of the time it was written, research and knowledge about medical and health
issues is constantly evolving and dose schedules for medications are being revised continually, with new side
effects recognized and accounted for regularly. Readers must therefore always check the product information
and clinical procedures with the most up-to-date published product information and data sheets provided by
the manufacturers and the most recent codes of conduct and safety regulation. The publisher and the authors
make no representations or warranties to readers, express or implied, as to the accuracy or completeness of this
material. Without limiting the foregoing, the publisher and the authors make no representations or warranties as
to the accuracy or efficacy of the drug dosages mentioned in the material. The authors and the publisher do not
accept, and expressly disclaim, any responsibility for any liability, loss, or risk that may be claimed or incurred as a
consequence of the use and/or application of any of the contents of this material.

1 3 5 7 9 8 6 4 2

Printed by Marquis, Canada

This book is dedicated to all palliative caretakers and health professionals throughout the world, in recognition of the remarkable compassion, love, and devotion they have for their cancer patients—regardless of the patients' origins, beliefs, or socioeconomic backgrounds—striving to alleviate suffering, for individuals and for society as a whole. In memory of my parents, Herbert and Marga-Miriam, whom I miss so much.

For my wife, Gisela, my friend and love,

For my brothers, Jonathan and Gadi, my children, Anat and Ronit, and my three grandchildren, Eliya, Hila and Keren, with whom so much of life has been shared.

To my friend and mentor in medical diplomacy, Dr. Donna Shalala, former Secretary of U.S. Health and Human Services, who was catalytic in the MECC odyssey and from whom so much was learned
—Michael Silbermann, Middle East Cancer Consortium, Haifa, Israel

To my spouse and children: Carl, Stephen and Rebecca, whose love and support have made my work possible
—Ann Berger, National Institute of Health, Bethesda, MD, USA

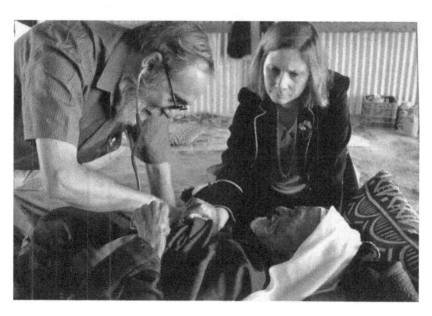

A visit of a palliative care team in a Bedouin tent in the Israeli Negev (desert)
Lt. Dr. Yehoram Zinger and Dr. Ann Berger

Contents

Foreword   xi
Preface   xiii
Contributors   xv

1. The Soul of Health Care: Caring for the Whole Person, United States   1
   Christina M. Puchalski

2. The How and Especially *Why* Clinicians Should Do a Spiritual
   Assessment, United States   10
   Joann B. Hunsberger, Thomas Y. Crowe II, Rhonda S. Cooper,
   and Thomas J. Smith

3. Caring at the Culture and Spirituality Interface: Case Studies from
   China, Taiwan, New Zealand, and Sub-Saharan Africa   22
   Richard A. Powell, Cheng-Pei Lin, Ping Guo, and Eve Namisango

4. Holistic Care of the Cancer Patient, United States:
   Identifying Unique Aspects of Palliative Care   33
   Phyllis Whitehead, Shereen Gamaluddin, Sarah DeWitt,
   Christi Stewart, and Kye Y. Kim

5. The Challenge of Truth-Telling in Cancer Care, United States   45
   Daniel B. Hinshaw

6. Cultural Challenges in Providing Psychosocial-Spiritual Support to
   Children with Cancer and Their Families, Turkey   57
   Rejin Kebudi, Fatma Betul Cakir, and Sema Bay Büyükkapu

7. Psychosocial Factors of Healthcare Professionals and Their Influence
   on Quality of Care for their Cancer Patient, United States   65
   Ora Nakash and Leeat Granek

8. Healing the Psychological and Emotional Aspects of Cancer, Jordan   75
   Mohammad Al Qadire

9. Nurses Providing Emotional Support and Spiritual Care to
   Patients and Families, Spain & Turkey   86
   Paz Fernández-Ortega, Sultan Kav, and Esther Arimón-Pagès

10. The Landscape of Loneliness: An Introspective Experience of Support
    and Depression in Older People Diagnosed with Cancer, Israel   99
    Lea Baider and Gil Goldzweig

11. The Psychosocial Burden of Cancer in Sexual and Gender Minority
Patients, United States   107
Yahya Almodallal and Aminah Jatoi

12. The Health-Care Team and Culture in an Israeli Cancer Center, Israel   117
Tzeela Cohen and Simon Wein

13. Mindfulness and Compassion Practices for Cancer Patients:
The Impact of Culture and Faith in Cancer Care, Italy   125
Simone Cheli and Nicola Petrocchi

14. Enhancing Dignity and Hope in Caring for Cancer Patients through
Palliative Care, Italy   132
Loredana Buonaccorso, Guido Miccinesi, and Carla Ida Ripamonti

15. Meaning-Making in Coping with Cancer: The Impact of Spirituality
and Culture among Cancer Patients in the Philippines   148
Maria Minerva P. Calimag

16. Spiritual and Religious Impacts on Advanced Cancer Care in Australia   163
Clare O'Callaghan, Natasha Michael, and David Kissane

17. The Influence of Spirituality on Quality of Life during Cancer, United
States   173
Jeannine M. Brant and Annette Brant Isozaki

18. Suffering and Compassion: The Role of Faith in the United States   187
Lodovico Balducci

19. The Role of Spirituality among Palliative Care Patients in
Poland, Poland   197
Jakub Pawlikowski, Małgorzata Krajnik, and
Aleksandra Kotlińska-Lemieszek

20. The Role of Faith in Coping with Cancer among Palliative Care
Patients in Turkey, Turkey   205
Adem Akcakaya and Gulbeyaz Can

21. The Impact of Culture and Beliefs on Cancer Care: Iranian
Perspectives, Iran   215
Maryam Rassouli, Azam Shirinabadi Farahan, Leila Khanali Mojen,
and Hadis Ashrafizadeh

22. Spiritual Healing in Cancer Care: A Hindu Perspective, India   229
Seema Rajesh Rao, Vidya Viswanath, and Srinagesh Simha

23. The Impact of Chinese Culture and Faith in Cancer Care, China   240
Lili Tang, Ying Pang, and He Yi

24. Sociocultural Influences on Cancer Care in Sub-Saharan Africa:
Use of Traditional and Complementary Medicines   249
Amos Deogratius Mwaka

25. Barriers to Addressing Emotional and Psycho-Social Needs in
Cancer Care, Turkey   261
Gülçin Şenel

26. A Jewish Israeli Case Study in End-of-Life Spiritual Care for a
Cancer Patient, Israel: "So that there will be one good and true
thing to say about me in my eulogy"   275
Michael Schultz

27. Existentialism and Spirituality in the Healing Process of
Cancer Patients, United Kingdom and United States   285
Eve Namisango, Lawrence Matovu, Richard Harding, and Ann Berger

28. Psychosocial-Spiritual Healing: An Impression of the Impact of Culture
and Faith in Cancer Care in Africa, Kenya, Sub-saharan Africa, Culture,
Beliefs, Traditional Healers, Herbal Treatment, Religion, Spirituality,
Ethnic Groups, Ancestors   295
John K. Weru and Esther W. Nafula

29. Psychosocial Aspects of Breast Cancer: The Turkish Experience, Turkey   302
Sedat Ozkan

30. Cancer Pain Care in French-speaking African Countries and Access to
Analgesics: Barriers and Cultural and Emotional Aspects, France   309
Yacine Hadjiat, Serge Perrot, Jallal Toufiq, and Christian Ntizimira

31. Support and Palliative Care for Cancer Patients in Mexico, Mexico   319
Maricela Salas Becerril and Noemi Hernández Cruz

32. Islamic Cultural-Spiritual Guidance in Caring for Cancer Patients, Iraq   329
Samaher A. Fadhil and Hasanein H. Ghali

33. The Impact of Latin American Cultural Values, Attitudes, and
Preferences on Palliative Cancer Care: An Overview from Patients'
and Families' Perspectives, Chile   340
Pamela Turrillas and Mariana Dittborn

34. The Impact of Culture and Belief on Cancer Care in
Costa Rica, Costa Rica   352
Ana Barrantes Ramírez and Isaías Salas Herrera

35. Reflections on Middle Eastern Cultural Perspectives in Cancer Care   357
*Manal A. Al-Zadjali, Anna E. Brown, Warda A. Al Amri,
Amal J. Al Balushi, Thamra S. Al Ghafri, and Nabiha S. Al Hasani*

36. Spirituality, Culture, Traditions, and Other Beliefs Affecting
    Cancer Care, Uganda   367
    Anne Merriman, Germans Natuhwera, and Eve Namisango

37. Sociocultural Context and Its Impact on Communication, India   382
    Naveen Salins and Srinagesh Simha

38. Emotional State, Spirituality, and Religion's Effect on the Acceptance
    of Cancer, Morocco   391
    Asmaa El Azhari and Abdellatif Benider

39. Breast Cancer Survivorship in Nigeria: The Experience of Survivors
    and Need for Development of Supportive Care, Nigeria & UK   401
    *Eme Asuquo, Omolola Salako, Therese Mbangsi, Kate Absolom, Bassey
    Ebenso, Kehinde Okunade, Temitope Adeleke, and Matthew J. Allsop*

40. Impact of Culture and Beliefs in Brain Tumor Patients' Care in
    Indonesia, Indonesia   414
    Tiara Aninditha, Feranindhya Agiananda, and Henry Riyanto Sofyan

41. The Contribution of Spiritual, Religious, and Customary Heritage to
    the Personalization of Modern Oncology in Multiethnic Societies of
    Developing Countries: The Model of Montenegro, Montenegro   422
    Nada Cicmil-Sarić, Milena Raspopović, and Damira Murić

42. Differences in Attitudes toward Advanced Cancer Care Planning
    through the Scope of Culture, Israel   432
    Gil Bar-Sela and Inbal Mitnik

43. Ugandan Culture: Spiritual Guidance in Caring for Cancer
    Patients, Uganda   441
    Emmanuel B. K. Luyirika

44. Cultural-Spiritual Guidance in Caring for Cancer Patients
    in the Dominican Republic, Dominican Republic   446
    Wendy C. Gómez García and Marleni R. Torres Núñez

45. Jamaican Cultural and Spiritual Guidance in Caring for
    Cancer Patients, Jamaica   454
    *Dingle Spence, Kari Brown, Steven Smith, Dorothy Grant, and
    David Picking*

46. Indian Cultural-Spiritual Guidance in Caring for Cancer Patients, India 475
    Aanchal Satija and Sushma Bhatnagar

Index   485

Foreword

Never has the world been more interconnected, geopolitically, by air travel, in cyberspace, genetically, and through generation of knowledge by transnational cooperation, and yet we often remain divided by an inability to understand the cultural mores of other nation states or ethnic groups. I have had the opportunity to practice cancer medicine in all five continents and would admit that while I was technically accomplished, I was culturally clumsy in wanting to apply the communication model based on fully informed consent, the gold standard in my own country.

Similarly, I come from a predominantly atheistic and deterministic point of view. As the Persian poet Omar Khayyam expressed in one of his quatrains: "And the first Morning of Creation wrote / What the Last Dawn of Reckoning shall read." This limited my capacity to engage more fully when patients wanted to explore and compare their religious and belief constructs. I could quote Ghandi: "Prayer is not an old woman's idle amusement. Properly understood and applied, it is the most potent instrument of action," and I would say that patients should consider any ancillary activity which they felt empowered them, returning their own sense of self.

Three simple, practical rules governed any alternative or additional approaches to healing:

- It shouldn't cost an arm or a leg; there are charlattans out there!
- It shouldn't get in the way of conventional therapy.
- It shouldn't cause distress/discomfort.

When clinical scholars of the stature and achievement of Michael Silbermann and Ann Berger join the expedition toward better health and health care, attention must be paid. I have had the pleasure of knowing both of them for over a decade, and I recognize and admire them as bridge-builders. Their talents and experience span the cultural and technical divide between the world of clinical care and the world of policy, and between both of those worlds and modern understandings of system dynamics.

They also understand as well as any other health care leaders why the pursuit of widening our understanding of the cultural nuances which determine how we deliver cancer care has become important. Arguably, it has become a moral duty in a time when we seek to apply a universal "rules-based" system of care that focuses on technical guidelines, which offer no real insights into how these might be adapted to cultural norms.

This excellent book provides an extraordinary collection of wisdom, across many cultures, religions, and geographies, underpinned by highly regarded authors from a wide range of backgrounds and viewpoints. I only wish that it had been available to me as a younger physician before I embarked on my own journey across the world. All the same, it has given the elder me much food for thought.

Patients, clinicians, policy and religious leaders, and the public at large all need to learn to ask about and discern the difference between what helps and what does not help, so that cancer care can help to its fullest potential. Michael Silbermann and Ann Berger typify the trustworthy scouts we need to find that path: healers above all who know how to read the map.

David J. Kerr, Professor of Cancer Medicine,
Oxford University

Preface

With cancer ranking as the primary or secondary cause of premature death in almost 100 countries worldwide, the World Health Organization recognized a high level of investment in cancer control and treatment (including palliative care) in 2019. At that time, governments at the World Health Assembly (WHA) unanimously adopted a new cancer resolution (Universal Health Coverage: Moving Together to Build a Healthier World). The resolution noted the potential for cancer prevention to reduce cancer burden in the future, while reducing the suffering from cancer in the communities.

As most countries are facing an overall increase in the absolute number of cancer cases, large geographical diversity in cancer occurrence and variations in the magnitude and profile of the disease still continue between and within world regions. Specific types of cancer dominate globally: lung, female breast, and colorectal cancer. The regional variations in common cancer types signal the extent to which societal, economic, and lifestyle changes interplay to differentially impact the profile of this most complex group of diseases.

Although survival rates for cancer have improved significantly over the past few decades, for each individual, the diagnosis and treatment of cancer are still devastating, affecting the family and community as well. The care of a person with cancer must be more than just the treatment of the cancer itself. Understanding the cultural, psychological, social, and spiritual dimensions of the cancer sufferer and their family and community will ensure the best care for the cancer.

In order to treat individuals with cancer and understand how to give the best possible care to underserved populations, we need to understand cultural diversity. Understanding that cultural aspects of a society may be intertwined with finances and other resources can improve adherence and access to care. Culture is made up of language, religion, cuisine, social norms, history, ancestry, music, arts, and spirituality. In order to improve cancer care outcomes, patients' diverse spiritual and cultural beliefs must be recognized. In addition, available methods must be utilized to improve access and adherence to treatment modalities and regimens.

In this book, we focus on numerous diverse cultures, traditions, and faiths. Many parts of the world are composed of indigenous cultures, with unique spiritual beliefs in addition to the region's primary religion. We present chapters on indigenous religions as well as indigenous traditional healers. People everywhere experience trouble, sorrow, need, and sickness, and they develop skills and knowledge in response to these adversities. This book provides insightful models of these parameters and serves as a valuable resource for health care providers and policymakers by taking a global approach to cultural diversity in the world. By understanding this multiculturalism and the many aspects of psychological, social, and spiritual dimensions of health and healing, we can learn from one another.

Contributors

Kate Absolom, PhD
University Academic Fellow
Leeds Institute of Medical Research at St
James's & Leeds Institute of Health Sciences
University of Leeds
Leeds, GB

Temitope Adeleke
PGDE in Education, PGDE in ECCE
Educator
Child of Promise School
Lagos

Feranindhya Agiananda, MD
Academic Staff
Department of Psychiatry
Universitas Indonesia
Jakarta, ID

Adem Akcakaya, MD
Professor
Head of General Surgery Department and
Palliative Care Center
Bezmialem Vakif University
Istanbul, TR

Warda A. Al Amri, PhD
Faculty
Department of Nursing
Oman College of Health Sciences
Al Azhaibah, OM

Amal J. Al Balushi, PhD
Lecturer
Department of Maternal and Child Health
Nursing
Oman Collage of Health Science
Al Wattayah-Muscat, OM

Thamra S. Al Ghafri, MD, MPH, PhD
Senior Consultant Public Health
Directorate General of Health Care Services
Oman Ministry of Health
Muscat, OM

Nabiha S. Al Hasani, BSN in Nursing
Oncology Nurse
Department of Oncology
Ministry of Health
Muscat, OM

Mohammad Al Qadire, PhD
Professor
Department of Oncology and Palliative Care
Nursing
Al Al Bayt University
Mafraq, JO

Matthew J. Allsop, BSc, PhD
University Academic Fellow
Academic Unit of Palliative Care
University of Leeds
Leeds, GB

Yahya Almodallal, MBBS
Pediatric Resident and Physician-Scientist
Trainee
Department of Pediatrics
University of Iowa
Iowa City, IA, USA

**Manal A. Al-Zadjali, PhD, Nursing &
Health Innovation**
Dean
Higher Institute of Health Specialties (HIHS)
Muscat, OM

Tiara Aninditha
Head of Neuro-Ooncology, Headache, and
Pain Division
Department of Neurology, Faculty of Medicine
University of Indonesia
Indonesia

Esther Arimón-Pagès, RNC, MSN, DM
Critical Care Nurse
Department of ICU
Hospital Clínic de Barcelona
Barcelona, ES

Hadis Ashrafizadeh, PhD
Candidate in Nursing
Nursing & Midwifery School
Ahvaz Jundishapur University of Medical
Sciences
Ahvaz, IR

Eme Asuquo
Lecturer
Department of Preventive & Social Medicine
University of Port Harcourt
Port Harcourt, Rivers State, NG

Lea Baider, MA, PhD
Full Professor of Medical and Clinical
Psychology
Director of Psycho-Oncology
Department of Oncology
Assuta Medical Center
Tel Aviv, Israel

Lodovico Balducci, MD
Senior Member Emeritus
Department of Interdisciplinary Oncology
Moffitt Cancer Center
Tampa, FL, USA

Gil Bar-Sela, MD
Associate Professor
Department of Oncology
Emek Medical Center
Afula, IL

Maricela Salas Becerril, BSc. Nursing
Department of Palliative Care
National Cancer Institute of Mexico (INCan)
Mexico City, Mexico

Abdellatif Benider, PhD
Professor
Department of Oncology
University Hassan II
Casablanca, MA

Ann Berger, MD, MSN
Chief Pain and Palliative Care
Bethesda, Maryland

Sushma Bhatnagar, MBBS, MD, MSc
Professor & HOD
Department of Onco-anaesthesia and
Palliative Medicine
Dr. B.R. Ambedkar, Institute Rotary Cancer
Hospital, All India Institute of Medical
Sciences
New Delhi, IN

**Jeannine M. Brant, PhD, APRN,
AOCN, FAAN**
Director and Oncology Clinical Nurse
Specialist
Department of Collaborative Science &
Innovation
Billings Clinic
Billings, MT, USA

**Anna E. Brown, MRes (Health Research),
MBA, DHSM, CMS, RM, RN**
Senior Sciences Tutor
Quality Assurance Section
Higher Institute of Health Specialties,
Ministry of Health
Muscat, OM

Kari Brown, MBBS, MSc
Research Associate
Jamaica Cancer Care & Research Institute
Kingston, JM

Loredana Buonaccorso, PsyD
Psycho-Oncology Unit
Azienda USL-IRCSS di Reggio Emilia
Reggio Emilia, IT

Sema Bay Büyükkapu
Medical Doctor
Doctor
Istanbul University, Oncology Institute
Istanbul, TR

Fatma Betul Cakir, MD
Professor
Department of Pediatrics, Division of
Pediatric Hematology and Oncology
Bezmialem Vakif University
Istanbul, TR

Maria Minerva P. Calimag, MD, PhD
Faculty of Medicine and Surgery
Research Center for Health Sciences
University of Santo Tomas
Manila, Philippines

Clare O'Callaghan, AM, PhD, MMus, BMus, BSW, RMT, RGIMT
Associate Professor
Music Therapist and Researcher
Caritas Christi Hospice
Department of Psychosocial Cancer Care, and Department of Medicine
St Vincent's Hospital, The University of Melbourne
Australia

Gulbeyaz Can, RN, PhD, Prof
Professor
Department of Medical Nursing
Istanbul University—Cerrahpasa Florence Nightingale Nursing Faculty
Istanbul, TR

Simone Cheli
University of Florence
Firenze, IT

Nada Cicmil-Sarić, MD
Internist, Medical Oncologist
Clinical Center of Montenegro
Institute of Oncology
Podgorica, ME

Tzeela Cohen, MD, MHA
Attending Physician
Department of Palliative Care Service at Davidoff Cancer Center
Rabin Medical Center
Petach Tikva, IL

Rhonda S. Cooper, MDiv, BCC
Cancer Center Chaplain
Department of Harry J. Duffey Patient and Family Services
The Johns Hopkins Hospital—Kimmel Cancer Center
Baltimore, MD, USA

Thomas Y. Crowe II, MDiv, BCC
Director
Department of Johns Hopkins Hospital Spiritual Care and Chaplaincy
Baltimore, MD, USA

Noemi Hernández Cruz, RN
National Cancer Institute of Mexico
Mexico City, Mexico

Sarah DeWitt, MD
Emergency Medicine Specialist
Carilion Roanoke Memorial Hospital
Roanoke, VA, USA

Mariana Dittborn, MSc
Research Associate
Centre for Bioethics
School of Medicine, Clínica Alemana de Santiago—Universidad del Desarrollo
Santiago, CL

Bassey Ebenso, MBBCh, MPH, PhD
Lecturer in International Public Health
Leeds Institute of Health Sciences
University of Leeds
Leeds, GB

Asmaa El Azhari
Specialist Doctor and Head of Palliative Care
Department of Palliative Care
Mohammed VI Center for the Treatment of Cancers UHC Ibn Rochd
Casablanca, MA

Samaher A. Fadhil, MD
Pediatric Hematology Oncology Consultant
Children Welfare Teaching Hospital
Baghdad Medical City
Baghdad, IQ

Azam Shirinabadi Farahan, PhD, RN
Assistant Professor
Department of Pediatric Nursing, School of Nursing & Midwifery
Shahid Beheshti University of Medical Sciences
Tehran, IR

Paz Fernández-Ortega, PhD, MSc, RN
Associate Professor, Nursing Research
Coordinator
Department of Public Health, Mental and
Maternal
University of Barcelona
Barcelona, ES

Shereen Gamaluddin, MD
Hospice and Palliative Medicine
Carilion Roanoke Memorial Hospital
Roanoke, VA, USA
Centra Lynchburg General Hospital
Lynchburg, VA, USA

**Hasanein H. Ghali, MBChB, DCH,
FICMS, Ped FICMS, HemOnc**
Assistant Professor of Pediatrics
Department of Pediatric Hematology
College of Medicine, University of Baghdad
Baghdad, IQ

Gil Goldzweig, PhD
Full Professor and Head of the Center for
Academia-Community Relations
School of Behavioral Sciences
The Academic College of Tel-Aviv Yaffo
Tel Aviv Jaffa, IL

Wendy C. Gómez García, MD
Oncology Unit Coordinator
Hematology-Oncology Service
Dr. Robert Reid Cabral Childrens Hospital
Santo Domingo, DO

Leeat Granek, PhD
Associate Professor
School of Health Policy and Management
and Department of Psychology
York University
Toronto, ON, Canada

Dorothy Grant, MDiv., BCC, CDP
Spiritual Care Coordinator
Treasure Coast Hospice
Port St Lucie, FL, USA

Ping Guo, PhD, MSc, BSc
Lecturer
School of Nursing, Institute of Clinical
Sciences, College of Medical and Dental
Sciences
University of Birmingham
Birmingham, GB

Yacine Hadjiat, MD
French National Institute of Health and
Medical Research (INSERM) U987
Paris-Saclay University (EDSP)
Paris, FR

Richard Harding
Professor and Director
Cicely Sanders Institute of Palliative Care,
Policy and Rehabilitation
Kings College
London, UK

Isaías Salas Herrera, MD
Office of Pain Control and Palliative
Care Unit
Plaza Médica del Este
San José, Costa Rica

Daniel B. Hinshaw, MD
Consultant in Palliative Medicine &
Professor Emeritus of Surgery
Department of Surgery, Section of General
Surgery
University of Michigan Medical School
Ann Arbor, MI, USA

Joann B. Hunsberger, MD, MS
Assistant Professor
Department of Anesthesiology and Critical
Care Medicine
Johns Hopkins University
Charlotte R. Bloomberg Childrens Center
Baltimore, MD, USA

Annette Brant Isozaki, RN, BSN
Clinical Registered Nurse
HCT, CAR T Cell Therapy, and
Investigational Research Therapy Unit
City of Hope National Medical Center
Duarte, CA, USA

Aminah Jatoi, MD
Mayo Clinic
Rochester, MN, USA

Sultan Kav, PhD, RN
Professor
Faculty of Health Sciences Department of
Nursing
Başkent University
Ankara, TR

Rejin Kebudi, MD, Prof
Professor and Chair
Department of Preventive Oncology and
Department of Clinical Oncology, Pediatric
Hematology-Oncology
Istanbul University, Oncology Institute
Istanbul, TR

Kye Y. Kim, MD
Professor
Department of Psychiatry and Behavioral
Medicine
Carilion Roanoke Memorial Hospital and
Palliative Care Service
Roanoke, VA, USA

**David Kissane, AC, MD, BS, MPM,
FRANZCP, FAChPM, FACLP**
Chair of Palliative Medicine Research
School of Medicine
University of Notre Dame Australia
St Vincent's Sydney
Darlinghurst, NSW, AU

**Aleksandra Kotlińska-Lemieszek,
MD, PhD**
Associate Professor
Chair and Department of Palliative Medicine
Poznań University of Medical Sciences
Poznań, PL

Małgorzata Krajnik
Full Professor
Department of Palliative Care
Nicolaus Copernicus University in Toruń,
Collegium Medicum
Bydgoszcz, PL

Cheng-Pei Lin, RN, MSc, PhD
Assistant Professor
Institute of Community Health Care
College of Nursing, National Yang Ming
Chiao Tung University
Taipei, TW

**Emmanuel B. K. Luyirika, M FAM MED,
MPA, BPA(Hons), MB, ChB**
Executive Director
African Palliative Care Association
Kampala, UG

Lawrence Matovu, MA
Psychologist
Department of Clinical
Hospice Africa Uganda
Kampala, Uganda, UG

**Anne Merriman, MBE, FRCPI,
FRCPEdin, MSc**
Director
International Programs at Hospice
Africa Uganda
Uganda, Kampala, UG

Guido Miccinesi, MD
Senior Researcher
Department of Clinical Epidemiology
Oncological Network, Prevention and
Research Institute-ISPRO
Florence, IT

**Natasha Michael, MBChB, FRACP,
FAChPM, MRCPI, MRCGP, MSc**
Associate Professor
Director of Palliative Medicine
Department of Palliative and Supportive Care
Cabrini Health
Melbourne, AU
University of Notre Dame
Australia
Monash University
Melbourne, AU

Inbal Mitnik, MA
Medical Psychologist
Oncology Division
RAMBAM Health Care Center
Haifa, IL

Leila Khanali Mojen, PhD, RN
Shahid Beheshti University of Medical
Sciences
Tehran, IR

Damira Murić, MS
Psychologist
Institute of Oncology
Podgorica

**Amos Deogratius Mwaka, MBChB,
MMed, MA, PhD**
Senior Lecturer
Department of Medicine
Makerere University College of Health
Sciences
Kampala, UG

**Esther W. Nafula, MSc (Palliative
Care), MBChB**
Palliative Care Specialist
Department of Medicine
Kenyatta National Hospital
Nairobi, KE

Ora Nakash
Professor
School for Social Work
Smith College
Northampton, MA, USA

Eve Namisango, Msc, PhD
Programmes and Research Manager
Department of Programmes and Research
African Palliative Care Association
Kampala, KS, UG

**Germans Natuhwera, MSc (Student), BSc,
DCMCH, PGCerts (BIOE1, BIOST, PH,
Epidemiol, Global Health)**
Palliative Care Clinician and Programs
Manager
Department of Clinical
Hospice Africa Uganda
Kampala, UG

Christian Ntizimira, MD, MSc
Executive Director
African Center for Research on End of Life
Care (ACREOL)
Kigali, RW

**Kehinde Okunade, MBBS,
FWACS, FMCOG**
Senior Lecturer
Department of Obstetrics and Gynaecology
College of Medicine, University of Lagos
Lagos, NG

Sedat Ozkan, MD
Institute of Oncology
Department of Psychosocial Oncology
University of Istanbul
Istanbul, Turkey

Ying Pang, MS
Clinical Psychologist
Department of Psycho-Oncology
Peking University Cancer Hospital
Beijing, CN

Jakub Pawlikowski, PhD, MD, MA, JD
Associate Professor
Department of Humanities and Social
Medicine
Medical University of Lublin
Lublin, PL

Serge Perrot, PhD
Professor, Head of Pain Center
Department of Pain Center
Cochin Hospital, Université de Paris
Paris, FR

Nicola Petrocchi, PhD, PsyD
John Cabot University
Rome, Italy
Compassionate Mind Italia
Rome, Italy

David Picking, PhD
Research Fellow
The Natural Products Institute
The University of the West Indies
Kingston, JM

Richard A. Powell, BA, MA, MSc
Project Evaluation Manager
Department of Primary Care and
Public Health
Imperial College London
London, GB

Christina M. Puchalski, MD, MS, FACP
Professor
Department of Medicine
Director, GW Institute for Spirituality
and Health
The George Washington University School of
Medicine
Washington, DC, USA

Ana Barrantes Ramírez
Doctor in Nursing
Departamento Onco-Hematología
Hospital México
San José, Costa Rica

**Seema Rajesh Rao, MBBS, DPM, MSc
(Palliative Medicine)**
Associate Director (Education & Research)
Department of Education and Research
Karunashraya Institute for Palliative
Care Education and Research (KIPCER),
Bangalore Hospice Trust—Karunashraya
Bangalore, Karnataka, IN

Milena Raspopović, MS
Psychologist
Institute of Oncology
Podgorica

Maryam Rassouli, PhD, RN
Professor
Cancer Research Center
Shahid Beheshti University of Medical
Sciences
Tehran, IR

Carla Ida Ripamonti, MD
Supportive Care Unit Department of Medical
Oncology & Haematology
Fondazione IRCCS, istituto Nazionale
dei Tumori
Milano, IT

Omolola Salako

Naveen Salins, MD, PhD, FRCP
Professor and Head
Department of Palliative Medicine and
Supportive Care
Kasturba Medical College, Manipal Academy
of Higher Education
Manipal, IN

Aanchal Satija, PhD
Research Scholar
Department of Onco-Anesthesia and
Palliative Medicine
Dr. B.R. Ambedkar, Institute Rotary Cancer
Hospital, All India Institute of Medical Sciences
New Delhi, IN

Michael Schultz
Director, Spiritual Care Service
Oncology Division
Rambam Health Care Campus
Haifa, IL

Gülçin Şenel, MD, Prof
Professor
Anesthesiology Clinic; Palliative Care Unit
University of Health Sciences, Dr. A.Y.
Ankara Oncology Education and Research
Hospital
Ankara, TR

Michael Silbermann, DMD, PhD
Executive Director
Middle East Cancer Consortium (MECC)
Haifa, IL

**Srinagesh Simha, MS (Gen Surg), MSc
Pall Med (Cardiff), FRCP (Lon)**
Medical Director
Department of Palliative Care
Hospice Karunashraya
Bangalore, IN

**Thomas J. Smith, MD, FACP, FASCO,
FAAHPM**
Director of Palliative Medicine
Johns Hopkins Medical Institutions
Professor of Oncology
Sidney Kimmel Comprehensive Cancer Center
Baltimore, MD, USA

Steven Smith, BMedsci, MBBS
Project Manager and Research Associate
Jamaica Cancer Care and Research Institute
Kingston, JM

Henry Riyanto Sofyan, MD
Neurologist, Clinical Lecturer, Chief of
Marketing & Health Promotion of RSCM
Universitas Indonesia - Dr. Cipto
Mangunkusumo National General Hospital
Jakarta, Indonesia

Dingle Spence, MBBS, FRCR
Senior Medical Officer
Hope Institute Hospital
Kingston, JM

Christi Stewart, MD
Carilion Roanoke Memorial Hospital and
Palliative Care Service
Roanoke, VA, USA

Lili Tang, MD
Chief Psychiatrist and Director
Department of Psycho-Oncology
Peking University Cancer Hospital
Beijing, CN

Marleni R. Torres-Núñez, MD
PL-2, Pediatric Resident
Department of Medical Education
Nicklaus Children's Hospital
Miami, FL, USA

Jallal Toufiq
Professor of Psychiatry, Rabat Faculty of
Medicine
Member of the International Narcotics
Control Board / Vienna
Director of the Ar-razi University Psychiatric
Hospital & the National Center on Drug
Abuse Prevention, Treatment and Research
Director of the Moroccan Observatory on
Drugs and Addictions

Pamela Turrillas, MD, MSc
Consultant in Internal Medicine
Department of Oncologic
Oncologic Supportive Care Unit
Clinica Alemana
Santiago of Chile, CL

Vidya Viswanath, MD, MSc Palliative
Medicine
Assistant Professor
Department of Palliative Medicine
Homi Bhabha Cancer Hospital and
Research Centre
Visakhapatnam-a Unit of Tata
Memorial Centre
Mumbai, IN
Consultant
Homi Bhabha Cancer Hospital and Research
Centre—a unit of Tata Memorial Centre
Visakhapatnam, IN

Simon Wein, MD
Director
Department of Pain and Palliative Care
Service
Davidoff Cancer Center, Beilinson Hospital
Petach Tikvah, IL

John K. Weru, MBCHB, MPC, PGD
Assistant Professor
Department of Hematology-Oncology
Aga Khan University Hospital
Nairobi, KE

Phyllis Whitehead, PhD, APRN, ACHPN,
PMGT-BC, FNAP, FAAN
Clinical Ethicist and Clinical Nurse Specialist
Palliative Medicine/Pain Management
Carilion Roanoke Memorial Hospital
Daleville, VA

He Yi, MD
Department of Psycho-Oncology
Peking University Cancer Hospital &
Institute
Beijing, China

1

The Soul of Health Care

Caring for the Whole Person, United States

Christina M. Puchalski

Introduction

Contemporary medical models focus predominantly on the technical and financial aspects of care. While these are important aspects of care, they fail to include what may be the most critical need of patients and families—that is, the whole-person approach to care where psychosocial and spiritual needs are viewed as essential and just as important as the physical. Cecily Saunders (1918–2005), the founder of the modern hospice movement, was one of the first to describe the concept of "total pain," which led to the biopsychosocial and spiritual model of care [1]. In 2014, the World Health Assembly for the World Health Organization (WHO) passed a resolution that included spiritual care as an essential domain of palliative care. The resolution stated that palliative care is an approach that improves the quality of life of patients "through the prevention and relief of suffering by means of early identification and correct assessment and treatment of pain and other problems, whether physical, psychosocial or spiritual" [2]. WHO also noted that "it is the ethical duty of health care professionals" to alleviate pain and suffering, whether physical, psychosocial, or *spiritual*. WHO further supported an interdisciplinary model by noting the need for collaboration between professional palliative care providers and support care providers, including spiritual support and counseling [3].

Many national and international guidelines have been developed for addressing spiritual care as part of whole-person care [4–7]. The clinical models described in these guidelines are based on addressing spirituality as part of wellness, but they also identify spiritual distress as part of symptom management. In these guidelines, spirituality is defined broadly as a "dynamic and intrinsic aspect of humanity through which persons seek ultimate meaning, purpose and transcendence, and experience relationship to self, family, others, community, society, nature and the significant or sacred. Spirituality is expressed through beliefs, values, traditions and practice" [4].

One key aspect of any whole-person model of care is the generalist specialist model of care [8,9]. While this model has been described more recently for spiritual care, with the clinicians being the generalists and spiritual care or chaplains being the specialists, this model also has to do with the way medical specialties function. Primary care physicians, for example, will refer patients to specialists—cardiologists, surgeons, and the like. Within the whole-person care model, any clinician should address the whole-person needs as described in the biopsychospiritual model. Part of that approach is recognizing when to refer the patient to specialists while still attending to all the needs of the patient and their families.

Let's examine the case of Maggie, a 48-year-old female who comes to the doctor after her breast biopsy. She is tense as she waits for the results of the biopsy. The physician tells her the biopsy is positive. She panics, is nervous, wriggles in her chair as the physician just keeps looking at the electronic health record and quickly runs through the list of next steps: see a surgeon and an oncologist, and surgery will likely be needed. Then the words get more confusing; she feels no one is listening. She starts to cry. The doctor offers her Valium and gives her a list of surgeons to see. The doctor then leaves the room.

Though efficient and correct in the technical aspects of care, the doctor's approach is missing a sense of connection and support for Maggie—connection and care that are important in Maggie's life as she faces a difficult diagnosis that has huge ramifications for her in the next days, month, and years. As the physician's words fade, Maggie experiences uncertainty, fear, and loneliness. Often, patients whom I have seen in palliative care don't even remember the details of what needs to be done next—they just tell me of the panic, fear, and confusion they feel about what to do next. Some express signs and symptoms of depression or anxiety. Many express spiritual and existential distress for which they have no words, except for a deep pain in their soul or spirit. Many talk about the impact of their diagnosis on their families, their work, and their friends. They also struggle with decisions that are complex: chemotherapy versus surgery; "what about a second opinion? who should I see that will listen to me and to all my concerns?"

Consider an alternative scenario: Maggie is tense while waiting for the doctor. The doctor arrives, asks how Maggie is doing, and then gently lets her know about the biopsy, sitting in silence while Maggie processes the information. Maggie wonders if this experience will be like her mother's breast cancer experience. The doctor listens to the whole story about her mother, showing real interest in Maggie. The doctor asks her what helped her during that time. Maggie talks of her garden, her faith and her family.

During that discussion, the doctor weaves in information about Maggie's illness with observations regarding her resources of strength. In this way, Maggie finds hope, possibility, and connection. The doctor suggests the next steps while pausing and allowing Maggie to ask questions. Maggie, in turn, can share her fears and concerns about all aspects of her life and how they might be affected by her illness. In recommending an oncologist and surgeon to Maggie, the physician asks about her preferences, for example, as to the type of person she might want to see and the location of the office. They work together on recommendations, next steps, and ways to navigate the complicated health care system. The physician offers to call Maggie at home that evening to see if she has more questions and to see if her partner may have questions.

What we see in the first scenario is a rapid, rushed visit with the focus on relaying the diagnosis and outlining the next steps. This truncated visit is likely due to the impact of the increases in health care costs, which are forcing health care professionals to see more and more patients in shorter time intervals, focusing mostly on acute, physical issues. Not surprisingly, the result is patient dissatisfaction with care: patients feel they are not being heard and that not all their issues are being addressed fully. This can mean poorer outcomes of care, stress for not only the patient and their family, but also for the clinicians, who may experience a high level of moral distress for their inability to be as thorough, and perhaps as thoughtful, as they would like to be. This may be the reason for the higher burnout rates among health care professionals: they are practicing medicine that is not congruent with their own beliefs and values, in addition to having to work in high-stress, rushed environments [10].

In the second scenario, we see patient-centered care delivery rooted in compassion and love. The physician is fully present to the patient and addresses the psychosocial and spiritual, as well as the physical, aspects of care. The patient feels less anxious and is more satisfied with her care. The physician is more gratified to be able to serve the patient in a more holistic way.

Recently, I was part of a presentation at a conference where another physician and I role-played the scenario with a "patient." The presentation of the physician who did the first scenario with Maggie lasted about 10 minutes. I played the physician in the second scenario, and it was only 2 minutes longer than the first. Even in the midst of a large conference room, as the patient talked of her suffering, for a few minutes I forgot the stage and was unaware of the audience of several hundred. During that time, I experienced a profoundly sacred moment of deep presence with the "patient." This was a window into compassionate presence, a critical aspect of spiritual care in whole-person care. Being able to establish a trusting connection with the patient, being intentional about addressing psychosocial and spiritual needs as well as the physical ones, and practicing compassionate presence actually may be more efficient and is certainly better care.

Whole-Person Assessment in Clinical Care

Whole-person care is gaining increasing attention as part of patient-centered care. While, for many years, it was still focused primarily on physical and emotional well-being, the concept of spiritual health is currently more widely recognized as an important part of whole-person care [11]. Whole-person assessment is grounded in the biopsychosocial and spiritual model of care. While initially a model in palliative care [12], more recently work has been done on a similar consensus-based model for a new definition of whole health [13]. In this later model, financial and intellectual health was also recognized. Table 1.1 shows the physical, emotional, social, and spiritual aspects of whole health. Distress would be the converse of whole health—for example, unmanaged pain, depression, social isolation, and lack of meaning.

The biopsychosocial-spiritual model assumes the totality of a patient's experience in the context of disease, which includes interdisciplinary management to address all dimensions of care.

The biological, psychological, social, and spiritual aspects of life are distinct dimensions of each person. No one aspect can be disaggregated from the whole. Each can be affected differently by a person's history and illness, and each can interact and affect other aspects of the person.

A comprehensive assessment includes all needs of the patient: physical, emotional, social, and spiritual. Input comes from the patient, family, and all members

Table 1.1 The BioPsychoSocial and Spiritual Model

Biological	Psychological	Social	Spiritual
Pain managed	Healthy emotional life	Strong community support	Meaning
Able to function physically	No chronic anxiety or managed	Appropriate roles/ relationships in personal/ professional life	Purpose
Sleeps well	No depression, or managed	No excessive financial burden	Dignity
Appetite good	No fear, anger, or managed		Hope
Minimal physical symptoms, or managed	No chronic sadness, fear, anger, or managed		Faith
			Community
			Connection
			Capacity to love
			Forgiveness
			Peace

of the interdisciplinary team and should be shared verbally as well as entered into the patient's written medical records. All of the above domains are evaluated in terms of strengths as well as symptoms of distress. As the symptoms are identified, they must be addressed, and, with ongoing assessment, the therapeutic plan must be adjusted accordingly. The physical assessment focuses on symptoms related to specific organ systems. The Palliative Performance Scale (PPS) is one measure used to determine functional status, including ambulation, activity and evidence of disease, self-care, intake, and consciousness level. The exam helps with making diagnoses and developing a treatment plan. The *psychological assessment* includes assessment of strengths (e.g., coping), as well as evaluation for psychopathology. The *social assessment* addresses many factors, including support systems, work satisfaction, work stress, and financial well-being. Finally, the *spiritual assessment* includes spiritual screening, history, and a full assessment performed by a spiritual care specialist. The goal of a spiritual screening is to identify spiritual distress and refer the patient to a spiritual care specialist. The goal of the spiritual history is to identify spiritual resources of strength and/or spiritual distress and to address them in the clinical visit as well as refer to appropriate specialists. Spiritual assessment done by chaplains is, in itself, a therapeutic intervention, but the chaplain also helps confirm or change the diagnosis of the type of spiritual distress identified by the clinician. Through compassionate listening and skilled reflective inquiry, the chaplain can help patients address and cope with distress.

While attention to physical and emotional issues is standard in medical care, addressing spiritual issues is of course less so. In the guidelines on spiritual care as an essential domain described earlier, spiritual distress is identified as a "clinical symptom" to be assessed and treated. Similar to the guidelines used for assessing the other domains, spiritual resources of strength are also identified. A spiritual issue becomes a diagnosis if the following criteria are met: (1) the spiritual issue leads to distress or suffering (e.g., lack of meaning, conflicted religious beliefs, inability to forgive); (2) the spiritual issue is the cause of a psychological or physical diagnosis such as depression, anxiety, or acute or chronic pain (e.g., severe meaninglessness that leads to depression or suicidal thoughts, guilt that leads to chronic physical pain); and (3) the spiritual issue is a secondary cause or affects the psychological or physical diagnosis (e.g., hypertension difficult to control as, due to religious beliefs, the patient refuses to take medications).

The National Cancer Comprehensive Network [14] developed diagnoses for spiritual distress that were used as a basis for spiritual distress diagnoses developed for the 2009 National Consensus Conference on Improving the Spiritual Domain of Palliative Care [15]. These spiritual distress diagnoses include: existential distress, feelings of abandonment by God or others, anger at God or others, concerns about relationship with the deity, conflicted or challenged belief systems, feelings of despair/hopelessness, grief/loss, guilt/shame, reconciliation, isolation, and religious-specific and religious/spiritual struggle. Once a clinician conducts a spiritual history, they can use communication strategies such as deep listening, presence, and reflective listening to invite the patient to share more about their spirituality. If the clinician identifies the spiritual distress and spiritual resources of strength and the means for coping, they should then integrate these resources into the patient treatment or care plan and document them in the patient's chart. The clinician must attend to spiritual distress with the same urgency as they would any other distress. The outcomes of patient spiritual care may present as the ability to come to an understanding of their suffering at a deeper level, perhaps finding an inner peace and sense of coherence, as well as a source or sources of meaning and purpose, and, perhaps reconnecting with a sense of transcendence or with whatever is sacred or significant in their lives.

In a clinical setting, one should also assess for spiritual health, including beliefs, values, and practices that support the well-being or inner life of patients. For some of them, that might be a connection with the transcendent; for others, it might be a connection to something sacred or significant. The act of seeking forgiveness or the willingness to forgive may be a spiritual strength. Other examples of spiritual strengths may include intrinsic values that enhance the patient's well-being; the ability to forgive and love others; participation in spiritual communities (e.g., church, synagogue, or mosque); or like-minded friends, family, or other spiritual support groups (for instance, a Parkinson's or cancer support group, which may be regarded as a spiritual support group). Spiritual practices, including meditation, prayer, mindfulness, connection with nature, music, or arts, may also help people find that sense of wholeness or healing. Spiritual strengths help patients cope, find hope in the midst of suffering, discover joy in life, and/or find the ability to be grateful. As with any other domain of care, it is important to identify patients' strengths and appropriately support and integrate these strengths within their care.

Spiritual care for patients may include practices such as reflective listening and being present. Treatment options might include referral to spiritual care professionals, art therapists, meaning-oriented therapists, and meditation. If the patient identifies specific spiritual or religious practices that are important to them, such as reconnecting with nature, prayer, meditation, community support, or rituals, then encouraging those practices might be appropriate. Part of wellness coping strategies might include spiritual coping strategies such as meditation or reestablishing priorities [16].

Whole-Person Assessment and Treatment Plan

Once a clinician does a complete assessment, including a spiritual history and a complete review of systems, and conducts a physical exam, a plan is developed with the participation of both the patient and the family. During the entire visit, the clinician uses communication strategies such as deep listening, presence, and reflective listening to invite the patient to share more about what they are experiencing or feeling and describe any distress, including spiritual. Several spiritual history tools are available, including the FICA© (Faith, Belief, Meaning/Importance and Influence/Community/Address and Action) tool, which we developed and is widely used in clinical settings [17].

In Maggie's case, the clinician's goal was to break the difficult news of a diagnosis of cancer and do a full assessment of her—psychosocial and spiritual as well as physical. Maggie's medical history was significant for hypertension and anxiety as a younger person. She is married to a man named Tom, they have one child, Susan, a dog named Jerry, and a cat named Sammy. She is a social worker and enjoys her work; she never smoked, drank alcohol, or took drugs. Her spiritual history was obtained with the FICA© spiritual history tool.

Maggie's FICA© spiritual history:

- F: Raised Episcopalian, was very involved in her faith community but is now more focused on personal spirituality that includes mindfulness practices and activities based in nature. She finds meaning in her family and her work. She wonders, "Why is this happening to me now?" as her life had been so full of joy.
- I: Her beliefs and practices are very important to her. During the "goals of care" discussion, she notes that she is very hopeful that surgery and chemotherapy will "cure" her cancer. She recognizes that, at some point, she will face end of life either from "old age, cancer, or both." She would like it noted in her chart that she would appreciate dying in hospice with a window looking out over nature.
- C: She has a strong spiritual community and is also a member of a woman's group that meets regularly for activities in nature and sharing with each other.
- A: At this point, Maggie feels supported by her physician but would be open to seeing a spiritual counselor to discuss her experience of "being a patient with cancer" and her struggles with uncertainty.

Maggie's review of systems is significant for some anxiety about the cancer diagnosis and some fear about the unknown, as well as for the insomnia she has experienced during the past few weeks since her cancer diagnosis. Otherwise, it is negative.

Table 1.2 Whole-Person Model Assessment and Plan

Maggie is a 48-year-old woman with history of hypertension and anxiety, recently diagnosed with breast cancer. Has struggled with anxiety since the diagnosis as well as existential and spiritual distress.

Physical	Breast cancer referrals made for oncology and surgery
	Elevated blood pressure may be secondary to anxiety and stress; patient will monitor at home, and we will adjust medications as needed. Discussed meditation practices as potentially helpful. Also discussed healthy nutrition and exercise, as tolerated
Emotional	Situational anxiety, recommended counselor as needed, and also reflected on connection with her spiritual community and meditation practices that lend her support
Social	Continue with strong support from family and friends
Spiritual	"Why me"? Existential distress, also facing uncertainty
	Recommended a spiritual counselor; continue with spiritual support group, spiritual practices

Her physical exam is significant for elevated BP 155/90 HR 70 and for a small mass in her left breast at the three o'clock position; the rest of the exam is normal. See Table 1.2 for her assessment and plan.

Maggie agreed with the plan and preferred to focus on meditation in order to deal with elevated systolic blood pressure and anxiety. She appreciated the referral to a spiritual counselor. She affirmed that her family was very supportive and says she will bring her husband to the next visit. Her physician gave her referrals and explained how to make the appointments, navigate the system, and set up a follow-up visit in 2 weeks.

Compassionate Gaze

Much has been written on the importance of presence and compassion in clinical care, particularly when attending to the suffering of another. Many definitions have been rendered, and some note the need for a contemplative practice in order to be able to enter into those moments of presence with the sufferer. Dr. Gerald Mays notes that "[c]ontemplation happens to everyone. It happens in the moments when we are open, undefended and immediately present" [18]. Thus, clinicians must use contemplative practices to enter into that compassionate space of deep silence, awareness, and love. In Maggie's case, the invitation to enter into those contemplative moments comes from the patient as she opens up about her pain and suffering. The response from the clinician begins with an awareness of this invitation and of the suffering and the ability to move into contemplation and, hence, deep presence. But it does not end there. It is important to know when to move from that space to the rest of the visit and, most importantly, to ensure ongoing connection and accompanying of the patient, particularly in the midst of the patient's difficulty and suffering. Practicing whole-person care does not end with checking off the biopsychosocial and spiritual boxes; it continues in our ongoing encounters with our patients on their health and life journeys.

Conclusion

Whole-person care recognizes not only the complexities of assessing and treating patients' distress and illness, but also their strengths. Each person reacts to a serious diagnosis in a different way, and each person has different ways of coping and accepting what is facing them. It is critically important to address and attend to all that is distressing the patient—the psychosocial and spiritual as well as the physical. While the treatment may vary depending on the illness, the patient, and their values, the approach is the same—to practice our skills as clinicians with humility, respect, compassion, and presence. We cannot provide the best clinical compassionate care unless we attend to the whole person. As clinicians, we use our scientific knowledge to provide the best medical care for our patients. As human beings accompanying our patients on their journeys through life, we provide connection, care, and the possibility of peace and healing in the midst of suffering. Caring for the whole person is the soul of health care.

References

1. Saunders. Embracing Cicely Saunders's concept of total pain. *BMJ*. 2005;331:576. doi: https://doi.org/10.1136/bmj.331.7516.576-d
2. Puchalski, CM, Vitillo, R. World Health Organization authorities promote greater attention and action on palliative care. *J. Palliat. Med.* 2014;17(9):988–989.
3. World Health Assembly 67. Strengthening of palliative care as a component of comprehensive care throughout the life course. https://apps.who.int/gb/ebwha/pdf_files/WHA67/A67_R19-en.pdf
4. Puchalski CM, Vitillo R, Hull SK, Reller N. Improving the spiritual dimension of whole person care: Reaching national and international consensus. *J. Palliat. Med.* 2014;17(6):642–656. doi:10.1089/jpm.2014.9427
5. Puchalski CM, Sbrana A, Ferrell B, et al. Interprofessional spiritual care in oncology: A literature review. ESMO Open. 2019; 4(1):e000465. doi:10.1136/esmoopen-2018-000465.
6. Meaningful Ageing Australia. *National Guidelines for Spiritual Care in Aged Care.* Parkville: Meaningful Ageing Australia;2016.
7. Handzo, G, Koenig, HG. Spiritual care: Whose job is it anyway? *Southern Med J.* 2004;97:1242–1244. http://dx.doi.org/10.1097/01.SMJ.0000146490.49723.AE
8. Puchalski C, Ferrell B, Virani R, et al. Improving the quality of spiritual care as a dimension of palliative care: The report of the consensus conference. *J Palliat Med.* 2009;12(10):885–904. doi:10.1089/jpm.2009.0142
9. Physician Burnout Agency for Healthcare Research and Quality https://www.ahrq.gov/sites/default/files/wysiwyg/professionals/clinicians-providers/ahrq-works/impact-burnout.pdf
10. Hutchinson, Tom. Whole person care. In *Whole Person Care*. New York: Springer; 2012, Chap. 1:1–8.
11. Puchalski, CM, Ferrell, B. *Making Healthcare Whole*. West Conshohoken, PA: Templeton Press;2010.
12. Sulmasy, DP. A biopsychosocial-spiritual model for the care of patients at the end of life. *Gerontologist.* 2002;42(Spec. No. 3):24–33.

13. Hubner, M, Knottnerus, JA, Green, L, van der Horst, H, Jadad, AR, Kromhout, D, ... Schnabel, P. How should we define health? BMJ(Online), 343;2011. https://tobacco.ucsf.edu/publications/how-should-we-define-health

14. https://jnccn.org/view/journals/jnccn/17/10/article-p1257.xml

15. Puchalski C, Ferrell B, Virani R, et al. Improving the quality of spiritual care as a dimension of palliative care: The report of the consensus conference. *J Palliat Med.* 2009;12(10):885–904. doi:10.1089/jpm.2009.0142

16. Kruizinga R, Scherer-Rath M, Schilderman HJBAM, Puchalski CM, van Laarhoven HHWM. Toward a fully fledged integration of spiritual care and medical care. *JPSM.* 2018;55(3):1035–1040.

17. Puchalski CM, Romer AL. Taking a spiritual history allows clinicians to understand patients more fully. *J Palliat Med.* 2000;3(1):129–137.

18. https://cac.org/wp-content/uploads/2015/11/2-CONTEMPLATION-AND-COMPASSION-THE-SECOND-GAZE.pdf

2

The How and Especially *Why* Clinicians Should Do a Spiritual Assessment, United States

Joann B. Hunsberger, Thomas Y. Crowe II, Rhonda S. Cooper, and Thomas J. Smith

Introduction

Cancer has seen rapid advances in diagnosis and treatment strategies, but it remains a deadly disease. At least half of all cancers are not caused by anything other than bad luck (and unfortunate changes in our DNA) [1]. The very mention of the word *cancer* can cause anxiety in a patient, with thoughts of death forefront in their mind [2]. The term most often conjures images of suffering, pain, punishment, and death. In addition, cancers always raise questions of causality and other significant issues [3]: Why me? Why at this time? What did I or my family do to deserve this? What is my future? What will dying look like? Will I die in pain? Is there life after death? [4,5] These existential questions lead to spiritual distress in seven domains: despair, dread, brokenness, helplessness, alienation, meaninglessness, and guilt/shame—which can then manifest in symptoms of depression, anxiety, and fatigue [5]. Health care providers (HCPs) are in a unique position to explore these issues, though the patient's questions may not be answered by medical science. HCPs are intimately involved in life processes and may have the opportunity to discern spiritual concerns or refer patients to team members better suited to answer spiritual or existential questions [3]. The HCP may need to realize that they should not answer all of a patient's questions with medical jargon and must allow space for spiritual concerns to be voiced when discussing treatment options and end-of-life (EOL) issues [6].

Spirituality can be defined as the collection of values, beliefs, and practices that an individual uses to give meaning and purpose to experiences and relationships [7–9]. According to the National Consensus Project for Quality Palliative Care (NCP Guidelines), spirituality is "a dynamic and intrinsic aspect of humanity, through which individuals seek meaning, purpose and transcendence, and experience relationship to self, family, others, community, society and the significant or sacred" [10]. It is important to understand that spirituality can be expressed through religious practices, but it is not the same as religion, and the two terms should not be used interchangeably [11]. In a spiritual assessment, it may be important to determine the patient's religious affiliation and also to recognize that a patient may practice religion and still have unmet spiritual needs. In the United States, 75% of the population identify religion as very important or fairly important in their lives. Fifty-eight percent report that they often pray to God outside of religious services, and 89% believe in God or a universal spirit [12]. During a health crisis, such as cancer or another potentially terminal disease, a patient's faith practice could become more important, as they seek to find meaning and cope with the life-limiting reality occasioned by the diagnosis and/or prognosis. At the same time, their medical condition may cause a measure of social isolation, which may hinder their ability to incorporate religious practices or receive direct support from their faith community [6].

The NCP has determined that spiritual care is one of eight clinical practice domains and recognizes spirituality as a fundamental characteristic of patient- and family-centered palliative care [10]. The Joint Commission in the United States requires an assessment of patients' cultural, religious, and spiritual practices on admission to the hospital, confirming its belief that these practices will affect a patient's perception of illness and approach to treatment [13]. In a study of cancer patients, those who identified as religious described fewer unmet psychosocial needs than those without a religious or faith framework [14]. Evidence also supports the idea that patients use religion and spirituality to cope with illness [15,16]. A majority of hospitalized patients believe that spiritual health is as important as physical health, and some may desire spiritual care involvement from their physician [17,18]. In this chapter, we explore how and why HCPs should perform spiritual assessments, recognizing the importance of spirituality in the lives of their patients.

Vignette

A woman in her early 90s is admitted to the hospital for heart failure. This is her third admission in five years, and before that, at age 80, she had coronary bypass surgery. On this admission, physicians note a mass on her lungs during her chest X-ray. Her providers are concerned that it might be cancer, given her significant smoking history. She is angry with almost all care providers and her family for "putting her in the hospital." The nursing staff is often offended at her brusqueness. Her mobility is waning, and she has barely been able to get around her own home or care for her own physical needs. When the hospitalist makes rounds during her hospitalization, she asks how the patient is doing. The woman tells her doctor that she NEVER wants to be admitted to the hospital again and that she just wants to be left home to die. The woman tells her doctor that her vision and hearing are failing her, so it is hard to watch TV, read a book, or even listen to the radio. She almost never goes out to do the things she loves, like going to church, playing Saturday night cards with her elderly brothers, or even getting out to her back patio to watch the birds. She can no longer sew or cook, hobbies that sustained her after her husband's death. She is sad much of the time and wonders why she is still alive after her husband died 30 years earlier. Surprised at this emotional outpouring and realizing after several attempts that the woman does not want any additional medical information, the physician sits down next to her and asks, "What is most important to you?" The woman shares that there is little meaning to her life since she can no longer do any "work" or take part in the hobbies that she has always enjoyed. She recounts, with pride, how she and her husband had successfully run several businesses prior to his death, which she continued after his death. She has three adult children and extended family who call and visit her several times per week. With some prompting, she also tells the physician how she misses her church and interactions with others. She is frustrated that no one from her church, especially her pastor, comes to visit. As a result, she now feels alienated from her church and is even angry with God for "taking her husband." After confirming with the woman that she truly never wants to be admitted to the hospital again, and because of her severe heart failure and likely cancerous lung pathology, the physician referred her to home hospice. With hospice, she was regularly visited by the chaplain, who explored areas of spiritual distress, including her grief, her resilience, and her beliefs about death. The chaplain helped her recognize her spiritual pain and revived her prayer life. With the woman's permission, the chaplain contacted her pastor and notified him of her request to be visited. The patient was able to receive an important ritual (communion) that helped her regain a sense of peace and decreased her anger at God. She began to pray daily with her full-time caregiver who lived in the home with her. The patient reconnected emotionally with her children, and they laughed and cried as they remembered their past. Some months later, the woman died after having made peace with God and her family, at home surrounded by loved ones.

HOW?

Conducting a spiritual assessment is as straightforward endeavor as asking appropriate and sometimes leading questions that can set the HCP in the right direction for receiving important and revealing answers about a patient's spirituality and religiosity. A typical spiritual assessment goes beyond the spiritual screening process that is often completed at admission. However, the Joint Commission does not specify the content and scope of spiritual assessments or determine who should perform them. A spiritual assessment can lead to a conversation that identifies spiritual needs and possible areas of distress, as well as spiritual beliefs, values, and practices of the patient and family [9]. HCPs can ask relevant questions by using a model that invites the patient to talk about their spirituality. Acronyms such as FICA (Faith, Importance/Influence, Community, Action in care) [19,20] and HOPE (Hope, Organized religion, Personal spirituality/Practices, Effects on medical care) [11], and the brief spiritual assessment model are guides available to the HCP.

An HCP can also enter into a conversation about spirituality by listening for the patient's cues when they mention words such as God, Creator, church, saints, faith, journey, guidance, or forgiveness [21]. The HCP maintains a communication posture of patient-centered empathetic listening and understanding, inwardly acknowledging that the patient's worldview may not match their own [22–24]. The act of empathetic listening and the patient's perception of being heard may allow the patient to feel validated and understood [24].

It is important to note the barriers to asking these questions. Three areas of concern that an HCP might have are: (1) What if I do not have enough time to devote to this level of conversation? (2) What if the patient brings up a spiritual question that I cannot answer and will ultimately make me uncomfortable? and (3) What if the questions about spirituality get turned back on me and the patient realizes that my personal approach to spirituality and religion doesn't match theirs? [25,26]

Once the HCP realizes that this conversation doesn't take as much time as presumed and that they have experts, such as hospital chaplains, to whom they can refer the patient for deeper spiritual concerns and distress, the spiritual assessments become easier to complete. An HCP may always have some level of anxiety associated with spiritual or religious topics and with the possibility that a patient may ask these questions. Therefore, it is beneficial for HCPs to reflect on their own spiritual or religious beliefs and practices as a way to become more conversant and comfortable in sharing and to acknowledge that religion and spirituality impact their clinical practice [27]. This level of sharing or disclosure tends to be helpful in building and sustaining trust between HCPs and their patients. The expectation that faith beliefs or practices must align is often unfounded, and the HCP should never impose their own personal beliefs on a patient [28].

Table 2.1 FICA Spiritual Assessment Tool ©™

F	Faith or beliefs	What is your **faith** or belief?
I	Importance and influence	Is it **important** in your life? How have your beliefs influenced your behavior during this illness?
C	Community	Are you part of a spiritual or religious **community**?
A	Address/Action in care	How would you like me, your health care provider, to **address** these issues in your health care?

The HCP uses the acronym FICA (see Table 2.1) to form questions such as: What is your faith and what does it mean to you? What brings meaning to you? How does your faith influence your choices, especially your medical choices? What/who is your faith community and how supportive are they? How will your faith ultimately impact your care? Answers to these questions allow the HCP to have a dialogue about the spiritual foundations of their patient. The information that emerges from this conversation often can shape medical choices and inspire new levels of trust, as mentioned above. Patients themselves might begin the conversation about spirituality with questions such as those listed in the following section. The HCP should become familiar with this type of patient-initiated question in order to anticipate an appropriate opening for further discussion about a patient's spirituality. Many questions about spirituality do not dwell on religion but rather stress the patient's hope for the future, sense of self-worth, and internal peace. Patient-initiated questions for religious or nonreligious or nondeistic patients revolve around their sense of meaning and purpose of their lives, connection and relatedness to others, grief, guilt, or regret about past experiences. The HCP can listen attentively with a response of reassurance which, while this takes practice, can be therapeutic to the patient's spiritual well-being.

Patient-initiated Questions

- Do you think every person has a purpose in life? If so, what if I have not discovered my purpose and it is too late?
- In my earlier days, I did something for which I still feel guilt. Is there a way to "make it right" with the person?
- I once did something that hurt my mother deeply. She has died. Can I ever be free of my feelings of guilt?

- My child died many years ago at age 4. I still weep every morning over his death. I don't believe in God or heaven, but do you think I will be reunited with my child after I have died?
- Do you think we all have a soul that lives on after our body has died?
- I feel utterly hopeless, and my friends say it is because I don't believe in God. What do you think?
- Where do I find hope in the face of such a poor prognosis?
- Do you think my family will still feel my presence after I have died?
- I just retired a year ago and had hoped to do a lot of things with my wife. Now I am sick, and I have so many regrets about this. I feel guilty that I always put her off when she asked me to go on vacation or fix things around the house.
- I had so hoped to see my grandchildren grow up. Do you think they will remember me?

As HCPs conduct these assessments, they should realize the importance of being open without judgment, listening without interrupting and talking less [29,30]. Sharing medical information with a patient is scientifically based and data-driven, offered as a one-way conversation that the HCP leads. Having a discussion about a patient's personal faith or beliefs, especially during hospitalization, requires sincerity, tact, and an acute listening posture. It is helpful when the HCP sits down, uses eye contact, and possibly even takes notes at the bedside. The more adept HCP will notice nuance and emotion and will have the ability to followup with curiosity and sincere interest, thus gaining important information about a patient's spiritual needs and possible areas of distress.

Another important function of any spiritual assessment is to determine if a referral should be made to the hospital chaplain or a patient's clergy. Hospital chaplains are equipped with the skills to assess spiritual needs and to provide interventions to help ease spiritual distress. The HCP who makes the general assessment can provide helpful information to the chaplain, and the chaplain can use this information during a follow-up, thus supporting the patient's continuity of care. In many cases, the HCP and the chaplain will work closely together to support the medical and spiritual issues the patient is facing.

Vignette

A young woman in her early 30s with an aggressive colon cancer is meeting with her palliative care physician via telemedicine after a recent hospitalization. It has been a tough few weeks for her, and she is becoming more aware of her own medical and physical decline. She is fatigued, barely eating, intermittently nauseous, and has abdominal pain, all managed by her outpatient palliative physician. She has been trying to continue to work so that she can maintain her health care coverage, but it is getting harder and harder, and she had to call out sick several days in a row. Tearfully, the patient admits that she is getting weaker and that it is harder to maintain her normal activities. She says that it was comforting in a way to be in the hospital, away from the eyes of her family and their expectations. She explains that she loves her husband, and together they long for children, though they know this will never be possible together. She feels he is angry with her, and she fears he will never forgive her. Her sister is always pressuring her to eat more so that she does not "starve" to death, not understanding how uncomfortable she becomes after eating too much food. She misses her family who live in another country, but she dreads talking to them, as they tell her she just needs to fight against the evil disease that is inside her. They tell her to get out of bed and eat more. She feels a sense of shame that she will never be a mother and that she is not doing enough to stop her inevitable death. She fears that her family will be angry with her after she dies. She wonders what meaning her life has had, especially since she had not lived up to the expectations of those around her. Together, the patient and physician lament the losses that she feels because of broken relationships with her family and for children that she will never have. The physician reassures the patient that she has shown incredible resilience through her disease process and that she has done everything humanly possible to fight off the aggressive cancer through chemotherapy, radiation, and surgery. Together, they reminisce about all of the patient's accomplishments in life, and they talk about emphasizing the moments of joy with her loved ones. She vows to talk to her husband about how much she loves him and that she is sad about not having children. She wants to ask him to forgive her for not being able to have children, so that they can enjoy each moment as much as possible. The patient, reminded of her own self-worth and meaning, is ready to face her family again, reassured that she is doing all that she can do and is hopeful for forgiveness.

WHY?

Most Americans report having religious and spiritual beliefs [12], and both patients and HCPs agree that spiritual care is an appropriate component of cancer care [31]. To best serve patients, HCPs need to recognize and inquire about their patients' beliefs. Interestingly, the spiritual needs of most patients with advanced cancer are not met by their religious communities or the medical system [6]. However, taking a detailed spiritual assessment may be a step out of an HCP's comfort zone [32]. In a U.S.-based cohort study, Balboni et al. enrolled 343 patients with advanced cancer from September 2002 through August 2008 and followed them until death at five diverse sites [31]. When they compared participants who felt well supported by their religious communities *and* received spiritual support from the medical team to those who did not receive it, they observed that the group that received spiritual support from their medical team had almost 2.5 times use of hospice and 81% fewer ICU deaths. Participants who had high spiritual support from their own religious communities were 63% less likely to use hospice, 2.62 times more likely to use aggressive measures at the end of life, and over five times more likely to die in the ICU. HCPs have generally not been trained to take such a history and so may feel inadequate or hesitant to do so [33,34]. HCPs may not wish to expose their own personal beliefs, may feel awkward inquiring about someone else's, or may have a negative perception of religiosity that affects their desire to explore spirituality [35].

A discussion about spiritual and religious beliefs might not change the disease course for a patient, but support for a patient's spiritual needs has been shown to improve quality of life in those with advanced cancer [6], despite physical limitations. Additionally, spiritual support can protect against EOL hopelessness and despair [36]. Discussions about spirituality can help the HCP understand the patient more completely and, therefore, enhance communication. During EOL conversations, this understanding can help the patient and HCP determine which goals of care are most important to the patient. As mentioned above, such a discussion could lead to spiritual growth for both the patient and the provider and help the HCP respond and anticipate the psychosocial needs of patients [14].

WHERE and WHEN?

For the comedian, timing is everything. Perhaps the same can be said for the timing of a spiritual assessment by the HCP. A complete spiritual assessment does not necessarily need to be conducted routinely [37]. A better approach may be to assess the spiritual well-being of patients during inflection points of stress or illness, such as early in a patient's diagnosis and after sudden decreases in functionality. It's likely better to wait until a trust relationship has been established, although some research shows that cancer patients are more comfortable having these discussions with someone other than their treating oncologist, even with someone new to them like a medical resident [38,39]. A spiritual assessment might also be helpful to determine reasons for misunderstanding of a prognostic mismatch or differing goals of care among patients, family members, and providers. The spiritual needs of the patient and family may actually change as the patient's medical needs change [9].

Patients don't always want providers to ask questions about spirituality, perhaps due to a concern that the provider will stop being concerned about the disease and focus only on the spiritual. Some evidence suggests that patients are less interested in a conversation about religion and spirituality in a routine office visit (19%) and become more interested in such a conversation during hospitalization (29%) and at EOL (50%) [36]. A patient and provider may see physical and spiritual health as being separate, instead of part of the same continuum, and thus they may be concerned that a conversation about religious/spiritual issues would mean a time trade-off in discussion of medical issues [36]. However, patients seem to welcome conversation about spiritual issues as health deteriorates, and some would even like physicians to accompany them in prayer at EOL [36]. Again, these findings support the thought that patients may not welcome or need inquiry into their spirituality and religiosity during a routine office visit, but, as they become more ill, are hospitalized, and certainly are at EOL, many do welcome such inquiries [36].

Vignette

A man in his late 60s receives a diagnosis of acute myeloid leukemia. The news is devastating to him, his wife, and his adult children. He wonders what he has done to cause his illness, thinks back on his transgressions throughout his lifetime, and worries that his bad genetics may cause the disease in his children. He is a professor at a university and has worked hard his entire life, spending extra hours at the office and teaching night classes. He is a loving husband and father and takes much joy in his young grandchildren, who live distant from him. He and his wife of 40 years have enjoyed their world travels and have been looking forward to a long retirement "full of adventure." They decide to aggressively move forward with a bone marrow transplant, even though they know that the rate of success with his disease is low. The couple does everything in their power to keep him healthy, and they continue to dream of their future together. After his transplant, he begins to improve, regains energy, and has better mobility. But a few months later, he begins to have worsening pulmonary issues and then a severe gastrointestinal bleed that requires acute hospitalization and intensive care. After blood transfusions and continuous use of noninvasive respiratory support, he has a massive heart attack overnight. His intensivist, who feels a commonality with this man, is frustrated and saddened at the news and is not sure what he will tell the family or what more he has to offer them. Dreading the conversation, he asks his team to set up a family meeting so that they can discuss goals of care. The intensivist is concerned that the family will want to continue with all treatment options, given their description of the man as the fighter of the family. At the family meeting, the man's wife insists that those present for the meeting pray with her. There is awkward shuffling in the room and glances that show the staff's discomfort with this idea. In the prayer, the man's wife asks for guidance, for peace, for strength, for healing, and for courage as the team goes forward with the man's care. She thanks God for the entire provider team, for their wisdom and their loving care of her husband. After the prayer, there is a sense of quietness in the room, with tears forming in the eyes of many. The intensivist struggles to say that he is concerned that any additional interventions will cause only more suffering, without lifesaving benefit. The wife of the man and their children agree without hesitation that he should suffer no more and say that they want to spend the remaining time at his bedside, with dignity and in celebration of his life.

WHO?

Studies have affirmed the interconnection between the physical and spiritual nature of humans [5], and patients have confirmed their desire for physicians to be aware of their spiritual beliefs. In a five-site survey, Balboni et al. found that 87% of patients had received no spiritual care from their nurses and 94% had received none from their physicians, despite 86% thinking it should be provided at least occasionally [31]. Eighty-eight percent of nurses and 86% of physicians reported *no* spiritual care training. Among those who had undergone spiritual care training, nurses were 11-fold and doctors were 7-fold more likely to provide it. The end of life discussion and spiritual care have been shown to correlate types of end of life care as seen in Figure 2.1. This leaves the question of who should perform the spiritual assessment. In the case of the FICA and HOPE assessments, the questions are focused on finding what is important to the patient and on what gives the patient meaning. Performing a spiritual assessment is not meant to be political or divisive, but rather to help the HCP understand the patient better and must be done in a culturally sensitive way [21]. Therefore, spiritual assessments can be performed by any HCP who seeks to better understand a patient and who wants to provide patient-centered care, including chaplains, social workers, physicians, and nurses [21]. In one study, physicians and nurses had some differing opinions about whose role it should be [40]. Nearly 100% of nurses and doctors thought that spiritual care was the domain of the chaplain or social worker. Nurses were somewhat more likely (73%) than doctors (about 50%) to think that spiritual care was part of their role. However, this belief did not translate into actually providing spiritual care. For physicians, a strong personal spiritual belief was highly associated with providing spiritual care to their last advanced cancer patient themselves (69% vs. 31%, $p < .001$) [40]. In the case of spiritual distress, or a patient requesting specific religious rituals, it is important to incorporate the expertise of the chaplain or appropriate clergy-person [4,41].

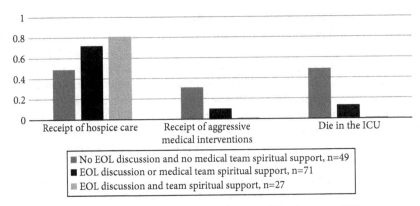

Figure 2.1 Relationship of EOL discussions and team spiritual care on EOL care
Adapted from Balboni TM, et al. JAMA Intern Med. 2013 Jun 24;173(12):1109-17

Summary

A patient with a serious illness such as advanced cancer may find it difficult to participate in religious activities that bring spiritual meaning, especially as EOL mobility worsens [42]. As their disease progresses, the patient's spiritual questions may increase as they seek to make meaning in their current situation [5]. It becomes the duty of HCPs who are responsible for the patient's well-being to assess spiritual needs as part of their overall care. Inherently, people are physical and spiritual. Therefore, the HCP needs to embrace and acknowledge the spiritual nature of their patients to truly provide holistic care. While providing holistic care and support of the patient, an HCP can improve quality of life and meet the psychosocial needs of their patient by including their faith and spiritual traditions into treatment plans and care goal discussions or even supporting spiritual practices like prayer or meditation, which can improve health outcomes [8]. Multiple tools exist to conduct a spiritual assessment, including the acronyms FICA and HOPE. Alternately, HCPs can simply ask patient-centered, open-ended questions, such as "What is your hope?" or "What gives your life meaning?"

Additional research is required to explore the best situational tools and appropriate timing for making a spiritual assessment and when or how to include questions on religiosity without trivializing faith traditions. Data are conflicting about whether patients want physicians to ask questions about spirituality. Therefore, more investigation is needed into the approach for inquiring about spiritual needs. We need to further understand why HCPs do not ask questions about religion and spirituality [43,44] and provide appropriate education to give them tools to assess this important part of a patient's ethos. Additionally, more research is needed into spiritual assessment tools appropriate for pediatric patients with cancer and their families.

Acknowledgments

The authors wish to acknowledge Claire F. Levine, MS, ELS Anesthesia and Critical Care Medicine, Johns Hopkins University, Baltimore, MD, for editing and critical review of this chapter.

References

1. Tomasetti C, Vogelstein B. Cancer etiology. Variation in cancer risk among tissues can be explained by the number of stem cell divisions. *Science*. 2015;347(6217):78–81. doi:10.1126/science.1260825
2. Lee, V. The existential plight of cancer: Meaning making as a concrete approach to the intangible search for meaning. *Support Care Cancer*. 2008;16:779–785. https://doi.org/10.1007/s00520-007-0396-7
3. Brown AE, Whitney SN, Duffy JD. The physician's role in the assessment and treatment of spiritual distress at the end of life. *Palliat Support Care*. 2006;4(1):81–86.
4. McClain CS, Rosenfeld B, Breitbart W. Effect of spiritual well-being on end-of-life despair in terminally-ill cancer patients. *The Lancet*. 2003;361(9369):1603–1607.
5. Hui D, de la Cruz M, Thorney S, Parsons HA, Delgado-Guay M., Bruera E. The frequency and correlates of spiritual distress among patients with advanced cancer admitted to an acute palliative care unit. *Am J Hosp Palliat Med*. 2011;28(4):264–270.
6. Balboni TA, Vanderwerker LC, Block SD, et al. Religiousness and spiritual support among advanced cancer patients and associations with end-of-life treatment preferences and quality of life. *J Clin Oncol*. 2007;25(5), 555.
7. Puchalski C, Ferrell B, Virani R, et al. Improving the quality of spiritual care as a dimension of palliative care: The report of the Consensus Conference. *J Palliat Med*. 2009;12(10):885–904.
8. Saguil A, Phelps K. The spiritual assessment. *Am Fam Phys*. 2012;86(6):546–550.
9. Ferrell B., Munevar C. Domain of spiritual care. *Progr Palliat Care*, 2012;20(2):66–71.
10. Ferrell BR, Twaddle ML, Melnick A, Meier DE. National consensus project clinical practice guidelines for quality palliative care guidelines. *J Palliat Med*. 2018;21(12), 1684–1689.
11. Anandarajah G, Hight E. Spirituality and medical practice: Using the HOPE questions as a practical tool for spiritual assessment. *Am Fam Phys*. 2001;63(1):81–88.
12. Gallup Religion. https://news.gallup.com/poll/1690/religion.aspx. Accessed September 9, 2020.
13. The Joint Commission. Advancing Effective Communication, Cultural Competence, and Patient- and Family-Centered Care: A Roadmap for Hospitals. Oakbrook Terrace, IL: The Joint Commission; 2010.
14. McIllmurray MB, Francis B, Harman JC, Morris SM, Soothill K, Thomas C. Psychosocial needs in cancer patients related to religious belief. *Palliat Med*. 2003;17(1):49–54.
15. Koenig HG. Religious attitudes and practices of hospitalized medically ill older adults. *Int J Geriatr Psychiatry*. 1998;13(4):213–224.
16. Fitchett G, Canada AL. The role of religion/spirituality in coping with cancer: Evidence, assessment, and intervention. In: Holland JC, Breitbard, WS Jacobson, PB. Lederberg, MS, Loscalzo MJ, McCorkle R. (eds). *Psycho-oncology*. 2nd ed. New York: Oxford University Press; 2010:440–446.
17. King DE, Bushwick B. Beliefs and attitudes of hospital inpatients about faith healing and prayer. *J Fam Pract*. 1994;39(4):349–352.
18. Ehman JW, Ott BB, Short TH, Ciampa, RC, Hansen-Flaschen J. Do patients want physicians to inquire about their spiritual or religious beliefs if they become gravely ill? *Arch Intern Med*. 1999;159(15):1803–1806.
19. Puchalski CM. The FICA spiritual history tool# 274. *J Palliat Med*. 2014;17(1):105–106.
20. Borneman T, Ferrell B., Puchalski, CM. Evaluation of the FICA tool for spiritual assessment. *J Pain Symptom Manage*. 2010;40(2):163–173.
21. Stewart M. Spiritual assessment: A patient-centered approach to oncology social work practice. *Soc work Health Care*. 2014;53(1):59–73.

22. Mundle RG, Smith B, Hospital chaplains and embodied listening: Engaging with stories and the body in healthcare environments. *Illn. Crisis Loss*, 2013;21(2):95–108.
23. Harvey K, Brown B, Crawford P, Sandlin S. "Elicitation Hooks": A discourse analysis of chaplain-patient interaction in pastoral and spiritual care. *J Past Care & Couns*. 2008;62(1–2):43–61.
24. Handzo GF, Flannelly KJ, Kudler T, et al. What do chaplains really do? II. Interventions in the New York Chaplaincy Study. *J Health Care Chaplaincy*. 2008;14(1):39–56.
25. Chibnall JT, Bennett ML, Videen SD, Duckro PN, Miller DK. Identifying barriers to psychosocial spiritual care at the end of life: A physician group study. *Am J Hosp Palliat Med*. 2004;21(6):419–426. https://doi.org/10.1177/104990910402100607
26. Balboni MJ, Sullivan A, Enzinger AC, et al. Nurse and physician barriers to spiritual care provision at the end of life. *J Pain Symptom Manage*. 2014;48(3):400–410.
27. Kelly EP, Hyer M, Payne N, Pawlik, TM. Does spiritual and religious orientation impact the clinical practice of healthcare providers? *J Interprofess Care*, 2020:1–8.
28. Puchalski C, Romer AL. Taking a spiritual history allows clinicians to understand patients more fully. *J Palliat Med*. 2000;3(1):129–137.
29. Ellis MR, Campbell JD. Patients' views about discussing spiritual issues with primary care physicians. *Southern Med J*. 2004;97(12):1158–1165.
30. Ospina NS, Phillips KA, et al. Eliciting the patient's agenda-secondary analysis of recorded clinical encounters; *J Gen Intern Med*. 2019;34:36–40.
31. Balboni MJ, Sullivan A, Amobi A, et al. Why is spiritual care infrequent at the end of life? Spiritual care perceptions among patients, nurses, and physicians and the role of training. *J Clin Oncol*. 2013;31(4):461.
32. Choudry M, Latif, A, Warburton KG. An overview of the spiritual importance of end-of-life care among the five major faiths of the United Kingdom. *Clin Med*. 2018;18(1):23.
33. Balboni TA, Balboni M, Enzinger AC, et al. Provision of spiritual support to patients with advanced cancer by religious communities and associations with medical care at the end of life. *JAMA Intern Med*. 2013;173(12):1109–1117. doi:10.1001/jamainternmed.2013.903
34. Atkinson HG, Fleenor D, Lerner SM, Poliandro E, Truglio, J. Teaching third-year medical students to address patients' spiritual needs in the surgery/anesthesiology clerkship. *MedEdPORTAL*. 2018;14:10784. doi:10.15766/mep_2374-8265.10784
35. Lennon-Dearing R, Florence JA, Halvorson H, Pollard JT. An interprofessional educational approach to teaching spiritual assessment. *J Health Care Chaplaincy*. 2012;18(3–4):121–132.
36. Maclean CD, Susi B, Phifer N., et al. Patient preference for physician discussion and practice of spirituality: Results from a multicenter patient survey. *J Gen Intern Med*. 2003;18(1):38–43.
37. Koenig, HG. Spiritual assessment in medical practice. *Am Fam Phys*, 2001;63(1):30.
38. Lamont EB, *Siegler M. Paradoxes in cancer patients' advance care planning. J Palliat Med*. 2000;3(1):27–35. doi:10.1089/jpm.2000.3.27
39. Dow LA, Matsuyama RK, Ramakrishnan V, et al. Paradoxes in advance care planning: The complex relationship of oncology patients, their physicians, and advance medical directives. *J Clin Oncol*. 2010;28(2):299.
40. Rodin D, Balboni M, Mitchell C, Smith PT, VanderWeele TJ, Balboni TA. Whose role? Oncology practitioners' perceptions of their role in providing spiritual care to advanced cancer patients. *Support Care Cancer*. 2015;23(9):2543–2550. doi:10.1007/s00520-015-2611-2
41. Hemming P, Teague PJ, Crowe T, Levine R. Chaplains on the medical team: A qualitative analysis of an interprofessional curriculum for internal medicine residents and chaplain interns. *J Relig Health*. 2016;55(2):560–571.

42. Ai AL, Ladd KL, Peterson C, Cook CA, Shearer M, Koenig, HG. Long-term adjustment after surviving open heart surgery: The effect of using prayer for coping replicated in a prospective design. *The Gerontologist*. 2010;50(6):798–809.
43. Ernecoff NC, Curlin FA., Buddadhumaruk P, White, DB. Health care professionals' responses to religious or spiritual statements by surrogate decision makers during goals-of-care discussions. *JAMA Int Med*, 2015;175(10):1662–1669.
44. Phelps AC., Lauderdale KE, Alcorn, S, et al. Addressing spirituality within the care of patients at the end of life: Perspectives of patients with advanced cancer, oncologists, and oncology nurses. *J Clin Oncol*. 2012;30(20):2538–2544.

3

Caring at the Culture and Spirituality Interface

Case Studies from China, Taiwan, New Zealand, and Sub-Saharan Africa

Richard A. Powell, Cheng-Pei Lin, Ping Guo, and Eve Namisango

Introduction

Premised on the keystone principle that "total pain" involves suffering in the potentially reciprocally impacting physical, psychological, social, and spiritual domains [1], palliative care addresses the relief of patients' serious health-related suffering in the totality of needs associated with severe illness [2], including their quality of life and those of families and caregivers.

It is, therefore, underpinned by a multidimensional, biopsychosocial-spiritual model of care provision [3]. Palliative care providers should not simply assess and manage these multiple domains of patient suffering holistically—including end-of-life spiritual concerns—but should do so with a cognisance of, and sensitivity to, prevailing cultural practices and expectations within which the patient, their family, and community exist [4].

In general, the ambiguous concept of "culture" entails what Spencer-Oatey described as "a fuzzy set of basic assumptions and values, orientations to life, beliefs, policies, procedures and behavioural conventions that are shared by a group of people, and that influence (but do not determine) each member's behaviour and his/her interpretations of the 'meaning' of other people's behaviour" [5]. Both resistant and predisposed to change, culture is composed of the varied universals of knowledge, belief, artifacts, morals, rules and law, custom and traditions of the groups and subgroups that compose a specific society.

"Spirituality" is one of the fundamental aspects of human existence, internationally defined as "a dynamic and intrinsic aspect of humanity through which persons seek ultimate meaning, purpose, and transcendence, and experience relationship to self, family, others, community, society, nature, and the significant or sacred. Spirituality is expressed through beliefs, values, traditions, and practices" [6]. As health care provision has transitioned toward a more holistic, person-centered approach, spiritual care has become increasingly important in patient care [7]. By finding solace in personal meaning, value, and connectedness, spirituality—and, more narrowly, religion—can exert a beneficial impact on individual physical and mental well-being, providing social support, existential meaning, a coherent belief system, and personal moral life codes [8]. Spiritual distress—the disruption of one's beliefs or value system [9]—can also occur, however, when a person is unable to find sources of meaning, love, and comfort or when conflict occurs between beliefs and life events [10].

Spirituality can be shaped by the sociocultural context in which it is practiced. As one of the core pain domains comprising the focus of palliative care [11], how spiritual care is delivered appropriately within differing cultural settings is critical. Understanding the intersection between culture and spirituality—for example, their influence on how patients cope and survive, perceive health and disease, pain and suffering, view death and their existential existence and mortality—is fundamental to determining how, when, where (e.g., home, hospitals, hospices as locales of death), and by whom palliative care and end-of-life services are delivered [3].

Patients are the complex product of their immediate and past social settings, histories, traditions, values and wishes, hopes and preferences, families and communities, and the roles they play within them, as well as their current age and stage in life. All factors can impact—directly and indirectly, spatially and temporally—on how the dying process and death itself is perceived, and its preferred experience, both individually—including managing physical pain, accepting and discussing the concept and prospect of impending death, and planning for its occurrence—but also in relation to patients' families [12].

Palliative care practitioners must be as aware of the cultural milieu that shaped individual patients as they are of their presenting problems, if care is to be person-centred. Some cultures disdain the disclosure of terminal diagnosis [13]—sometimes to avoid emotional suffering or preserve hope—and evade discussing death aloud to circumvent tempting fate [12,14,15], and some religions eschew the teachings of euthanasia and medications that confuse the mind before, or hasten the onset of, death [16], and mourn familial losses publicly, or privately, in open display, stoically or discreetly [17]. Service providers should, therefore, make every effort to sensitise themselves to existing cultural and spiritual beliefs, customs and rituals, and accommodate them as much as possible, especially at the end of life. Failure to understand and, at least, empathise with the diverse spiritual-cultural values and beliefs of patients and families in multicultural societies—negotiating with them when these values and beliefs compromise care provision [18]—can have a deleterious affect on the patient–provider relationship. They can impact the services provided and received and, ultimately, their effectiveness in managing their patients—as well as their family and friends—and help them adjust to the dying process.

This chapter explores this intersection between culture and spirituality in four brief illustrative settings: China, Taiwan, New Zealand (specifically in Māori culture) and sub-Saharan Africa.

Palliative Care in China

Palliative care was first introduced to China with the establishment of the End-of-Life Care Research Centre at Tianjin Medical University in 1988 [19]. Since then, the approach has developed slowly, and the country's poor performance in palliative care provision—(ranked 71st among 80 countries across the globe in the Quality of Death Index [20])—has raised concern about its quality.

With a rapidly ageing population and increased incidence of chronic diseases and cancer, China faces a high demand for palliative care [21]. Responding to this challenge, the Chinese government issued palliative and hospice care guidelines in 2017 and selected pilot areas to promote services and improve quality-of-life for patients and families needing palliative and hospice care [22]. Despite progress—the country is now rated as being at a preliminary stage of integration [23]—palliative care needs to advance further and confront many obstacles hindering its development, including limited national policy and guidelines, lack of financial support, limited professional training, and, most importantly, the public's misunderstanding of death and palliative care [19].

Traditionally, most Chinese people believe that if there is a glimmer of hope for living a few days longer, it is worth paying a significant price, even their dignity, for it. This is reflected in a famous Chinese saying: *To live is better than to die*. A cross-sectional survey conducted to quantify current awareness of palliative care among patients across mainland China found that out of 549 respondents, only 68 (12%) reported awareness of palliative care. Of the 481 without prior awareness, 326 (68%) wanted more information, demonstrating the urgent need of raising public awareness of palliative care and promoting death education at all levels through public health education programs [24].

A systematic literature review conducted in the Greater China region (including Mainland China, Hong Kong, Macau, and Taiwan) suggested that spiritual care can promote perceived healing, provide life wisdom, and the search for belonging in the future world, while playing a pivotal role in death preparation and continuing bonds with ancestors. In traditional Chinese culture, relatives' views play an important role in end-of-life care decisions [25]. This tradition creates a major challenge for health care providers when the views of patients' family members are at odds with the recommendations of professionals. The literature review also highlighted the gaps remaining in our understanding. Further research is needed into palliative care for patients with nonmalignant diseases and identifying partnerships between specialist palliative care and community services.

Palliative Care in Taiwan

Taiwan is an island country located in East Asia, with a population of 23.5 million. Hospice and palliative care was first introduced to Taiwan in 1983, the first organization (MacKay Memorial Hospital) providing palliative care services built in 1990 [26]. Today, Taiwan is categorized as a Group 4b typology country, with hospice and palliative care services at an advanced stage of integration into mainstream service provision [23]. It was ranked sixth across 80 countries (first place in Asia) in the 2015 Quality of Death Index [20].

Taiwan is the first Asian country to adopt legislation honoring patients' care values and decision making regarding end of life. The Hospice-Palliative Care Act (also known as the Natural Death Act) of 2000 enabled terminally ill patients' self-determination on end-of-life care (i.e., signing Do Not Resuscitate [DNR] orders and appointing medical surrogates to speak for them once they lose capacity). In 2019,

Taiwan also adopted the Patient Right to Autonomy Act, extending access to palliative care by legalizing advance care planning and decision making for more diagnostic populations (persistent vegetative states, irreversible coma, and severe dementia, etc.) [27].

Understanding individual cultural backgrounds, life values, future goals, religious beliefs, as well as spiritual needs, and providing responsive health care are generally crucial in palliative care provision [28]. In Taiwan, this provision is heavily influenced by social norms and cultural and religious/spiritual beliefs that indirectly affect patients' well-being.

Key factors to be taken into account in this regard, while providing palliative care include (1) the notion of filial piety (i.e., an important virtue and a primary duty of respect and care of one's parents or family members); (2) patriarchal tradition (i.e., a society based on a male-dominated power structure throughout organized society and in individual relationships); (3) family-centered decision making, and (4) religion-guided life value [15,29].

For example, truth-telling a deteriorating cancer prognosis to a patient is forbidden, as it is considered to deprive them of hope and cause depression [30]. Family-led discussion regarding a patient's end-of-life care decision making is common—as is the subordination of patient autonomy to physician authority [31]—as family want to be filial children by protecting patients from distressing end-of-life care decision making [32]. This phenomenon was evident in Huang et al. [33], who found that the majority of DNR patient forms were signed by family members (82.1%); only around 20% of patients completed the forms themselves. Additionally, health care professionals tend to communicate with family members—including nurses with terminally ill patients [34], a finding echoed in Japan and South Korea [35]—and leave patients no opportunity to engage with their own future palliative care plan before they lose capacity [36]. Decision makers in Taiwan are usually not patients, but male family members (often the patient's elder son), resulting from patriarchal traditions [15], despite legislation honoring individual patients' right to end-of-life care self-determination.

In Taiwan, traditional religions (such as Taoism, Confucianism, and Buddhism) affect Taiwanese people's daily lives, particularly their thoughts on death and dying [15,37]. Older patients presume death and dying is a natural process of life; they should not so presume, and they have no right to act against nature. Therefore, cancer patients are reluctant to discuss end-of-life care issues and make their own palliative care decisions, often authorizing the right to family members, the medical team, or God [32]. One striking example is patients' belief that an individual's end of life tends to be predetermined by their actions in their present and past lives. This was influenced by the cause and effect of Karma (the sum of a person's actions in this and previous states of existence, viewed as deciding their fate in future existences) and Samsara (the cycle of death and rebirth to which life in the material world is bound) beliefs in Buddhism [15]. This situation is exacerbated by difficulties reported among physicians and nurses in addressing spiritual care concerns, including its definition in practice, who instead base their perceptions and practices on patients' emotional and physical needs [38].

Palliative Care in New Zealand

Palliative care service provision was initiated in 1979 when the Mary Potter Hospice was opened in Wellington, followed by Te Omanga Hospice in Lower Hutt and Saint Joseph's Mercy Hospice in Auckland. Twenty-five years later, the hospice movement had grown to 42 programs [39]. Today, palliative care services are rated at an advanced stage of integration into mainstream health care services [23]. Despite currently being based on the *Te Whare Tapa Whā Māori* model of health that compares it to the four walls of a house—physical health; extended family well-being, belonging, caring and sharing; mental health, including the inseparability of mind and body; and spiritual health, including unseen and unspoken energies [40]—the extent to which how, and how successfully, these services are sensitive to and incorporate indigeonous Māori people's cultural and, especially, spiritual belief systems is underresearched [41].

Comparative research across Australia, Canada, the United States, and New Zealand has highlighted commonalities in palliative care practices delivered to indigenous populations. Service users' preferences include: dying close to or at home; involving family members; and integrating cultural practices. Reported barriers include: services' inaccessibility and affordability; lack of awareness of services offered; perceptions of palliative care; and inappropriate services [42]. However, while usefully providing insights into generic similarities across disparate cultural settings, such research can obscure the rich diversity of experiences, beliefs, and practices that exist within varied indigenous populations.

Derived from Eastern Polynesian roots, *Māori* culture—also known as *Māoritanga*—comprises the customs, practices, and beliefs of the *Māori* people of New Zealand (*Aotearoa* in *Māori*). While there is growing appreciation of the importance of spirituality and spiritual care among hospice patients, families and staff—as a search for meaning, peace of mind, and a degree of uncertainty in an uncertain world [43]—and nursing staff more generally [44], notions of spirituality (including concerns and resilience) among *Māori* populations are multidimensional, complex, and relatively neglected in palliative care services [41].

In contrast to Western individualistic models of bioethics—with an emphasis on death locale that has underpinned palliative care policy and practice—end-of-life priorities among *Māori* peoples are much more nuanced. Extending beyond the physical location of expiration, central to *Māori* beliefs is "preparing the spirit" for transition to the next life, as they confront their own mortality and spiritual journey [45], providing family, including older men and women, (*kaumātua*) with an opportunity to move toward the *arai* (veil).

This movement needs support from *whānau* (family, including extended family) carers. Everything that occurs on the journey to the *arai* either adds to, or diminishes, the spiritual experience and well-being of *kaumātua*. *Whānau* contribute positively to this process, strengthening their *wairua* (spirit), by intentionally providing care as an expression of *whanaungatanga* (connectedness), *aroha* (love, care, concern), *awhi* (affection, support), and *manaakitanga* (reciprocal care) [46].

This entails healing, connecting, and protecting to realize what people want at the end of their life [45], considerations that persist despite the assumed negative impact of urban drift—cultural disenfranchisement, ethnic diversity, changing *whānau* (given closer contact with *Pākehā* [New Zealanders of European/colonial descent]) and living in *te ao hurihuri* (the ever-changing world)—upon cultural care traditions [47]. *Māori* cultural practices provide spiritual and physical connections with *whānau*, the land, ancestors and with a greater force than self which, in turn, provide strength and comfort for the final journey [45].

The primary end-of-life concern of *kaumātua* is for their *whānau* and subtribe (*hapu*) or tribe (*iwi*); specifically their well-being after they have died, and not consituting a burden to them before their demise, followed by being at peace with their God and, third, feeling their life is complete. Good holistic care—embodied in the *Whare Tapa Whā* Older Person's Palliative Care Model [48]—is therefore relationship-orientated, upholding older people's *mana* (authority, status, spiritual power) across four domains: *whānau* (social/family); *hinengaro* (emotional/mental); *tinana* (physical); and *wairua* (spiritual).

Palliative care services should help identify barriers to, and facilitators of, these four domains in different care settings (home, hospice, hospital, and residential care home). Part of this entails appreciating the relational, contextual, and circumstantial contexts of care in relation to *Māori* diversity by building understanding, challenging stereotypes, appreciating the necessity of different approaches; communicating (avoiding jargon); having two-way information exchanges; having conversations around advance care planning; and, critically, extending health workers' knowledge of *Māori* values and care customs and their potential adaptation, among other factors [49], in ways that are culturally sensitive [50].

Sub-Saharan Africa

In most sub-Saharan African countries, health care systems are composed of biomedical and traditional treatments, the choice usually depending on belief, cost, proximity and guidance from significant others. The traditional realm of care consists of herbalists, bone setters, diviners, and ritual specialists; the last-named are mediums with spirits and ancestors. Some practitioners specialize in various afflictions (e.g., love, financial prosperity), identifying causes and curses and breaking complex yokes [51]. Patients are at liberty to consult care providers from any cultural group.

A cancer diagnosis is a typical example of a complex situation, as it comes with the "Why me?" existential/spiritual questions and mysteries regarding its metaphysical cause and what it is. Most patients and families believe that a higher power decides and controls a person's fate. Consequently, many have unresolved questions in the face of adversity. They tend to blame the higher power, or they may attach the adversity to a curse or a punishment for their own sins or for those of their ancestors. Others link it to witchcraft or ancestral punishments for breaking traditional taboos and other forms of transgressions [52]. This causes anger and spiritual distress that negatively impacts on their quality of life and that of their loved ones. Some patients denounce treatment because the wishes of the higher power must be realized. Reassurance that developing cancer is an accident is, therefore, encouraged in palliative cancer care to alleviate bitterness and spiritual distress and potentially to help with healing.

Cancer treatment is an extended journey, and, at times, cure is impossible, especially for the majority of patients reporting with advanced-stage disease who have diminished curative options [53]. Many patients believe that cancer is incurable and are less willing to seek Western treatment options, interpreting it as a death sentence; this mindset negatively impacts care outcomes. Consequently, many resort to divine interventions, while others consider herbal options as they believe Western medicine will be futile. Moreover, some patients focus on looking for a cure and refuse to accept that palliation is the feasible goal of care. Failure to reconcile care goals can result in service dropouts, poor outcomes, and less satisfaction with the quality of services [54]. For instance, in Cameroon, examples of learned professionals refusing Western options in preference for spiritual or traditional options have been noted and may be explained by attachment to cultural customs and beliefs [55]. Most sub-Saharan African cultures consider any discussion about death and dying as taboo [14]. Advance care planning is, therefore, not commonly practiced, which compromises patients' ability to express their end-of-life preferences. Research in Uganda (Namisango et al., unpublished) shows that bereaved caregivers rate the quality of death and dying as good if patients had an opportunity to express their end-of-life wishes and these wishes were fulfilled. Opportunities to celebrate a religious service and to have end-of-life rites were also indicators of a quality death and dying process. If service providers don't feel comfortable to break bad news and inform patients and their caregivers that cure is not an option or that the end of life is close, it is difficult to realize these goals.

Future Research Agenda

This chapter demonstrates the relevance of culture and spirituality in palliative care and the progress made in integrating them into care approaches. Further research is, however, required to address the culture–spirituality–palliative care nexus. Insufficient research exists on culture and culturally safe approaches to palliative care, especially among indigenous populations [56]. Cultural traditions, especially in diverse multicultural settings, are heterogeneous rather than homogeneous, dynamic rather than static, and ungeneralizable to all families and generations. Cultural traditions and practices need to be investigated as determinants of expectations and experiences of service users, and how those services are organized and delivered [57], to develop culturally appropriate models of care provision.

Similarly, spirituality has been relatively neglected in palliative care services, where the understandable immediate priority concern—especially in low-income countries—is management and relief of physical pain. Research should explore and evaluate different models of spiritual care provision, underpinned by an understanding of how death and the dying process are understood, how people find meaning in illness, and the preferred communication and rituals surrounding and planning for death. While attempts have been made to develop a taxonomy of spiritual care interventions to enable their operationalization and evaluation [58], spiritual care assessment and outcome measures remain a nascent field [59], with minimal attempts to validate what exists in varied cultures and countries [60]. This evidence is essential to guide services in the provision of culturally and spiritually appropriate, and cost-effective, care that meets patients' needs [61].

Conclusions

For some patients, spirituality is a search for a purpose and connectedness to the sacred [62], finding meaning in death's journey and helping to cope with what can be a distressing experience [63]. Providing compassionate and effective palliative care to patients and their families, especially toward the end of life, is premised on practitioners who are competent in their understanding of, and empathy with, patients' spiritual beliefs and cultural backgrounds, values, rituals, needs, and preferences. It is also imperative that they comprehend spiritual care in its wider sense, as encompassing not simply religious guidance but also support with existential concerns. The assessment of spiritual needs should explore the content of patient and family members' beliefs rather than simply their source. By being sensitive to patients' spiritual and cultural needs and wants, palliative care practitioners acquire the insights and understanding necessary to provide holistic care for the whole person and to address their suffering in its totality, in accord with the biopsychosocial-spiritual model of care provision, as well as helping ensure that their dignity, right to self-determination and autonomy are respected [64].

At a time of global reflection on ethnic and racial inequalities, North–South power differentials, and the decolonization of historical legacies, this sensitivity is more pertinent and demanded than ever, especially among indigenous populations who have directly experienced the impact of colonization, discrimination, and racism. Palliative care services should seek to forge meaningful partnerships— through sharing power and decision making—in care delivery that is not only culturally sensitive and competent but also culturally safe, involving patients and families in service planning, reflecting on individual and systemic racism, community ownership of services, and recognizing distinct worldviews that shape care [56]. As Moeke-Maxwell et al. remarked: "it is *how* we care that ultimately matters at the end of life. Culturally informed care practices bring quality of life to the dying and dignity to death" [65:150].

References

1. Ong C-K, Forbes D. Embracing Cicely Saunders's concept of total pain. *BMJ*. 2005;331:576–577.
2. Radbruch L, De Lima L, Knaul F, et al. Redefining palliative care—A new consensus-based definition. *J Pain Symptom Manage*. 2020;60:754–764.
3. Staudt C. Whole-person, whole-community care at the end of life. *Virtual Mentor*. 2013;13:1069–1080.
4. Clark D. Cultural considerations in planning palliative and end of life care. *Palliat Med*. 2012;26:195–196.
5. Spencer-Oatey H. *Culturally Speaking: Culture, Communication and Politeness Theory*. 2nd ed. London: Continuum; 2008.

6. Puchalski CM, Vitillo R, Hull SK, Reller N. Improving the spiritual dimension of whole person care: Reaching national and international consensus. *J Palliat Med.* 2014;17: 642–656.
7. Rogers M, Wattis J. Understanding the role of spirituality in providing person-centred care. *Nurs Stand.* 2020;35:25–30.
8. Eckersley RM. Culture, spirituality, religion and health: Looking at the big picture. *Med J Aust.* 2007;186:S54–56.
9. Richardson P. Spirituality, religion and palliative care. *Ann Palliat Med.* 2014;3:150–159.
10. Anandarajah G, Hight E. Spirituality and medical practice: Using the HOPE questions as a practical tool for spiritual assessment. *Am Fam Phys.* 2001;63:81–89.
11. Clark D. "Total pain," disciplinary power and the body in the work of Cicely Saunders, 1958-1967. *Soc Sci Med.* 1999;49:727–736.
12. Lanre-Abass B. Cultural issues in advance directives relating to end-of-life decision making. *Prajna Vihara J Philos.* 2008;9:23–49.
13. Zahedi F. The challenge of truth telling across cultures: A case study. *J Med Ethics Hist Med.* 2011;4:11.
14. Ekore RI, Lanre-Abass B. African cultural concept of death and the idea of advance care directives. *Indian J Palliat Care.* 2016;22:369–372.
15. Lee H-TS, Cheng S-C, Dai Y-T, Chang M, Hu W-Y. Cultural perspectives of older nursing home residents regarding signing their own DNR directives in Eastern Taiwan: A qualitative pilot study. *BMC Palliat Care.* 2016;15:45.
16. Magaña D. Praying to win this battle: Cancer metaphors in Latina and Spanish women's narratives. *Health Commun.* 2020;35:649–657.
17. Kagawa-Singer M. The cultural context of death rituals and mourning practices. *Oncol Nurs Forum.* 1998;25:1752–1756.
18. Taylor EJ. Spirituality, culture, and cancer care. *Semin Oncol Nurs.* 2001;17:197–205.
19. Liu W, Guo P. Exploring the challenges of implementing palliative care in China. *Eur J Palliat Care.* 2017;24:12–17.
20. The Economist Intelligence Unit. The 2015 Quality of Death Index Ranking palliative care across the world. Singapore: LIEN Foundation, 2015.
21. Lu Y, Gu Y, Yu W. Hospice and palliative care in China: Development and challenges. *Asia-Pacific J Oncol Nurs.* 2018;5:26–32.
22. The National Health and Family Planning Commission of the People's Republic of China. 2017. Notice of the General Office of the National Health and Family Planning Commission on printing and distributing the practice guidelines for hospice care. (Trial in Chinese). [Online]. Available: http://www.nhc.gov.cn/yzygj/s3593/201702/3ec857f8c4a244e69b233 ce2f5f270b3.shtml. Accessed April 19, 2021.
23. Clark D, Baur N, Clelland D, et al. Mapping levels of palliative care development in 198 countries: The situation in 2017. *J Pain Symptom Manage.* 2020;59:794–807.
24. Yan Y, Zhang H, Gao W, et al. Current awareness of palliative care in China. *Lancet Glob Health.* 2020;8:e333–e335.
25. Chung H, Harding R, Guo P. Palliative care in the Greater China region: A systematic review of needs, models, and outcomes. *J Pain Symptom Manage.* 2021;61:585–612.
26. Lai YL. Taiwan Hospice Palliative Care—A step by step development. *Taiwan J Hospice Palliat Care.* 2006;11:404–415. (in Mandarin)
27. Laws & Regulations Database of The Republic of China. Hospice-palliative care act, 2013. http://law.moj.gov.tw/LawClass/LawAll.aspx?PCode=L0020066.
28. McDermott E, Selman LE. Cultural factors influencing advance care planning in progressive, incurable disease: A systematic review with narrative synthesis. *J Pain Symptom Manage.* 2018;56:613–636.

29. Lin C-P, Evans CJ, Koffman J, Sheu S-J, Hsu S-H, Harding R. What influences patients' decisions regarding palliative care in advance care planning discussions? Perspectives from a qualitative study conducted with advanced cancer patients, families and healthcare professionals. *Palliat Med.* 2019;33:1299–1309.

30. Wang SY, Chen CH, Chen YS, Huang H-L. The attitude toward truth telling of cancer in Taiwan. *J Psychosom Res.* 2004;57:53–58.

31. Cheng S-Y, Lin C-P, Chan HY-L, Martina D, Mori M, Kim S-H, Ng R. Advance care planning in Asian culture. *Jpn J Clin Oncol.* 2020;50:976–989.

32. Lee H-TS, Cheng C-Y, Hu W-Y. Advance care planning and elderly autonomy among long-term care facilities residents under Chinese filial piety and familism culture. *Taiwan J Hosp Palliat Care.* 2012;17:187–199. (in Mandarin)

33. Huang CH, Hu W-Y, Chiu T-Y, Chen C-Y. The practicalities of terminally ill patients signing their own DNR orders—a study in Taiwan. *J Med Ethics.* 2008;34:336–340.

34. Lin Y-H, Lin MH, Chen C-K, et al. The differences in nurses' willingness to discuss palliative care with patients and their family members. *J Chin Med Assoc.* 2021;84:280–284.

35. Yamaguchi T, Maeda I, Hatano Y, et al. EASED investigators: Communication and behavior of palliative care physicians of patients with cancer near end of life in three East Asian countries. *J Pain Symptom Manage.* 2021;61:315–322.e1.

36. Lin C-P, Evans CJ, Koffman J, Chen P-J, Hou M-F, Harding R. Feasibility and acceptability of a culturally adapted advance care planning intervention for people living with advanced cancer and their families: A mixed methods study. *Palliat Med.* 2020;34:651–666.

37. Lee H-TS, Cheng S-C, Huang C-F, Wu Y-M, Hu W-Y. Implementation and barriers for elderly nursing home residents in signing their own advance directives in Taiwan: From culture perspectives of Taoism, Confucianism, and Buddhism. *Taiwan J Hosp Palliat Care.* 2015;20:154–165. (in Mandarin)

38. Tao Z, Wu P, Luo A, Ho T-L, Chen C-Y, Cheng S-Y. Perceptions and practices of spiritual care among hospice physicians and nurses in a Taiwanese tertiary hospital: a qualitative study. *BMC Palliat Care.* 2020;19:96.

39. McCabe M. The hospice movement in New Zealand—25 years on. The Nathaniel Centre: The New Zealand Catholic Bioethics Centre. Issue 13, 2004. Source: http://www.nathaniel.org.nz/bioethics-politics-and-slovenly-language-lessons-from-history/16-bioethical-issues/bioethics-at-the-end-of-life/114-the-hospice-movement-in-new-zealand-25-years-on. Accessed April 6, 2021.

40. Ministry of Health. Te Ara Whakapiri: Principles and guidance for the last days of life. 2nd ed. Wellington, New Zealand: Ministry of Health. 12 April 2017.

41. Nelson-Becker H, Moeke-Maxwell T. Spiritual diversity, spiritual assessment, and Māori end-of-life perspectives: Attaining Ka Ea. *Religions.* 2020;11:536.

42. Shahid S, Taylor EV, Cheetham S, Woods JA, Aoun SM, Thompson SC. Key features of palliative care service delivery to Indigenous peoples in Australia, New Zealand, Canada and the United States: A comprehensive review. *BMC Palliat Care.* 2018;17:72.

43. Egan R, MacLeod R, Jaye C, et al. Spiritual beliefs, practices, and needs at the end of life: Results from a New Zealand national hospice study. *Palliat Support Care.* 2017;15:223–230.

44. Egan R, Llewellyn R, Cox B, MacLeod R, McSherry W, Austin P. New Zealand nurses' perceptions of spirituality and spiritual care: Qualitative findings from a national survey. *Religions.* 2017;8(5):79. https://doi.org/10.3390/rel8050079

45. Duggleby W, Kuchera S, MacLeod R, et al. Indigenous people's experiences at the end of life. *Palliat Support Care.* 2015;13:1721–1733.

46. Moeke-Maxwell T, Mason K, Toohey F, Dudley J. Pou Aroha: An indigenous perspective on Māori palliative care. In: MacLeod RD, Van den Block L (eds). *Textbook of Palliative Care.* Oxford: Oxford University Press; 2019:1247–1263.

47. Moeke-Maxwell T. Growing closer to death: Māori spirituality and ageing. School of Nursing Conference, the University of Auckland, September 17, 2015.

48. Laws and Regulations Databases of the Republic of China. Patient Right to Autonomy Act, 2016. http://www.6law.idv.tw/6law/law/%E7%97%85%E4%BA%BA%E8%87%AA%E4 %B8%BB%E6%AC%8A%E5%88%A9%E6%B3%95.htm. Accessed August 18, 2017.

49. Moeke-Maxwell T. Palliative care: How can we do things better for Māori? Indigenous people and cancer; A shared agenda for Aotearoa, Australia and Pacific nations. New Zealand: University of Otago; February 20, 2018.

50. Foliaki S, Pulu V, Denison H, Weatherall M, Douwes J. Pacific meets west in addressing palliative care for Pacific populations in Aotearoa/New Zealand: A qualitative study. *BMC Palliat Care.* 2020;19:100.

51. Geschiere P. *The Modernity of Witchcraft: Politics and the Occult in Postcolonial Africa.* 1998. Charlottesville, VA: University of Virginia Press.

52. Kinsman J. "A time of fear": Local, national, and international responses to a large Ebola outbreak in Uganda. *Global Health.* 2012;8:15.

53. Brand NR, Qu LG, Chao A, Ilbawi AM. Delays and barriers to cancer care in low- and middle-income countries: A systematic review. *Oncologist.* 2019;24:e1371–e1380.

54. van Laarhoven HWM, Henselmans I, de Haes JHC. To treat or not to treat: Who should decide? *Oncologist.* 2014;19:433–436.

55. Ngwang M. Grief in Cameroon society—a blog. International Children's Palliative Care Network, 2021. Source: https://www.icpcn.org/grief-in-cameroon-society-a-blog-by-ngwang-menang

56. Schill K, Caxaj S. Cultural safety strategies for rural Indigenous palliative care: a scoping review. *BMC Palliat Care.* 2019;18:21.

57. Gott M, Moeke-Maxwell T, Williams L, et al. Te Pākeketanga: Living and dying in advanced age—a study protocol. *BMC Palliat Care.* 2015;14:74.

58. Massey K, Barnes MJD, Villines D, et al. What do I do? Developing a taxonomy of chaplaincy activities and interventions for spiritual care in intensive care unit palliative care. *BMC Palliat Care.* 2015;14:10.

59. Emanuel LL, Powell RA, Handzo G, et al. Validated assessment tools for psychological, spiritual and family issues. In: Cherny N, Fallon M, Kaasa S, Portenoy RK, Currow DC (eds). *Oxford Textbook of Palliative Medicine,* 5th ed. Oxford: Oxford University Press; 2015:398–406.

60. Selman L, Harding R, Gysels M, Speck P, Higginson IJ. The measurement of spirituality in palliative care and the content of tools validated cross-culturally: A systematic review. *J Pain Symptom Manage.* 2011;41:728–753.

61. Harding R, Powell RA, Downing J, et al. Generating an African palliative care evidence base: The context, need, challenges and strategies. *J Pain Symptom Manage.* 2008;36:304–309.

62. Drutchas A, Anandarajah G. Spirituality and coping with chronic disease in paediatrics. *Rhode Island Med Soc.* 2014;97:26–30.

63. Murray SA, Kendall, M, Boyd K, Worth A, Benton TF. Exploring the spiritual needs of people dying of lung cancer or heart failure: A prospective qualitative interview study of patients and their carers. *Palliat Med.* 2004;18:39–45.

64. Moss EL, Dobson KS. Psychology, spirituality and end-of-life care: An ethical integration? *Can Psychol.* 2006;47:284–299.

65. Moeke-Maxwell T, Nikora LW, Awekotuku NT. End-of-life care and Māori whānau resilience. *Mai J.* 2014;3:140–152.

4

Holistic Care of the Cancer Patient, United States

Identifying Unique Aspects of Palliative Care

*Phyllis Whitehead, Shereen Gamaluddin, Sarah DeWitt,
Christi Stewart, and Kye Y. Kim*

Palliative Care versus Hospice Care

Patients with a serious illness may hear the terms *palliative care* and *hospice* during the course of their illness and treatment. These terms are often mistaken for the same type of care provided to patients at the end of life. While the two are commonly thought of as the same type of care, they are in fact different.

Palliative care is a type of medical care given to patients with a serious or life-threatening illness, such as cancer. The goal of this type of care is improving quality of life by providing relief of symptoms and the stress of illness, in addition to identifying patient goals and advanced care planning. Palliative care is an approach to care that addresses not only a patient's disease process, but the person as a whole, including physical, emotional, and spiritual suffering. It is provided by a specialty-trained team of physicians, nurses, social workers, chaplains, and therapists who work together to provide an additional layer of support to patients and their families. It is care that is provided at any stage of a patient's illness, including during curative treatment, and it is not dependent on prognosis. It can be provided in the hospital setting, as an outpatient model of care, as well as in the home [1].

Hospice care is compassionate comfort care for those facing a terminal illness with an expected prognosis of six months or less if their disease were to follow its natural and expected progression. It is delivered in an interdisciplinary team approach addressing physical, emotional, and spiritual pain as well. It is an insurance benefit that is paid for by Medicare, Medicaid, and private insurance, and it includes medications, medical equipment, access to care no matter the time of day, nursing services, social services, chaplains, and grief support for families. Hospice has traditionally been cared that is provided at home, but it can also be provided in a nursing home setting outside of the hospital [2].

Numerous studies show that palliative care and hospice significantly improve patients' quality of life and lowers symptom burden. Previous studies have shown that the majority of Americans, approximately 80%, would prefer to die at home if possible. A recent article in the *New England Journal of Medicine*, published December 2019, revealed that for the first time in decades, more people are dying at home as opposed to in the hospital; the percentage increased from 23% in 2003 to 30% in

2017 [1]. Although no causality has been established, it is likely that the increase in palliative and hospice services over the past decade has been instrumental in this change, allowing patients to have the dignity and ability to die at home with less suffering.

Unique Challenges for Cancer Patients

Palliative medicine is meant to serve patients living with chronic, and possibly terminal, illnesses by addressing the needs of the entire mind, body, and spirit. Its aims involve a comprehensive and compassionate approach toward the alleviation of suffering. This suffering includes not only physical symptoms, but also psychosocial, spiritual, and existential symptoms for those whose illness impacts their daily lives. Cancer patients, especially, are susceptible and vulnerable to this impact.

The physical symptoms of cancer are often debilitating and life altering. Pain is often prevalent and affects all parts of a person's life. Pain, however, is not always related to the cancer itself. Pain may be due to direct disease burden, such as a tumor pressing on organs, bones, or nerves. However, often the diagnosis of cancer involves painful testing and procedures, such as biopsies or more invasive imaging. Surgeries are often part of the treatment for cancer that grows as a solid tumor, which can cause pain during and after the operation. Even treatments for cancer are often associated with painful side effects. Chemotherapy can induce peripheral neuropathy, leading to chronic nerve pain and debility. Mouth sores and abdominal pain can accompany many forms of treatment. Radiation used to reduce tumor size can induce mucositis (mouth sores), external skin burning, and irritation and scarring—all of which can cause pain [3].

Physical symptoms other than pain can also manifest in those with cancer, either from the disease process itself or from testing and treatments for the cancer. Shortness of breath (dyspnea), either at rest or with any form of exertion, is not uncommon. Nausea can be chronically debilitating, with or without vomiting. Nausea is often associated with chemotherapies but may be due to cancer burden independently of treatments. Changes in bowel habits, either constipation or diarrhea, can be caused by cancer and/or cancer-related treatments, and aside from causing pain or discomfort, can lead to functional decline and social isolation. Loss of appetite with associated weight loss can lead to weakness and further debility. Some treatments may even cause extensive weight gain due to internal fluid shifts and edema.

Sleep changes are often associated with cancers and cancer-related treatments. Fatigue is found in 90% of patients diagnosed with cancer and is one of the most common and debilitating symptoms that can cause significant distress for patients. All the above symptoms are common and well documented, and can cause physical, emotional, and spiritual distress for those who suffer from cancer and cancer treatments. A large part of the field of palliative medicine involves monitoring, assessment, and treatment for the physical symptoms of cancer and cancer-related therapies. Due to the high physical symptom burden, palliative medicine is recommended per national quality guidelines to be a part of a patient's cancer treatment team from the time of diagnosis and throughout the course of treatment for holistic care [4].

While physical symptoms of cancer and cancer treatments may be easier to identify, the diagnosis of cancer has been shown to impact a person on a much deeper, comprehensive level than physical symptoms alone could represent. Fear is very common. This fear may manifest for a variety of reasons: death, debility, loss of independence, pain or physical symptoms, debility, financial strain, and becoming a burden to others. Even after patients have achieved remission of their cancer, they often report continued fear of recurrence. For those experiencing cancer, the times that others would associate with relief and joy, such as the anniversary date of remission or discontinuation of long-term treatments, are often associated with fear [5].

The diagnosis, treatments, and management of cancer in all stages also involve fundamental losses. Patients grieve loss of health, but many other losses can follow. Grief can impact sex drive and sexual relationships. Fertility is often sacrificed for younger persons undergoing cancer treatments. The physical side effects of cancer and its treatment often result in an increased dependence on others, and this loss of physical independence may cause anger and grief for patients, as well as those supporting them. Grief over the changes in body image during and after cancer is common, as many cancer treatments are associated with amputations, scarring, hair loss, lymphedema or limb swelling, weight changes, and disfigurement.

Beside fear and grief, cancer can influence the psyche and sense of self. Descriptions of feeling hopeless, powerless, uncertain, exposed, vulnerable, and useless are found throughout the literature. Loss of sense of purpose is something many people living with chronic illness suffer and is an independent risk factor for social isolation, depression, and even cognitive impairment and debility. Depression is present in 70% of persons diagnosed with cancer, and this concurrent depression can escalate emotional distress, as well as increase the difficulty of compliance with treatment plans and maintaining functional independence. Additionally, depression may persist even after remission of cancer. Therefore, it is critical to have palliative care counselors and chaplains to explore, validate, and work with patients through the symptoms of fear and grief. The emotional impact of the disease process can be just as, or even more, debilitating for a person's daily life than even the more apparent physical manifestations of cancer [6].

The spirituality of an individual diagnosed with cancer can often be strengthened, but for some it can be deeply shaken. Different from, but inclusive of, faith and religion, spirituality is the relationship people have with a force or power beyond themselves that helps them feel connected and can often involve a search for the meaning of life. Alternatively, religion is defined as a specific set of beliefs concerning the cause, nature and purpose of the universe. For most, cancer is a first opportunity for a person to confront and examine their mortality. This can lead to a deeper sense of connection with their spirituality or religion. Some return to religious groups or organizations in which they had once participated. This reconnection can improve their social and spiritual support system and allow them to find new opportunities to cope with the physical and emotional suffering that often accompanies cancer diagnosis and treatment. Studies have shown that a connection with one's spirituality helps patients experience more hope, optimism, and satisfaction with life. Spirituality can lead to decreased rates of anxiety and depression, decreased feelings of loneliness, decreased alcohol and drug abuse, lower blood pressure, and better control of pain and nausea. For some, a diagnosis of cancer allows deeper evaluation and discovery of life's meaning and connection with their spirituality [7].

For others, as suggested earlier, cancer has the opposite effect on their sense of spirituality. The diagnosis can make them doubt their beliefs and religious values or challenge their faith. This can cause significant spiritual distress. Up to half of patients with advanced cancer have reported some level of spiritual distress. Sometimes a person's anger and grief over a diagnosis can be pointed toward a spiritual or religious entity. Some wonder if they are being punished for past actions, a questioning that leads them to take a distrustful and antagonistic approach to their religion or spirituality. Spiritual distress can also lead to a sense of alienation and isolation from a spiritual entity that previously gave them comfort and promote social isolation from their previously established religious group. In order to provide comprehensive relief of suffering, a spiritual assessment as an individual and ongoing process through diagnosis and treatment of cancer, and through end of life, is a critical component of holistic palliative care. A chaplain often takes part in a comprehensive palliative care team, providing ongoing spiritual assessment, evaluation, and support to those diagnosed with long-term illnesses and cancer [7].

The physical, emotional, and spiritual impact of cancer can also impact the social system of an individual. Cancer patients often talk about feeling "alone in a crowd." Those who have never had cancer often have difficulty interacting with those who are diagnosed, unsure of what to say or do in their presence. Some pull back from interactions entirely, and those who attempt to interact are often accused of treating the cancer patient differently than prior to the diagnosis. Physical strength and stamina decline, both with the disease process itself, throughout the course of treatment, and at end of life. This makes it difficult to engage with others in and outside the home, make appointments, and seek additional support and counsel.

Workplace relationships often change as well, with performance fatigue being common, and some people being unable to work at all during or after treatments. This can also escalate financial distress, both directly and through loss of insurance. Body disfigurement is common, with weight loss, skin changes, hair and tooth loss due to treatment, and even amputations for solid tumors. This can lead to embarrassment and increased difficulty in matters of social interaction and intimacy. There is often immune system compromise with cancer treatments, with social interaction posing a risk and fear of contracting an infection. Some patients, now experiencing increased emotional and physical care needs, fear the burden they will place on those around them. A diagnosis and treatment of cancer will not just impact the individual with the diagnosis, but the entire family and community that surround them, leading to increased stress and distress for all parties involved [1].

Coping is defined as a process of dealing with stressful events by means of cognitive appraisal, purposeful efforts, and use of available supports and resources in order to achieve physiological and psychological adjustment. Palliative care is devoted to the holistic care of the individual at all stages of their disease. Palliative specialists understand that both the disease and the treatments for it can cause suffering on every level. They work alongside other members of the medical care team to provide an additional layer of support for relief of pain, symptoms, and emotional, spiritual, and social stress for people with cancer, their families, and their community.

Defining Total Pain

Total pain is defined as the suffering that affects the physical, psychological, social, and spiritual dimensions of persons diagnosed with cancer. Cancer can influence an individual emotionally, psychologically, socially, and spiritually, as we have discussed. It is consistent with other current theories of pain that recognize cancer pain from a holistic perspective. The consequences of total pain for the physical, social, and spiritual functioning of patients suggest there may also be a bidirectional influence between all these dimensions [8].

Cancer pain is distinguished from other types of pain that result from other illnesses because of its unpredictable course, which can vary dramatically in severity and duration, depending on the type of treatment and disease progression. Most patients with advanced cancer also report more than one type of pain, which means that, although patients may present initially with an acute episode of pain, it can progress to be acute and chronic in unpredictable ways [3].

Clinicians cannot properly manage cancer pain without approaching it holistically, including pharmacological and nonpharmacological interventions. Using the total pain model (see Figure 4.1), clinicians need to assess for all four dimensions of pain and devise holistic treatment plans.

Nonpharmacological Interventions

Recent advances in psychosocial interventions addressing pain offer huge potential for providing holistic care in caring for cancer patients. Multimodal therapy is considered the standard of care for cancer pain, and the utilization of these potentially opioid-sparing modalities is more critical in the face of the existing opioid crisis.

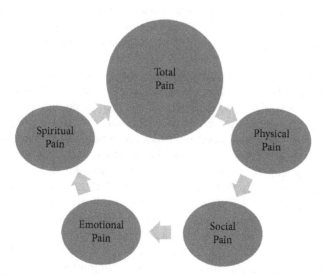

Figure 4.1 Total Pain Experience

Multimodal interventions are the use of at least two different analgesic medications and nonpharmacologic therapies with different mechanisms of action to provide more effective pain relief compared with single-modality interventions. Underutilized in both acute and chronic cancer pain management, these nonpharmacologic interventions can reduce pain, minimize suffering, and provide beneficial effects on functionality up to one year after completion of the therapy [9].

Stress-reducing psychosocial interventions have been developed and shown to improve immune function. Psychosocial treatments in palliative care are categorized into cognitive-behavioral therapy (CBT), mindfulness-based interventions, life review or meaning-centered interventions, and creative-arts based therapies.

CBT has been shown to improve depression, sleep disturbances, and quality of life in patients with advanced cancer. Arts and music in creative-arts-based therapies can also be used to facilitate feelings of meaning and a psychospiritual integration of life experiences in seriously ill patients and caregivers. Music therapy is generally defined as a systematic process of intervention wherein a music therapist helps the client promote health, using music experiences and the relationships that develop through them as dynamic forces of change. Music therapy has been frequently associated with pain reduction and enhancement of physical comfort [10–14]. Mindfulness is defined as the act of paying attention on purpose, in the present moment, and nonjudgmentally. Mindfulness-based interventions have been shown to improve health outcomes in different settings and to reduce anxiety, depression, sexual difficulties, stress, and sleep disturbances in various oncological conditions [5,10]. Mindfulness promotes spirituality that allows a person to experience a transcendent meaning in life and is increasingly being recognized as an important factor in maintaining health, well-being, and symptom management [9, 15–17].

Additionally, biofield therapies, also known as energy therapies, include Therapeutic Touch (TT), Reiki, Healing Touch (HT), and Qigong; these therapies have existed among many traditional cultures for centuries. In the 1970s, their use resurfaced within the nursing discipline. TT, for example, was created by two nurses in the 1970s and was incorporated into nursing curricula. TT is based on the ancient practices of Qigong and Reiki and is a distinct-phase process that results in an exchange of energy to facilitate healing and relaxation. HT also developed out of nursing in the late 1980s and involves restoring the free flow of energy by opening blockages that contribute to disease and imbalance. Biofield healing conducted by Fazzino et al., which was part of a trend toward effectiveness, was detected for Reiki, TT, and HT and provided pain relief in addition to either decreasing the amount of opioids participants required or increasing the time span between opioid dosages for those receiving biofield treatments [18,19]. Additionally, interpersonal touch has been found to have physiological and psychological effects, influencing neuroendocrine functioning and reducing stress, pain, and ultimately promoting comfort and well-being. TT, HT, Reiki, and other Complementary and Alternative Medicine (CAM) modalities, which involve touch, may allow clinicians to further improve cancer experiences for patients and their families in a cost-effective manner, whether administered directly or indirectly through caregiver education.

Exercise has proven to be an efficient supportive therapy to counteract disease and treatment-associated side effects (e.g., fatigue, lymphedema) and to increase patients' emotional wellness [20]. Yoga is known to reduce expressive suppression and to develop calmness and mindfulness, which increases body awareness and emotion regulation, thereby helping to decrease patients' anxiety and pain.

Hypnosis has three major components, which can influence cognition and emotional regulation: (1) absorption, which is the involvement in a perceptual, imaginative, or ideational experience; (2) dissociation, which is the mental separation of different components of experience that would usually be processed; and (3) suggestibility, which is the responsiveness to social clues, enhancing the propensity to comply with hypnotic instructions and suspending critical judgment. These hypnotic suggestions can facilitate mind–body connection and lead to physical, emotional, and behavioral changes, which could explain the impact of that intervention on patients' emotional distress, fatigue, and anxiety [20–22].

It is crucial to recognize the healing potential of the above-mentioned interventions. Healing is the aspect of humanity that refers to the way individuals seek and express meaning and purpose and the way they experience their connectedness to the moment, to self, to others, to nature, and to the significant or sacred [23–25]. The choice of which modality to use and which clinician to work with involves many factors, including what sort of clinicians are available in any given community, whether the patient is ambulatory or hospitalized, and whether financial resources exist since many integrative clinicians are not covered by standard health insurance or Medicare. Ultimately, healing represents an inner process of transformation that may occur at a level beyond a patient's everyday awareness. It is our responsibility to assess, encourage, and support cancer patients during this journey [23–25].

Interprofessional Approach to the Care of the Cancer Patient

Palliative care gives support to patients with chronic and/or life-limiting disease. It has developed into a multifocus discipline, with attention given to symptom management, psychosocial and spiritual care, caregiver support, patient–clinician communication, complex decision making, and end-of-life care. The collaboration of different health care professionals working as a team from different care perspectives can help improve patient experiences, access to resources, and overall care.

According to the National Coalition for Hospice and Palliative Care, an interdisciplinary team (IDT) provides care that encompasses the individual's physical, functional, psychological, social, spiritual, and cultural needs. An IDT can include physicians, nurses, psychologists, social workers, chaplains, pharmacists, physiotherapists, occupational therapists, Speech Language Pathologist (SLP)s as well as other health professionals. An IDT encourages team members to maximize their professional skills for the benefit of patients and families, allowing each member to contribute their unique expertise to patient care

The components of the care needs of patient and caregiver are complex and can include

1. Information—prognosis, treatment risks, benefits
2. Spiritual support—hope, faith and religion, dignity

3. Physical needs—pain, fatigue, nausea, dyspnea, function
4. Emotional support—anxiety, depression
5. Social—role of caregivers, family, relationships, finances [1]

Recognizing these needs, the IDT members can support patients and their families by their strength and expertise. Physicians can focus on illness, prognosis, and medical treatments. They can provide direct patient care while collaborating with advanced practice registered nurses and physician assistants to address the care needs of cancer patients.

Nurses provide direct patient care, patient advocacy, and care coordination as well as immediate assessment and reassessment of patient needs. Advanced practice providers (physician assistants and advanced practice registered nurses) expand the ability to deliver complex and/or direct care. Social workers attend to family dynamics, assess and support coping mechanisms and social determinants of health, identify and facilitate access to resources, and mediate conflict. Chaplains assess and address spiritual needs and help facilitate continuity with the patient's faith community.

The strengths of this interdisciplinary approach include shared decision making and responsibility to support patients and families. As not all members are required at all times, this approach can give an added benefit of helping to prevent provider burnout [26].

Cultural Influences on Palliative Care and the Cancer Patient

A culture is a group of people's way of life—the behaviors, belief, values, and symbols that accept and are passed along by communication and imitation from one generation to the next. The role of culture has become significantly relevant in health care. Given the demographic changes in many countries, health care providers increasingly have come to care for patients of diverse cultural backgrounds. Palliative care has become well recognized as one area wherein care must be shaped according to the unique physical, emotional, social, cultural, and spiritual needs of individuals. Again, culture plays a critical role in different perceptions of end-of-life needs by patients, their families, and health care providers [27]. Therefore, contemporary palliative care should be an approach that improves the quality of life of patients and their families facing problems associated with serious illness through the prevention and relief of suffering by means of early identification and impeccable assessment and treatment of pain and other physical, psychosocial, and spiritual problems [28].

Culture provides a framework of expectations for patients that include communication concerns with health care professionals, dynamics of decision making, the dying process itself, as well as expectations about the role of health care professionals, family members, and patients [29]. The important role of culture is also reflected in the Joint Commission's new standards for culturally competent patient care and assessment in American hospitals [30], but specific assessment questions for the patient in palliative care should be added, for instance, "Who makes the decisions about treatment options at the end of care?"

Werth et al. [31] clearly summarized guidelines for encouraging more culturally sensitive end-of-life care by emphasizing that each patient must be treated as a unique participant from different belief systems concerning specifically:

1. Documented differences in the cultural interpretations of the ethical meta principles (e.g., autonomy and respect).
2. Provision of medical service in general and pain management in particular to different groups.
3. Attitudes toward various end-of-life interventions and the use of advance directives.

In the United States, advance directives, do not resuscitate (DNR) orders, and durable power of attorneys Medical Power of Attorney (MPOA) are ways to reflect patients' autonomy in situations where patients can no longer make decisions for themselves. However, non-Western cultures believe that communities and families, not patients alone, are affected by serious illnesses and the accompanying medical decisions [32]. Some cultures view discussion of serious illness and death as disrespectful or impolite (Singer). In most Asian cultures, it is perceived as unnecessarily cruel to inform a patient of a cancer diagnosis [12,33], and more so with elderly patients [12,32]. In Chinese, Native American, Filipino, and Bosnian cultures, it is emphasized that words should be carefully chosen because once spoken, they may become self-fulfilling or a reality [34,35].

Locus of decision making is another culturally sensitive issue in end-of-life care and cancer patients. Compared with individuals of African and European descent, Koreans and Mexican Americans were more likely to consider family members rather than the patient alone, as holding the decision-making power regarding life support [36]. African descendants view an overly individualistic focus as disrespectful to their family heritage [37].

Interestingly, significantly lower rates of advance directives completion were found among Asians, Hispanics, and African Americans [24,38]. According to Searlight [39], the low rate of advance directive completion among nonwhites may reflect distrust of the health care system, health care disparities, cultural perspectives on death and suffering, and family dynamics such as parent–child relationships [39]. Searlight wisely advises that health care professionals' partnership with their patients and their families provide unique insight into their values, spirituality, and relationship dynamics, and may be especially helpful during end-of-life care.

Conclusion

Palliative medicine is a comprehensive care model that serves patients living with chronic and possibly terminal illnesses. It addresses the needs of the entire person: mind, body, and spirit. Palliative care is devoted to the holistic care of the individual at all stages of their disease. Palliative specialists work alongside other members of the medical care team to provide an additional layer of support for relief of pain, symptoms, and emotional, spiritual, and social stress for people with cancer, their families, and their community.

Those living with chronic illness are at risk for suffering from not only physical symptoms, but psychosocial, spiritual, and existential symptoms as well. Cancer patients are especially at risk and vulnerable to the potential impact of this type of suffering on their daily lives. Physical symptoms can also cause significant burden to those with cancer and are caused not only by the disease process itself but by testing and treatments of cancer. Treatment for physical symptoms should include pharmacological and nonpharmacological interventions. Palliative medicine is provided by an interdisciplinary team. This interprofessional approach to physical and nonphysical symptom management is crucial to holistically care for those living with cancer. It is the hallmark of the specialty of palliative medicine.

References

1. Budhwani S, Wodchis WP, Zimmermann C, Moineddin R, Howell D. Support needs and interventions in advanced cancer: A scoping review. BMJ Supportive & Palliative Care, 2019, 9(1):12–25. doi:10.1136/bmjspcare-2018-001529
2. Clinical Practice Guidelines for Quality Palliative Care, 4th Edition. National Coalition for Quality Palliative Care. Richmond, VA; 2018. https://www.nationalcoalitionhpc.org/ncp
3. Mehta A, Chan LS. Understanding of the concept of "total pain": A prerequisite for pain control. J Hosp Palliat Nurs. 2008;10(1):26–34. doi:10.1097/01.NJH.0000306714.50539.1a
4. Palliative care versus hospice. nhpco.org/wp-content/uploads/2019/04/PalliativeCare_ VS_Hospice.pdf. Published 2019.
5. Pan-Weisz TM, Kryza-Lacombe M, Burkeen J, Hattangadi-Gluth J, Malcarne VL, McDonald CR. Patient-reported health-related quality of life outcomes in supportive-care interventions for adults with brain tumors: A systematic review. Psychooncology. 2019;28(1):11–21. doi:10.1002/pon.4906
6. Teo I, Krishnan A, Lee GL. Psychosocial interventions for advanced cancer patients: A systematic review. Psychooncology. 2019;28(7):1394–1407. doi:10.1002/pon.5103
7. Martins H, Caldeira S. Spiritual distress in cancer patients: A synthesis of qualitative studies. Religions. 2018;9(10):1–17. doi:10.3390/rel9100285
8. Relieving pain in America fostering a cultural transformation pain as a public health challenge. Natl Acad Sci. 2012;June, 1–4. www.iom.edu/relievingpain. Accessed July 29, 2017.
9. O'Brien MR, Kinloch K, Groves KE, Jack BA. Meeting patients' spiritual needs during end-of-life care: A qualitative study of nurses' and healthcare professionals' perceptions of spiritual care training. J Clin Nurs. 2019;28(1–2):182–189. doi:10.1111/jocn.14648
10. Warth M, Koehler F, Weber M, Bardenheuer HJ, Ditzen B, Kessler J. "Song of Life (SOL)" study protocol: A multicenter, randomized trial on the emotional, spiritual, and psychobiological effects of music therapy in palliative care. BMC Palliat Care. 2019;18(1):1–11. doi:10.1186/s12904-019-0397-6
11. Araw AC, Araw AM, Pekmezaris R, et al. Medical orders for life-sustaining treatment: Is it time yet? Palliat Support Care. 2014;12(02):101–105. doi:10.1017/S1478951512001010
12. Rodin G. From evidence to implementation: The global challenge for psychosocial oncology. Psychooncology. 2018;27(10):2310–2316. doi:10.1002/pon.4837
13. Bradley N, Lloyd-Williams M, Dowrick C. Effectiveness of palliative care interventions offering social support to people with life-limiting illness—A systematic review. Eur J Cancer Care (Engl). 2018;27(3):1–12. doi:10.1111/ecc.12837

14. Ben-Arye E, Preis L, Barak Y, Samuels N. A collaborative model of integrative care: Synergy between anthroposophic music therapy, acupuncture, and spiritual care in two patients with breast cancer. *Complement Ther Med.* 2018;40(April 2018):195–197. doi:10.1016/j.ctim.2018.04.002

15. Kang KA, Han SJ, Lim YS, Kim SJ. Meaning-centered interventions for patients with advanced or terminal cancer: A meta-analysis. *Cancer Nurs.* 2019;42(4):332–340. doi:10.1097/NCC.0000000000000628

16. Yong J, Park J, Kim J, Kim P, Seo IS, Lee H. The effects of holy name meditation on spiritual well-being, depression, and anxiety of patients with cancer. *J Hosp Palliat Nurs.* 2018;20(4):368–376. doi:10.1097/NJH.0000000000000451

17. Nedjat-Haiem FR, Carrion I V., Gonzalez K, Ell K, Thompson B, Mishra SI. Exploring health care providers' views about initiating end-of-life care communication. *Am J Hosp Palliat Med.* 2017;34(4):308–317. doi:10.1177/1049909115627773

18. Henneghan AM, Schnyer RN. Biofield therapies for symptom management in palliative and end-of-life care. *Am J Hosp Palliat Med.* 2015;32(1):90–100. doi:10.1177/1049909113509400

19. Lehto RH. Psychosocial challenges for patients with advanced lung cancer: Interventions to improve well-being. *Lung Cancer Targets Ther.* 2017;8:79–90. doi:10.2147/LCTT.S120215

20. Ferrell BR, Temel JS, Temin S, et al. Integration of palliative care into standard oncology care: American Society of Clinical Oncology clinical practice guideline update. 2018;35(1):96–112. doi:10.1200/JCO.2016.70.1474

21. Grégoire C, Bragard I, Jerusalem G, et al. Group interventions to reduce emotional distress and fatigue in breast cancer patients: A 9-month follow-up pragmatic trial. *Br J Cancer.* 2017;117(10):1442–1449. doi:10.1038/bjc.2017.326

22. Lichtenstein AH, Berger A, Cheng MJ. Definitions of healing and healing interventions across different cultures. *Ann Palliat Med.* 2017;6(3):248–252. doi:10.21037/apm.2017.06.16

23. Steinhorn DM, Din J, Johnson A. Healing, spirituality and integrative medicine. *Ann Palliat Med.* 2017;6(3):237–247. doi:10.21037/apm.2017.05.01

24. Sloan DH, BrintzenhofeSzoc K, Kichline T, et al. An assessment of meaning in life-threatening illness: Development of the Healing Experience in All Life Stressors (HEALS). *Patient Relat Outcome Meas.* 2017;8:15–21. doi:10.2147/prom.s118696

25. Koh S-J, Kim S, Kim J, et al. Experiences and opinions related to end-of-life discussion: From oncologists' and resident physicians' perspectives. *Cancer Res Treat.* 2017;50(2), 614–623. doi:10.4143/crt.2016.446

26. Zhao X, Zhang D, Wu M, et al. Loneliness and depression symptoms among the elderly in nursing homes: A moderated mediation model of resilience and social support. *Psychiatry Res.* 2018 Oct;268, 143–151. doi:10.1016/j.psychres.2018.07.011

27. Lee P-C, Lo C, Ko W-J, Huang S-J, Lee P-H. When and how should physicians determine the need for palliative and hospice care for patients with end-stage liver disease?: An experience in Taiwan. *Am J Hosp Palliat Care.* 2014;31(4):454–458. doi:10.1177/1049909113495707

28. Organization WH. Palliative care definition. August 5, 2020. http://www.who.int/cancer/palliative/definition/en

29. Blackhall LJ. The Treatment of Suffering in Patients with Advanced Cancer. Handbook of Psychiatry in Palliative Medicine. In: Chochinov HM, Breitbart W, eds. *Handbook of Psychiatry in Palliative Medicine.* 2nd ed. New York: Oxford University Press; 2009:186–187.

30. Foglia MB, Lowery J, Sharpe VA, Tompkins P, Fox E. A comprehensive approach to eliciting, documenting, and honoring patient wishes for care near the end of life: The Veterans Health Administration's Life-Sustaining Treatment Decisions Initiative. *Jt Comm J Qual Patient Saf.* 2019;45(1):47–56. doi:10.1016/j.jcjq.2018.04.007

31. Werth, JL J, Blevins D, Toussaint K. The influence of cultural diversity on end-of-life care and decision. *Am Behav Sci*. 2002;46:204–219.
32. Candib L. Truth telling and advance planning at the end of life: Problems with autonomy in a multicultural world. *Fam Syst Heal*. 2002;20:213–228.
33. Matsumura S, Bito S, Liu H, et al. Acculturation of attitudes toward end-of-life care: A cross-cultural survey of Japanese Americans and Japanese. *J Gen Intern Med*. 2002;17:531–539.
34. Bussmann S, Muders P, Zahrt-Omar CA, et al. Improving end-of-life care in hospitals: A qualitative analysis of bereaved families' experiences and suggestions. *Am J Hosp Palliat Care*. 2015;32(1):44–51. doi:10.1177/1049909113512718
35. Carrese J, Rhodes L. Western bioethics on the Navajo reservation: Benefit or harm? *JAMA*. 1995;274:826–829.
36. Beauchamp T, Childress J. *Principles of Biomedical Ethics*. 4th ed. New York: Oxford University Press; 1994.
37. Waters C. Understanding and supporting African Americans' perspectives of end-of-life care planning and decision making. *Qual Heal Resour*. 2001;11:385–398.
38. Pietch J, Braun K. Autonomy, advance directives, and the patient self-determination act. In: Braun K, Pietch J, Blanchette P (eds). *Cultural Issues in End-of-Life Decision-Making*. Thousand Oaks, CA: SAGE Publications; 2000:37–53.
39. Searlight H, Gafford J. Cultural diversity as the end-of-life: Issues and guidelines for family physicians. *Am Fam Physician*. 2005;71(3):515–522.

5

The Challenge of Truth-Telling in Cancer Care, United States

Daniel B. Hinshaw

"Even in our most decent society, you meet with the wish to lie with the purpose of making your neighbor happy, for we all suffer from this unrestraint of the heart."

—Fyodor Dostoevsky [1]

"I hold that it is an excellent thing for a physician to practice forecasting. For if he discover and declare unaided by the side of his patients the present, the past, and the future, and fill in the gaps in the account given by the sick, he will be the more believed to understand the cases, so that men will confidently entrust themselves to him for treatment."

— Hippocrates [2]

"You shall know the truth and the truth shall make you free."

—John 8:32

Introduction and Historical Background

"You just don't understand our culture." This objection, or something very similar to it, often presents itself when I am teaching in different countries and cultural settings about the need for truth-telling in communicating bad news to patients. Typically, two reasons are offered in support of this objection to truth-telling in communicating bad news. First, it is claimed that the compassionate practice of medicine at times requires intentional deception of the patient facing an advanced illness, such as cancer, or at least necessitates withholding significant information regarding the diagnosis and prognosis to prevent the loss of hope, which is assumed will occur upon full disclosure. Second, the claim is often made that the given culture in which nondisclosure is commonly practiced is more oriented toward communal decision making in which family members often control the flow of information in order to protect their loved one. In such cultures, it appears that there is often willing collusion between physicians and families in the deception, with the declared intention of preserving hope.

There is an interesting irony in such claims regarding the lack of cross-cultural understanding. Certainly, it is quite appropriate to challenge any outsider who comes from another culture making claims that transcend and appear to contradict local cultural values and traditions. However, it is important to ponder some fundamental questions at this point. Are the forces driving collusion entirely cultural? Is it not possible that something more fundamental to human nature is operative here? Besides these questions, it is important to note that at least two cultures are involved in this phenomenon. Not only is there the dominant shared culture of the patient, family, physician and country in which they reside, but there is also the culture of medicine itself.

Human beings are the one species with the capacity to anticipate their mortality [3]. Coupled closely with the ability to contemplate one's mortality is the attendant dread of the antecedent suffering and progressive debility that often characterize a death due to advanced illnesses like cancer. Even though many malignant neoplasms are now amenable to curative treatment, the word *cancer,* in the public mind, still almost reflexively evokes images of intense suffering and death. Physicians and other members of the healing professions are not immune to this same sense of awe mixed with dread that is conjured up by mere mention of the word. For physicians who conscientiously inform their patients of a cancer diagnosis, it may not be unusual to have the disconcerting experience of receiving an angry response from the distraught recipient of the bad news—for example, "I was fine until you spoke to me. Now, you have given me cancer!"

It is this very human ability to anticipate suffering and death that has likely given expression in turn to the cultural responses, both in the wider culture but also in the medical subculture, in which the fear and denial of death drive the process of collusion. The desires to avoid naming the *unmentionable* and to protect the sick person from such distressing information have not been the unique province of any given culture. Until recently, even in the United States, it was common practice for oncologists to avoid disclosure of a cancer diagnosis to their patients [4]. The same survey study, first performed in 1961 and later repeated in 1979, revealed a remarkable shift in which 90% of physicians in the United States routinely did *not* disclose a cancer diagnosis to their patients to one of frank disclosure by 97% in just 18 years [5]. What could possibly account for such a rapid and dramatic reversal of physician behavior?

A number of possible explanations have been offered to account for this rapid, enormous frameshift in physician behavior. Multiple currents converged to effect profound change: from a culture in the 1960s in which it became normative to question authority to a growing movement advocating consumer rights and patient autonomy in health care, and both in turn compounded by several scandals in which human subjects were abused in clinical research. The most egregious of these abuses was the Tuskegee Syphilis experiment in which male African American subjects were intentionally deceived and thereby kept from effective treatment (i.e., penicillin) that became available during the course of the study [6]. Thus, the protections embodied in the principle of informed consent that were subsequently afforded to human subjects, coming as a response to the research scandals, were also extended to patients in general. Physicians who only recently had practiced a medicine characterized by condescension and paternalism now were cognizant of an increasing need for transparency in their communication with patients. To highlight the truly profound nature of the change transforming American medicine in the latter part of the 20th century, it is helpful to quote extensively from the American Medical Association's Code of Medical Ethics written in the mid-19th century:

A physician should not be forward to make gloomy prognostications, because they savour of empiricism, by magnifying the importance of his services in the treatment or cure of the disease. But he should not fail, on proper occasions, to give to the friends of the patient timely notice of danger when it really occurs; and *even to the patient himself, if absolutely necessary. This office, however, is so peculiarly alarming when executed by him, that it ought to be declined whenever it can be assigned to any other person of sufficient judgment and delicacy. For, the physician should be the minister of hope and comfort to the sick*; that, by such cordials to the drooping spirit, he may smooth the bed of death, revive expiring life, and counteract the depressing influence of those maladies which often disturb the tranquility of the most resigned in their last moments. The life of a sick person can be shortened not only by the *acts*, but also by the *words* or the *manner* of a physician. It is, therefore, a sacred duty to guard himself carefully in this respect, and to *avoid all things which have a tendency to discourage the patient and to depress his spirits*. [7]

Review of this statement makes it readily apparent that all of the reasons still given by physicians and family members within many cultures to justify avoiding disclosure of a cancer diagnosis and/or poor prognosis were also expressed and endorsed by organized American medicine in the mid-nineteenth century. For all practical purposes, these same codes of physician behavior were still normative within American culture and its medical subculture until the transition in the 1960s and 1970s to an increasing emphasis on the principle of autonomy or right of self-determination. Although responses to human suffering and mortality may indeed acquire features unique to a given culture, the issue of whether truth-telling occurs in the context of bad news (e.g., a cancer diagnosis) appears to be not so much a function of culture per se as it is a culturally conditioned indicator of the pervasive presence and power of human anxieties related to death and dying. To better understand the interplay of cross-cultural issues with the basic human anxieties about mortality, the remainder of this chapter will review the challenges of communicating bad news in the physician–patient encounter in different cultural settings, the meaning of hope in advanced illness, the ethics of truth-telling in relation to "compassionate" lying, and the role of informed consent in this process. Finally, an approach to compassionate truth-telling integrating the process of informed consent will be proposed that eliminates the perceived need for deception while respecting the desire to preserve hope in a culturally sensitive manner.

Physician–Patient Communication in Advanced Cancer: Should Preserving Hope Create an Ethical Conflict?

As noted in the 1847 AMA Code of Medical Ethics, physicians have traditionally perceived a major aspect of their professional role to be ministers "of hope and comfort to the sick" [8]. This perception has been used to justify avoidance, vague language, or even frank deception in their communication with very ill patients to honor what has been seen as a higher duty of nonmaleficence, the Hippocratic principle of *do no harm*. A major concern stated so well in the Code of Medical Ethics, and perhaps the most compelling reason to exercise caution in communicating bad news to the sick, is the observation that the "life of a sick person can be shortened not only by the *acts*, but also by the *words* or the *manner* of a physician" [9]. Here is a succinct description of the crucial balance that must exist between the physical interventions (*acts*) and the communication, both verbal and nonverbal (*words* and *manner*), of the physician that constitute the therapeutic encounter. Often medical interventions are primarily understood as being either pharmacological or procedural, while the powerful role of the communication that accompanies such interventions is forgotten or minimized.

Two aspects of communication between physicians and their patients should be emphasized here. First, although tremendous efforts have been made to move away from paternalism through such models as shared decision making [10], the unequal nature of the relationship remains. The physician has specialized knowledge and expertise to offer that the patient does not have and is seeking. This inequality in the encounter between physician and patient can take on powerful, even intimidating, dimensions, especially when a patient comes to a physician in the context of an advanced life-threatening illness. Second, human beings are generally considered to be rational beings, capable of thoughtful deliberation when presented with factual information. However, they are also emotional beings who, when confronted by a threat to their survival, may no longer react in rational ways. This observation applies not only to patients with a life-threatening illness but also to their physicians. This same unequal relationship places a hidden emotional burden on physicians, who consciously (or unconsciously) assume the role of "savior" for their increasingly desperate patients when advanced cancers progress. As they contemplate whether to offer second- and third-line therapies of dubious benefit to their patients, the professional ethos embodied in the admonition from the 1847 AMA Code of Ethics to be *ministers of hope and comfort* challenges them. Is treatment, even when it is only palliative (i.e., intended to relieve symptoms), a source of hope and comfort to their patients? Is it easier emotionally for oncologists to continue to offer more treatment, albeit of questionable benefit, as the disease progresses than to initiate painful and difficult conversations about goals of care in the face of worsening prognosis? Weeks and colleagues in their study [11] of the expectations of over 1,000 patients with advanced cancer who were receiving palliative chemotherapy provided important insights into these questions while raising additional questions.

When patients who at the time of diagnosis presented with stage IV lung or colorectal cancer and were offered palliative chemotherapy, there was a surprisingly high prevalence of the expectation that their treatment might be curative—69% in lung and 81% in colorectal cancer patients [12]. Of particular interest and concern, patients who gave a higher rating to their physician's communication skills were more likely to have inaccurate expectations about the effect of their chemotherapy. This study underscores the challenges created when emotion and reason collide in conversations between physicians and their seriously ill patients. Informed consent that would be obtained before administering chemotherapy requires a full disclosure of the risks and benefits of the proposed intervention with their implicit comprehension by the patient. In a situation (advanced stage IV cancer) where the treatment that is being offered by definition has no curative potential, full disclosure of the patient's prognosis would be expected. The disconnect in this study between patients' higher ratings of their physicians' communication skills and those same patients' inaccurate expectations regarding the effect of their chemotherapy likely reflects reciprocal problems in physician–patient communication occurring on competing planes governed either by reason or emotion. If one party (e.g., the physician) is engaged purely on a rational level while the other (e.g., the patient) is primarily responding on the emotional level or vice versa, meaningful communication may be difficult.

For the physician–patient relationship to be effective, especially in the context of life-threatening illness, it is critically important for physicians to be able to engage empathically with their patients' *cognitive* and *emotional* states [13]. Clinical empathy in this context is understood to be distinct from compassion or sympathy for the patient's suffering. One good working definition of clinical empathy is: "(i) to understand the patient's situation, perspective and feelings (and their attached meanings), (ii) to communicate that understanding and check its accuracy and (iii) to act on that understanding with the patient in a helpful (therapeutic) way" [14]. In other words, the cultivation and practice of clinical empathy may provide a helpful corrective balancing the rational (cognitive) and emotional aspects of physician–patient communication.

While noting that physician prognostication generally tends to be overly optimistic, Christakis and Lamont further observed that the longer and better a physician knows a patient, the more likely that the physician will overestimate the patient's survival [15]. The competing emotional and rational goals of such exchanges challenge physicians' ability to balance truthful and accurate disclosure of critical clinical information with their patients' dual need to be both informed and comforted. To a great degree, physicians' emotions and emotional relationships with their patients are powerful determinants of how they present the bad news regarding a cancer diagnosis and its prognosis. The temptation to avoid personal emotional distress provides a strong motivation for physicians to downplay or minimize the true nature of diagnostic and especially prognostic information for their patients facing terminal illness. An additional challenge to this process is the frequent insertion of the good intentions of family members who insist on protecting their loved one from the adverse clinical information, which they are convinced will harm the patient by reducing or even eliminating hope. These two factors —physicians' and family members' desire to protect the patient from distressing diagnostic and prognostic information and physicians' temptation to avoid the intense anxiety associated with giving bad news—appear to be the primary catalytic agents for collusion regardless of the given culture in which it occurs. They create potential barriers to the necessary exchange of information that is fundamental to the process of informed consent.

Consciously or unconsciously, physicians may use the manner of their truth-telling as a means of exerting control in the patient encounter. By limiting the information shared, they may reduce the level of distress in a given encounter, not only the patient's but also their own. A recent study from Greece confirmed that intense physician anxiety does occur with giving bad news to patients [16]. In a simulated patient encounter (a young brain tumor patient with a poor prognosis), medical students who were assigned in the experiment to give accurate prognostic information experienced significantly greater stress than their colleagues who were instructed to not disclose the prognostic information but still refer the patient for chemotherapy.

An extensive literature has documented the many cultures that continue to engage in various levels of collusion [17–29], in which physicians and family members agree to either withhold all or significant portions of diagnostic and prognostic information from cancer patients and in some cases engage in frank deception, all in an effort to maintain the hope of the patient. A growing dissent among international investigators provides a counterpoint to the still highly prevalent practice of collusion. Several provocative studies emanating from countries and cultures that have been assumed to endorse the practice of collusion between physicians and family members in deceiving cancer patients about their diagnosis and prognosis document a growing interest, even demand, from cancer patients for full disclosure of diagnostic and prognostic information related to their disease. For example, a large study from Taiwan surveyed 195 respondents about their attitudes toward knowing a cancer diagnosis [30]. The vast majority (92.3%) of the respondents indicated that they would want to know their cancer diagnosis, particularly younger, better educated, and employed persons. Similarly, other studies from Asian countries are also revealing the same trend toward a desire among cancer patients for full disclosure [31]. A major finding in these studies, which probably reflects an enduring cultural difference from many Western cultures that are so heavily invested in individual autonomy, has been the clearly expressed desire for the oncologist to include patients' family members in the process of communication. The desire for strong family involvement, so prevalent in more traditional cultures, is evolving into a desire expressed by cancer patients for full disclosure to facilitate more honest and meaningful support by their loved ones. Indeed, one recent study from Taiwan emphasized that rather than causing despair, awareness of their terminal condition was felt to facilitate patients' spiritual preparation for death as well as enhance their conversations with loved ones about spiritual and practical concerns (e.g., expressing their last will and testament) [32].

A growing focus on individual autonomy extending to the realm of health care decision making seems to be an inevitable consequence as the world becomes more connected through the Internet and as levels of education and incomes rise. Regardless of the cultural context (i.e., Eastern Europe, the Middle East, East Africa, or the United States), it has been the custom of the author to query his students about their own personal preferences regarding full disclosure of a cancer diagnosis and prognosis; the response has always been a resounding *yes* to full disclosure. When the same question is then applied to their patients, varying levels of resistance are raised to applying their own personal standard of full disclosure to others. The old concern articulated so clearly in the 1847 AMA Code of Medical Ethics about physicians being *ministers of hope and comfort* is raised in one form or another. This invites a brief exploration of the nature of truth-telling, even when full disclosure is advocated.

Hardly anyone who has cared for the sick would deny the useful insights contained within this sentence from the 1847 AMA Code of Medical Ethics. "The life of a sick person can be shortened not only by the *acts*, but also by the *words* or the *manner* of a physician" [33]. However, it is not clear that mere *words* spoken by a physician, even if they are true and accurate descriptions of a patient's serious condition, will necessarily cause harm to the patient. A critical distinction to be made here is between the manner in which information is presented as opposed to the actual content of that information. Great strides have been made in recent years in developing kinder, gentler means of conveying bad news to cancer patients [34] and educating physicians in the process [35]. A growing body of evidence refutes the common assertion that being informed of a cancer diagnosis or terminal prognosis destroys hope and shortens life.

Temel et al. demonstrated that patients presenting with advanced non-small cell lung cancer who received palliative care from the time of diagnosis lived longer with better quality of life and less depression [36]. Patients receiving palliative care are usually well informed and aware of the terminal nature of their condition. In the *Coping with Cancer* study [37], patients with advanced cancer who were "peacefully aware" of their diagnosis had less psychological distress and better quality of death, and their surviving caregivers had better bereavement outcomes. In a recent study of 87 cancer patients with poor prognosis (estimated less than six months survival), psychological well-being was assessed as a function of prognostic understanding before, immediately after, and at a subsequent follow-up visit, approximately six weeks later. Psychological well-being initially declined in those patients with a better understanding of their prognosis but they quickly recovered, while patients with poor understanding of their prognosis had initial increases but later experienced decrements in psychological well-being [38].

Miyaji's study [39] of American physicians' attitudes regarding disclosure of a cancer diagnosis and prognosis, though more than 25 years old, still has many insights to offer in parsing out the various shades of truth that physicians are willing to share with their cancer patients. In his analysis, Miyaji identified three styles of truth-telling by physicians in America: telling what patients want to know, telling what patients need to know, and translating information into terms that patients can take [40]. Although physicians insisted that they were committed to telling the truth to their patients, they were not averse to being selective in what "truth" was presented and when.

More recently, an American oncologist has attempted to justify this selectivity in communication on ethical grounds invoking the inherent uncertainty that complicates prognostication. He has defined collusion as "the spoken or unspoken agreement we sometimes enter into with some patients to avoid or delay discussing a definitive, numerical prognostic estimate of life expectancy" [41]. In his justification for collusion, Helft relies on an old argument—that the physician's role is ultimately to be healer and that, in the case of terminal cancer, preserving hope is the essential element in healing where cure is no longer possible [42]. This begs the question: hope for what? In a commentary on Helft's essay [43], it was observed that an accurate prognosis must be provided so that oncology patients can make informed decisions about their future—either to pursue additional antineoplastic treatment or to fully embrace palliative care, making the practical and spiritual preparations for their death.

While preservation of hope is usually cited as the justification for nondisclosure or overt deception of patients facing a terminal illness, the nature of the hope to be preserved is rarely defined. Etymologically, hope is closely related to expectation, a *desired* expectation [44]. Discussions of hope and truth-telling in advanced illness often avoid placing the discussion in the realistic context of the universal nature of human mortality—a reality that may not be hoped for *now* or *ever* but certainly should be an expectation as the horizon of one's life approaches. Any hope (and expectation) for cure of a cancer, though cherished for as long as possible, must be balanced by a sober appreciation of this limit to human aspirations. Throughout the trajectory of care for a progressive cancer, the primary goal of a patient's expectation or hope, of necessity, must gradually shift from cure to other goals (e.g., achieving reconciliation in relationships, planning funeral arrangements) that are bound by temporal limits. Hope must dialogue with expectation based in reality, where ultimately hope bifurcates into a hope related to the *quality* of the time remaining and to a hope *transcending* mortality.

In reviewing the ethics of truth-telling to cancer patients, Surbone [45] has suggested that more is involved than merely a conflict between the Hippocratic principle of nonmaleficence (*do no harm*) used to justify compassionate nondisclosure or deception regarding distressing prognostic information and the right of self-determination (*autonomy*) invoked in support of full disclosure. Based on a broad clinical experience in multiple cultural settings, Surbone has urged a recognition that truth is not static but emerges through an unfolding process within the dynamics of human relationships existing not only between physicians and patients but also between their families and the wider culture within which they live and interact.

Collusion and nondisclosure of prognostic information, no matter how compassionate the intent, deny terminally ill cancer patients access to essential information that they need as part of their journey toward death. They also produce moral wounds in physicians who use them in their practice. In considering the challenge that uncertainty poses to suffering patients and their physicians, Eric Cassell has noted the critical nature of trust in the therapeutic relationship. "Trust in others is one of the central human solutions to the paralysis of unbearable uncertainty. For these reasons the sick put their trust in doctors. The requirement for trust adds to the relationship between doctor and patient" [46]. Deception can never provide a solid foundation for an enduring relationship between physicians and their patients who are facing a terminal illness. How can oncologists encourage and sustain hope in their patients with advanced cancer while, at the same time, nourish a relationship of trust based on truth-telling that fully respects their patients' autonomy and cultural context?

A Proposal for Compassionate Truth-Telling in Cancer Care

In summary, several observations can be made (see Box 5.1 for a summary of key elements in compassionate truth-telling). Although *enduring* cultural differences have been invoked to explain and justify nondisclosure and collusion regarding cancer diagnoses and poor prognoses, a historical analysis suggests that the strong motivation to conceal bad news is more likely a universal human phenomenon present in all cultures. The enduring difference that remains between cultures lies in the nature of how information is shared and how decisions are made. In Western societies where a heavy emphasis is placed on the individual, communication of bad news and medical decisions are centered in the dyad of physician and autonomous patient. In other more traditional cultures, there is still a strong communal commitment to

---

Box 5.1 Compassionate Truth-Telling

- **Informed consent**—establish ground rules for disclosure of clinical information with the patient's permission: Does the patient want to be the primary recipient of clinical information? What role does the patient want family members or others to have in the disclosure/receipt of the information? How much does the patient want to know now?
- **Process**—understand that the disclosure of the truth about the illness is a process that will unfold through multiple encounters, as the situation and considerations affecting treatment decisions change over time.
- **Trust**—reassure the patient that no lies will be told, but the patient's right to refuse to hear more information will also be respected. If the patient refuses to hear the disclosure of diagnostic and/or prognostic information that are essential for informed consent regarding proposed treatment, the patient may need to authorize a surrogate decision maker to receive the information and make treatment decisions on the patient's behalf. As the disease progresses, gently *offer* information about the prognosis repeatedly without forcing the issue. It is reasonable to say, "I respect your wish to avoid hearing more about your illness, but I also believe that the information is so important for you to hear and consider that I will keep offering to tell you."
- **Hope**—encourage and support hope based on a *realistic* assessment of the *current* condition and *likely prognosis* of the patient. Understand that the patient may misinterpret offers of further disease-focused treatment, even though explicitly "palliative." Balance the patient's expectations with the use of language such as: "we will hope for the best, but also prepare for the worst."

---

include the patient's family support system in the process. What is rapidly changing as a result of greater levels of education and access to the Internet across many cultures is an insistence by cancer patients of knowing their diagnosis and prognosis—and that collusion is increasingly unacceptable.

A crucial aspect of truth-telling in advanced cancer that cannot be emphasized enough is that, ideally, it is a *process* centered in a *relationship of trust* between physician and patient. Lies have no place in this process. However, the truth of the disease during its evolution and its impact on the life of a cancer patient can only be revealed to the fullest extent possible over time with the consent of the patient. This allows for the possibility of patients receiving as much information as they desire at a given time, but does not obviate the need for the fullest disclosure possible at an opportune moment. Such information should never be forced on patients. Truth-telling becomes a mutual journey of discovery for patients and their physicians, which can and should include other persons depending on the wishes of patients in a given cultural context.

Physicians may benefit from additional training in compassionate communication of bad news and must avoid the use of confusing medical jargon. It is a part of the art of medicine to differentiate what is essential from what is nonessential. In informed consent, patients need to know enough to appreciate the risks and potential benefits of a given course of action, which also means they need to understand the context in which they are making such decisions. Certainly, prognostication is limited by uncertainty. However, when the likelihood of cure is essentially nil or the probability of death in months or less is quite real, patients can understand this reality and plan accordingly. A way of offering balance in conversations with patients struggling with advanced cancer is to frame the conversation with the commonly used aphorism: "Hope for the best, but also prepare for the worst" [47]. Just stating the aphorism opens up the possibility for patients and their loved ones to ask for further clarification of what the *best* and *worst* are at this point in the illness. This can foster a realistic discussion of diagnosis and prognosis appropriate to the circumstances and, in turn, focus goal setting on achievable goals. Hope for a cure can be replaced with hope for excellent pain and symptom relief, hope for reconciliation and healing in relationships and, ultimately, hope for transcendence.

References

1. Dostoevsky, F. *The Adolescent*. Pevear R, Volokhonsky L. (trans). New York: Vintage Classics; 2003:205.
2. Hippocrates, Prognostic. *Volume II, Hippocrates*. Jones, WHS (trans). Cambridge, MA: Harvard University Press, Loeb Classical Library; 1923:7.
3. For an excellent discussion of the existential fear inherent in the human condition, see discussion, especially pages 26 and 27, in Becker, E. *The Denial of Death*. New York: Free Press Paperbacks; 1973.
4. Oken, D. What to Tell Cancer Patients: A Study of Medical Attitudes. *JAMA*. 1961; 175(13):1120–1128.
5. Novack, DH, Plumer, R, Smith, RL, Ochitill, H, Morrow, GR, Bennett, JM. Changes in physicians' attitudes toward telling the cancer patient. *JAMA*. 1979;241(9):897–900.
6. For excellent reviews, see Sisk, B, Frankel, R, Kodish, E, Isaacson, JH. The truth about truth-telling in American medicine: A brief history. *Perm J*. 2016;20(3):74–77 and Sokol, D. How the doctor's nose has shortened over time; A historical overview of the truth-telling debate in the doctor-patient relationship. *J R Soc Med*. 2006;99:632–636.
7. *American Medical Association Code of Medical Ethics 1847*, pp. 8–9; accessed on August 25, 2020 at: http://ethics.iit.edu/ecodes/sites/default/files/Americaan%20Medical%20Association%20Code%20of%20Medical%20Ethics%20%281847%29.pdf (italics added)
8. *American Medical Association Code of Medical Ethics 1847*, pp. 8–9.
9. *American Medical Association Code of Medical Ethics 1847*, pp. 8–9.
10. See, for example: Frosch, DL, Kaplan, RM. Shared decision making in clinical medicine: past research and future directions. *Am J Prev Med*. 1999;17(4): 285–294; Kon, AA. The shared decision-making continuum. *JAMA*. 2010;304(8):903–904; and Elwyn, G, Frosch, D, Thomson, R, et al. Shared decision making: A model for clinical practice. *J Gen Intern Med*. 2012;27(10):1361–1367.
11. Weeks, JC, Catalano, PJ, Cronin, A, et al. Patients' expectations about effects of chemotherapy for advanced cancer. *N Engl J Med*. 2012;367:1616–1625.
12. Ibid. For further discussion of the significance of this study for other forms of cancer treatment (i.e., surgical oncology) see Pawlik, TM, Devon, KM, Fields, CA, Hinshaw, DB. What are patients' expectations about the effects of chemotherapy for advanced cancer? *J Am Coll Surg*. 2014;219(3):587–590.

13. Neumann, M, Bensing, J, Mercer, S, Ernstmann, N, Ommen, O, Pfaff, H. Analyzing the "nature" and "specific effectiveness" of clinical empathy: A theoretical overview and contribution towards a theory-based research agenda. *Patient Educ Couns.* 2009;74:339–346.
14. Mercer SW, Reynolds WJ. Empathy and quality of care. *Br J Gen Pract.* 2002;52:S9–13.
15. Christakis NA, Lamont EB. Extent and determinants of error in doctors' prognoses in terminally ill patients: prospective cohort study. *Br Med J.* 2000; 320: 469–72.
16. Panagopoulou, E, Mintziori, G, Montgomery, A, Kapoukranidou, D, Benos, A. Concealment of information in clinical practice: Is lying less stressful than telling the truth? *J Clin Oncol.* 2008;26(7):1175–1177.
17. For general reviews of culture and truth-telling see: Fallowfield, LJ, Jenkins, VA, Beveridge, HA. Truth may hurt but deceit hurts more: Communication in palliative care. *Palliat Med.* 2002;16:297–303.
18. Bruera E, Neumann CM, Mazzocato C, Stiefel F, Sala R. Attitudes and beliefs of palliative care physicians regarding communication with terminally ill cancer patients. *Palliat Med.* 2000;14: 287–298.
19. Surbone A. Cultural aspects of communication in cancer care. *Support Care Cancer.* 2008;16: 235–240.
20. Kazdaglis GA, Arnaoutoglou, C, Karypidis, D, Memekidou, G, Spanos, G, Papadopoulos, O. Disclosing the truth to terminal cancer patients: A discussion of ethical and cultural issues *EMHJ.* 2010;16(4):442–447.

For reviews of cultural aspects of communicating bad news with children:

21. Die Trill, M, Kovalcik, R. The child with cancer: Influence of culture on truth-telling and patient care. *Ann NY Acad Sci.* 1997;809(1):197–210.
22. Rosenberg, AR, Starks, H, Yoram Unguru, Y, Feudtner, C, Diekema, D. Truth-telling in the setting of cultural differences and incurable pediatric illness *JAMA Pediatr.* 2017;171(11):1113–1119.

The following references are representative of the great interest in this topic by specific country/culture:

23. From **Iran**: Tavakol M, Murphy R, Torabi S. Educating doctors about breaking bad news: An Iranian perspective. *J Cancer Educ.* 2008;23:260–263.
24. From **Turkey**: Ozdogan M, Samur M, Artac M, Yildiz M, Savas B, Bozcuk HS. Factors related to truth-telling practice of physicians treating patients with cancer in Turkey. *J Palliat Med.* 2006;9(5):1114–1119.
25. From **Greece**: Oikonomidou, D, Anagnostopoulos F, Dimitrakaki C, Ploumpidis D, Stylianidis S, Tountas Y. Doctor's perceptions and practices of breaking bad news: A qualitative study from Greece. *Health Communication.* 2017;32(6):657–666 and Mystakidou K, Liossi C, Vlachos L, Papadimitriou J. Disclosure of diagnostic information to cancer patients in Greece. *Palliat Med.* 1996;10:195–200.
26. From **Italy**: Locatelli C, Piselli, P, Cicerchia, M, Repetto L. Physicians' age and sex influence breaking bad news to elderly cancer patients. Beliefs and practices of 50 Italian oncologists: The G.I.O. Ger study *Psycho-Oncology.* 2013;22:1112–1119.
27. from **Mexico**: Torrecillas, L. Communication of the cancer diagnosis to Mexican patients: Attitudes of physicians and patients *Ann NY Acad Sci.* 1997;809(1):188–196.
28. From **China**: Li S, Chou J-L. Communication with the cancer patient in China *Ann NY Acad Sci* 1997; 809(1):243–248.

29. From **Japan**: Uchitomi, Y, and Yamawaki, S. Truth-telling practice in cancer care in Japan *Ann NY Acad Sci*. 1997;809(1):290–299.

30. Wang S-Y, Chen C-H, Chen Y-S, Huang, H.-L. The attitude toward truth-telling of cancer in Taiwan *J Psychosom Res*. 2004;57:53–58.

31. Jiang Y, Liu C, Li J-Y, et al. Different attitudes of Chinese patients and their families toward truth telling of different stages of cancer. *Psychooncology*. 2007;16:928–936. Fielding RG, Hung J. Preferences for information and involvement in decisions during cancer care among a Hong Kong Chinese population. *Psychooncology*.1996;5:321–329; Rao A, Sunil B, Ekstrand M, Heylen E, Raju G, Shet A. Breaking Bad News: Patient preferences and the role of family members when delivering a cancer diagnosis *APJCP*. 2016;17(4):779–1784; and Leung K-K, Chiu T-Y, Chen, C-Y. The influence of awareness of terminal condition on spiritual well-being in terminal cancer patients. *J Pain Symptom Manage*. 2006;31:449–456.

32. Leung K-K, Chiu T-Y, Chen C-Y. The influence of awareness of terminal condition on spiritual well-being in terminal cancer patients *J Pain Symptom Manage*. 2006;31:449–456.

33. *American Medical Association Code of Medical Ethics 1847*, pp. 8–9; accessed on August 25, 2020 at: http://ethics.iit.edu/ecodes/sites/default/files/Americaan%20Medical%20Association%20Code%20of%20Medical%20Ethics%20%281847%29.pdf (italics added)

34. For example, the SPIKES Protocol: Baile, WF, Buckman, R, Lenzi, R, Glober, G, Beale, EA, and Kudelka, AP. SPIKES—A Six-Step Protocol for Delivering Bad News: Application to the Patient with Cancer. *The Oncologist*. 2000;5:302–311.

35. Online resource for educating physicians in communication with seriously ill patients, Vital Talk at: https://www.vitaltalk.org

36. Temel JS, Greer JA, Muzikansky A, et al. Early palliative care for patients with metastatic non–small-cell lung cancer *N Engl J Med*. 2010;363:733–742.

37. Ray A, Block SD, Friedlander RJ, Zhang B, Maciejewski PK, Prigerson, HG. Peaceful awareness in patients with advanced cancer. *J Palliat Med*. 2006;9(6):1359–1368.

38. George LS, Maciejewski PK, Epstein AS, Shen M, Prigerson HG. Advanced cancer patients' changes in accurate prognostic understanding and their psychological well-being. *J Pain Symptom Manage*. 2020;59:983–989.

39. Miyaji, NT. The power of compassion: Truth-telling among American doctors in the care of dying patients. *Soc SciMed*.1993;36(3):249–264.

40. Miyaji. The power of compassion.

41. Helft, P. Necessary collusion: Prognostic communication with advanced cancer patients. *J Clin Oncol*. 2005;23(13):3146–3150.

42. Helft. Necessary collusion.

43. Kalemkerian, GP. Is collusion necessary? A commentary on necessary collusion. *J Clin Oncol*. 2005;23(13):3153–3154.

44. In Classical Greek, ελπις – elpis, the word commonly translated as hope also meant expectation. Liddell HG, Scott R. *A Greek-English Lexicon*. Oxford: Oxford University Press, 1968:537.

45. Surbone, A. Telling the truth to patients with cancer: What is the truth? *Lancet Oncol*. 2006;7:944–950.

46. Cassell, EJ. *The Nature of Suffering and the Goals of Medicine*. 2nd ed. Oxford: Oxford University Press; 2004:71.

47. Common aphorism with one version attributed to the 19th-century British Prime Minister Benjamin Disraeli (1804–1881): "I am prepared for the worst but hope for the best." Accessed on August 31, 2020 at: https://www.brainyquote.com/quotes/benjamin_disraeli_154186

6

Cultural Challenges in Providing Psychosocial-Spiritual Support to Children with Cancer and Their Families, Turkey

Rejin Kebudi, Fatma Betul Cakir, and Sema Bay Büyükkapu

Introduction

Although survival rates for pediatric cancer have improved significantly over the past few decades, the diagnosis and treatment of pediatric cancer is still challenging. Childhood cancer has been described as a "family disease" affecting the entire family and all those in the child's close environment, including their friends in school [1,2]. The care of a child with cancer must be family-centered, and consideration of the family's cultural background is of the utmost importance [1–3]. Families of children with cancer struggle with an acute life-altering disease as well as with possible long-term chronic complications. The cultural background of the family influences the treatment and followup for pediatric cancer patients [3–5]. Influential cultural factors include socioeconomic status, education, traditions, religion, and other moral values.

Communication and Breaking the Bad News

Communicating with the child and family can be challenging at all stages: at diagnosis, during treatment, and, in terminal cases, at the end of life. Cultural differences must be respected and should guide how the information of the cancer diagnosis is presented to the family and patient. Nonverbal communication deserves special attention in populations that might encounter difficulties with the local spoken language.

The word "cancer" has a significant emotional impact on families. In Turkey, in pediatric oncology, all parents are informed, in detail, of the diagnosis and prognosis at the initial diagnosis [3–5]. Despite the significant increase in survival rates for children with cancer [6], many people in the community think of cancer as a fatal disease. Thus, most families do not want physicians to use the word "cancer" when informing their children of the diagnosis. Physicians may explain to the parents that, rather than lie to the child, they will at least use the word "tumor" at the first session and will add details in further sessions. According to the age of the child, physicians may describe the condition as "the uncontrolled growth of some cells that form a lump" (in cases of a solid tumor) or that "invade the bone marrow" (in cases of leukemia). The cells may be described as "naughty" cells to young children [3–5]. Older children, especially adolescents, can use the Internet and easily read about their "cancer" diagnosis. They usually also prefer not to use the word "cancer." Even in Western cultures, where full disclosure is a common practice, it has been reported that parents often find it difficult to tell their child about the disease [7–9].

In Japan, as in Turkey, the trend of parents making a full disclosure of the child's diagnosis has slowly progressed [7,10,11]. Families initially find it emotionally difficult to accept the diagnosis and possibility of a poor prognosis; therefore, good communication skills are needed to counter high levels of anxiety, depression, and probable denial [12].

Psychosocial Status of Families, Associated Risk Factors, and Solutions

An integrative review of 19 articles reported between 1997 and 2017 analyzed the psychosocial status of families of pediatric cancer patients in Turkey and concluded that status varies according to the specific type of cancer, treatment, and individual and environmental factors [13]. Kostak and Avci [14] and Bayat et al. [15] reported that, for parents, there is a strong relationship between hopelessness and depressive symptoms; that is, the higher the degree of hopelessness, the higher the magnitude of depression and anxiety. Other factors may have an affect on depression in patients. Demirtepe-Saygılı and Bozo [16] added that mothers who were unable to cope emotionally and who received less social support were at higher risk of developing depressive symptoms. Kudubes et al. [17] found that the higher the frequency of symptoms in children, the more their mothers' physical and psychological health, spiritual wellness, and quality of life decreased. This review also showed that mothers are more affected psychosocially than fathers [13]. For example, Gülses et al. [18] found that fathers of children (with either cancer or other chronic illnesses) had higher scores when measuring general and mental health than mothers. The same article also showed that cancer, as a chronic disease, affects the quality of life of parents and their children more adversely than other chronic diseases [18]. Yalug et al. [19] reported that parents whose children receive a poor prognosis and require high-intensity treatments have significantly higher anxiety scores. Guilt-arousing thoughts such as, "I am being punished," are also more frequent in mothers who suffer from posttraumatic stress disorder after their child undergoes cancer surgery [20]. However, mothers who have social support, for example, mothers living in extended families, were reported to have lower depression scores than those living in nuclear families [21]. Eyigor et al. [22] stated that mothers found social support to be very important as they were, generally, more comfortable talking to other mothers experiencing similar situations. This review also showed that the diagnosis of a child with pediatric cancer profoundly affects all family members, especially parents and siblings, who are at risk for developing psychosocial problems [23–25]. Adaptation to "cancer" can be difficult, and family members may experience psychological problems that negatively impact their quality of life [13,25–28].

A study in Turkey [29] of parents of pediatric patients who were in remission reported that 46% of the mothers experienced serious psychological problems during and after treatment and 41% of the families embraced religious practices more frequently during the treatment period to cope with the psychological implications. There is a common global tendency for patients and their caregivers to use spiritual and religious measures and to rely on their spirituality and faith in order to better cope with cancer [1,3–5,13,30–33]. Patients and their caregivers have reported less depression and anxiety and better health and quality of life with the intervention of spirituality and religious beliefs [30–36].

From the children's perspective, factors that negatively affect their quality of life and may lead to depression include disclosure of the disease, inability of adults to communicate effectively using simple language, frequent hospitalization, physical symptoms such as pain, nausea, and vomiting, and psychosocial problems related to cancer treatment, such as the inability to attend school and separation from friends [13,17]. These factors may also result in reduced compliance to treatment, especially in adolescents [13,17,37]. It is reported that as the severity and frequency of the child's symptoms increase, parents find it more difficult to deal with these symptoms and feel helpless [38,39]. Psychosocial support for patients, caregivers, and the health care staff is very important, but unfortunately the number of centers in Turkey that have a liaison psychological support team is limited. It is recommended that every center have a permanent psychological support team [3–5].

These children and their families also need socialization. These families reportedly prefer to communicate with other families that have children with cancer rather than their own close relatives, as they share common feelings of anxiety, hope or hopelessness, or depression. Some nongovernmental organizations and other volunteer groups offer psychosocial support, especially to children, by organizing parties, picnics, and celebrations, which are very much appreciated by both patients and parents. These groups also sometimes make home visits to these patients [3–5]. Psychosocial support should be provided to children with cancer, their siblings and their parents, especially the mothers. One reason explaining why mothers have more anxiety and feelings of hopelessness than fathers do is the simple fact that they spend more time with their ill children. Mothers reported that, with increasing levels of anxiety, the levels of despair and hopelessness also increased [13,15].

For schoolchildren, attending school is very important. Major pediatric cancer centers in Turkey therefore offer "hospital schools/classes" and teachers provided by the Ministry of Health. Children enjoy attending school/class, despite the hospital setting. Knowing that they will attend the same class with their peers when their treatment is over helps them to adapt to their life while in the hospital and when treatment is over.

In Turkey, all children diagnosed with cancer receive the appropriate oncological treatment, which is completely funded by the government [3–5]. In a recent study, significant factors were found to increase the level of hope, notably: advances in technology, cancer treatment and supportive care, adequate family support, and the availability of governmental health insurance [5,40,41]. Financial problems were reported to cause psychological distress and thus, adversely affect the level of hope [29,40,42]. Bozkurt et al. [29] reported that the average monthly income in 80% of families was below the level that would meet the family's needs. Additional economic support from extended family members or relatives was obtained in 93% of these cases. One-fourth of the families had to sell their house or private car during the treatment. Forty-nine percent of the families had borrowed money from acquaintances and relatives or had taken a bank loan.

Traditional Attitudes, Moral Values, and Current Health Status

In urban areas, traditions and religious practices play an even more vital role in decision making regarding treatment. In some communities where socioeconomic and literacy levels are low, families may obey the decision of the oldest community leader, consult traditional healers when their children experience health issues, and use alternative treatment or some herbal treatment [4,5]. However, this consultation leads to a delay in diagnosis and decreased survival rates. Many patients use herbal medicines during treatment; the most commonly used herbal agents are stinging nettle [*Urtica dioica*], honey, pollens, garlic, olive oil, or *pekmez* (a traditional syrup obtained primarily from boiled grape juice or other fruits) [4,43]. Physicians should remain open-minded so that the families feel free to ask about the benefits or potential harm of these complementary medicines. Alternative or complementary treatment is used mostly when the disease is refractory or has relapsed.

Universal health insurance coverage and increasing awareness about cancer in the community facilitate early diagnosis and adherence to proper treatment and, therefore, lead to increased survival rates.

Turkey underwent health care system reform in 2002, which gives all citizens easier access to health care services, Specifically, it allows all pediatric patients to have free universal health insurance coverage, thus enabling all children to be admitted to tertiary health centers for diagnosis and treatment, free of charge [4,44,45]. According to the cancer registry data obtained from the Turkish Pediatric Oncology Group (TPOG), the five-year survival rate in childhood malignancies diagnosed in all the centers in Turkey was 65% between 2002 and 2008 and increased to 69.5% during 2009–2016 [46,47]. In some centers, such as the Istanbul University Oncology Institute, the five-year survival rate of all patients diagnosed between 1990 and 2012 was reported to be 74.4% [6].

The cultural aspects of Turkish society are a blend of both Eastern and Western societies. There is a common myth about cancer treatment among Turkish communities; namely, patients who have a tumorous mass in their viscera are often reluctant to undergo surgery because they believe "a cut made through a cancerous mass will cause it to spread all over the body" [4,5,30]. Although this misbelief has changed in recent years with the success of advances in medicine and increased awareness about cancer and its treatment in the society, some families continue to resist surgery.

End-of-Life Care and Palliative Care

For many metastatic/refractory/relapsed patients, the prognosis is still dismal despite salvage therapies such as chemotherapy, radiotherapy, stem cell transplantation, and immunotherapy. The terminal stage is challenging for both patients and families, as well as for physicians and nurses. Palliative care (PC) is a set of approaches that aims to decrease symptoms, to improve physical, social, and psychological well-being, and to provide a good quality of life for both the patient and the family. PC is provided not only at the terminal stage but should begin at diagnosis and continue throughout treatment until the end of life [3–5,40,45]. Cultural differences should be recognized when providing PC. In Turkey, end-of-life care is provided mostly in the inpatient setting, as the country still has no hospices. Although, in rural areas, most patients and family members prefer to stay at home at their end-of-life period, in urban areas most patients and most families of children with cancer prefer to stay in the hospital during the terminal stage, contrary to many countries in the Middle East where the patients or families prefer the patients to die at home where they can be cared for by their family [3–5,40]. For pediatric cases, sending the child home to die is frequently considered by the families as "giving up on us," and the hospital sometimes becomes more of a "home" for the sick child than the child's own home [3–5]. However, if hospice or home care were available, they would prefer it. As a result, the pediatric patient and the family should be offered an integrated model of palliative care that continues throughout the course of the illness, regardless of the outcome [3–5]. The families can sometimes misunderstand palliative care consultation because it may symbolize evidence of the patient's deterioration, which may be difficult to face. Many families prefer the term *supportive care* to *palliative care*. All cancer care must be provided with respect for families' spiritual and cultural backgrounds. Spiritual and religious practices may become more important, particularly during end of life [30,48,49]. Health care professionals should be sensitive and tolerant of traditions and religious beliefs in order to meet the unique spiritual needs of patients and families and ensure a "good death" and healthy bereavement [3–5,13,30,35,36,48,49]. The rights of dying patients have not yet been established by law in Turkey; "do-not-resuscitate" orders and practices of euthanasia for patients suffering from refractory symptoms are not legal [3–5].

Good communication skills are essential at the terminal phase of the disease. Some health professionals, especially if they are new in their career, may face difficulties talking about death to patients and their families [3–5]. Training programs for improving communication skills include teaching clinicians to respond in a sensitive way, to listen with empathy, and to respect the wishes of the patients and their families.

Conclusion

The way health care professionals relay information to children with cancer and their families, whether it be at diagnosis, during treatment, or at end of life, is paramount and should demonstrate respect and consideration for cultural differences, traditions, spirituality, beliefs, and all aspects that the family considers important. Cultural challenges in providing psychosocial support to children and their families is of the utmost importance in pediatric oncology.

References

1. Thibodeaux AG, Deatrick JA. Cultural influence on family management of children with cancer. *J Pediatr Oncol Nurs*. 2007;24(4):227–233.
2. Cincotta N. Psychosocial issues in the world of children with cancer. *Cancer Supplement*. 1993;17:3251–3260.
3. Kebudi R, Cakir FB, Gultekin M. Palliative care to the cancer patient in Turkey. In: Silbermann M (eds). *Palliative Care to the Cancer Patient: The Middle East as a Model for Emerging Countries*. New York: Nova Publishers; 2014, pp. 193–210.
4. Kebudi R, Cakir FB. Cancer care in a country undergoing transition: Turkey, current challenges and trends for the future. In: Silbermann M (ed). *Cancer Care in Countries and Societies in Transition*. New York: Springer; 2016, pp. 193–208.
5. Kebudi R, Cakir FB. Cultural challenges in implementing palliative services in Turkey. *Palliat Med Hosp Care Open J*. 2017;SE(1):S10–S14.
6. Kebudi R, Alkaya DU. Epidemiology and survival of childhood cancer in Turkey. *Pediatr Blood Cancer*. 2021;68(2):e28754. doi: 10.1002/pbc.28754.
7. Nakajima-Yamaguchi R, Morita N, Nakao T, et al. Parental post-traumatic stress symptoms as predictors of psychosocial problems in children treated for cancer. *Int J Environ Res Public Health*. 2016;13(8):812.
8. Chesler MA, Paris J, Barbarin OA. "Telling" the child with cancer: Parental choices to share information with ill children. *J. Pediatr Psychol*. 1986;11:497–516.
9. Clarke S, Davies H, Jenney M, Glaser A, Eiser C. Parental communication and children's behaviour following diagnosis of childhood leukaemia. *Psychooncology*. 2005;14:274–281.
10. Holland JC, Geary N, Marchini A, Tross S. An international survey of physician attitudes and practice in regard to revealing the diagnosis of cancer. *Cancer Investig*. 1987;5:151–154.
11. Parsons S, Saiki Craighill S, Mayer D, et al. Telling children and adolescents about their cancer diagnosis: Cross-cultural comparisons between pediatric oncologists in the US and Japan. *Psychooncology*. 2007;16:60–68.
12. You JJ, Downar J, Fowler RA, et al. Barriers to goals of care discussions with seriously ill hospitalized patients and their families. A multicenter survey of clinicians. *JAMA Intern Med*. 201;175(4):549–556.
13. Ay MA, Akyar I. Psychosocial status of Turkish families of pediatric cancer patients. *J Transcult Nurs*. 2020;31(3):227–241.
14. Kostak MA, Avci G. Hopelessness and depression levels of parents of children with cancer. *APFCP*. 2013;14:6833–6838.
15. Bayat M, Erdem E, Gül KE. Depression, anxiety, hopelessness, and social support levels of the parents of children with cancer. *J Pediatr Oncol Nurs*. 2008;25:247–253.
16. Demirtepe-Saygılı D, Bozo Ö. Predicting depressive symptoms among the mothers of children with leukaemia: A caregiver stress model perspective. *Psychol Health*. 2011;26:585–599.
17. Kudubes AA, Bektas M, Ugur O. Symptom frequency of children with cancer and parent quality of life in Turkey. *APJCP*. 2014;15:3487–3493.
18. Gülses S, Yildirim ZK, Büyükavci M. Does the quality of life of children with cancer and their parents differ from that of patients with other diseases? *Cocuk Sagligi ve Hastaliklari Dergisi*. 2014;57:16–23 [in Turkish].
19. Yalug I, Corapcioglu F, Fayda M, et al. Posttraumatic stress disorder and risk factors in parents of children with a cancer diagnosis. *Pediatr Hematol Oncol*. 2008;25:27–38.
20. Karadeniz Cerit K, Cerit C, Nart Ö, et al. Post-traumatic stress disorder in mothers of children who have undergone cancer surgery. *Pediatr Int*. 2017;59:996–1001.

21. Altay N, Kilicarslan E, Sari Ç, Kisecik Z. Determination of social support needs and expectations of mothers of children with cancer. *J Pediatr Oncol Nurs.* 2014;31:147–153.
22. Eyigor S, Karapolat H, Yesil H, Kantar M. The quality of life and psychological status of mothers of hospitalized pediatric oncology patients. *Pediatr Hematol Oncol.* 2011;28:428–438.
23. Bahadir A, Kurucu N. Evaluation of psycho-social status in mothers of children with cancer. *Fırat Üniversitesi Sağlık Bilimleri Tıp Dergisi.* 2015;29(3):131–134 [in Turkish].
24. Guggemos A, Juen F, Engelmann L, Diesselhorst V, Henze G, Di Gallo A. Siblings of children with cancer: The price they pay to function. *Support Care Cancer.* 2015;23:1837–1839.
25. Kobayashi K, Hayakawa A, Hohashi N. Interrelations between siblings and parents in families living with children with cancer. *J Fam Nurs.* 2015;21:119–148.
26. Kohlsdorf M, Costa Junior ÁL. Psychosocial impact of pediatric cancer on parents: A literature review. *Paidéia (Ribeirão Preto).* 2012;22(51):119–129.
27. Mavrides N, Pao M. Updates in paediatric psychooncology. *Int Rev Psychiatry.* 2014;26:63–73.
28. Williams LK, McCarthy MC, Eyles DJ, Drew S. Parenting a child with cancer: Perceptions of adolescents and parents of adolescents and younger children following completion of childhood cancer treatment. *J Fam Stud.* 2013;19:80–89.
29. Bozkurt C, Ugurlu Z, Tanyıldız HG, et al. Economic and psychosocial problems experienced by pediatric with cancer patients and their families during the treatment and follow-up process. *Turk Pediatr Ars.* 2019;54(1):35–39.
30. Daher M. Cultural beliefs and values in cancer patients. *Ann Oncol.* 2012;23(Suppl 3):66–69.
31. Ashing-Giwa KT, Padilla G, Tejero J, et al. Understanding the breast cancer experience of women: A qualitative study of African American, Asian American, Latina and Caucasian cancer survivors. *Psychooncology.* 2004;13:408–428.
32. Koenig HG. Religion, spirituality and medicine: Application to clinical practice. *JAMA.* 2000;284:1708.
33. Tix AP, Frazier PA. The use of religious coping during stressful life events: Main effects, moderation, and mediation. *J Consult Clin Psychol.* 1997;66:411–422.
34. Bowie J, Sydnor KD, Granot M. Spirituality and care of prostate cancer patients: A pilot study. *J Natl Med Assoc.* 2003;95:951–954.
35. Kashani FL, Vaziri S, Akbari ME, et al. Spiritual interventions and distress in mothers of children with cancer. *Procedia—Soc Behav Sci.* 2014;159:224–227.
36. Yesilbakan OU, Özkütük N, Ardahan M. Comparision quality of life of Turkish cancer patients and their family caregivers. *APJCP.* 2010;11(6):1575–1579.
37. Bergkvist K, Wengstrom Y. Symptom experiences during chemotherapy treatment-with focus on nausea and vomiting. *Eur J Oncol Nurs.* 2006;10:21–29.
38. Karasuya RT, Poglar B, Takeuchi R. Caregiver burden and burnout. *Postgrad Med.* 2000;108:119–123.
39. Hoekstra-Weebers JE, Jaspers JP, Kamps WA, Klip EC. Psychological adaptation and social support of parents of pediatric cancer patients: A prospective longitudinal study. *J Pediatr Psychol.* 2001;26:225–235.
40. Ozgul N, Gultekin M, Koc O, Goksel F, Bayraktar G, Ekinci H, et al. Turkish community-based palliative care model: A unique design. *Ann Oncol.* 2012;23(Suppl 3):76–78.
41. Kavradim ST, Ozer SC, Bozcuk H. Hope in people with cancer: a multivariate analysis from Turkey. *J Adv Nurs.* 2012;69(5):1183–1195.
42. Durusoy R, Karaca B, Junushova B., Uslu R. Cancer patients' satisfaction with doctors and preferences about death in a university hospital in Turkey. *Patient Educ Couns.* 2011;85(3):285–290.

43. Samur M, Bozcuk HS, Kara A, Savas B. Factors associated with utilization of nonproven cancer therapies in Turkey: A study of 135 patients from a single center. *Support Care Cancer*. 2001;9:452–458.

44. Atun R, Aydın S, Chakraborty S, et al. Universal health coverage in Turkey: Enhancement of equity. *The Lancet*. 2013;382(9886):65–99.

45. Kebudi R, Cakir FB. Pediatric palliative care in the community: The Turkish experience. In: Silbermann M (eds). *Palliative Care for Chronic Cancer Patients in the Community: Global Approaches and Future Applications*. New York: Springer Nature Switzerland AG 2020, pp. 407–412.

46. Kutluk T, Yesilipek MA. Turkish national pediatric cancer registry 2002–2008 (Turkish Pediatric Oncology Group and Turkish Pediatric Hematology Society). *Pediatr Blood Cancer*. 2009;53(5):e22015.

47. Kutluk MT, Yesilipek A. Pediatric cancer registry Turkey: 2009–2016 (TPOG & TPHD). *J Clin Oncol*. 2017;35(15 Suppl):e22015.

48. Hexem KR, Mollen CJ, Carroll K, Lanctot DA, Feudtner C. How parents of children receiving pediatric palliative care use religion, spirituality, or life philosophy in tough times. *J Palliat Med*. 2011;14:39–44.

49. Bar-Sela G, Schultz MJ, Elshamy K, et al. Training for awareness of one's own spirituality: A key factor in overcoming barriers to the provision of spiritual care to advanced cancer patients by doctors and nurses. *Palliat Support Care*. September 6, 2018;17(3):1–8.

7

Psychosocial Factors of Healthcare Professionals and Their Influence on Quality of Care for their Cancer Patient, United States

Ora Nakash and Leeat Granek

People with cancer are at an increased risk for mental health distress, as documented in studies showing higher prevalence of common mental disorders among cancer patients compared to the general population [1,2]. Approximately 20% of patients with cancer will suffer from depression, and 10% will experience anxiety compared with a past-year prevalence of 5% and 7% respectively, in the general population [3]. Cancer patients are also at increased risk for suicidal ideation [4], suicide attempts [5], and suicidal acts [3], with standardized mortality ratios ranging from 1.2 to 1.9 among cancer patients compared with the general population [3,6].

Studies to date have largely focused on identifying sociodemographic and clinical factors that are associated with increased mental health morbidity and suicidality among cancer patients [7]. For example, fewer years of formal education, poverty, and unemployment are associated with increased suicide risk among cancer patients [8]. Similarly, pre-cancer psychiatric history [9], as well as disease-specific attributes such as type, stage, tumor site, and intervention, have also been associated with increased risk for mental health distress and suicidality [10,11].

While accurate diagnosis of mental health distress is the basis for designing appropriate intervention, research on how health care providers identify mental health distress and suicidality among cancer patients is sparse [7].

Large-scale entities such as the American College of Surgeons' Commission on Cancer and the National Comprehensive Cancer Network have made multiple efforts to establish standard guidelines for management of mental health distress in oncology practice [12–14]. Despite these efforts, health care providers often fail to identify and treat mental health distress and suicidal ideation among their cancer patients [15,16]. A study by Fallowfield et al. [17] assessing the sensitivity and specificity of oncologists' evaluation of mental health distress in their patients found that less than a third of the patients were correctly classified as having a psychiatric morbidity. Similarly, a study by Zebrack et al. [14] found that providers documented contact with, or referral of, cancer patients suffering from clinically significant mental health distress only 50–63% of the time. Additional literature has established that one-fifth to one-third of health care providers fail to evaluate oncology patients regularly for mental health distress, and of those who do conduct mental health assessments, even fewer adhere to use of standardized screening instruments [12,13]. These findings are important because health care providers occupy a pivotal role in the mental health care of cancer patients. Another study, one by Aboumrad et al. [18] of the U.S. Veterans Health Administration National Center for Patient Safety Root Cause Analysis database, found that most patients' cancer-related suicides occurred within one week of a medical visit. As such, understanding and addressing oncology practitioners' barriers to appropriate identification of mental health distress and suicidality among cancer patients is of critical concern.

Barriers to Identifying Mental Health Distress and Suicidality

Multiple barriers to health care providers' identification of mental health distress and suicidality among oncology patients have been identified in the literature. Impediments to accurate assessment range from systematic obstacles and psychosocial factors that hinder decision making under time pressure and limited resources to issues related to providers' own culturally diverse contexts [16,19,20].

Systemic Barriers

Systemic barriers to accurate identification of mental health distress and suicidality include: absence of training, a dearth of standard protocols, awareness of increased risk among the oncology population, and insufficient resources to cope with distressed and/or suicidal patients [7,12,15,16,21,22]. A study among a national sample of social workers who work in oncology settings found the most common structural barriers to identifying distress included a lack of explicit practices and guidelines for identifying and treating patients and a lack of involvement of mental health professionals in developing such protocols [12]. Additional obstacles include overcomplexity of screenings (e.g., administrative burden, redundant forms for patients and caregivers) and providers' limited availability and lack of control in scheduling assessments [12,13]. In addition, lack of administrative support, limited staff, employee turnover, absence of interdisciplinary oncology teams, and substandard electronic medical systems that failed to help integrate mental health status screening procedures contributed to the gap in assessment and treatment of mental health concerns among cancer patients [12,22,23].

Psychological Barriers

Variables related to providers' own beliefs and attitudes toward mental health can also impede assessment [7,24]. Providers' subjective perception of the appropriateness and relevance of mental health care in routine oncology care and their individual role in providing it may affect their assessment and treatment [20,24]. Further, providers' perception of mental health topics such as suicidal ideation (i.e., viewing it as a cry for help, as an attempt to seek attention, or as a means of expressing distress) or explanatory models of such behavior (i.e., viewing suicide as a biological disease, a consequence of mental disorder, an aberration, or an act of impulsiveness) may alter the way such topics are discussed and addressed with patients [25].

In addition to the variable way providers perceive mental health distress among oncology patients, they can also endorse myths about mental health and suicidality that may undermine their assessment process [13,19]. Pirl and colleagues [13] surveyed a thousand oncologists and found that misconceptions such as believing patients are reluctant to discuss mental health distress were a key limitation to routine mental health screenings. In line with the above findings, additional studies have found that oncology health care providers harbor certain myths regarding mental health distress and suicidality, such as a fear that discussing it will make mental health distress worse or that talking about suicide will encourage it [19]. Our own research team found that oncologists, nurses, and social workers could endorse myths around suicide that included the belief that talking about suicide will lead to or encourage suicidality in patients; that suicide is not something that cancer patients often think about; that bringing up suicide with patients might make them angry; that suicide attempts are a way to receive attention; and that suicide is an act of weakness [26]. A review of 25 studies on the patient and the provider's barriers to delivery of mental health care found that such attitudes contribute to limited communication about mental health distress and, consequently, fewer referrals to mental health services [19].

Health care providers' personal worldviews further augment the gap in identifying and addressing mental health distress among oncology patients [24]. Granek, Nakash, et al. [25] reported that oncology health care providers generally held three types of moral views on suicide, each with implications for how oncology providers approach suicidality among their patients: (1) accepting attitudes toward suicidality (i.e., perceiving it to be a reasonable decision or encouraging it as a personal choice); (2) rejecting views (i.e., perceiving it as wrong, incomprehensible, and a sign of weakness of societal failure); and (3) ambivalent considerations where providers' oscillated between their sense of commitment to prolonging life and protecting patients, while simultaneously seeing and empathizing with their patients' suffering and their rationale in wanting to end their life and misery [25]. These varying personal approaches may lead to discrepancies in care and should be further studied.

Cultural Barriers

The lack of a systematic approach to assessing mental health distress and suicidality is even more pronounced when providing care to culturally diverse populations [27–29]. Broadly speaking, research on oncology care has documented the effects of cultural diversity on communication and care [30,31]. For example, racial disparities in treatment are associated with miscommunication between patients and providers that is affected by attitudes and perceptions both members of the dyad endorse about their own and the other's race/ethnicity [30,32–35]. Communication between patients and providers across racial/ethnic and nativity backgrounds (e.g., white provider with black patient) has been found to be poorer than among racially concordant pairs [30,36]. For example, a study among Australian-born and immigrant oncology patients found that providers tended to communicate differently with native versus immigrant patients; Oncologists provided fewer hopeful messages and used greater medical jargon with immigrants compared with native patients [37]. Jean-Pierre et al. [35] found nonwhite cancer patients were more likely than their white counterparts to express concern about understanding their diagnosis and treatment plan and to indicate a wish for more information. A mixed-method systematic review of 18 studies on implementation of oncological care to ethnic minorities found that linguistic obstacles as well as ambiguity and assumptions regarding cultural matters were a major hindrance to providing appropriate care [31]. Brown et al. [38] provided an integrative review of 35 studies investigating themes of providing culturally competent care to adult cancer patients; key motifs included skills needed for culturally competent communication and assessment, awareness of providers' personal beliefs, conscientiousness of their own and their patients' culture, and their knowledgeability of their patients' culture.

Despite findings pointing to the importance of cultural factors related to mental health care, limited research has focused on health care providers themselves. A recent qualitative study documented that health care providers felt more comfortable and open talking to patients who came from the same ethnic/racial background as their own about mental health distress and suicidality [27]. This suggests that a mismatch between patient and provider cultural backgrounds can potentially lead to impediments in managing and understanding mental health distress, specifically, among cancer patients. This hypothesis requires further study. For example, providers' incompetence in patients' native language (i.e., lack of fluency in language and limited understanding of linguistic nuances) may hinder discussions of mental health distress [27,39]. Religiosity and religious taboos may serve as a further obstacle to identifying distress, broadly, and suicidality, specifically. Patients may be uncomfortable discussing suicidal ideation, and health care providers may be similarly hesitant to bring it up based on their own background or their perception that it may an inappropriate topic to bring up with certain ethnic/religious groups [27,31].

Other research, mostly in the United States, has documented oncologists' biases in interactions with patients of diverse backgrounds and their influence on treatment disparities among minority populations [40]. A study among 18 oncologists and over 100 black identified patients in the United States found that providers' implicit racial bias led to shorter interactions between patients and providers and less patient-focused and supportive communication, and affected patient's perceptions of treatment recommendations [40]. Additional research has identified substantial disparities in exchange of information in interactions with racial minorities such as black cancer patients. Studies have documented differences in the amount of information clinicians provided and in patients' understanding of it [41]. Further inequities are apparent in the quality of cancer treatment given to racial minorities. A recent study among 957 breast cancer patients found that nonstandard treatment regimens were used more frequently with black patients [42]. Another study found systematic biases in administration of chemotherapy to African American women [43]. Research has identified a key cause of differences in treatment and diagnosis of minority patients: poor quality of care between patients and physicians designated by low patient health literacy and biases in physician communication [44]. Thus far, research on clinician bias has focused mainly on cancer treatment. More research is needed to explore whether provider bias may also impact assessment of mental health distress in oncology settings.

In contrast to the scarcity of literature on cultural factors of oncology health care providers in identifying mental health distress among cancer patients, a plethora of research exists on patients' cultural characteristics and their contribution to cancer patients' risk for mental health distress and suicidality [10,20,39,45]. A large majority of studies have focused on documenting ethnic/racial disparities in mental health risk in cancer patients. For example, studies have documented increased risk for mental health disorders such as depression among racial/ethnic minorities diagnosed with cancer compared to majority group patients [39,46,47]. A recent review of over 20 articles found that cancer patients of minority status (i.e., immigrants, ethnic, linguistic, or religious minorities) experienced greater mental health distress and rates of depression and poorer health-related quality of life [46]. Other research has documented the effect of patients' racial/ethnic backgrounds on their communication with their providers. For example, a study among Chinese immigrant breast cancer survivors found they were less likely than U.S.-born Chinese and non-Hispanic white breast cancer survivors to articulate their wishes to providers due to cultural norms and their culturally specific means of expression [48]. An additional study evaluating over 100 oncologist–patient–companion interactions found that black patients in the United States asked fewer and less direct questions than their white counterparts [32]. Thus, the cancer patient's cultural background may affect not only their risk for mental health outcomes but also their ability to communicate with their providers.

Clinical Implications and Recommendations for Best Practices

While an immense amount of literature has documented the increased risk for mental health distress and incidence of suicide among cancer patients, research on how health care professionals identify this risk is scarce. Health care providers face multiple barriers to identifying mental health distress and suicidality in cancer patients that include systemic and organizational factors as well as psychosocial and cultural barriers. Health care providers tend to use ad-hoc strategies to identify mental health distress and suicide risk that may lead to underdiagnosis, with concerning repercussions for people who could benefit from psychosocial support during their cancer trajectory [7].

Screening for mental health distress and suicide risk in cancer patients must be systematic and context-specific, recognizing that cancer patients are a unique population with unique risk factors [49]. Ongoing training and education for health care providers who work in the oncology setting are urgently needed. Reliable and valid universal screening for mental health distress and suicidality can be a cost-effective way to engage in mental health assessment of cancer patients and help health care providers accurately diagnose their patients' suffering. Correct diagnosis is the basis for appropriate treatment planning, including referral to specialized mental health providers when needed. Importantly, untreated mental health distress affects patients' quality of life as well as treatment adherence and prognosis [50,51]. Thus, effective screening for distress is not only cost-effective for the health care system, but it also has a significant impact on both patients' and their providers' well-being.

Clinical decisions in oncology care are often made in overburdened and severely resource-constrained environments. As a result, diagnostic decisions are often made with limited and, at times, missing clinical information. One possible approach to mitigate this issue is to increase efficiency in diagnosis for the most common mental disorders in cancer patients (e.g., major depressive disorder) [3]. Though more research is needed to identify the best screening probes in oncology care, these can include questions assessing the presence of depressed mood and diminished interest or pleasure, which have been shown to significantly improve the accuracy of diagnostic decisions for major depression in psychiatric care [52].

Alternative approaches should consider systematic utilization of reliable and valid measures for screening mental health distress such as the Hospital Anxiety and Depression Scale (HADS) [53] and the Distress Thermometer [54,55]. Similarly, the Columbia-Suicide Severity Rating Scale (C-SSRS), which can be used for both screening and in-depth assessment of suicide ideation and behaviors, has received growing support for implementation in the field, as it offers improved conceptual uniformity and clinical utility [56,57]. Prior to implementing universal screening for mental health distress for patients with cancer, health care providers must receive appropriate training on identification and management of mental health distress and suicide. Training should include modules about the frequency of mental health distress and suicide in patients and outline the risk factors for these occurrences. Moreover, health care providers should receive training in the protocols of what to do when risk is identified. Raising awareness to their personal attitudes and potential bias toward mental health distress, as well as practicing the clinical skills needed, should also be part of ongoing training.

Identifying mental health distress and suicidality in oncology care should be culturally competent. Such an approach includes engaging in culturally sensitive communication [58,59], using culturally sensitive assessment tools [60], being attuned to culturally appropriate nonverbal communication [59], and avoiding stereotypes and bias. Moreover, there is a shift among clinicians who are calling to move away from the cultural competence framework, which emphasizes a "way of doing" and places the provider as the expert in the room, to embracing a cultural humble approach, which refers to the providers' "way of being" with the patient and values mutuality and patient-centered care [61,62]. Cultural humility offers an approach to care that acknowledges the differential power that characterizes medical encounters and addresses structural forces that result in inequity in the quality of care. In their landmark paper distinguishing between cultural competence and cultural humility in physician training, Tervalon and Murray-García [63] suggested that "cultural humility incorporates a lifelong commitment to self-evaluation and critique, to redressing the power imbalances in the physician- patient dynamic, and to developing mutually beneficial and non-paternalistic partnerships with communities on behalf of individuals and defined populations" (p. 123). Maintaining a culturally humble stance requires a degree of curiosity and openness to others' experiences and preferences. It centers the patient's voice and adopts a humble approach that maintains respect and strives for mutuality when communicating with a patient [64].

References

1. Grassi L, Caruso R, Sabato S, Massarenti S, Nanni MG. Psychosocial screening and assessment in oncology and palliative care settings. *Front Psychol.* 2015;5:1485.
2. Nakash O, Levav I, Aguilar-Gaxiola S, et al. Comorbidity of common mental disorders with cancer and their treatment gap: Findings from the World Mental Health Surveys. *Psychooncology.* 2014;23(1):40–51.
3. Pitman A, Suleman S, Hyde N, Hodgkiss A. Depression and anxiety in patients with cancer. *BMJ.* 2018;361:k1415. DOI: 10.1136/bmj.k1415.
4. Henry M, Rosberger Z, Bertrand L, et al. Prevalence and risk factors of suicidal ideation among patients with head and neck cancer: Longitudinal study. *Otolaryngol Head Neck Surg.* 2018; 159(5):843–852.
5. Sun LM, Lin CL, Hsu CY, Kao CH. Risk of suicide attempts among colorectal cancer patients: A nationwide population-based matched cohort study. *Psychooncology.* 2018;27(12):2794–2801.
6. Ravaioli A, Crocetti E, Mancini S, et al. Suicide death among cancer patients: New data from northern Italy, systematic review of the last 22 years and meta-analysis. *Eur J Cancer.* 2020;125:104–113.
7. Granek L, Nakash O. Prevalence and risk factors for suicidality in cancer patients and oncology healthcare professionals' strategies in identifying suicide risk in cancer patients. *Curr Opin Support Palliat Care.* 2020; 14(3):239–246.
8. Abdel-Rahman O. Socioeconomic predictors of suicide risk among cancer patients in the United States: A population-based study. *Cancer Epidemiol.* 2019;63:101601.
9. Choi JW, Park E-C. Suicide risk after cancer diagnosis among older adults: A nationwide retrospective cohort study. *J Geriatr Oncol.* 2020;11(5):814–819.
10. Guo Z, Gan S, Li Y, et al. Incidence and risk factors of suicide after a prostate cancer diagnosis: A meta-analysis of observational studies. *Prostate Cancer Prostatic Dis.* 2018;21(4):499–508.
11. Caruso R, Nanni MG, Riba M, et al. Depressive spectrum disorders in cancer: prevalence, risk factors and screening for depression: A critical review. *Acta oncologica.* 2017;56(2):146–155.
12. BrintzenhofeSzoc K, Davis C, Kayser K, et al. Screening for psychosocial distress: A national survey of oncology social workers. *J Psychosoc Oncol.* 2015;33(1):34–47.
13. Pirl WF, Muriel A, Hwang V, et al. Screening for psychosocial distress: A national survey of oncologists. *J Support Oncol.* 2007;5(10):499–504.
14. Zebrack B, Kayser K, Sundstrom L, et al. Psychosocial distress screening implementation in cancer care: An analysis of adherence, responsiveness, and acceptability. *J Clin Oncol.* 2015;33(10):1165–1170.
15. Granek L, Nakash O, Ariad S, Shapira S, Ben-David M. Oncologists' identification of mental health distress in cancer patients: Strategies and barriers. *Eur J Cancer Care.* 2018;27(3):e12835.
16. Granek L, Nakash O, Ben-David M, Shapira S, Ariad S. Oncologists', nurses', and social workers' strategies and barriers to identifying suicide risk in cancer patients. *Psychooncology.* 2018;27(1):148–154.
17. Fallowfield L, Ratcliffe D, Jenkins V, Saul J. Psychiatric morbidity and its recognition by doctors in patients with cancer. *Br J Cancer.* 2001;84(8):1011–1015.
18. Aboumrad M, Shiner B, Riblet N, Mills PD, Watts BV. Factors contributing to cancer-related suicide: A study of root-cause analysis reports. *Psychooncology.* 2018;27(9):2237–2244.
19. Dilworth S, Higgins I, Parker V, Kelly B, Turner J. Patient and health professional's perceived barriers to the delivery of psychosocial care to adults with cancer: A systematic review. *Psychooncology.* 2014;23(6):601–612.

20. Neumann M, Galushko M, Karbach U, et al. Barriers to using psycho-oncology services: a qualitative research into the perspectives of users, their relatives, non-users, physicians, and nurses. *Support Care Cancer.* 2010;18(9):1147–1156.
21. Granek L, Nakash O, Ariad S, Shapira S, Ben-David M. Oncology nurses' strategies and barriers in identifying mental health distress in cancer patients. *Clin J Oncol Nurs.* 2019; 23(1), 43–51.22.
22. Ercolano E, Hoffman E, Tan H, Pasacreta N, Lazenby M, McCorkle R. Managing psycho-social distress comorbidity: Lessons learned in optimizing psychosocial distress screening program implementation. *Oncology* (Williston Park, NY). 2018;32(10):488..
23. Knies AK, Jutagir DR, Ercolano E, Pasacreta N, Lazenby M, McCorkle R. Barriers and facilitators to implementing the commission on cancer's distress screening program standard. *Palliat Support Care.* 2019;17(3):253–261.
24. Lee J. Health workers' perceptions of psychosocial support services for cancer patients in rural Victoria. Paper presented at: Cancer Forum, 2007;253–261.
25. Granek L, Nakash O, Ariad S, Shapira S, Ben-David J. Oncology healthcare professionals' perceptions, explanatory models, and moral views on suicidality. *Support Care Cancer.* 2019;27(12):4723–4732.
26. Granek L, Nakash O. Oncologists, nurses, and social workers endorsement of suicide myths. Unpublished manuscript.
27. Granek L, Nakash O, Ariad S, Shapira S, Ben-David MA. The role of culture/ethnicity in communicating with cancer patients about mental health distress and suicidality. *Cult Med Psychiatry.* 2020: 44(2):214–229.28. Alegría M, Nakash O, NeMoyer A. Increasing eq-uity in access to mental health care: A critical first step in improving service quality. *World Psychiatry.* 2018;17(1):43–44.
29. Nakash O, Saguy T. Social identities of clients and therapists during the mental health in-take predict diagnostic accuracy. *Soc Psychol Personal Sci.* 2015;6(6):710–717.
30. Hamel LM, Moulder R, Albrecht TL, Boker S, Eggly S, Penner LA. Nonverbal synchrony as a behavioural marker of patient and physician race-related attitudes and a predictor of out-comes in oncology interactions: protocol for a secondary analysis of video-recorded cancer treatment discussions. *BMJ Open.* 2018;8:e023648.
31. van Eechoud IJ, Grypdonck M, Beeckman D, Van Lancker A, Van Hecke A, Verhaeghe S. Oncology health workers' views and experiences on caring for ethnic minority patients: A mixed method systematic review. *Int J Nurs Stud.* 2016;53:379–398.
32. Eggly S, Harper FW, Penner LA, Gleason MJ, Foster T, Albrecht TL. Variation in question asking during cancer clinical interactions: A potential source of disparities in access to in-formation. *Patient Educ Couns.* 2011;82(1):63–68.
33. Song L, Hamilton JB, Moore AD. Patient-healthcare provider communication: Perspectives of African American cancer patients. *Health Psychol.* 2012;31(5):539.
34. Gordon HS, Street Jr RL, Sharf BF, Souchek J. Racial differences in doctors' information-giving and patients' participation. *Cancer.* 2006;107(6):1313–1320.
35. Jean-Pierre P, Fiscella K, Griggs J, et al. Race/ethnicity-based concerns over understanding cancer diagnosis and treatment plan. *J Natl Med Assoc.* 2010;102(3):184–189.
36. Gordon HS, Street RL, Sharf BF, Kelly PA, Souchek J. Racial differences in trust and lung cancer patients' perceptions of physician communication. *J Clin Oncol.* 2006;24(6):904–909.
37. Butow PN, Sze M, Eisenbruch M, et al. Should culture affect practice? A comparison of prognostic discussions in consultations with immigrant versus native-born cancer pa-tients. *Patient Educ Couns.* 2013;92(2):246–252.
38. Brown O, Ham-Baloyi Wt, Rooyen Dv, Aldous C, Marais LC. Culturally competent pa-tient–provider communication in the management of cancer: An integrative literature re-view. *Glob Health Action.* 2016;9(1):33208.

39. Butow PN, Aldridge L, Bell ML, et al. Inferior health-related quality of life and psychological well-being in immigrant cancer survivors: A population-based study. *Eur J Cancer.* 2013;49(8):1948–1956.

40. Penner LA, Dovidio JF, Gonzalez R, et al. The effects of oncologist implicit racial bias in racially discordant oncology interactions. *J Clin Oncol.* 2016;34(24):2874–2880.

41. Penner LA, Eggly S, Griggs JJ, Underwood III W, Orom H, Albrecht TL. Life-threatening disparities: The treatment of black and white cancer patients. *J Soc Iss.* 2012;68(2):328–357.

42. Griggs JJ, Culakova E, Sorbero ME, et al. Social and racial differences in selection of breast cancer adjuvant chemotherapy regimens. *J Clin Oncol.* 2007;25(18):2522–2527.

43. Griggs JJ, Sorbero ME, Stark AT, Heininger SE, Dick AW. Racial disparity in the dose and dose intensity of breast cancer adjuvant chemotherapy. *Breast Cancer Res Treat.* 2003;81(1):21–31.

44. Daly B, Olopade OI. Race, ethnicity, and the diagnosis of breast cancer. *JAMA.* 2015;313(2):141–142.

45. Samawi H, Shaheen A, Tang P, Heng D, Cheung W, Vickers M. Risk and predictors of suicide in colorectal cancer patients: A surveillance, epidemiology, and end results analysis. *Curr Oncol.* 2017;24(6):e513.

46. Luckett T, Goldstein D, Butow PN, et al. Psychological morbidity and quality of life of ethnic minority patients with cancer: a systematic review and meta-analysis. *The Lancet Oncol.* 2011;12(13):1240–1248.

47. Sheppard VB, Llanos AA, Hurtado-de-Mendoza A, Taylor TR, Adams-Campbell LL. Correlates of depressive symptomatology in African-American breast cancer patients. *J Cancer Surviv.* 2013;7(3):292–299.

48. Wang JH-y, Adams I, Huang E, Ashing-Giwa K, Gomez SL, Allen L. Physical distress and cancer care experiences among Chinese-American and non-Hispanic white breast cancer survivors. *Gynecol Oncol.* 2012;124(3):383–388.

49. Granek L, Nakash O, Ariad S, et al. From will to live to will to die: Oncologists, nurses, and social workers identification of suicidality in cancer patients. *Support Care Cancer.* 2017;25(12):3691–3702.

50. Kennard BD, Stewart SM, Olvera R, Bawdon RE, Lewis CP, Winick NJ. Nonadherence in adolescent oncology patients: Preliminary data on psychological risk factors and relationships to outcome. *J Clin Psychol Med Set.* 2004;11(1):31–39.

51. Pasquini M, Biondi M. Depression in cancer patients: A critical review. *Clin Prac Epidemiol Ment Health.* 2007;3(1):2.

52. Nakash O, Nagar M, Kanat-Maymon Y. The clinical utility of DSM categorical diagnostic system during the mental health intake. *J Clin Psychiatry.* 2015;76(7):e862–e869.

53. Zigmond AS, Snaith RP. The hospital anxiety and depression scale. *Acta Psychiatr Scand.* 1983;67(6):361–370.

54. Roth AJ, Kornblith AB, Batel-Copel L, Peabody E, Scher HI, Holland JC. Rapid screening for psychologic distress in men with prostate carcinoma. *Cancer.* 1998;82(10):1904–1908.

55. Holland JC, Bultz BD. The NCCN guideline for distress management: A case for making distress the sixth vital sign. *JNCCN.* 2007;5(1):3–7.

56. Interian A, Chesin M, Kline A, et al. Use of the Columbia-Suicide Severity Rating Scale (C-SSRS) to classify suicidal behaviors. *Arch Suicide Res.* 2018;22(2):278–294.

57. Thom R, Hogan C, Hazen E. Suicide risk screening in the hospital setting: A review of brief validated tools. *Psychosomatics.* 2020;61(1):1–7.

58. Surbone A. Cultural aspects of communication in cancer care. *Recent Results Cancer Res.* 2006;168:91–104.

59. Kagawa-Singer M, Dadia AV, Yu MC, Surbone A. Cancer, culture, and health disparities: Time to chart a new course? *CA Cancer J Clin.* 2010;60:12–39.

60. Huang YL, Yates P, Prior D. Factors influencing oncology nurses' approaches to accommodating cultural needs in palliative care. *J Clin Nurs.* 2009;18:3421–3429.

61. Hook JN, Farrell JE, Davis DE, DeBlaere C, Van Tongeren DR, Utsey SO. Cultural humility and racial microaggressions in counseling. *J Couns Psychol.* 2016;63:269–277.

62. Ndiwane AN, Baker NC, Makosky A, Reidy P, Guarino AJ. Use of simulation to integrate cultural humility into advanced health assessment for nurse practitioner students. *J Nurs Educ.* 2017;56:567–571.

63. Tervalon M, Murray-Garcia J. Cultural humility versus cultural competence: A critical distinction in defining physician training outcomes in multicultural education. *J Health Care Poor and Underserved.* 1998;9:117–125.

64. Hook JN, Davis DE, Owen J, Worthington Jr EL, Utsey SO. Cultural humility: Measuring openness to culturally diverse clients. *J Couns Psychol.* 2013;60(3):353.

8

Healing the Psychological and Emotional Aspects of Cancer, Jordan

Mohammad Al Qadire

Introduction

Cancer is a devastating and burdensome disease affecting all aspects of patients' and their families' lives. It is estimated that the number of newly diagnosed cases worldwide will reach 21.6 million by 2030 and that cancer-related deaths will reach 12 million in the same year [1]. At the same time, early detection and advancements in cancer treatment have led to an increase in the number of people surviving with cancer. Patients with cancer are subjected to various types of treatment modules including, but not limited to, surgery, chemotherapy, radiotherapy, immunotherapy and hormonal therapy. Such treatments cause many annoying and difficult-to-treat symptoms that may also result from the disease itself [2,3,4,5]. In addition, cancer changes patients' physical status as it declines with the progression of the disease trajectory from the time of diagnosis, throughout the treatment and until the end of life [6]. For the past few decades, cancer treatments have remained focused mainly on the physical aspects of disease with less attention paid to the psychological and emotional dimensions of the cancer experience [1]. Psychological aspects are usually compromised by the diagnosis and treatment of cancer. At the time of diagnosis, patients may experience adjustment disorder, anxiety and depression. Furthermore, cancer treatment may cause the loss of a patient's organ and/or limb, and a change in appearance may lead to impaired self-image and self-esteem and increase the occurrence of anxiety, depression, and feelings of helplessness among patients and their families. In addition, facing a life-threatening disease such as cancer may cause patients to feel the inevitability of death and hence may cause them to lose their fighting spirit and give up on the treatment [7–9]. These feelings may lead to suicidal thoughts and even actual attempts at suicide. Therefore, the patient with cancer should not be treated as a "tumor carrier" but rather as a whole person, taking into consideration the physical, psychological, and emotional aspects of their experience.

Another factor that may contribute to physicians' primary focus on treating the cancer itself and underestimating the psychological and emotional aspects is the adoption of a biomedical approach to health care that is currently the most prevalent medical system worldwide. As the goal of biomedicine is to cure physical suffering, in this module, psychological and emotional aspects receive lower priority [9]. It is postulated that once the physical disease is cured, the suffering will be eliminated. However, this is not realistic as many diseases have no available cure and these patients are left to suffer. In addition, most of the psychological and emotional symptoms may not only be caused by the physical disease but also by the patient's reaction to a life-threatening and debilitating disease such as cancer [9]. Spiritual, cultural, religious, philosophical, and financial factors have a crucial role in the nature and severity of psychological distress experienced by cancer patients and their families. Therefore, the psychological aspect of cancer care should be dealt with at the very beginning of the cancer trajectory. This chapter aims to highlight the most commonly experienced psychological issues among cancer patients.

Spiritual and Cultural Considerations in Cancer Care

Spirituality and culture are correlated with human well-being and perception of their health status [10]. Cancer patients may use their spiritual and cultural beliefs to understand, accept, and adapt to their disease [5,11]. Spirituality and culture are core components of the holistic care approach that calls for comprehensive management of physical, psychological, spiritual, emotional, and cultural aspects of cancer care. In comparison to the biomedical approach, it aims to treat patients as whole persons, reduce suffering, and promote healing rather than cure [12]. This gives the value to cancer patients' quality of life, with more focus on their spiritual needs and their cultural background.

Spirituality may be defined as "those beliefs, values and practices that relate to the human search for meaning in life. For some people, spirituality is expressed through adherence to an organized religion, while for others it may relate to their personal identities, relationships with others, secular, ethical values or humanistic philosophies" [13, p. 6]. Thus, having a life-threatening disease such as cancer may intensify patients' search for the meaning of life and reasons of existence. Also, this may lead to spiritual distress, which is manifested by patients expressing loss of hope, rage, and misunderstanding of their health condition and its related consequences [5,11].

Health care providers (i.e., physicians and nurses) should understand that spiritual care is a crucial component of patients' daily care and is not a mere accessory. Hence, patients' spiritual needs must be assessed and evaluated [12]. This demands building a trust relationship with the patients, possessing high communications skills, and being active listener. Including family members in care planning is not less important than involving other health care team members. Further, religious clerics are important players on the team and should be made available, for they hold the main responsibility to speak, listen, and support patients. But they should understand that their mission is to support patients rather than convert them. Nevertheless, relatives, friends, and significant others may provide spiritual and emotional support [12].

Spiritual care cannot be provided in isolation from patients' cultural background. Culture may represent a way of living for a certain group of people who may/may not live in the same geographical area [14]. This way of living forms our understanding, our method of adapting to life events, and our approach to dealing with persons or other cultures. Both spirituality and culture affect each other as well as the nature of patients' response to cancer diagnosis, treatment, death, and dying [14]. For example, some Muslim cancer patients with pain may refuse to take opioids because they know that Islam prohibits use of drugs (and perhaps that is the case in other religions as well) [15,16]. Thus, Islamic clerics may need to explain to the patient that opioid use for medical purposes is allowed. Other patients may refuse opioids for fear of being stigmatized within their local communities as addicts [15,16]. So, a physician or a nurse should emphasize to patients and their families that the addiction rate from taking opioids for health reasons is very low, and it is even less likely to occur among patients with cancer pain. This brings us back to the holistic care approach where all patients' concerns should be assessed and addressed. Ignoring this fact and focusing on the physical and physiological aspects could result in several avoidable consequences and a compromised quality of life for patients.

Consequences of Unmanaged Psychological and Psychiatric Disorders

The psychological well-being of cancer patients is affected by the diagnosis of cancer, and this effect continues throughout the trajectory of the disease [17]. Unattended psychological disorders limit patients' adaptability and their ability to cope with the disease, which may lead to inadequate compliance with treatment plans and negatively affect their quality of life [2,17]. Having a high level of anxiety, for example, is usually combined with several somatic symptoms, which may distract health care providers from the planned treatment. Furthermore, depression has been found to be correlated with the reduced response to chemotherapy, the increased risk of recurrence, and suicide attempts among cancer patients [9].

Aside from patients who may experience psychological disorders, family caregivers tend to experience psychological distress in the form of anxiety and depression, thereby increasing their suffering and burden. A recent survey of 222 parents of children with cancer reported that 178 of them had moderate to severe symptoms of anxiety and 209 had depressive symptoms [18]. Several studies have revealed that the families of cancer patients usually suffer from psychological problems such as depression, feelings of helplessness, and anxiety during the course of diagnosis and treatment [19,20]. Fearing recurrence of the disease after treatment and the prospect of death are other serious concerns [21,22].

Families of cancer patients who have limited financial resources tend to report an especially high level of stress and depressive symptoms [22]. They have more days of absence from work, reducing their opportunity for employment and increasing their inability to pay for cost of treatment, which in turn increases the family's burden and suffering [20,23–25]. Family members caring for children with cancer are more likely to have physical and mental health problems and to develop illnesses due to the multiple responsibilities and hard work involved in meeting all of their responsibilities [23,24,20]. Other studies have found that most family caregivers complain of many physical symptoms such as fatigue, heart problems, increased body weight, back and shoulder pain, arthritis, high blood pressure, sleep disturbance, loss of energy, and loss of appetite [26–28]. This is a call for health care providers to consider family caregivers when planning the care for cancer patients.

Psychological Disorders among Cancer Patients

Psychological abnormalities can occur at any time throughout the cancer trajectory, but there are certain points in time that mark a high probability of its occurrence. These points in time include the instance when an alarming symptom is detected (e.g., a breast lump), the period of diagnosis, confirmation of the diagnosis, start of the treatment, failure of or change in treatment, the follow-up diagnostic workup, recurrence or progression of the disease, and the period of advanced cancer when end of life is approaching [7,8,11]. Thus, it is important to understand that continuous assessment of the patients' psychological and emotional status is crucial to identifying at-risk patients and then treating or referring them to specialized psychiatric care.

In the context of cancer, patients could experience a vast range of normal (e.g., feelings of fear) or more severe emotions (e.g., depression), with a variety of psychological and emotional responses. The three most common disorders are highlighted in this chapter: adjustment disorders, anxiety, and depression.

Adjustment disorders are emotional responses to a stressor (i.e., cancer) that are worse than normal and result in functional disability, interfering with the patients' lives [7,9]. Patients with adjustment distress may experience symptoms such as anxiety, worry, loss of hope, and loss of appetite. Adjustment disorders are the mildest form of psychological reactions to cancer. Because its symptoms are of a generic nature, adjustment disorders are difficult to detect and diagnose [8,9]. However, other symptoms may help detect adjustment disorders; these symptoms include insomnia, muscle weakness, dyspnea, palpitation, sweating, mood swings, and crying, the last of which can provide emotional relief. Adjustment disorders can be acute or chronic when they present for six months or longer [8].

Adjustment disorder treatment should support patients in their attempt to regain their ability to cope with and adapt to life stressors. Also, treatment should aim at enhancing patients' physical ability to perform their daily living activity. Further, physical symptoms (e.g., insomnia) need to be eliminated [7,9]. One of the effective treatment options is group therapy, which allows patients to understand and recognize the sources of their stress. In addition, it helps patients find meaning in their lives and revives their hope and motivation to live and adapt. This approach requires giving the patients adequate information regarding their diagnosis, prognosis, and available treatment modules [7]. They will then have a better understanding of their situation and can share their experience with others. Nevertheless, cognitive-behavioral therapy along with pharmacological treatment may be prescribed as per patients' needs [8,29,30].

Anxiety can be defined as a feeling of worry or apprehension about uncertain future events; it is a normal sensation that everyone experiences at some time in their lives [31]. A feeling of anxiety helps people to adapt to minor stressors such as sitting for an examination or attending an interview. However, if the anxiety becomes persistent and severe, it can develop into a mood disturbance and negatively affect quality of life. Persistent anxiety usually occurs when an individual is diagnosed with a life-threatening illness such as cancer [31]. It is a subjective symptom associated with other symptoms such as fatigue, tachycardia, headache, muscle spasm, dizziness, and sleep problems, continuing for at least six months and causing decreased social functioning

[32]. It is estimated that about 20–60% of cancer patients experience anxiety at some stage of their illness and after completion of treatment [7,33]. Anxiety negatively affects patients' quality of life, interferes with daily living activities, distorts treatment plans, and increases patients' and families' suffering [2,7,11,17,18].

Depression is defined as "a mood disorder incorporating both psychological and somatic symptoms that alter mood, affect personality and result in loss of interest or pleasure in nearly all activities" [42, p. 436]. It is the most common disease burden worldwide and results in significant functional impairment, increasing the risk of suicide and comorbid physical health problems [34]. Depression is prevalent and is the fourth-leading cause of disability worldwide [35]. Although published reports differ, it is estimated that approximately 20–35% of patients with cancer reported having experienced depression [7].

Depression is associated with many symptoms, such as feelings of guilt, changes in appetite and sleep, difficulty concentrating, and attempted suicide [7]. It is a common psychiatric phenomenon and has a variety of causes relating to biological, social, physical, and psychological aspects [32]. It can interfere with the efficacy of cancer treatment as it may cause patients to refuse treatment, delay treatment, or reduce the frequency of treatment. Thus, the assessment and management of psychological disorders is crucial in oncology, no less important than treating the cancer itself.

Assessment of Anxiety and Depression

Screening as a Golden Standard of Practice

Screening for psychological disorders should be an integral part of health care providers' daily practice. According to the National Comprehensive Cancer Network (NCCN), the term *distress*, in the context of cancer, indicates a wide range of psychiatric conditions, ranging from normal feelings of fear to the formal diagnosis of depression [36]. Use of this term is meant to increase awareness of the necessity for regular screening for psychological disorders in cancer patients. In addition, psychiatric care should be integrated within the regular care of patients with cancer, along with conventional treatment modules and should not be ignored or underestimated [36]. Hence, "distress" has been declared to be the sixth vital sign when detecting at-risk patients who must then receive prompt treatment either by primary health care providers or by psychiatric consultation [36]. Despite this, the assessment and management of distress among cancer patients is still inadequate and not well integrated into clinical practice.

Assessment Is the Cornerstone

Anxiety and depression should be assessed on a regular basis using a valid assessment tool. Assessments must integrate depression as one of the six vital signs and should be the responsibility of the oncology team; oncologists and oncology nurses are in the best position to perform this task. In addition, it should be noted that assessment tools are used to recognize at-risk patients but are not a replacement for psychiatric interviews for establishing a formal diagnosis and to set treatment plans. Holistic assessment is the gold standard that practitioners should aim to achieve. It requires excellent interpersonal communication skills with the patient, the family, and the multidisciplinary team; excellent listening skills; and the ability to develop a trusting therapeutic relationship whereby patients can express their needs.

Anxiety

Anxiety is initially assessed by reviewing the patient's medical history and possible causes of this disorder, along with a physical examination for tachycardia, tachypnea, and rapid speech. It is very important for oncologists and oncology nurses to listen to patients in order to build trust and the good rapport necessary to facilitate future assessment and treatment.

Of the various measurement tools that are available, the Hamilton Anxiety Rating Scale (HAM-A) was one of the first tools to measure the severity of anxiety symptoms [37]. It consists of 14 items, each defined by a series of symptoms, and it measures both mental anxiety (agitation and psychological distress) and somatic anxiety (physical complaints related to anxiety). Each item is scored on a scale of 0 (not present) to 4 (severe), with a total score range of 0–56; a score of less than 17 indicates mild severity, 18–24 mild to moderate severity, and 25–30 moderate to severe anxiety [37]. The Anxiety Sensitivity Index (ASI), another self-reporting questionnaire, consists of 16 items and measures the level of fear related to feelings of anxiety, and again it is rated from 0 to 4 [38]. Finally, the Beck Anxiety Inventory (BAI) Scale is a self-reporting measure of anxiety that consists of 21 items [11]: 0–21 represents a low level of anxiety, 22–35 moderate anxiety, and 36 and above indicates a high level of potential concern [39].

Depression

Several tools are available for the assessment of depressive symptoms for either clinical or research purposes. First, the Beck Depression Inventory (BDI) is composed of 21 self-reporting items that assess depression [40]. Each item is rated with four options and scores between 0 and 3. Then, based on the total score, respondents can be classified into one of three categories; mild depression (10–18), moderate depression (19–29), and severe depression (30–63). Second, the Hamilton Depression Rating Scale (HAM-D) consists of 21 items, developed from the original version, which had 17 items [1]. Eight items are scored on a 5-point scale, ranging from 0 (not present) to 4 (severe); and nine are scored from 0 to 2 [41]. A total score of 0–6 is considered normal, 7–17 mild, 18–24 moderately severe, and a score greater than 24 major depression.

Finally, both anxiety and depression are assessed together by HADS. It is composed of 14 items, 7 of which refer to anxiety and 7 to depression [42]. Patients are required to rate their responses on a scale of 0 to 3 for each item. Therefore, the total score for each subscale ranges from 0 to 21: a total score of 0–7 is considered normal, 8–10 is borderline-abnormal, and 11–21 is considered abnormal [42].

The Management of Anxiety and Depression

The assessment of anxiety and depression is a primary step in providing adequate mental health care management. Pharmacological measures are the most common but not the only available approach to treatment. In addition, evidence demonstrates the efficacy of a nonpharmacological approach in the management of anxiety and depression [43–45]. Further, an interdisciplinary approach is most effective in the management of anxiety and depression and may enhance response to treatment.

Pharmacological Intervention

Several groups of anxiolytic medications are currently used; however, benzodiazepines are the drug of choice for the treatment of anxiety. Of the benzodiazepines, Alprazolam is short-acting, while the other medications in this group, such as Clonazepam and Diazepam, have longer half-lives. In addition, azapirones (i.e., Buspirone), antidepressants (e.g., selective serotonin reuptake inhibitors [SSRIs]), antipsychotics (e.g., Olanzapine), and antihistamines (e.g., Hydroxyzine) can also be used in the treatment of anxiety.

Depression can be treated with SSRIs, which are considered to be the first line of treatment. Dopaminergic antidepressants (Bupropion) are also used. Further, tricyclic antidepressants (TCAs) can be used.

Nonpharmacological Intervention

Anxiety and depression are frequently associated with tension and stress. Relaxation is the natural answer to stress, and the many ways to relax include yoga, reading, or going away for a short holiday. Relaxation exercises can also be used to help people prepare for sleep. For moderate and severe anxiety and depression, there are two broad approaches to treatment: antidepressant medication and formal psychological treatment. The type of psychological therapy recommended depends on the patient's personality and the severity and duration of their symptoms [46].

Cognitive-behavioral therapy (CBT) is a talking treatment that helps people recognize their problems and overcome emotional difficulties [46]. It aims to help them develop practical skills, which can then be utilized to follow a more positive and constructive way of life, therefore improving their mood. CBT may not always address the underlying causes behind a problem, but it can provide the tools required to help manage their symptoms. In addition, for mild to moderate cases of anxiety and depression, complementary therapy may include treatment such as reducing the patient's daily caffeine and alcohol intake. Stress and pain management programs, relaxation techniques, massage, touch, distraction, music therapy, and psychotherapy such as guided imagery and hypnosis are frequently used [43,44,46]. The current evidence on the use of nonpharmacological interventions suggests a synergic effect, in conjunction with the available medication, but more research is needed in order to recommend its sole usage in the treatment of anxiety and depression [43,45].

A Framework for Clinical Practice

To maximize the management of the psychological aspects of cancer, health care providers must be aware that psychological symptoms tend to occur in clusters among cancer patients. This mean that patients may have anxiety, depression, and/or a combination of other symptoms at the same time. It is reported that psychological cluster symptoms are the most common cluster symptoms experienced by cancer patients. Furthermore, adopting a multidisciplinary approach is highly recommended.

To optimally manage psychological symptoms, three main components are needed: comprehensive assessment and reevaluation, effective treatment, and knowledgeable and skillful health care providers. In order to manage a psychological symptom, it first must be recognized and therefore can only be achieved through comprehensive and regularly scheduled screening and assessment. Health care providers should be cognizant that patients' cultural backgrounds and beliefs affect their presentation of symptoms; this relationship with culture and religion has been corroborated by the patients themselves. Thus, when using assessment tools or conducting a diagnostic interview, it should be designed with the patient's cultural and religious beliefs in mind. Then, once treatment is initiated, a reevaluation assessment should be conducted to measure how effective the intervention has been and whether the patient is satisfied with the treatment; if not, the intervention needs to be modified or replaced.

The second important component is the availability of the required pharmacological and nonpharmacological interventions. Without them, it is not possible to treat patients' symptoms and reduce their suffering. Furthermore, guidelines on the use of interventions need to be developed and implemented in clinical practices.

Finally, conducting a comprehensive assessment and using the appropriate intervention requires knowledgeable and skilled health care providers (e.g., physicians and nurses). This can be achieved by adequate education and training at either the undergraduate or postgraduate level. It may take several forms, such as regular workshops, online courses, and simulation scenarios. However, this suggested model remains to be expanded, critiqued, and tested for its effectiveness and outcome. We believe it will provide insights to advance the clinical aspects of psychological symptom management.

References

1. Luigi G, Spiegel D, Riba M. Advancing psychosocial care in cancer patients. F1000Research. 2017;6. 2083. https://doi.org/10.12688/f1000research.11902.1
2. Al Qadire M, Al Khalaileh M. Prevalence of symptoms and quality of life among Jordanian cancer patients. Clin Nurs Res. 2016;25(2):174–191.

3. Al Qadire M. Chemotherapy-induced nausea and vomiting: Incidence and management in Jordan. Clin Nurs Res. 2018;27(6):730–742.

4. Don, ST, Butow PN, Costa D, Lovell MR, Agar, M. Symptom clusters in patients with advanced cancer: A systematic review of observational studies. J Pain Symptom Manage. 2014;48(3):411–450.

5. Gudenkauf LM, Clark MM, Novotny PJ, et al. Spirituality and emotional distress among lung cancer survivors. Clin Lung Cancer. 2019;20(6):e661–e666.

6. Russell J, Wong ML, Mackin L, et al. Stability of symptom clusters in patients with lung cancer receiving chemotherapy. J Pain Symptom Manage. 2019;57(5):909–922.

7. Bail JR, Traeger L, Pirl WF, Bakitas MA. Psychological Symptoms in Advanced Cancer. Seminars in oncology nursing; 2018;34(3):241–251.

8. McFarland DC, Holland JC. The management of psychological issues in oncology. Clin Adv Hematol Oncol. 2016;14(12):13–16.

9. Berger AM, Shuster L, Von Roenn JH. Principles and Practice of Palliative Care and Supportive Oncology. 4th ed. Baltimore, MD: Lippincott Williams & Wilkins; 2013.

10. Musa AS, Al Qadire MI, Aljezawi M, et al. Barriers to the provision of spiritual care by nurses for hospitalized patients in Jordan. Res Theory Nurs Prac. 2019;33(4):392–409.

11. Bovero A, Leombruni P, Miniotti M, Rocca G, Torta R. Spirituality, quality of life, psychological adjustment in terminal cancer patients in hospice. Eur J Cancer Care. 2016;25(6):961–969.

12. Rosser M, Walsh H. Fundamentals of Palliative Care for Student Nurses: Hoboken, NJ: John Wiley; 2014.

13. NHS. Draft spiritual support and bereavement quality markers and measures for end of life care NHS National End of Life Care programme Retrieved November 30, 2020, from file:/// C:/Users/m.alqadire/Downloads/Draft-spiritual-support-and-bereavement-care-quality-markers-and-measures-for-end-of-life-care.pdf. 2011.

14. Hughes CR, van Heugten K, Keeling S. Cultural meaning-making in the journey from diagnosis to end of life. Austr Soc Work. 2015;68(2):169–183.

15. Al Khalaileh M, Al Qadire M. Barriers to cancer pain management: Jordanian nurses' perspectives. Int J Palliat Nurs. 2012;18(11):535–540.

16. Al Qadire M. Patient-related barriers to cancer pain management in Jordan. J Pediatr Hematol/Oncol. 2012;34:S28–S31.

17. Mosleh SM, Alja'afreh M, Alnajar MK, Subih M. The prevalence and predictors of emotional distress and social difficulties among surviving cancer patients in Jordan. Eur J Oncol Nurs. 2018;33:5–40.

18. Al Qadire M, Al-Sheikh H, Suliman M, et al. (2018). Predictors of anxiety and depression among parents of children with cancer in Jordan. Psychooncology. 2018;1:3.

19. Masa'Deh R, Collier J, Hall C, Alhalaiqa F. Predictors of stress of parents of a child with cancer: A Jordanian perspective. Glob J Health Sci. 2013;5(6):81.

20. McDonnell GA, Salley CG, Barnett M, et al. Anxiety among adolescent survivors of pediatric cancer. J Adolesc Health. 2017;61(4):409–423. doi: https://doi.org/10.1016/j.jadohealth.2017.04.004

21. Aghdam AM, Rahmani A, Nejad ZK, Ferguson C, Mohammadpoorasl A, Sanaat Z. Fear of cancer recurrence and its predictive factors among Iranian cancer patients. Indian J Palliat Care. 2014;20(2):128.

22. Lim SM, Kim, HC, Lee S. Psychosocial impact of cancer patients on their family members. Cancer Res Treat. 2013;45(3):226–233.

23. Al-Gharib RM, Abu-Saad Huijer H, Darwish H. Quality of care and relationships as reported by children with cancer and their parents. Ann Palliat Med. 2015;4(1):22–31.

24. Haimour AI, Abu-Hawwash RM. Evaluating quality of life of parents having a child with disability. Int Interdiscip J Educ. 2012;1(2):37–43.

25. Al Qadire M, Aloush S, Alkhalaileh M, Qandeel H, Al-Sabbah A. Burden among parents of children with cancer in Jordan: Prevalence and predictors. Cancer Nurs.2019;43(5):396–401.

26. Stenberg U, Ruland, CM, Miaskowski C. Review of the literature on the effects of caring for a patient with cancer. Psychooncology. 2010;19(10):1013–1025.

27. Girgis A, Lambert S, Johnson C, Waller A, Currow D. Physical, psychosocial, relationship, and economic burden of caring for people with cancer: a review. J Oncol Prac. 2013;9(4):197–202.

28. Santo EA, Gaíva MAM, Espinosa MM, Barbosa DA, Belasco AGS. Taking care of children with cancer: Evaluation of the caregivers' burden and quality of life. Revista Latino-Americana de Enfermagem. 2011;19(3):515–522.

29. Mosher CE, Ott MA, Hanna N, Jalal SI, Champion VL. Coping with physical and psychological symptoms: A qualitative study of advanced lung cancer patients and their family caregivers. Support Care in Cancer. 2015;23(7):2053–2060.

30. de la Torre-Luque A, Gambara H, López E, Cruzado JA. Psychological treatments to improve quality of life in cancer contexts: A meta-analysis. Int J Clin Health Psychol. 2016;16(2):211–219.

31. Combes S. Nursing assessment of anxiety and mood disturbance in a palliative patient. End of Life J. 2016;6(1):e000026.

32. Sherman DW. Palliative Care Nursing: Quality Care to the End of Life. New York: Springer; 2010.

33. Maass SW, Roorda C, Berendsen AJ, Verhaak PF, de Bock GH. The prevalence of long-term symptoms of depression and anxiety after breast cancer treatment: A systematic review. Maturitas. 2015;82(1):100–108.

35. Labonté B, Engmann O, Purushothaman I, et al. Sex-specific transcriptional signatures in human depression. Nat Med. 2017;23(9):1102.

36. Holland JC, Bultz BD. The NCCN guideline for distress management: A case for making distress the sixth vital sign. J Natl Compr Canc Netw. 2007;5(1):3–7.

37. Hamilton M. The assessment of anxiety states by rating. Br J Med Psychol. 1959;32(1):50–55.

38. Peterson RA, Heilbronner RL. The anxiety sensitivity index: Construct validity and factor analytic structure. J Anxiety Disord. 1987;1(2):117–121.

39. Ulusoy M, Sahin NH, Erkmen H. The Beck Anxiety Inventory: Psychometric properties. J Cogn Psychother. 1998;12(2):163–172.

40. Beck AT, Steer RA, Carbin MG. Psychometric properties of the Beck Depression Inventory: Twenty-five years of evaluation. Clin Psychol Rev. 1988;8(1):77–100.

41. Aben I, Verhey F, Lousberg R, Lodder J, Honig A. Validity of the Beck Depression Inventory, Hospital Anxiety and Depression Scale, SCL-90, and Hamilton Depression Rating Scale as screening instruments for depression in stroke patients. Psychosomatics. 2012;43(5):386–393.

42. Zigmond AS, Snaith RP. The hospital anxiety and depression scale. Acta psychiatrica scandinavica. 1983;67(6):361–370.

43. Buckman J, Underwood A, Clarke K, et al. Risk factors for relapse and recurrence of depression in adults and how they operate: A four-phase systematic review and meta-synthesis. Clini Psychol Rev. 2018;64:13–38.

43. Coutiño-Escamilla L, Piña-Pozas M, Garces AT, Gamboa-Loira B, López-Carrillo L. Non-pharmacological therapies for depressive symptoms in breast cancer patients: Systematic review and meta-analysis of randomized clinical trials. Breast. 2019; 44:135–143.

44. Zweers D, de Graaf E, Teunissen SC. Non-pharmacological nurse-led interventions to manage anxiety in patients with advanced cancer: A systematic literature review. Int J Nurs Stud. 2016;56:102–113.
45. Okuyama T, Akechi T, Mackenzie L, Furukawa TA. Psychotherapy for depression among advanced, incurable cancer patients: A systematic review and meta-analysis. Cancer Treat Rev. 2017;56:16–27.
46. Haddad M, Buszewicz M, Murphy B. Supporting people with depression and anxiety: A guide for practice nurses; 2011. London: Mind. Available online: chrome-extension://efa idnbmnnnibpcajpcglclefindmkaj/viewer.html?pdfurl=https%3A%2F%2Fopenaccess.city. ac.uk%2Fid%2Feprint%2F1689%2F3%2FMIND_ProCEED_Training_Pack.pdf&clen= 3620128&chunk=true

9

Nurses Providing Emotional Support and Spiritual Care to Patients and Families, Spain & Turkey

Paz Fernández-Ortega, Sultan Kav, and Esther Arimón-Pagès

Introduction

Nursing is regarded as a caring profession that takes a holistic approach to the total care of a patient; we are speaking of healing for the individual as a whole, including the body, mind, and soul. This is particularly relevant when one becomes critically sick and suffers; in addition to physical pain, what some call "pain of the soul"—the pain that involves the fear, sadness, loneliness, and dejection people feel when facing mortality. If anything defines human beings, it is the ability to transcend and analyze their own lives and goals. Hope and faith are linked with people's earliest instincts of relying on the world around them, in their beliefs and in their own self-efficacy [1].

Although every culture expresses this pain of the soul in different ways, bereavement is a universal natural phenomenon for which patients and family members must adapt and prepare. In recent decades, our society has seen some drastic changes as many patients have become reluctant to die at home because they perceive it to be a burden on the family. In the same manner, according to researchers, the external manifestations of the pain of the soul in the face of the death of a loved one have been modified. These changes present an added difficulty to overcome during this period of farewell or end of life. The current accelerated pace of life has resulted in shortened funeral rituals and religious ceremonies. This has been even more the case during the COVID-19 pandemic when some ceremonies have been completely omitted or prohibited. This unnatural process of grieving has led to exacerbated mental health problems [2].

Expressing one's spirituality and emotions, though proven to be therapeutic for all involved, has long been suppressed in health systems. At times, this suppression has been related to sociodemographic factors, but it has also been influenced by cultural patterns. For instance, emotional labor has traditionally been undervalued and was historically viewed as "women's work." It was perceived to be a natural tendency for women, contrary to men, to show compassion, care, and understanding for the suffering of others [3].

In addition, in regions with racial and social minority populations such as migrants or refugees, where power relations in gender and income are unequal, occultism of cancer, social rejection, and familial isolation are more likely to develop when disease appears [4]. For example, with regard to breast cancer, the meaning of the cancer itself is strongly influenced by women's spiritual, religious, and fatalistic beliefs [5]; the stigma it brings can be related to body image changes, hair loss, or disfigurement. In lower-income populations, fear of the unknown prevails: they cling to God as savior, use rituals to achieve a peaceful state of being and turn to natural and traditional healing remedies.

The attention of health care professionals to the spiritual sphere can be ascribed to the assessment of the emotional sphere, which is difficult to assess and address from a scientific or biomedical paradigm. In general, keeping in mind that healing is a holistic process, health care professionals should not dismiss either the achievements of medicine nor the soul. In this framework, patients and health care workers are equally vulnerable to the negative impacts of emotional overexposure [6] and to the lack of spiritual support.

Medical staff usually have a more distant approach and nurses a closer one. Although nurses are the health care professionals that manage patient emotions and their spiritual concerns every day, in our cultural environment, nurses are often required to mask their personal feelings in order to evoke a certain emotional response in others. Regarding emotional intelligence, Goleman [7,8] classified emotions as being basic or primary, but other authors, such as Bizquerra [9], classified them as being positive, negative, or ambiguous.

Challenges in the Context of Palliative Care

The goal of palliative care is to relieve the suffering of patients and their families, first by performing a comprehensive assessment and followed with a mutual decision process pertaining to treating the physical, psychosocial, and spiritual symptoms [10]. As is true of many severe conditions, it is crucial that cancer and palliative care address not only the physical burden stemming from the treatments or the disease, but also the emotional and spiritual components of all those effected. The palliative care unit is perceived to be an emotionally intense workplace, requiring additional support to patients. Some of the negative emotions that professionals endure, deriving from interactions during the provision of care, have been widely presented in the literature. However, health care workers on nonpalliative units also experience grief and need support. In developed countries, even in palliative care units, grief still tends to be viewed as an emotion that must be contained and suppressed in some way.

A 2017 study by Funk et al. [11] explained that professionalism is a powerful organizational norm in the health system and may provide the staff and other members of the team with a means to rationalize maintaining an emotional distance from patients and families while caring in order to protect themselves from emotional distress. However, there is little evidence to suggest that this is the best strategy. Participants' narratives revealed complex, ambivalent, and even conflicting interpretations regarding the appropriateness and meaning of feeling and displaying grief and sadness at work [11]. Working with dying patients and their families was characterized as emotionally difficult, and so the belief was that health care employees needed the time and space, either at work or at home, to manage their emotions [12].

Contrary to most of the studies performed in the United States, Europe published less research on spiritual care within palliative care. Gijsberts et al. [13] reviewed 53 articles that reported the benefits of easing discomfort—presence, empowerment, and bringing peace—and described the competencies required in order to provide spiritual care to patients. In their systematic review, the Spanish authors Pinedo Velazquez and Jimenez [14] presented nurses' perceptions regarding the emotional attention given to patients and observed that emotions such as anxiety, fear, depression, anger, and dissatisfaction present a high emotional and spiritual burden for nurses, although they are not part of patients' care plan.

A qualitative study from Denmark revealed that hospice nurses experienced emotional challenges due to their exposure to suffering and death, as well as an increased awareness of their own mortality [15]. Oncology unit nurses in particular have expressed their desire to leave the unit [16]. The participants in the study described their emotional challenges as being simultaneously draining and enriching experiences, leading to personal and professional growth and development. In this study, different situations involving various exposures and emotions brought about dynamic fluctuations between identifying with and separating themselves from the suffering of patients and their relatives. Through preconceptions, expectations, and the demand for what being professional implies, the nurses' perception of their own professionalism was challenged. Adopting a positive attitude and perceiving suffering, pain, and death as part of a natural human process are some of the coping mechanisms they used to deal with their emotions [16]. The nurses were also emotionally challenged by the dichotomy of being enriched in their own lives as a consequence of facing the dying [15].

It should be emphasized that healing suffering does not involve forgetting; overcoming grief fundamentally shows that, while this state of suffering is natural following a loss, it eventually ceases to dominate our lives. Several interesting initiatives for dealing with spiritual and emotional suffering and grief have been introduced, such as complementary mind and body treatments, targeting those aspects that conventional health systems do not attend to.

From the psychotherapy standpoint, the most effective methods for coping are grief support and bereavement groups, even online [17]. Assisting a bereaved person means admitting one's own vulnerability and exposing oneself to the awakening of one's own anxiety and unresolved feelings of grief and loss. In Spain, over the last 15 years and even earlier, professionals have developed groups to help others; together, patients, family members, and professionals participate in dealing with spiritual needs and managing their grief [18]. Payás, in her work "How to Be Prepared for Grief" [19], emphasizes that health care professionals need to enhance their basic abilities and skills, such as empathy, listening, validation, understanding, accompaniment, and respect. Although health care professionals [20] now have better training in grief counseling, if they have not regularly practiced these skills during their education, they may cause additional pain to people already experiencing grief due to their loss.

Another interesting approach is art therapy, which can help adults and especially children to express their emotional pain. Since time immemorial, people have often found art and the creative process as ways to cushion the pain of loss, helping to express or overcome grief. In many palliative, oncological, and geriatric units, art has been introduced to reconsolidate memory in patients with dementia or to combat and neutralize trauma [21]. Rieger et al.'s review [22] studied the use of art as a pedagogic tool for student or new nurses. This was seen as an effective method for teaching professional behavior required for the emotional work, reflective practice, and self-transcendence that can aid in attending to spiritual needs. Other ways to connect with patients' deep emotions and spiritual distress are music therapy, writing, praying in groups or individually, practicing spiritually focused meditation [23], or mindfulness, which can bring about positivity, spiritual well-being, and recognition of God's healing power, which many patients describe as a global spiritual growth.

Religion and Spirituality Support in Spanish and Turkish Societies

When asked, nurses working in palliative care units in Spain often reported that patients provide invaluable "lessons for living." This helps nurses value their own lives and work, although sparse resources, insufficient staff, and lack of adequate training and informational support are common in many palliative units. Nurses often explain that it is a privilege to be able to share these final experiences with palliative patients. In some ways, they state, it recharges their energy to continue with their caring. This reaction is clearly related to the spiritual meaning nurses find in their profession and their sense of coherence with their daily activities.

In a macro context, governments and health care systems worldwide have revised their laws to ensure the provision of spiritual dimensions. Accordingly, the National Consensus Project's Clinical Practice Guidelines for Quality Palliative Care [24] in the United States regulates the practice and training of professional chaplains. The Scientific Multidisciplinary Society (MASCC), identifying spirituality as an essential part of supportive care, asked its members how they provide spiritual care. The majority recognized that they do not directly deliver spiritual care, and only half of them offered spiritual care as part of addressing the psychosocial need to help alleviate existential suffering [25]. The Palliative Care Strategy of National Health System of the Spanish Ministry of Health, Social Services, and Equality, which was set up in 2011, recognized that spiritual care is within the lines of action, and has become mandatory for all health professionals as a quality standard [26].

Similarly to many other studies around the world, dimensions of spirituality and hope are predictors of quality-of-life satisfaction in elderly patients [27]. A questionnaire was developed to evaluate spirituality at the end of life. The Spiritual Group of the Spanish Palliative Care Society (SECPAL) ran a study to explore spirituality in 121 patients within three levels: intrapersonal, interpersonal, and transpersonal, and the study found a positive correlation between spirituality and resilience and a negative correlation between lack of spirituality and anxiety and depression [28]. Thus, health care professionals' attention to patients' religious or spiritual beliefs is vital to support individuals' efforts to accept their circumstances at the end of life [29].

In the study, 202 palliative care workers were asked about heath care professionals' perceptions and what proportion of their patients expressed some spiritual needs. Only half of the 202 professionals responded, and they reported that on very few occasions, only a minority of their patients' spirituality was taken into account. Regarding participants' religious beliefs, one-third believed in life after death, and regarding perceived competencies, one-half of the participants showed a poor ability to respond to patients' spiritual concerns [30]. Apparently, professionals tend to separate the cancer patient's physical needs from their spiritual needs, confirming that spirituality is addressed on only a very intimate level and that holistic care is seldom achieved.

Many studies agree about the important role of nursing in spiritual interchanges at the end of life. However, religious and spiritual needs are not initially addressed in the assessment interview with advanced or palliative patients. Often, if a patient does not express or initiate the conversation, neither do the nurses. Likewise, family members as well do not initiate such conversations, and, as in many countries in southern Europe such as Portugal, Italy, Croatia, and Cyprus, families in Spain are afraid to start those conversations because of the "fear of death." Catholicism, the majority religion in the nation, marks an imprint on their lives, urging them to leave these things in "God's hands." Patients and family members put up a defensive wall, and no one talks about their unique and common worry—death [31]. In one study conducted in Spain [27], only one-third of patients expressed spiritual concerns.

Understanding culture and religion is important because of the unique characteristics ethnocultural groups bring to approaches of palliative care [10]. Different ethnicities and cultures possess their own particular meaning for illness, suffering, and dying, and this defines the theoretical underpinnings on which patients and health care draw in their relations. Culture and religion also affect communication, decision making, response to symptoms, treatment choices, and emotional expression at the end of life [32].

The meaning attributed to death, as well as cultural and religious practices at the time of death, are different for all individuals. While death is easily discussed by health care professionals in some cultures, inasmuch as it is an inevitable fact in their work, in other cultures not talking about death is predominant. For example, in Muslim and other traditional societies, as in Turkey, discussing death is regarded as taboo [33]. Studies on Turkish nurses' attitudes toward death and caring for the dying showed generally positive attitudes toward death [34]. In addition, Karadag et al. [33] found that in two regions of Turkey, the attitude of nurses to death was positively affected by cultural and religious beliefs, and, hence, they did not have problem. However, it was determined that nurses experienced feelings of grief, despair, and anxiety while caring for a dying patient, did not talk to patients about death, and found the training they received to be insufficient [28,32].

Other cultural differences are apparent in the external manifestations of fear and spiritual and emotional distress [35]. Some cultures tend to hide their feelings, whereas others are very expressive [32]. A qualitative study from Sweden acknowledged that every encounter with a crying person should be unique and that individualized care should be provided. The results of this study [36] showed that physical closeness and touch are important but should be used with great sensitivity. The nurses' ability to strike a balance between closeness and physical contact is essential for effective support, and showing compassion and being responsive is critical in a situation where a patient is crying [36]. Physical closeness may undermine the relationship when the person does not want to be touched or feels uncomfortable with proximity. The nurse can be emotionally and spirituality supportive to the crying person by being present and affirmative, displaying empathy, offering an opportunity to talk, and showing respect for the individual's beliefs, values, and needs, regardless of their expressions or crying, with or without tears [36]. Knowledge of cultural differences and how to switch between closeness and distance with a palliative patient is an important part of the nurses' invisible professional role.

How Nurses Provide Spiritual and Emotional Support

An important part of nursing focuses on emotional care and spiritual support for patients and their families. Due to the lack of clarity regarding the terms used to describe emotional care and support [37], Watson [38] analyzed the concepts of spiritual and emotional support for patients requiring palliative care. A total of eight defining attributes of emotional support were reported (Table 9.1) [38].

Patients and nurses agree that the first issue in humanizing care is kindness. Nurses state that they demonstrate "kindness, love and care," understand how patients and relatives feel, and try, as much as possible, to be warm and respectful. The level of their care is displayed by giving a kind reception, a pat on the shoulder, and by clarifying any doubts patients and relatives may have. Patients valued as essential their being made to feel welcome and comfortable, and receiving spiritual support during the entire process.

Figure 9.1 presents all the components essential for emotional support during care, ranging from understanding feelings to communicating information, or simply just being there.

Table 9.1 Defining Attributes of Emotional Support

Defining Attributes	Nurses' Skills and Behaviors
1. Feelings and emotions	Providing emotional support and enable patients and families to express their feelings and emotions
2. Communication	Facilitating a discussion by using effective communication skills to enable patients to express their feelings
3. Understanding	Demonstrating concern, showing empathy, and recognizing and respecting individuals
4. Caring	Demonstrating behaviors such as comforting gestures, kindness, and compassion, and having a caring attitude
5. Providing information	Dealing with questions, providing explanations, and offering advice
6. Being there	Finding the time to spend with patients; understanding the importance patients attach to the presence of the nurse
7. Listening	Maintaining an active listening attitude
8. Support	Providing comfort and encouragement to the patient

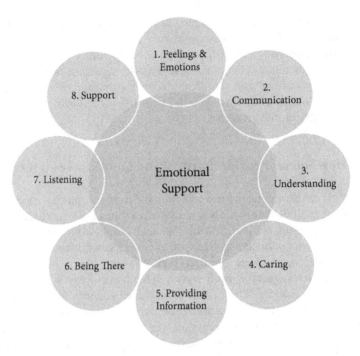

Figure 9.1 Defining attributes of the term "emotional support" in palliative care nursing, based on Watson [38]

In a qualitative meta-synthesis describing the nurse's role in providing palliative care, the essential dimensions have been defined as being available, coordinating care, being attentive and dedicated, and functioning well in demanding situations. No doubt these situations involve controlling emotions when working in an emotionally demanding environment and managing every aspect in the most effective way possible [39].

The way in which a patient understands the role of the nurse also defines how their relationship is established. Patients expect a nurse to always be available and in all situations. However, many nurses explain that it is not always easy or possible to offer the spiritual and emotional support that patients or families require [40].

The end-stage cancer patient is a vulnerable being who may suffer from the existential dilemma of "imminent death" and may need support in strengthening their faith and religious beliefs. Many patients who are in the final stages of their disease feel a compelling need to become closer to God and to resume their religious beliefs and feelings, which in their busy daily lives, they may have previously neglected. Even some patients who do not profess to be part of any formal religion, however, describe a need for a broader spirituality that prioritizes the pending issues they have in their lives. Nurses should consider each patient's and each family's circumstances as a unique entity requiring a sensitive approach.

Spiritual distress has been defined as the state of suffering related to one's impaired ability to experience meaning in life through connections with self, others, the world,

---

Box 9.1 NIC—Nursing Intervention in Spiritual Support [41]

Definition: to help the patient achieve balance through their beliefs.

Activities:

- Be open to the patient's expressions of loneliness and helplessness.
- Encourage attendance at religious services, if desired.
- Encourage the use of spiritual resources, if desired.
- Provide spiritual objects, according to the patient's preferences.
- Refer to the patient's chosen spiritual advisor.
- Use value clarification techniques to help the patient clarify their beliefs and values, when appropriate.
- Be willing to listen to the patient's/family's feelings.
- Express sympathy with the patient's/family's feelings.
- Facilitate the patient's use of meditation, prayer, and other religious traditions and rituals.
- Listen attentively to patients and develop an opportunity for prayer or spiritual rituals.
- Assure the patient that the caregiver will be available to support him or her in times of suffering.
- Be open to the patient's feelings about illness and death.
- Help the patient to express and release anger in an appropriate manner.

---

or a superior being. It can cause anxiety, insomnia, fear, and questioning of identity and the meaning of suffering. A nursing specialist, counselor, religious chaplain, or psychologist can usually help cancer patients to overcome their emotional angst and suffering as well as their spiritual distress.

The NANDA-I [40], formerly known as the North American Nursing Diagnosis Association, is the ultimate tutorial and nursing diagnosis list that has been used in clinical practices in many countries, including Spain and Turkey. It identifies diagnoses and nursing interventions and relates to spiritual needs as life principles. Nursing activities for spiritual support are presented in Box 9.1.

Developing Competencies in Supporting Patients and Their Families

When asked, many palliative patients often stress that one of the most important skills they expect from a health professional should be empathy. Empathy is a complex construct with four constituents: cognitive (identification and understanding another's feelings); emotional (experiment with and share feelings); moral/spiritual (internal encouragement to empathize); and relationship (communicative response to understanding). This ability to connect with the patient's feelings and emotions has been shown to have therapeutic benefits and has a direct impact on the patient's health outcome. Bas–Sarmiento et al. [31] performed a randomized controlled study in 2019 that simulated clinical interviews for student nurses in order to train them in empathy and self-esteem. The results showed significant statistical differences between the experimental group and the control group [31]. Empathy improves the quality of information relayed between the professional and the patient, as well as the quality of care, impact on staff, and patients' and families' satisfaction.

Nurses receive only limited training regarding these complex scenarios beyond what occurs in on-the-job training. A patient's transition from acute care to palliative, supportive, or comfort care is a critical moment requiring that nurses help patients and families cope [42]. Although emotional and spiritual education is scarcely offered in universities, hospitals, or palliative units, it has been highly demanded by nurses. One of the major conclusions from a study by Arimon et al. [43], with nurses working in cancer units, shows a high correlation between level of compassion fatigue and need for specific training on the subject of emotional labor.

Students may not be aware of palliative patients' feelings and experiences prior to their working in a clinical environment. The skills essential to be an effective professional can be learned during the training process [7]. Without doubt, in order to be successful as a nurse or a doctor, one must acquire specialized skills to perform clinical tasks; it is equally important that nurses and doctors learn how to manage their own and others' emotions, especially if the others are palliative patients or family members. This personal attribute can be modeled with an educational program targeted and attentive to the needs of each nursing student.

A recent systematic review from Singh et al. [44] demonstrated that there is a positive correlation not only between emotional intelligence (EI) and communication skills, but also between EI and the academic success of nursing, medical, or dental students. The ability to focus on "attention to feelings" and to train for how to modulate one's own emotions was shown in some studies to have an impact on general cognitive ability [44]. Medical staff usually take a more distant approach and nurses a closer one.

Recently included in the International Classification of Diseases (11th Revision) is the phenomenon of "burnout" as "a negative occupational occurrence," which has been investigated over the past 45 years. Christine Maslach, in 1981, was the first to define occupational burnout, and her scale remains one of the most widely used tools to assess professionals who are feeling emotionally drained or experiencing emotional exhaustion, depersonalization, or lack of confidence to do their job well. Burnout often occurs in a stressful working environment and relates to how people handle the pressures of work. Palliative care units, or any other unit with difficult working conditions, are usually understaffed, with insufficient resources to cope with highly emotional cases. Health care professionals are often pushed to the limit and are left feeling exhausted, dissatisfied with their job, and wanting to quit [45].

Compassion fatigue (CF) is a wide-ranging concept that results from the sum of burnout, plus the emotional burden that nursing and medical professionals assume. Dall'Ora proffered that a positive work environment decreases the risk of these outcomes [40,46]. Recognition at work, sharing expertise and experiences, and interprofessional training among physicians and nurses could optimize the work environment, even when dealing with difficult clinical cases [47]. The excessive emotional labor required to provide patients with adequate support also leads to compassion fatigue and burnout. Palliative care nurses function under high emotional stress, but if the focus of care is clear and end-of-life management focuses more on comfort than on cure, the CF scores are lower [48]. A recent systematic review among health professionals working in palliative care revealed only a 17.3% prevalence of burnout [48]. While burnout occurs among nurses, physicians, and social workers, it is even more common in the context of homecare [49]. Nurses have higher levels of emotional exhaustion and depersonalization [50]. The literature suggests work-setting interventions, including staff retreats, grief teams, support groups, get-togethers, debriefings, and rituals such as attending funerals, sending sympathy cards, and making memory books as opportunities to express grieving [6].

Based on scientific evidence, men and women were found to display emotions differently [51], and other personal characteristics such as self-esteem [35] are enhanced by appropriate training in social skills or social interactions, modulated by cultural conditions that are present in different parts of the world. Age was also a variable that correlated with the capacity for empathy. In their study, Batt-Rawden et al. [52] found that younger students have higher levels of empathy than their elders.

In 2020, during the beginning of the COVID-19 pandemic, the mental health system took note that the general population, as well as health care professionals, have had increased psychological challenges, including anxiety, depression, and stress [2]. Nurses working with geriatric patients and palliative patients in intensive care and oncology units have been especially affected. Their resilience has primarily been sustained by peer support. Internet platforms have devised new models of expert–coach–teacher collaborations integrating physicians, psychiatrists, psychologists, and social workers to carry out psychological interventions for patients and their families, in addition to health care staff.

In the same way that education provides an effective tool for nurses to learn how to manage emotions, taking care of oneself, both mentally and physically, also provides clear benefits [53]. For nurses to be able to successfully adapt in their work and in their private lives, a positive mental health attitude is essential, as routine work or "automatism" (becoming emotionally numb) can turn off positive emotions, cause frustration, and increase compassion fatigue, emotional exhaustion, and burnout. "The more I take care of myself, the better I feel" and "the better I feel, the more I take care of myself"—this is a circular action with continual positive effects. In summary, spiritual and emotional support is more necessary than ever, and attention should always be paid to patients' spiritual and emotional needs in the context of care.

References

1. Carni E. Issues of hope and faith in the cancer patient. *J Relig Heal*. 1988;27(4):285–290. doi:10.1007/BF01533196
2. Duan L, Zhu G. Psychological interventions for people affected by the COVID-19 epidemic. *The Lancet Psychiatry*. 2020;7(4):300–302. doi:10.1016/S2215-0366(20)30073-0
3. Elliott C. Emotional labour: Learning from the past, understanding the present. *Br J Nurs*. 2017;26(19):1070–1077. doi:10.12968/bjon.2017.26.19.1070
4. Williamson TJ, Ostroff JS, Martin CM, et al. Evaluating relationships between lung cancer stigma, anxiety, and depressive symptoms and the absence of empathic opportunities

presented during routine clinical consultations. *Patient Educ Couns*. 2021;104(2):322–328. doi:10.1016/j.pec.2020.08.005

5. Gullatte MM, Brawley O, Kinney A, Powe B, Mooney K. Religiosity, spirituality, and cancer fatalism beliefs on delay in breast cancer diagnosis in African American women. *J Relig Health*. 2010;49(1):62–72. doi:10.1007/s10943-008-9232-8

6. Houck D. Helping nurses cope with grief and compassion fatigue: An educational intervention. *Clin J Oncol Nurs*. 2014;18(4):454–458. doi:10.1188/14.CJON.454-458

7. Alconero-Camarero AR, Sarabia-Cobo CM, González-Gómez S, Ibáñez-Rementería I, Lavín-Alconero L, Sarabia-Cobo AB. Nursing students' emotional intelligence, coping styles and learning satisfaction in clinically simulated palliative care scenarios: An observational study. *Nurse Educ Today*. 2018;61:94–100. doi:10.1016/j.nedt.2017.11.013

8. Singh N, Kulkarni S, Gupta R, Singh N, Kulkarni S. Is emotional intelligence related to objective parameters of academic performance in medical, dental, and nursing students: A systematic review. *Educ Heal Chang Learn Pract*. 2020;33(1):8–12. doi:10.4103/efh.EfH_208_17

9. Bizquerra Alzina R. *Educacion Emocional y Bienestar*. 6th ed. Madrid: Wolkers Kluwer; 2006.

10. Cain CL, Surbone A, Elk R, Kagawa-Singer M. Culture and palliative care: Preferences, communication, meaning, and mutual decision making. *J Pain Symptom Manage*. 2018;55(5):1408–1419. doi:10.1016/j.jpainsymman.2018.01.007

11. Funk LM, Peters S, Roger KS. The emotional labor of personal grief in palliative care: Balancing caring and professional identities. *Qual Health Res*. 2017;27(14):2211–2221. doi:10.1177/1049732317729139

12. Lehto RH, Heeter C, Allbritton M, Wiseman M. Hospice and palliative care provider experiences with meditation using mobile applications. *Oncol Nurs Forum*. 2018;45(3):380–388. doi:10.1188/18.ONF.380-388

13. Gijsberts M-JHE, Liefbroer AI, Otten R, Olsman E. Spiritual care in palliative care: A systematic review of the recent European literature. *Med Sci*. 2019;7(2):25. doi:10.3390/medsci7020025

14. Pinedo Velázquez MT, Jiménez Jiménez JC. Cuidados del personal de enfermería en la dimensión espiritual del paciente. Revisión sistemática. *Cult los Cuid Rev Enfermería y Humanidades*. 2017;21(48):110–118. doi:10.14198/cuid.2017.48.13

15. Ingebretsen LP, Sagbakken M. Hospice nurses' emotional challenges in their encounters with the dying. *Int J Qual Stud Health Well-being*. 2016;11(0130):1–13. doi:10.3402/qhw.v11.31170

16. Greer JA, Applebaum AJ, Jacobsen JC, Temel JS, Jackson VA. Understanding and addressing the role of coping in palliative care for patients with advanced cancer. *J Clin Oncol*. 2020;38(9):915–925. doi:10.1200/JCO.19.00013

17. Robinson C, Pond R. Do online support groups for grief benefit the bereaved? Systematic review of the quantitative and qualitative literature. Published online 2019. doi:10.1016/j.chb.2019.06.011

18. Melguizo-Garín A, Hombrados-Mendieta I, Martos-Méndez MJ. La experiencia de un grupo de apoyo en el proceso de duelo de familiares de niños con cáncer. Un estudio cualitativo. *Psicooncología*. 2020;17(1):117–129. doi:10.5209/psic.68245

19. Payás Puigarnau A. *Las Tareas Del Duelo. Psicoterapia de Duelo Desde Un Modelo Integrativo-Relacional, Barcelona, Paidós Ibérica*, 2010, 447 Pp. ISBN: 978-84-493-2423-9-Dialnet. Accessed March 3, 2021. http://dx.doi.org/10.33776/erebea.v6i0.2977

20. Fernández-Alcántara M, Pérez-Marfil MN, Catena-Martínez A, Cruz-Quintana F. Duelo, pérdida y procesos de final de vida. *Estud Psicol*. 2017;38(3):553–560. doi:10.1080/02109395.2017.1342941

21. Nicol J, Pocock M. Memento Mori: Can art assist student nurses to explore death and dying? A qualitative study. *Nurse Educ Today*. 2020;89:104404. doi:10.1016/j.nedt.2020.104404

22. Rieger KL, Chernomas WM, McMillan DE, Morin FL, Demczuk L. Effectiveness and experience of arts-based pedagogy among undergraduate nursing students: a mixed methods systematic review. *JBI Database Syst Rev Implement Reports*. 2016;14(11):139–239. doi:10.11124/jbisrir-2016-003188

23. Agarwal K, Fortune L, Heintzman JC, Kelly LL. Spiritual experiences of long-term meditation practitioners diagnosed with breast cancer: An interpretative phenomenological analysis pilot study. *J Relig Health*. 2020;59(5):2364–2380. doi:10.1007/s10943-020-00995-9

24. Handzo GF, Atkinson M-M, Wintz SK. National Consensus Project's Clinical Practice Guidelines for Quality Palliative Care, Fourth Edition: Why Is This Important to Chaplains? *Journal of health care chaplaincy*. 2020;26(2):58–71. Published online 2019. doi:10.1080/08854726.2019.1582212

25. Ramondetta LM, Sun C, Surbone A, et al. Surprising results regarding MASCC members' beliefs about spiritual care. *Support Care Cancer*. 2013;21(11):2991–2998. doi:10.1007/s00520-013-1863-y

26. *Palliative Care Strategy of the National Health System*. Update 2010–2014. Estrategia en Cuidados Paliativos del Sistema Nacional de Salud. Actualización 2010-2014. Edited 2011 Spanish Ministry of Health and Social Policy and Equality. Accessed: 2021-03-29 https://www.mscbs.gob.es/organizacion/sns/planCalidadSNS/docs/paliativos/cuidadospaliativos.pdf

27. Galiana L, Oliver A, Benito E, Sansó N. Cuestionarios de atención espiritual en cuidados paliativos: Revisión de la evidencia para su aplicación clínica. *Psicooncologia*. 2016;13(2–3):385–397. doi:10.5209/PSIC.54443

28. Barreto P, Fombuena M, Diego R, Galiana L, Oliver A, Benito E. Bienestar emocional y espiritualidad al final de la vida. *Med Paliativa*. 2015;22(1):25–32. doi:10.1016/j.medipa.2013.02.002

29. Wittenberg E, Ragan SL, Ferrell B. Exploring Nurse Communication About Spirituality. *Am J Hosp Palliat Med*. 2017;34(6):566–571. doi:10.1177/1049909116641630

30. Payás Puigarnau A, Jesús BG, Bayés Sopena R, et al. *Como perciben los profesionales de paliat ivos las necesidades espirituales del paciente al final de la vida?*; 2008;15(4):225–237. Accessed November 29, 2020. https://www.researchgate.net/publication/287118822

31. Bas-Sarmiento P, Fernández-Gutiérrez M, Díaz-Rodríguez M, et al. Teaching empathy to nursing students: A randomised controlled trial. *Nurse Educ Today*. 2019;80:40–51. doi:10.1016/j.nedt.2019.06.002

32. Busolo D, Woodgate R. Palliative care experiences of adult cancer patients from ethnocultural groups: A qualitative systematic review protocol. *JBI Database Syst Rev Implement Reports*. 2015;13(1):99–111. doi:10.11124/jbisrir-2015-1809

33. Karadag E, Parlar Kilic S, Ugur O, Akyol MA. Attitudes of nurses in Turkey toward care of dying individual and the associated religious and cultural factors. *J Relig Health*. 2019;58(1):303–316. doi:10.1007/s10943-018-0657-4

34. Cevik B, Kav S. Attitudes and experiences of nurses toward death and caring for dying patients in Turkey. *Cancer Nurs*. 2013;36(6):E58–E65. doi:10.1097/NCC.0b013e318276924c

35. Cetinkaya-Uslusoy E, Paslı-Gürdogan E, Aydınlı A. Professional values of Turkish nurses: A descriptive study. *Nurs Ethics*. 2017;24(4):493–501. doi:10.1177/0969733015611072

36. Rydé K, Hjelm K. How to support patients who are crying in palliative home care: An interview study from the nurses' perspective. *Prim Heal Care Res Dev*. 2016;17(5):479–488. doi:10.1017/S1463423616000037

37. Skilbeck J, Payne S. Emotional support and the role of clinical nurse specialists in palliative care. *J Adv Nurs*. 2003;43(5):521–530. doi:10.1046/j.1365-2648.2003.02749.x

38. Watson FCT. *Emotional Support in Palliative Care Nursing: A Concept Analysis.*; 2010. Robert Gordon University, MRes thesis. http://hdl.handle.net/10059/559

39. Sekse RJT, Hunskår I, Ellingsen S. The nurse's role in palliative care: A qualitative meta-synthesis. *J Clin Nurs.* 2018;27(1–2):e21–e38. doi:10.1111/jocn.13912

40. Dall'Ora C, Griffiths P, Ball J, Simon M, Aiken LH. Association of 12 h shifts and nurses' job satisfaction, burnout and intention to leave: Findings from a cross-sectional study of 12 European countries. *BMJ Open.* 2015;5(9):e0088331. doi:10.1136/bmjopen-2015-008331

41. Butcher, H. K., Bulechek, G. M., Dochterman, J. M. M., & Wagner, C. M. (2018). *Nursing interventions classification (NIC)-E-Book.* Spiritual Support. Pages 323. Elsevier Health Sciences.

42. Canzona MR, Love D, Barrett R, et al. "Operating in the dark": Nurses' attempts to help patients and families manage the transition from oncology to comfort care. *J Clin Nurs.* 2018;27(21–22):4158–4167. doi:10.1111/jocn.14603

43. Arimon-Pagès E, Torres-Puig-Gros J, Fernández-Ortega P, Canela-Soler J. Emotional impact and compassion fatigue in oncology nurses: Results of a multicentre study. *Eur J Oncol Nurs.* 2019;43:101666. doi:10.1016/j.ejon.2019.09.007

44. Singh N, Kulkarni S, Gupta R. Is emotional intelligence related to objective parameters of academic performance in medical, dental, and nursing students: A systematic review. *Educ Heal Chang Learn Pract.* 2020;33(1):8–12. doi:10.4103/efh.EfH_208_17

45. Dobrina R, Chialchia S, Palese A. "Difficult patients" in the advanced stages of cancer as experienced by nursing staff: A descriptive qualitative study. *Eur J Oncol Nurs.* 2020;46(October 2019):101766. doi:10.1016/j.ejon.2020.101766

46. Cleary M, Visentin D, West S, Lopez V, Kornhaber R. Promoting emotional intelligence and resilience in undergraduate nursing students: An integrative review. *Nurse Educ Today.* 2018;68:112–120. doi:10.1016/j.nedt.2018.05.018

47. Engberink AO, Mailly M, Marco V, et al. A phenomenological study of nurses experience about their palliative approach and their use of mobile palliative care teams in medical and surgical care units in France. *BMC Palliat Care.* 2020;19(1):1–10. doi:10.1186/s12904-020-0536-0

48. Cross LA. Compassion fatigue in palliative care nursing: A concept analysis. *J Hosp Palliat Nurs.* 2019;21(1):21–28. doi:10.1097/NJH.0000000000000477

49. Dall'Ora C, Ball J, Reinius M, Griffiths P, Griffiths P. Burnout in nursing: A theoretical review. *Hum Resour Health.* 2020;18(1):1–17. doi:10.1186/s12960-020-00469-9

50. Parola V, Coelho A, Cardoso D, Sandgren A, Apóstolo J. Prevalence of burnout in health professionals working in palliative care. *JBI Database Syst Rev Implement Rpts.* 2017;15(7):1905–1933. doi:10.11124/JBISRIR-2016-003309

51. Rahat E, İlhan T. Coping styles, social support, relational self- construal, and resilience in predicting students' adjustment to university life. *Kuram ve Uygulamada Egit Bilim.* 2016;16(1):187–208. doi:10.12738/estp.2016.1.0058

52. Batt-Rawden SA, Chisolm MS, Anton B, Flickinger TE. Teaching empathy to medical students: An updated, systematic review. *Acad Med.* 2013;88(8):1171–1177. doi:10.1097/ACM.0b013e318299f3e3

53. Fragkos KC, Crampton PES. The effectiveness of teaching clinical empathy to medical students: A systematic review and meta-analysis of randomized controlled trials. *Acad Med.* 2020;95(6):947–957. doi:10.1097/ACM.0000000000003058

10

The Landscape of Loneliness

An Introspective Experience of Support and Depression in Older People Diagnosed with Cancer, Israel

Lea Baider and Gil Goldzweig

Beginning

"The eternal quest of the individual human being is to shatter his loneliness" [1]

"Then the LORD God said, "It is not good for the man to be alone; I will make him a helper suitable for him."

—Genesis 2:18, King James Version)

Introduction

Hades, the god of the Underworld, tired of his loneliness, glanced up at the world above and saw Persephone.

The tale of Hades and Persephone is more than an ancient myth of love and abduction. It is a representation of the subjective experience of being and feeling alone. The lonely Hades falls in love with Persephone and decides to kidnap her. According to the myth, he leaves the Underworld—one of the rare times he does so—comes aboveground into a field where she is gathering flowers, and captures her.

Hades had seized the earth as his domain, and Zeus, Persephone's father, had taken the heavens. Because all things are born beneath the sky and all things return to the earth, the kingdoms of both grew in concert and unity, and the power of neither ever diminished.

Ancient Greece marked the disappearance and subsequent return of Persephone with several major festivals. One was known as the Eleusinian Mysteries, the most famous of the civilization's religious rites, whose secrets were so closely guarded that little is known about them today. Experts believe that the Eleusinian rites fostered the idea of a more perfect life following death, helping lay the foundations for the coming of Christianity and its belief in everlasting life in total communion with the universe [2].

An Epidemic of Loneliness

Philosophers have long made a careful and crucial distinction between solitude and loneliness. In *The Republic* (c. 380 BCE), Plato proffered a parable in which Socrates celebrates the solitary philosopher. In his allegory of the cave, the philosopher escapes from the darkness of an underground den and the company of human beings into the sunlight of contemplative thought. Alone but not lonely, the philosopher attunes to his inner self and to the world. The soundless dialogue that the soul holds with itself becomes audible [3].

Individuals, however, may grow lonely in their solitude. They are surely at grave risk of becoming isolated. Hannah Arendt [4], echoing Plato, observes that thinking is a solitary but not a lonely experience. Solitude is a human condition in which individuals keep themselves company. Loneliness differs. It is when company is desired but cannot be found.

For Arendt [4], solitude also entails the capacity to think and to judge in privacy. It empowers individuals to contemplate their actions, develop their consciences, and, away from the cacophony of the crowd, finally to hear, to listen to, to think, and to analyze self.

In the same year that Arendt's book [4] was published, D. W. Winnicott published his paper on the "capacity to be alone" [5]. Winnicott described the capacity to be alone as a sign of mature emotional development. Nevertheless, he distinguishes this capacity from actually being alone, feelings of loneliness, and withdrawal. The capacity to be alone is based on the undemanding presence of a mother, who allows her infants to experience fully their own personal lives [5].

In 2018, in an article in the magazine *1843*, Maggie Fergusson, the literary editor of *Tablet*, referred to loneliness as "the leprosy of the 21st century" [6]. U.S. Surgeon General Vivek Murthy refers to loneliness as a pathology more common than heart disease or diabetes that kills more people than obesity [7]. Dr. Murthy treats loneliness as a public health crisis. In his recent *Together: The Healing Power of Human Connection in a Sometimes Lonely World*" [8], he brings evidence that loneliness was found to be associated with greater risk of coronary heart disease, high blood pressure, stroke, dementia, depression, and anxiety. Dr. Murthy argues for a link between social and emotional health that has implications for physical health. He emphasizes that, in the modern era, there are more elderly people than ever before and that the fact that they are living longer is a double-edged sword. Many of these elderly people have outlived friends, relatives, and even children. This problem is more acute in developing countries where elderly people rapidly lose their traditional place of respect and honor, and feel abandoned and betrayed. Based on these insights, Murthy makes a powerful, compassionate, and convincing argument for building a more connected world [8].

There are certainly people who can live alone without being lonely, and there are people who are lonely without living alone—but the two states are closely linked, which makes lockdowns and sheltering in place harder to bear. In her *Biography of Loneliness* [9], cultural historian F. B. Alberti claims that loneliness is a modern epidemic created by social and demographic shifts toward individualized secular society. She points toward the relation between living alone and loneliness. Whether living alone makes people lonely, or whether people are living alone because they are lonely is hard to say, but Alberti's analysis supports the former. It is the force of history, not the exertion of choice, that leads people to live alone. This is a clash in the battle against the epidemic of loneliness because the force of history is relentless.

Alberti [9] defines loneliness not as the state of being alone, but rather as a subjective experience, a conscious, cognitive feeling of estrangement or social separation from meaningful other—an emotional lack that concerns a person's place in the world. Before the 19th century, it was not possible to survive without living among others, bonded to them by ties of affection, loyalty, and obligation. People were dependent on others in such a way that loneliness was, at most, a passing experience. A state of continuous or chronic loneliness was akin to dying. These ideas were supported by the pioneering work of J. Cacioppo in the field of neuroscience. Cacioppo and his team [10,11] described being alone and loneliness as different but related. Social isolation is the objective physical separation from other people (living alone), while loneliness is the subjective distressed feeling of being alone or separate. It is possible to feel lonely in the company of others and to be alone without feeling lonely. Loneliness is a state of hypervigilance stemming from our evolutionary past where being alone or with strangers evoked a fight-or-flight response [12]. Further, loneliness is a highly subjective experience to which meaning and interpretation are attached by individuals driven by their own expectations, values, and beliefs. These are both personal and shaped by the cultural values they have developed, interjected, assimilated, and integrated into their own experience. Any theoretical model that approximates loneliness more fully must weigh the contributing role of individual subjective meaning-making as well as social value systems and context. While this is true for all sociodemographic groups, it is especially true for the elderly and the chronically ill [11].

When loneliness takes hold in old age, how the elderly perceive themselves and how they respond to growing old are heavily influenced by how they confront the reality of aging. It is a reality that inevitably impairs their individualism, the subjective value placed on their independence, and their ability to accept social-family support during the bleak trajectory of illness and death. Chronic feelings of isolation can drive a cascade of psychological events that may accelerate the aging process [13]. Cacioppo and colleagues [11,14] drive home the severity of loneliness by describing it as a condition that makes individuals irritable, depressed, and self-centered. They found it to be associated with a 26% increase in risk of premature mortality, affecting one in every three people in industrialized countries—one in twelve of them severely—and they noted that these proportions are steadily increasing. Loneliness is often stigmatized, trivialized, or ignored, but with the rapidly growing number of older adults in developed countries, and increased depression and premature mortality, loneliness has emerged as a major public health problem.

Research Outcomes: Cancer, Old Age, and Loneliness

Research repeatedly reports the widespread and significant impact of loneliness on the health of older people. A vast body of evidence demonstrates the negative effects of loneliness on the physical and psychological health of older people, including higher risk of mortality [15]. The close association between loneliness and aging may be a consequence of multiple losses: loss of abilities, loss of and changes in personal relationships, loss of familiar environments, and altered contact with friends and relatives. All this combines into a paucity of kinship connections [16].

Loss of "full self-identity" through unwelcome retirement not only affects the socioeconomic independence of older people, it also forces them to relinquish their dignity and the established social roles that meaningfully connect them to society. If unaddressed, this alienation from society can transmute into ostracism. Stillman and colleagues [17] argue that this is reflected in chronic loneliness and manifests as depleted meaning in life.

In 1985, when researchers asked a cross section of North Americans how many confidants each had, the most common answer was three. In 2004, when researchers repeated the question, 25% of respondents indicated that they had no confidant. That is, one quarter of these 21st-century North Americans answered that they had no one at all with whom to talk openly and intimately [18].

A recent national survey by the American Association of Retired Persons (AARP) examined loneliness among adults aged 45 and older. Loneliness was defined as the subjective experience of lack of connections, companionship, or sense of belonging. Social isolation, on the other hand, was defined as an objective measure of the size of the social network, availability of transportation, and ability to utilize support resources [19]. The survey revealed that 35% of adults aged 45 and older in the United States are lonely (based on validation of self-report measures), and older adults with lower income were at the greatest risk of loneliness. The top predictors of loneliness were the size of the social network and physical isolation. Both the public and healthcare providers unaware of the magnitude of the problem and of the connections between loneliness and adverse physical and mental health. Only a few people have discussed their feeling of loneliness with their healthcare providers [19]. The survey indicated that social media and the internet have benefits only for individuals who did not feel lonely, but only amplified the difficulties of older adults who experienced themselves as lonely.

Almost 30% said they socialized with friends, family, or neighbors once a week at most, and often less frequently. Of those who claimed to feel socially isolated, 28% reported fair or poor physical health, compared with 13% of those who did not feel isolated. In addition, 17% of people who saw themselves as socially isolated rated their mental health as fair or poor, compared with only 2% of those who rarely felt isolated [19].

Our own research interest in loneliness among older adults diagnosed with cancer started more than a decade ago as a result of research focused on perceived social support, coping, and distress. Participants included more than 300 older adults (above age 60) at least two years after active treatment [20]. We found that participants who did not live with a partner at the time of our study reported significantly higher levels of distress than older people diagnosed with cancer who did live with a partner. This effect was much stronger among men than women and was independent of levels of perceived social support reported by the participants.

Research demonstrates a link between age, loneliness, perceived social support, and depression, each of which has a complex relationship with the others. It is a common finding in psycho-oncology literature that older patients adjust to and cope more competently with their illness than younger patients [21,22]. Recent studies, however, indicate that this linear relation (older age related to lower levels of depression) holds true only until a certain age [23,24]. For those aged 65 and older, this relationship is reversed, and older age is related to higher levels of depression, even after controlling for all medical variables. Higher levels of depression among people diagnosed with cancer have been found to correlate with higher levels of subjective feelings of loneliness and lower levels of perceived social support.

What is the underlying mechanism of the relationship between depression and age, perceived social support and loneliness? Is the sense of loneliness a subjective state of mind that is part of the process of aging, and is it expressed through a reduction of perceived social support and higher levels of depression? Or, alternatively, is depression in old age the result of a sense of loneliness and reduced perceived social support?

Our findings indicate that the role of social support as a protective factor against depression declines with age. In a study involving 45 patients aged 86 years and older, living at home and being treated for active disease, it was found that the predictors of depression were hope and age rather than social support. The patients reported high perceived levels of support from their spouses and families (a mean of more than 4.3 on a Likert-type scale of 1–5), together with "high hope" as an internal self-reliance resource. The fact that older age and lower hope were related to higher levels of depression among older patients may express a process of their turning inward toward internal resources [23]. In another study [25] of 58 elderly patients (aged 86 years and older), our research again found no negative link between social support and distress or depression. Nor was any interdependence found between depression or distress in patients or their caregivers, while controlling for perceived social support. Interestingly, there was some corroboration of the hypothesis that perceived social support is related to depression, but only through hope as a mediator [25]. It could be that elderly patients direct their attention inward and rely on social support to enhance hope (strengthen their inner resources) and, through hope, reduce their distress levels. This thesis is supported by other research [26], which indicates that age may be related to depression, independent of social support. Our team compared levels of depression and distress (measured, respectively, by the Five Items Geriatric Depression Scale, and the Distress Thermometer) among three groups of older patients receiving treatment for active disease. Participants were grouped by age: younger-old, 65–74 years ($n = 125$); old, 75–84 years ($n = 49$); and elderly, ≥ 85 years ($n = 69$). After controlling for all medical variables and social support, participants in the elderly group reported significantly higher levels of distress and depression compared with those in the other two groups [26]. Depression levels in the elderly group were found to be as much as four times higher than those in the younger-old group. Eighty-six years of age was identified as the optimal cutoff for predicting clinical levels of both depression and distress. Also of interest, perceived social support was lower among the elderly group compared with that reported by the young-old group. Even after controlling for this, however, age was found to be significant in predicting depression [26]. Based on these results, it can be hypothesized that cultural aspects and self-perception of being old, along with declining mental and physical health extenuated by the cancer diagnosis, play a crucial role in the relationship between age and depression.

In a study of more than 600 patients (mean age 63.1 years), we found significant but only moderately negative relationships between perceived social support and loneliness (Pearson's R-values of −0.13 to −0.35) [27], indicating that a subjective sense of loneliness (but not perceived social support) may be directly related to depression.

In contrast to these findings in patients, it seems that perceived social support has an important role for caregivers of older people diagnosed with cancer. In a study of 242 spousal caregivers to patients aged 65 and above diagnosed with cancer, perceived social support, especially from the spouse (that is, support the caregiver perceives to be getting from the patient), plays an important role in protecting the caregiver from depression [28]. The impact of social support in reducing depression among caregivers may be more prominent in women than in men [22].

In summary, one of the main conclusions of our research is that age correlates with depression among older patients, whereas perceived social support does not. These results should, however, be considered as no more than preliminary steps toward understanding the complex relationship between depression, loneliness, and social support.

Ahead

Further studies of the daily lives and networks of social support in older adults who are lonely and feel alone are required to understand the processes underway. Sensitive interventions must then be designed to improve their wellbeing, health situation, social integration, and community involvement [29].

At the pivot of loneliness in older people is the innate desire to embed and connect. Humankind has evolved as a bonding community, to forge lasting attachments with others, to support one another through crisis, illness, and aging, and to share and integrate into daily living. Simply put, people are integral parts of humanity, and they fare better together than sundered, in every sense.

I miss me . . .
The old me . . .
The smiling me . . .
The friendly me . . .
The social me . . .
Now, the loneliness has eroded my soul.
Support is forever gone.
And me? . . . Where is the "me" within myself? . . .
Total silence . . .
Total loneliness . . .
—85-year-old woman with cancer

References

1. Cousins N. *The Celebration of Life: A Dialogue on Immortality and Infinity*. New York: HarperCollins; 1974.
2. Hard R. *The Routledge Handbook of Greek Mythology*. London: Routledge; 2019.

3. Sachs D. A fallacy in Plato's Republic. *Philos Rev.* 1963;72(2):141–158.

4. Arendt H. Part II: The public and the private realm, Chapter 9: The social and the privet. In: *The Human Condition.* Chicago: University of Chicago Press; 1958, pp. 68–73.

5. Winnicott D, W. The capacity to be alone. *Int J Psycho-Anal.* 1958;39:416–420.

6. Fergosson M. How Does It Really Feel to Be Lonely? *1843 Stories of Extraordinary World*.2018;Society. https://www.economist.com/1843/2018/01/22/how-does-it-really-feel-to-be-lonely. Accessed December 7, 2021

7. Murthy V. Work and the loneliness epidemic. *Harv Bus Rev.* 2017;9:3–7.

8. Murthy VH. *Together: The Healing Power of Human Connection in a Sometimes Lonely World.* First edition. New York: Harper Wave, an imprint of HarperCollins; 2020.

9. Alberti FB. *A Biography of Loneliness: The History of an Emotion.* New York: Oxford University Press; 2019.

10. Cacioppo JT, Cacioppo S, Boomsma DI. Evolutionary mechanisms for loneliness. *Cogn Emot.* 2014;28(1):3–21.

11. Cacioppo JT, Patrick W. *Loneliness: Human Nature and the Need for Social Connection.* New York: W. W. Norton; 2008.

12. Hawkley LC, Cacioppo JT. Aging and loneliness: Downhill quickly? *Curr Dir Psychol Sci.* 2007;16(4):187–191.

13. Holt-Lunstad J, Smith TB, Baker M, Harris T, Stephenson D. Loneliness and social isolation as risk factors for mortality: A meta-analytic review. *Perspect Psychol Sci.* 2015;10(2):227–237.

14. Cacioppo JT, Cacioppo S. The growing problem of loneliness. *Lancet.* 2018;391(10119):426.

15. Wong A, Chau AK, Fang Y, Woo J. Illuminating the psychological experience of elderly loneliness from a societal perspective: A qualitative study of alienation between older people and society. *Int J Environ Res Public Health.* 2017;14(7):824.

16. Roos V, Malan L. The role of context and the interpersonal experience of loneliness among older people in a residential care facility. *Glob Health Action.* 2012;5(1):18861.

17. Stillman TF, Baumeister RF, Lambert NM, Crescioni AW, DeWall CN, Fincham FD. Alone and without purpose: Life loses meaning following social exclusion. *J Exper Soc Psychol.* 2009;45(4):686–694.

18. McPherson M, Smith-Lovin L, Brashears ME. Social isolation in America: Changes in core discussion networks over two decades. *Am Sociol Rev.* 2006;71(3):353–375.

19. Anderson GO, Thayer C. *Loneliness and Social Connections: A National Survey of Adults 45 and Older.* Washington, DC: AARP Foundation; 2018. https://www.aarp.org/content/dam/aarp/research/surveys_statistics/life-leisure/2018/loneliness-social-connections-2018.doi.10.26419-2Fres.00246.001.pdf Accessed December 7, 2021 doi.org/10.26419/res.00246.001

20. Goldzweig G, Andritsch E, Hubert A, et al. How relevant is marital status and gender variables in coping with colorectal cancer? A sample of middle-aged and older cancer survivors. *Psychooncology.* 2009;18(8):866–874.

21. Goldzweig G, Andritsch E, Hubert A, et al. Psychological distress among male patients and male spouses: What do oncologists need to know? *Ann Oncol.* 2010;21(4):877–883.

22. Goldzweig G, Merims S, Ganon R, Peretz T, Baider L. Coping and distress among spouse caregivers to older patients with cancer: An intricate path. *J Geriatr Oncol.* 2012;3(4):376–385.

23. Goldzweig G, Baider L, Andritsch E, Pfeffer R, Rottenberg Y. A dialogue of depression and hope: Elderly patients diagnosed with cancer and their spousal caregivers. *J Cancer Educ.* 2017;32(3):549–555.

24. Goldzweig G, Merims S, Ganon R, Peretz T, Altman A, Baider L. Informal caregiving to older cancer patients: Preliminary research outcomes and implications. *Ann Oncol.* 2013;24(10):2635–2640.

25. Goldzweig G, Baider L, Andritsch E, Rottenberg Y. Hope and social support in elderly patients with cancer and their partners: An actor-partner interdependence model. *Future Oncol.* 2016:12(24):2801–2809.

26. Goldzweig G, Baider L, Rottenberg Y, Andritsch E, Jacobs JM. Is age a risk factor for depression among the oldest old with cancer? *J Geriatr Oncol.* 2018;9(5):476–481.

27. Goldzweig G, Hasson-Ohayon I, Meirovitz A, Braun M, Hubert A, Baider L. Agents of support: psychometric properties of the Cancer Perceived Agents of Social Support (CPASS) questionnaire. *Psychooncology.* 2010;19(11):1179–1186.

28. Goldzweig G, Schapira L, Baider L, Jacobs JM, Andritsch E, Rottenberg Y. Who will care for the caregiver? Distress and depression among spousal caregivers of older patients undergoing treatment for cancer. *Support Care Cancer.* 2019;27(11):4221–4227.

29. Portacolone E, Perissinotto C, Yeh JC, Greysen SR. "I feel trapped": The tension between personal and structural factors of social isolation and the desire for social integration among older residents of a high-crime neighborhood. *Gerontologist.* 2018;58(1):79–88.

11

The Psychosocial Burden of Cancer in Sexual and Gender Minority Patients, United States

Yahya Almodallal and Aminah Jatoi

Introduction

Over 200,000 patients with cancer in the United States identify as belonging to a sexual and gender minority (SGM) group [1,2]. This term refers to individuals whose sexual orientation, gender identity or expression, or reproductive development differs from that of the general population at large, although definitions are rapidly evolving. Currently, this group encompasses lesbian, gay, bisexual, transgender, queer/questioning, asexual, two-spirit, intersex as well as other individuals who do not identify with one of these terms, but whose self-identification, behavior, and/or cultural beliefs about sex, gender, or reproduction are nonbinary [3].

The number and proportion of SGM patients with cancer might increase in the future for at least two reasons. First, based on increasing societal acceptance, younger individuals are more likely to identify as belonging to an SGM group, thus shifting cancer projections to include more patients in the future [4]. Second, because of the AIDS epidemic, many older SGM patients have died, further shifting the percentage of SGM patients toward a younger age and resulting in larger overall percentages with time [5]. Nonetheless, for some patients—whether young or old—discussing their SGM status with health care providers continues to be met with reluctance [6–8], thus artifactually bringing down the above estimate. In actuality, today the true percentage of cancer patients who identify as belonging to an SGM subgroup remains unknown.

This challenge of acquiring accurate estimates detracts from the ability of health care providers to know these patients, to serve them, and to generate relevant research to help them [8]. Illustrative of this limitation, Kent and others performed a review of medical databases through 2017 for articles on cancer care delivery among SGM patients; this search yielded only 37 publications [9]. The lack of sufficient data on SGM cancer patients is more pronounced among transgender people; in surveying the published literature for transgender patients with breast cancer, Stone and others found only 18 publications, which focused on only 39 patients [10,11]. Although one cannot cite all the factors for this dearth of publications and data, explanations include an absence of demographic data that serve to identify SGM patients, as alluded to above, and perhaps, in a related manner, limited interest on the part of the health care providers to study these groups because of the inherent challenges in identifying these patients [2,12–14].

From the standpoint of understanding the psychosocial burden these cancer patients face, much remains unknown because of limited published data [15]. Indeed, it appears that SGM patients are more likely than some others to have no health insurance and no personal physician [16,17]. Yet SGM patients appear to have higher rates of cancer and fare worse after a cancer diagnosis [18–23]. These unfavorable cancer statistics are bound to be both resultant and reflective of a high psychosocial burden in these groups of patients. Of parenthetical note, however, in the absence of data, health care providers should not conclude that SGM patients represent a monolithic group or even sets of monolithic subgroups. This chapter highlights the available data, comments on the presumed psychosocial implications and ramifications of the published data, suggests ways to improve outcomes for these patients in the near future, and, perhaps most importantly, increases awareness that not all patients are the same and that acceptance is a key aspect of lessening the psychosocial burden of cancer among all patients.

Specific Cancer Risk, Incidence Rates, and Outcomes

Because of specific risk factors, SGM patients appear to be at higher risk for certain cancers [19,21]. Along similar lines, because many SGM patients have limited engagement in health care systems, they appear at higher risk for cancers that are more advanced at diagnosis likely because of suboptimal screening and limited health care visits [24–31]. Saliently, negative experiences during health care—presumably overt discrimination or perceived discrimination—account in part for this lack of engagement with health care systems and demonstrate how this psychosocial burden might directly and negatively impact cancer outcomes [32,33].

To be more specific, men who have sex with men are at a higher risk for developing anal cancer than the general population [34]. Lesbians and bisexual women are less likely to obtain pap smears and therefore are more likely to suffer the negative ramifications of poor screening rates [17,24,26,35]. Sandoval and Obstein concluded that fewer than 30% of the SGM patients are screened for colorectal cancer with colonoscopies compared to 69% of the general population. This observation suggests that colorectal cancers in these patients might be more advanced at diagnosis [36]. Higher smoking and drinking rates suggest the possibility of higher rates of lung, pancreas, and liver malignancies [37–40]. Finally, in part because of higher risks of sexually transmitted diseases, SGM persons face greater rates of Hodgkin's disease, non-Hodgkin's lymphoma, and Kaposi sarcoma [41–45].

Going beyond specific cancers, Gonzales and Zinone reported that gay men are more likely to have been diagnosed with cancer in general compared to heterosexual men [20]. Similarly, data from the California Health Interview Surveys showed higher cancer rates in gay compared to heterosexual men and poorer cancer outcomes in lesbian and bisexual women compared to heterosexual women [18]. In line with what has been observed with specific cancers, it also appears that SGM patients fare worse after a cancer diagnosis in general. For example, Cochran and Mays reported worse cancer-related mortality at nine years in women who were in a same-sex relationship [22].

Understanding the Psychosocial Burden of Cancer

Previous studies suggest that distress is high among SGM cancer patients [46–48]. For example, Hart and others reported on greater fear of cancer recurrence in gay men with prostate cancer compared to published normative data [49]. In a study that attempted to catalogue the needs of SGM cancer patients, over 50% of patients reported unmet needs related to sadness, depressed mood, and cancer-related fears [50]. One patient with a history of prostate cancer stated, "It's hard really to get a positive out of being transformed from a fit, healthy, happy life loving (man) ... [to] a changed being who is depressed, full of stress and a lot of anxiety" [51].

The fallout of such physical changes from cancer and its treatment is likely to manifest in the form of psychosocial burden. Boehmer and others surveyed over 70,000 cancer patients, of whom 2,000 were SGM patients and reported the latter group described worse quality of life [16]. Hart and others described how gay men with a history of prostate cancer described urinary, bowel, and hormonal symptoms that appeared far worse than those in heterosexual men [49]. Commenting on this treatment-induced incontinence, one SGM patient with a history of prostate cancer commented, "Going to the supermarket is a struggle" [52].

Cancer treatment can alter body image, and health care providers, at times, appear inadvertently to provide undue pressure to patients, recommending conventional interventions and failing to acknowledge individual preferences. For example, among 68 SGM breast cancer patients, as many as 25% opted against breast reconstruction after bilateral mastectomies [53]. At times, patients' individual decisions appear to go against the norm, presumably creating a higher level of stress for the patient. A 56-year-old lesbian with breast cancer underwent reconstruction, noting "I felt that if I have both ... taken out, why do I need reconstruction? She said no, the doctor, because of this, that, and whatever, you know. Trying to convince me. And finally she did" [54]. Another SGM patient explained, "I really resented assumptions about my priorities. There's a hell of a lot of emphasis in the breast cancer awareness movement and in group oncology practices about helping women look stereotypically feminine ... it irked me that I was automatically referred to a plastic surgeon.... It irked me that reconstruction was so pushed in the patient ed materials" [55]. The above quotations seem to suggest some level of stress as a result of conversations with and recommendations from health care providers and seem to suggest that forced, undesired clinical outcomes can also be a source of undue stress.

Similarly, SGM cancer patients have also described a disruption of their sexual lives, a situation perhaps made worse by health care providers' lack of acknowledgment. Brown and McElroy found that among 68 SGM cancer patients, cancer treatment had a negative impact on their sexual lives with, for example, one patient commenting, "I have no sex drive—AIs [aromatase inhibitors] have taken care of that. I have no breasts so no sense of pleasure there" [56]. Similarly, Thomas, Wootten, and Robinson described the experience of gay and bisexual men with prostate cancer, illustrating how loss of erectile function, decreased penile length, and altered sexual function negatively impacted these patients' sense of masculinity, with associated anxiety and mood disturbances [51]. In another study, one patient commented, "You've got scars on your abdomen where the robot ... did the surgery.... For me, it was all about confidence approaching other gay men for sex, that was really sort of the thing, because of all that sort of emphasis on the body and not having an erection" [57]. These changes in sexual function likely lead to a heavier psychosocial burden for these patients.

Many SGM patients have limited social and family support, having been alienated from family and having had no children, thus making a diagnosis of cancer perhaps even more isolating [6,58,59]. Older single SGM women appear to have lower levels of social support overall [60], but, in general, SGM cancer patients are more likely to face challenges in their relationships in the setting of a cancer diagnosis compared to heterosexual patients [46]. Even when a relationship with a partner is strong and durable, SGM cancer patients must sometimes justify the strength of their relationship with a partner in a manner that a heterosexual couple would not have to do. Such need for justification likely generates psychosocial tension with health care providers. For example, one patient explained, "At the time, my biggest concern was that, under the law, my partner had no standing, so we went through this process.... How would she be treated? Would her wishes be respected? Would my wishes regarding her presence be respected?" [61] Another SGM patient noted, "We experienced [the nurse] being extremely resistant to talking with or acknowledging my partner" [62]. Such circumstances result in undue stress that is presumably unique to SGM patients.

A manifestation of this psychosocial anxiety is observed in what many SGM cancer patients have clearly articulated: a need for cancer support groups [62,63]. However, SGM patients appear to need cancer support groups that enable them to be comfortably forthcoming with respect to their SGM status. Matthews and others reported that rates of participation in support groups were initially similar regardless of whether or not patients belonged to an SGM group, but, over time, SGM patients' attendance dropped off, presumably because of diminishing levels of comfort. Multiple studies have examined SGM cancer patients' perspective on general support groups, with some describing homophobia as a reason for lack of or short-lived participation [56,60,62]. One SGM patient with breast cancer noted, "I felt like a fish out of water. I was becoming unraveled, and everything was so heterocentric. Talk of gender issues, non-conformity seems to be threatening. Straight, happy talk is acceptable" [56].

A key source of stress among SGM patients appears to be whether or not to disclose SGM status. As one gay man with prostate cancer described it, "You fear, you're frightened of the judgmental attitude of the doctor. You're frightened that he might not have your best interest at heart. Better to be silent about it all, and not create waves" [57]. Health care providers typically do not ask patients about SGM status, putting the onus on the patient about whether or not to disclose [7]. Although sexual dysfunction with cancer therapy is common and distressing, fewer than one in four health care providers ask cancer patients about sexual orientation and fewer than one in ten about gender identity [64,65]. Such fear of discrimination—whether actual or perceived on the part of the patient—must be acknowledged. One transgender cancer patient described their wife's experience with end-of-life care, "My wife died horribly in pain and terror from overt homophobic physical abuse and denial of treatment for infection in a nursing home while I was incapacitated by serious complications following my double mastectomy for breast cancer, and unable to visit her to monitor her care and well-being" [66]. Durso and Meyer as well as other investigators, have reported worse psychological health in SGM patients who had not disclosed their SGM status—but it is important to acknowledge that disclosure in an unwelcoming environment may very well lead to even higher levels of distress [50]. Such findings and logical assumptions suggest that the willingness of health care providers to create an accepting environment for SGM patients might make the diagnosis of cancer, its treatment, and long-term follow -up much easier for patients.

Recommendations

The Institute of Medicine, the National Summit of Cancer in the LGBT communities, the American Cancer Institute, and the American Society of Clinical Oncology have all recognized that SGM cancer patients face disparities in health care [67–70]. These and other organizations have called for more equitable health care, summoning better educational materials for patients, better education of health care providers, cultural competency on the part of health care providers, the creation of a more welcoming health care environment for SGM patients, the mandate of policies that prohibit discrimination, the creation of a safe environment that allows for disclosure of SGM status, and the generation of further research to understand how to address the needs of SGM patients. As mentioned earlier, SGM groups and subgroups are likely not monolithic groups, and certainly such changes and resources would need to be analyzed over time for their efficacy.

In concrete terms, measures—such as "all-gender" signage over restrooms; health care staff who are trained in diversity issues, understand it, and welcome it; and the existence of diversity among health care staff themselves—can all contribute to making the stress of cancer somewhat easier for patients. Furthermore, over time and with continued receptiveness and willingness to listen to patients, cancer health care providers will learn more about how to enhance comfort and how to improve cancer outcomes for these SGM patients and for many others.

References

1. Cancer Statistics—National Cancer Institute [Internet]. [cited November 21, 2020]; [last updated September 25, 2020]. Available from: https://www.cancer.gov/about-cancer/understanding/statistics
2. Quinn GP, Alpert AB, Sutter M, Schabath MB. What oncologists should know about treating sexual and gender minority patients with cancer. *JCO Oncol Pract.* June 2020;16(6):309–316.
3. NOT-OD-19-139: Sexual and gender minority populations in NIH-supported research [Internet]. [cited November 19, 2020]. Available from: https://grants.nih.gov/grants/guide/notice-files/NOT-OD-19-139.html
4. In U.S., Estimate of LGBT Population Rises to 4.5% [Internet]. [cited November 16, 2020]. Available from: https://news.gallup.com/poll/234863/estimate-lgbt-population-rises.aspx
5. The HIV/AIDS Epidemic in the United States: *The Basics* | KFF [Internet]. [cited December 12, 2020]. Available from: https://www.kff.org/hivaids/fact-sheet/the-hivaids-epidemic-in-the-united-states-the-basics/

6. Kamen CS, Smith-Stoner M, Heckler CE, Flannery M, Margolies L. Social support, self-rated health, and lesbian, gay, bisexual, and transgender identity disclosure to cancer care providers. *Oncol Nurs Forum* [Internet]. January 1, 2015 [cited November 28, 2020];42(1):44–51. Available from: /pmc/articles/PMC4360905/?report=abstract

7. Boehmer U, Case P. Physicians don't ask, sometimes patients tell. *Cancer* [Internet]. October 15, 2004 [cited November 12, 2020];101(8):1882–1889. Available from: http://doi.wiley.com/10.1002/cncr.20563

8. Cathcart-Rake E, O'Connor JM, et al. Querying patients with cancer about sexual health and sexual and gender minority status: A qualitative study of health-care providers. *Am J Hospice Palliat Med.* 2020;37:1–6.

9. Kent EE, Wheldon CW, Smith AW, Srinivasan S, Geiger AM. *Care Delivery, Patient Experiences, and Health Outcomes among Sexual and Gender Minority Patients with Cancer and Survivors: A Scoping Review.* Vol. 125, *Cancer.* Hoboken, NJ: John Wiley; 2019:4371–4379.

10. Hartley RL, Stone JP, Temple-Oberle C, Hartley RL, Temple-Oberle C. Breast cancer in transgender patients: A systematic review. Part 2: Female to male. *Eur J Surg Oncol,* 2018;44(10):1455–1462.

11. Hartley RL, Stone JP, Temple-Oberle C. Breast cancer in transgender patients: A systematic review. Part 1: Male to female. *Eur J Surg Oncol.* 2018;44(10):1455–1462.

12. Bowen DJ, Boehmer U. The lack of cancer surveillance data on sexual minorities and strategies for change. *Cancer Causes and Control* [Internet]. May 2007 [cited November 13, 2020];18(4):343–249. Available from https://pubmed.ncbi.nlm.nih.gov/17325829

13. Taneja A, Stark S, Chokshi B, Alhusain R. A knowledge, attitudes and practices survey for medical trainees about cancer in the LGBTQ community. *J Clin Oncol.* 2020;20:38(Suppl 15):e19073–e19073.

14. Tamargo CL, Quinn GP, Sanchez JA, Schabath MB. Cancer and the LGBTQ population: Quantitative and qualitative results from an oncology providers' survey on knowledge, attitudes, and practice behaviors. *J Clin Med.* 2017;6(10):93.

15. Watters Y, Harsh J, Corbett C. Cancer care for transgender patients: *Systematic Literature Review* [Internet]. Vol. 15, *Int J Transgend. Routledge.* 2014 [cited November 22, 2020]:136–145. Available from: https://www.tandfonline.com/doi/abs/10.1080/15532739.2014.960638

16. Boehmer U, Gereige J, Winter M, Ozonoff A. Cancer survivors' access to care and quality of life: Do sexual minorities fare worse than heterosexuals? *Cancer* [Internet]. 2019 [cited November 24, 2020];125(17):3079–3085. Available from: https://onlinelibrary.wiley.com/doi/abs/10.1002/cncr.32151

17. Buchmueller T, Carpenter CS. Disparities in health insurance coverage, access, and outcomes for individuals in same-sex versus different-sex relationships, 2000–2007. *Am J Public Health* [Internet]. March 1, 2010 [cited November 12, 2020];100(3):489–495. Available from: http://ajph.aphapublications.org/doi/10.2105/AJPH.2009.160804

18. Boehmer U, Miao X, Ozonoff A. Cancer survivorship and sexual orientation. *Cancer.* 2011;117(16):3796–3804.

19. Silverberg MJ, Nash R, Becerra-Culqui TA, et al. Cohort study of cancer risk among insured transgender people. *Ann Epidemiol.* 2017;27(8):499–501.

20. Gonzales G, Zinone R. Cancer diagnoses among lesbian, gay, and bisexual adults: results from the 2013–2016 National Health Interview Survey. *Cancer Causes Control;*29(9):845–854.

21. Boehmer U, Miao X, Maxwell NI, Ozonoff A. Sexual minority population density and incidence of lung, colorectal and female breast cancer in California. *BMJ Open* [Internet].

March, 2014 [cited November 19, 2020];4(3):4461. Available from: http://bmjopen.bmj.com/

22. Cochran SD, Mays VM. Risk of breast cancer mortality among women cohabiting with same sex partners: Findings from the national health interview survey, 1997–2003. *J Women's Health* [Internet]. May 1, 2012 [cited November 12, 2020];21(5):528–533. Available from: www.liebertpub.com

23. Lehavot K, Rillamas-Sun E, et al. Mortality in postmenopausal women by sexual orientation and veteran status. *The Gerontologist* [Internet]. February 1, 2016 [cited November 12, 2020];56(S1):S150–162. Available from: https://academic.oup.com/gerontologist/article/56/Suppl_1/S150/2605481

24. Charlton BM, Corliss HL, Missmer SA, et al. Reproductive health screening disparities and sexual orientation in a cohort study of U.S. adolescent and young adult females. *J Adolesc Health*. 2011;49(5):505–510.

25. Charlton BM, Corliss HL, Missmer SA, et al. Influence of hormonal contraceptive use and health beliefs on sexual orientation disparities in Papanicolaou test use. *Am J Public Health* [Internet]. February 16, 2014 [cited November 24, 2020];104(2):319–325. Available from: http://ajph.aphapublications.org

26. Power J, McNair R, Carr S. Absent sexual scripts: Lesbian and bisexual women's knowledge, attitudes and action regarding safer sex and sexual health information. *Cult, Health Sex* [Internet]. 2009 [cited November 24, 2020];11(1):67–81. Available from: https://www.tandfonline.com/doi/abs/10.1080/13691050802541674

27. Weyers S, Villeirs G, Vanherreweghe E, Verstraelen H, Monstrey S, van den Broecke R, et al. Mammography and breast sonography in transsexual women. *Eur J Radiol*. June 1, 2010;74(3):508–513.

28. Bazzi AR, Whorms DS, King DS, Potter J. Adherence to mammography screening guidelines among transgender persons and sexual minority women. *Am J Public Health*. November 1, 2015;105(11):2356–2358.

29. Kiran T, Fcfp C, Davie S, et al. Cancer screening rates among transgender adults Cross-sectional analysis of primary care data [Internet]. *Can Fam Phys* 65[Le Médecin de famille canadien]. 2019;65(1):e30–e37. [cited November 25, 2020]. Available from: www.cfp.ca.

30. Gorbach PM, Cook R, Gratzer B, et al. Human papillomavirus vaccination among young men who have sex with men and transgender women in 2 US cities, 2012–2014. *Sex Transm Dis* [Internet]. 2017 [cited November 24, 2020];44(7):436–441. Available from: /pmc/articles/PMC5553567/?report=abstract

31. Nadarzynski T, Smith H, Richardson D, Pollard A, Llewellyn C. Perceptions of HPV and attitudes towards HPV vaccination amongst men who have sex with men: A qualitative analysis. *Br J Health Psychol* [Internet]. May 1 [cited November 24, 2020];22(2):345–361. Available from: http://doi.wiley.com/10.1111/bjhp.12233

32. Burns ZT, Bitterman DS, Perni S, et al. Clinical characteristics, experiences, and outcomes of transgender patients with cancer. *JAMA Oncol* [Internet]. 2021;7(1):e205671. November 12, 2020 [cited 2020 November 16, 2020]. Available from: https://jamanetwork.com/journals/jamaoncology/fullarticle/2772836

33. Gerend MA, Madkins K, Phillips G, Mustanski B. Predictors of human papillomavirus vaccination among young men who have sex with men. *Sex Transm Dis* [Internet]. 2016 [cited November 24, 2020];43(3):185–191. Available from: /pmc/articles/PMC4748724/?report=abstract

34. Machalek DA, Poynten M, Jin F, et al. Anal human papillomavirus infection and associated neoplastic lesions in men who have sex with men: A systematic review and meta-analysis. *The Lancet Oncol*. May 1, 2012;13(5):487–500.

35. Solazzo AL, Gorman BK, Denney JT. Cancer screening utilization among U.S. women: How mammogram and Pap test use varies among heterosexual, lesbian, and bisexual women. *Pop Res Policy Rev* [Internet]. June 1, 2017 [cited November 24, 2020];36(3):357–377. Available from: https://link.springer.com/article/10.1007/s11113-017-9425-5

36. Sandoval G, Obstein KL. Tu1116 disparities in health: Lower colorectal cancer screening rates among LGBTQ patients. *Gastrointest Endo* [Internet]. June 1, 2020 [cited November 16, 2020];91(6):AB552. Available from: www.giejournal.org

37. Roberts L, Heyworth B, Gilliver A, Mackereth P. Smoking and vaping among lesbian, gay, bisexual and trans people: results of a Proud2BSmokefree survey. *Cancer Nurs* Pract. December 7, 2017;16(10):35–41.

38. Wheldon CW, Watson RJ, Fish JN, Gamarel K. Cigarette smoking among youth at the intersection of sexual orientation and gender identity. *LGBT Health*. July 1, 2019;6(5):235–241.

39. Shahab L, Brown J, Hagger-Johnson G, et al. Sexual orientation identity and tobacco and hazardous alcohol use: Findings from a cross-sectional English population survey. *BMJ Open*. October 1, 2017;7(10):e015058.

40. EP Gruskin SHNGLA. Patterns of cigarette smoking and alcohol use among lesbians and bisexual women enrolled in a large health maintenance organization. *Am J Public Health*. 2001;91:976–979.

41. Silverberg MJ, Lau B, Justice AC, et al. Risk of anal cancer in HIV-infected and HIV-uninfected individuals in North America. *Clin Infect Dis* [Internet]. 2012 April 1, 2012 [cited 2020 November 24, 2020];54(7):1026–1034. Available from: https://academic.oup.com/cid/article/54/7/1026/297148

42. Robbins HA, Pfeiffer RM, Shiels MS, Li J, Hall HI, Engels EA. Excess cancers among HIV-infected people in the United States. *J Natl Cancer Inst* [Internet]. April 1, 2015 [cited November 24, 2020];107(4):503. Available from: https://academic.oup.com/jnci/article/107/4/dju503/893667

43. Gorgos LM, Marrazzo JM. Sexually transmitted infections among women who have sex with women. *Clin Infect Dis* [Internet]. December 15, 2011 [cited November 24, 2020];53(Suppl 3):S84–891. Available from: https://academic.oup.com/cid/article/53/suppl_3/S84/312345

44. Smith TW. Adult sexual behavior in 1989: Number of partners, frequency of intercourse and risk of AIDS. *Fam Plan Perspect*. 1991;23(3):102–107.

45. Clark H, Babu AS, Wiewel EW, Opoku J, Crepaz N. Diagnosed HIV infection in transgender adults and adolescents: Results from the National HIV Surveillance System, 2009–2014. *AIDS Behav* [Internet]. September 1, 2012 [cited November 25, 2020];21(9):2774–2783. Available from: https://link.springer.com/article/10.1007/s10461-016-1656-7

46. Kamen C, Mustian KM, Dozier A, Bowen DJ, Li Y. Disparities in psychological distress impacting lesbian, gay, bisexual and transgender cancer survivors. *Psychooncology* [Internet]. November 1, 2015 [cited November 30, 2020];24(11):1384–1391. Available from: /pmc/articles/PMC4517981/?report=abstract

47. Kamen C, Heckler C, Janelsins MC, et al. A dyadic exercise intervention to reduce psychological distress among lesbian, gay, and heterosexual cancer survivors. *LGBT Health* [Internet]. February 27, 2016 [cited November 14, 2020];3(1):57–64. Available from: http://www.liebertpub.com/doi/10.1089/lgbt.2015.0101

48. Desai MJ, Gold RS, Jones CK, et al. Mental health outcomes in adolescent and young adult female cancer survivors of a sexual minority. *J Adolesc Young Adult Oncol* [Internet]. July 27, 2020 [cited November 16, 2020];jayao.2020.0082. Available from: https://www.liebertpub.com/doi/10.1089/jayao.2020.0082

49. Hart TL, Coon DW, Kowalkowski MA, et al. Changes in sexual roles and quality of life for gay men after prostate cancer: Challenges for sexual health providers. *J Sex Med.* 2014;11(9):2308–2317.

50. Seay J, Mitteldorf D, Yankie A, Pirl WF, Kobetz E, Schlumbrecht M. Survivorship care needs among LGBT cancer survivors. *J Psychosoc Oncol.* July 4, 2018;36(4):393–405.

51. Thomas C, Wootten A, Robinson P. The experiences of gay and bisexual men diagnosed with prostate cancer: Results from an online focus group. *Eur J Cancer Care.* July 2013;22(4):522–529.

52. Torbit LA, Albiani JJ, Crangle CJ, Latini DM, Hart TL. Fear of recurrence: The importance of self-efficacy and satisfaction with care in gay men with prostate cancer. *Psychooncology* [Internet]. June 1, 2015 [cited December 1, 2020];24(6):691–698. Available from: http://doi.wiley.com/10.1002/pon.3630

53. Brown MT, McElroy JA. Sexual and gender minority breast cancer patients choosing bilateral mastectomy without reconstruction: "I now have a body that fits me." *Women Health.* April 21, 2018;58(4):403–418.

54. Rubin LR, Tanenbaum M. "Does That Make Me a Woman?" *Psychol Women Q* [Internet]. September 3, 2011 [cited December 3, 2020];35(3):401–414. Available from: http://journals.sagepub.com/doi/10.1177/0361684310395606

55. Margolies L, Kamen C. Needs of LGBT cancer survivors. In: *Cancer and the LGBT Community: Unique Perspectives from Risk to Survivorship.* Springer International Publishing; 2015:203–226.

56. Brown MT, McElroy JA. Unmet support needs of sexual and gender minority breast cancer survivors. *Support Care Cancer.* April 1, 2018;26(4):1189–1196.

57. Filiault SM, Drummond MJN, Smith JA. Gay men and prostate cancer: voicing the concerns of a hidden population. *J Men's Health.* December 2008;5(4):327–332.

58. Ryan C, Huebner D, Diaz R, Pediatrics JS-, 2009 undefined. Family rejection as a predictor of negative health outcomes in white and Latino lesbian, gay, and bisexual young adults. *Am Acad Pediatrics* [Internet]. [cited November 30, 2020]. Available from: https://pediatrics.aappublications.org/content/123/1/346?sso=1&sso_redirect_count=2&nfstatus=401&nftoken=00000000-0000-0000-0000-000000000000&nfstatusdescription=ERROR:%20No%20local%20token&nfstatus=401&nftoken=00000000-0000-0000-0000-000000000000&nfstatusdescription=ERROR:+No+local+token

59. Savin-Williams RC. Verbal and physical abuse as stressors in the lives of lesbian, gay male, and bisexual youths: Associations with school problems, running away, substance abuse, prostitution, and suicide. *J Consult Clin Psychol.* 1994;62(2):261–269.

60. Paul LB, Pitagora D, Brown B, Tworecke A, Rubin L. Support needs and resources of sexual minority women with breast cancer. *Psychooncology* [Internet]. May 1, 2014 [cited November 30, 2020];23(5):578–584. Available from: http://doi.wiley.com/10.1002/pon.3451

61. Katz A. Gay and lesbian patients with cancer. *Oncol Nurs Forum.* March 2009;36(2):203–207.

62. Carr E. The personal experience of LGBT patients with cancer. Vol. 34, *Seminars in Oncology Nursing.*:W.B. Saunders;2018:72–79.

63. Capistrant BD, Torres B, Merengwa E, West WG, Mitteldorf D, Rosser BRS. Caregiving and social support for gay and bisexual men with prostate cancer. *Psychoncology.* November 1, 2016;25(11):1329–1336.

64. Melisko ME, Narus JB. Sexual function in cancer survivors: Updates to the NCCN guidelines for survivorship. In: *JNCCN J Natl Compr Cancer Netw* [Internet]. 2016 [cited November 30, 2020]:685–689. Available from: https://jnccn.org/view/journals/jnccn/14/5S/article-p685.xml

65. Cathcart-Rake EJ, Zemla T, Jatoi A, et al. Acquisition of sexual orientation and gender identity data among NCI Community Oncology Research Program practice groups. *Cancer* [Internet]. April 15, 2019 [cited November 11, 2020];125(8):1313–1318. Available from: https://onlinelibrary.wiley.com/doi/abs/10.1002/cncr.31925

66. Witten TM. End of life, chronic illness, and trans-identities. *J Soc Work End-of-Life Palliat Care.* 2014;10(1):34–58.

67. Griggs J, Maingi S, Blinder V, et al. American Society of Clinical Oncology Position Statement: Strategies for Reducing Cancer Health Disparities Among Sexual and Gender Minority Populations. *J Clin Oncol.* July 1, 2017;35(19):2203–2208.

68. Graham R, Berkowitz B, ... RB-, Of DI, 2011 U. The health of lesbian, gay, bisexual, and transgender people: Building a foundation for better understanding. nationalacademies. org [Internet]. 2010 [cited November 19, 2020]; Available from: https://www. nationalacademies.org/hmd/reports/2011/the-health-of-lesbian-gay-bisexual-and-transgender-people.aspx

69. Burkhalter JE, Margolies L, Sigurdsson HO, et al. The National LGBT Cancer Action Plan: A White Paper of the 2014 National Summit on Cancer in the LGBT Communities. *LGBT Health.* February 2016;3(1):19–31.

70. Wender R, Sharpe KB, Westmaas JL, Patel A v. The American Cancer Society's approach to addressing the cancer burden in the LGBT community. *LGBT Health* [Internet]. February 2016 [cited December 9, 2020];3(1):15–18. Available from: https://pubmed.ncbi.nlm.nih. gov/26789399

12

The Health-Care Team and Culture in an Israeli Cancer Center, Israel

Tzeela Cohen and Simon Wein

"*Cultures, functioning as shared symbolic conceptions of reality, not only give meaning and order to existence, but also provide a venue for expanding and perpetuating oneself in a larger beyond. In other words, cultures carry within themselves the prospect that death can be transcended, either literally or symbolically perpetuating oneself in a larger beyond. In other words, cultures carry within* [1].

"*When a group of people makes something sacred, the members of the cult lose the ability to think clearly about it. Morality binds and blinds*" [2].

Introduction

Of what value is culture? What is the significance of different cultures—or are all cultures the same? What would the world look like without culture? Is culture genetically ingrained, for example, like the waggle dance of the bees?

The issue of what constitutes the culture of a country is compounded by the many different subcultures found in that country. There may be a dominant culture, but in the practice of medicine, it is the culture of the particular patient that is relevant.

Many of the serious ethical and clinical problems in health care reflect a conflict between the individual and the culture. Is the experience of the individual facing death similar in all countries, or do cultures influence how an individual dies?

Culture

There is no universal definition of culture. Hence, the word "culture" is best described as a set of common characteristics that have not yet coalesced sufficiently in order to achieve the high degree of integrity required to be labeled a definition.

Reviewing the literature suggests three core characteristics of culture: symbols, sharing, and groups.

1. Symbols represent values, attitudes, and beliefs and may be an idea, a graphic illustration, or a city. Culture, through these accumulated symbols, is imprinted

onto the individual's mind as a blueprint that shapes thinking and behavior. Jerusalem and the Star of David are symbols of Israeli culture.

2. Culture is shared by transmitting these symbols across and down through generations. Educational systems and communal celebrations, such as Independence Day, serve these purposes.

3. As a result of the symbols and the sharing, groups are formed and individuals are brought into line. Thus, culture serves to distinguish one group from another, for better and for worse.

Culture, however, is a two-way street. Individuals, through their unique creativity, can break free from the confines of their culture-programmed minds and change the culture. Just think of Gershwin and Rembrandt; or Abraham and Buddha. Each of us ordinary folk has a personal life story, which is separate from the ambient culture but is, of course, deeply indebted and intertwined. Tension between the individual and the culture—be it the ethics of abortion or end-of-life resuscitation—is universal and is a source of much disquiet and, paradoxically, of suffering. It touches on the tug of war between autonomy and paternalism.

Culture, with its symbols, sharing, and groups, provides meaning to people and helps them make sense of and cope with their suffering and loss [1]. Culture, unfortunately, does not always successfully teach us how to live with suffering. For example, unproven therapies may worsen pain with ineffective herbs; minority cultures may clash with the majority culture; or the individual may not know how to use their group's set of shared symbols and values. And what of the modern West which seems to have discarded its traditional culture throughout the course of the previous century. What has come in its stead?

The Demographics of Israel

According to the 2020 Israel Central Bureau of Statistics, of the 9.2 million people living in Israel, 75% are Jews and 21% are Arabs. Among the Arabs, 85% are Muslims and the other 15% are composed of Christians and Druze. Among the Jewish population, 48% are second-generation Israelis, 29% are immigrants, and 22% are first-generation Israelis. Most Jewish immigrants originated either from Europe, the former Soviet Union, or Arab countries in Asia and Africa. According to data from 2016, approximately 47.5% of Israelis over the age of 20 lead a secular lifestyle, 26% traditional, 14% orthodox and 8.6% ultraorthodox. Among Arabs of the same age, only 12% lead a secular lifestyle, 55% are traditional, and 30% are orthodox [3].

This varied panoply of peoples represents a plethora of cultures and values by which medical decisions are made, especially at the end of life.

Clinical Case 1: The Ethical Unit

Mr. A., a 33-year-old orthodox religious Jewish man, married with three children, was diagnosed with Crohn's disease at the age of 9. He endured a host of medical and surgical treatments to relieve his symptoms. His last bout of nonremitting abdominal pain led to the diagnosis of disseminated abdominal cancer. Since he was totally obstructed, a venting gastrostomy was placed and total parenteral nutrition (TPN) commenced. After a year of chemotherapy, and in the face of advancing disease, his oncologist recommended best supportive care. Seven weeks before his death he was hospitalized with jaundice, anasarca, abdominal pain, and dyspnea, requiring continuous intravenous morphine in escalating doses. The family refused an inpatient hospice because of its symbolism and the necessity to stop TPN. As the dyspnea increased, we discussed advanced directives. He requested to be ventilated, recalling that he had previously survived intubation following postoperative sepsis. His breathing deteriorated. We explained to him that, once intubated, he would be sedated until death and unable to communicate. He could not decide what to do. His secular brother and orthodox father quietly asked for supportive care only, while his wife and orthodox brother were in favor of intubation. At this point, his mother suggested consulting his rabbi. With the family on speaker-phone and the patient and staff present, the rabbi stated that, according to Jewish law, he should be intubated. He was sedated and intubated and succumbed to cancer 24 hours later.

Issues

1. Autonomous discussion versus rabbinical dictate
2. Sanctity of life versus quality of life
3. Patient's beliefs versus medical futility and scarce resources

Clinical Case 2: The Value of Life

Mrs. R., a secular Jew married with two children, was a 87-year-old retired secretary and artist. She was diagnosed with cancer of the upper esophagus, which caused difficulty swallowing and narrowed the airway. Aware of the grave prognosis, she completed advanced medical directives as per the Israeli Dying Patient Act [4] (detailed below), stating she did not want her life prolonged. However, after lengthy discussions with oncologists and family, she consented to radiotherapy and a feeding gastrostomy to avoid the risk of suffocation and to survive long enough to attend her granddaughter's wedding. Radiotherapy was physically and mentally excruciating. A few weeks after completing radiotherapy, she was hospitalized with stridor and dyspnea. The surgeons recommended an urgent tracheostomy. However, the patient, who was fully alert and supported by her children, declined the procedure and wished to be allowed to die without further interventions; (according to the Israeli Dying Patient Act, it is permitted to withhold lifesaving treatment from a patient who is compos mentis or has advanced directives to that effect, only if the prognosis is estimated to be 6 months or less.) The institutional Ethics Committee was urgently summoned because the oncologist thought cure was still possible. The committee interviewed the patient and deemed it reasonable to respect her wishes for supportive measures only.

Over the next 10 days, despite increasing dyspnea and anxiety, the surgical staff resisted administering sufficient morphine lest it hasten her death. As dyspnea worsened, *and pressured by her anxious children, she consented to a tracheostomy which provided a couple of weeks of relief. A major upper-airway bleeding episode led to her transferal to hospice were she died a week later.*

Issues

1. Autonomy versus paternalism
2. Prolonging life versus relief of suffering

Israel's Dying Patient Act 2006

Based on the recommendations of a culturally diverse expert committee:

- A terminal patient (defined as life expectancy < 6 months) can refuse the initiation of life-prolonging treatments, including mechanical ventilation.
- Active euthanasia or physician-assisted suicide is prohibited.
- Withdrawing or interrupting ongoing treatment is morally unacceptable.
- At the request of the patient or the patient's surrogate decision maker, life support can be discontinued indirectly, for example, by stopping a respirator or using a timer (this is currently a theoretical option only).
- Withholding nutrition and hydration is prohibited except for during the final stages of life (last weeks) when a patient may refuse nutrition and fluid sustenance.
- Patients have the right to receive maximal pharmacologic analgesia, even when such treatment may shorten life.

General Discussion on Culture

Is a function of culture to provide support and meaning in the face of suffering?

Death creates anxiety. Becker posited that people expend much effort to avoid this anxiety by creating cultural items that provide meaning in our lives in the face of death. Sometimes we create these elements to outlive ourselves (e.g., the pyramids of Egypt, a great novel) in order to achieve symbolic immortality [5,6].

Kellehear proposed that "the anticipation of death and dying for people in the Stone Age may have been the single biggest impetus for culture-building: for the development of laws, technologies and sciences," as opposed to the fear and neurosis that psychoanalysis emphasizes in anticipation of the ego's death [7].

Culture and the Individual: Our Cases

The cases we have recounted here describe two different clashes within the Israeli culture. One clash occurred between two dominant subcultures: the scientific norm and religious law; the second was between an individual and the culture of medicine.

The scientific norm aims to cure, but it also seeks to understand the limits of medical intervention and, hence, prognosis; whereas, in the first clinical case, the religion to which the mother and son adhered answered a different question: how do we value life? Curiously, regarding the question of intubation, while it probably did prolong the patient's life by 24 hours, it also rendered him symptom-free. So, other than the cost of intubation and dying *in tubus*, it was a reasonable compromise. We must never forget that the family lives on with those decisions taken at the end of life. The mother, who had treated and worried about her son's Crohn's disease since he was 9, could live on with her loss and say, "I did everything possible."

The second clinical case leaves us with the uneasy impression that culture failed the individual. The medical culture aims to cure. The individual, at age 87, felt at peace with dying after a rich and rewarding life; however, she was fearful of the cure-at-all-cost culture. Sadly, she died not in the manner of her choosing and the medical culture failed to cure.

Jewish Law

There is an extensive bibliography on Jewish Medical Law with a few guiding principles. It is noted that these principles are primarily encountered within the religious community, however their influence on the Jewish population at large is apparent, albeit diminished. It is beyond the scope of this chapter to analyze other cultural and faith groups, although Islamic law generally holds beliefs and views similar to those of Jewish law. The religious-cultural "sanctification of life" is a mechanism that helps us cope with the fear of death.

The first guiding principle is that the value of life is absolute, except for three specific circumstances where one's life may be forfeited (idolatry, incest, murder). This leads to the conclusion that quantity of life is more important than quality of life. Hence, in the first clinical case, the rabbi felt morally justified in intubating the young man, as living for a further 24 hours was a sanctification of life. However, the majority of rabbinical authorities rule that one should allow natural death to take its course and that one is not required (and according to some, is even forbidden) to intervene in such a case [8,9].

The second principle is that only God can heal and that medical workers are merely agents sanctioned by God. As a result, the concept and belief in miracles is often raised to extort more futile medicine. Conversely, futility represents a loss of faith in God.

The third principle is that our soul is "on loan" from God—it is not ours—and we are not morally free to shorten the soul's passage on earth. Hence, suicide and self-harm are prohibited. We must act to preserve the soul on earth for as long as possible until God decides otherwise. Yet, the leading authorities allow for significant autonomy in deciding whether or not to proceed with a risk-laden treatment, or even a potentially curative treatment, if it will cause distress [10].

Rabbinical Medical Broker

Rabbis in Israel play three roles within the health care system. The first is to provide religious advice on whether a particular medical decision is legally (hence, ethically) permissible, for example, organ transplantation. The second role is to help people navigate the medical system. This might include advising who they think the best doctor is for a particular problem, providing medical equipment, or connecting a patient with medical institutions overseas. The third role is to offer spiritual support to community members. This function is far less common in Israel than in Jewish communities outside of Israel.

It should be noted that Christian or Muslim clerical brokers are uncommon.

Greenfield showed that the rationale of all rabbinical brokers is based on the religious concept—both Jewish and Islamic—that only God is the ultimate healer, the final arbiter of life and death [11]. Therefore, the rabbi, as a conduit of God, is best placed to direct the patient. Whether this is true, a belief or a talisman does not matter, except when it brushes up awkwardly against the medical profession, for two reasons:

1. Professional jealousy: that is, how can a nondoctor know better than a doctor?
2. Faith versus science: similar to alternative therapy practitioners: there is the concern that bad advice is being given.

A survey found that 63–77% of pediatricians agree to a patient's request for rabbinical consultation on medical decisions. But in cases where the rabbi's advice diverges from accepted medical practice, especially in emergencies, almost all stated they would resist the rabbi's advice. A quarter of the doctors said they would contact the rabbi to clarify decision making [12].

Given patients' deep cultural acceptance of both rabbinical medical brokers in Israel (in one survey 32% used a rabbinical broker [13]), and doctors alike, most interviewees thought that guidelines should be established to demarcate "norms for rabbi–physician collaborations." Due to patterns of referral, many doctors would prefer to be on the rabbis' referral lists.

Doctors should understand that patients have freedom to make decisions regarding their own medical care, be it rabbinical or alternative medicine, even if the outcome is adverse. The patient has the right to be wrong [1,2].

The concept of a clerical medical broker is almost unique to the Jewish community of Israel. What has led to this? This has not been studied; however, experience suggests the following: a sense of moral imperative to save lives; it provides them with a sense of heroism and, therefore, protects them against their own fear of death (also for doctors); empowers the shepherd over the flock; gives them a power over life and death, to be like God; frustrated doctors; to attempt to influence the secular world with their religious beliefs; and finally, there is an unstated belief that illness is a punishment for breaching God's law. For example, in the Old Testament, Miriam was punished with "leprosy" for speaking against her brother, Moses.

Autonomy, Paternalism, and the Ethical Unit

The standard viewpoint in Western medical ethics today is that the individual's right to decide for themselves is sacrosanct. In the Near East, as well as in Israel, this viewpoint is not so clear. The Israeli courts strongly uphold the rights and autonomy of the individual. Paradoxically, many individuals choose to hand over the authority of medical decision making to other members of the family; this is usually done informally or presumptively. The family will enter the doctor's office and everyone will speak with equal authority in the presence of the apparently consenting patient. The ethical unit for making medical decisions is often the family and, occasionally, is extended to include the rabbi.

It is important to ensure that the individual patient agrees with the ethical arrangement. It does not have to be done formally, but a summary of the discussion should be recorded in the medical chart along with who was present at the meeting, especially for family meetings where the patient is not always present.

In Israel it is not uncommon for a family member to ask the doctor not to discuss the prognosis with the patient. Notwithstanding the presumed good intentions of the family member, this is unacceptable without the patient's explicit consent.

Thus, in Israel, the ethical unit for making the medical decisions is usually the patient, but it is often extended to include family members.

Improving Our Culture-biased Care

1. Early identification of the potential conflicts between an individual and their culture. Societal culture changes slowly over decades, whereas in a hospital changes may take just months or a few years. Palliative care, psycho-oncology, and integrative medicine are best placed to develop interventions designed to change institutional culture.
2. Family meetings with the patient need to take place early and regularly, especially where problems are anticipated.
3. In medical meetings, differences of opinion need to be proactively sought and voiced by the leader. "We should not expect individuals to produce good, open-minded, truth-seeking reasoning, particularly when self-interest or reputational concerns are in play. But if . . . individuals (have) some common bond or shared fate you can create a group that ends up producing good reasoning as an emergent property of the social system" [2].
4. Patients should have advocates in their journey through the medical system.
5. Morality differs around the world and within societies and their subcultures. How much I value life might not be the same as how much patients value their lives. The question then becomes: how much difference and dissent are we able to tolerate?
6. Staff should receive psychosocial education, which includes in-depth psychology (anger, heroism, courage, cowardice, hope, angst) and philosophy (what is the meaning of my life?).

Conclusion

Should we not spend more of our lives embracing our culture to anticipate our death? To use literature, theater, music, religion, science, sport, spirituality as a stimulus, an irritant, to think about failure; about loss, love and hate; about problematic human relationships; about the journey and not just the destination; about the aging process and loss of youthful powers; about retirement and about our nonfuture? All this should be part and parcel of our day-to-day culture, like the medieval *Ars moriendi*—the art of dying—to prepare and teach—the patient, the family, and the health care staff—to prepare for loss and death.

References

1. Kesebir P. Existential functions of culture: The Monumental Immortality Project. March 2011:1–23. doi: 10.1017/CBO9780511779374.010
2. Haidt J. *The Righteous Mind: Why Good People Are Divided by Politics and Religion.* New York: Knopf Doubleday Publishing Group; 2012.
3. Israel Central Bureau of Statistics. https://www.cbs.gov.il/HE/Pages/default.aspx, 2020.
4. Steinberg A, Sprung CL. The Dying Patient Act, 2005: Israeli innovative legislation. *Isr Med Assoc J.* 2007 Jul;9(7):550–552.
5. Becker E. *The Denial of Death.* New York: The Free Press; 1979.
6. Lifton RJ. On death and the continuity of life: a "new" paradigm. *HEQ.* 1974;1(4):681–696.
7. Kellehear A. *A Social History of Dying.* Cambridge: Cambridge University Press; 1970.
8. Bleich JD. *Judaism and Healing: Halakhic Perspectives.* New York: Ktav Publishing; 1981.
9. Pan CX, Costa BA, Yushuvayev EK. Can orthodox Jewish patients undergo palliative extubation? A challenging ethics case study. *JPSM.* 2020;60(6):1260–1265.
10. Linzer D. Treatment of terminally ill patients according to Jewish law. *AMA J Ethics.* 2013;15(12):1081–1087.
11. Greenfield G, Pliskin JS, Wientroub S. Orthopedic surgeons' and neurologists' attitudes towards second opinions in the Israeli healthcare system: A qualitative study. *Isr J Health Policy Res.* 2012;1:30:1–12.
12. Shuper A, Zeharia A, Balter-Seri J. The paediatrician and the rabbi, *J Med Ethics.* 2000;26(6):441–443.
13. Sapir R, Catane R, Kaufman B. Cancer patient expectations of and communication with oncologists and oncology nurses: the experience of an integrated oncology and palliative care service. *Support Care Cancer.* 2000;8:458–463.

13

Mindfulness and Compassion Practices for Cancer Patients

The impact of Culture and Faith in Cancer Care, Italy

Simone Cheli and Nicola Petrocchi

Introduction

A patient's journey through cancer is studded with visible and invisible constraints. Once diagnosed, the patient's life seems to be driven by urgencies, deadlines, and duties; the weekly calendar is marked by visits, pills, and appointments, and what was once a daily routine no longer exists. One's entire existence appears guided and controlled by external forces, which have turned body image, career, relationships, and one's whole identity upside down. People feel less able to control, predict, and understand their own lives, and these feelings, in turn, are accompanied with an impaired capacity to cope with the treatments and their side effects.

Indeed, hopelessness [1], demoralization [2], and a general loss of the purpose of life [3] are associated with several psychosocial factors such as depression, death anxiety, and maladaptive coping. These factors seemingly activate a vicious cycle where "the more I experience side effects, the more I tend to isolate myself; and the more I isolate myself, the more I run the risk of experiencing side effects." From a broader point of view, demoralized people recurrently act under a sense of threat that activates and is perpetuated by a progressive maladjustment [4] and a downregulation of positive affect systems [5].

For example, Salma (fictional name), a 41-year-old breast cancer patient facing a recurrence, turned her life and her treatments upside down once radiotherapy was over. Since her cancer was recurring, she decided not to start hormone therapy again. And now that there was a new scar on her breast, she decided to end her current romantic relationship without explanation. Because her family members lived abroad and, in her eyes, had not been able to handle the first diagnosis, she did not tell anyone about the recurrence. Salma was a perfectionist; a self-critical and overcontrolled woman with a high, even if deeply hidden, sensitivity to shame and guilt. She was born and raised in North Africa but had lived in Italy for many years. The only reason why she asked for a single psycho-oncology consultation was to get a second opinion about stopping hormone therapy. She considered it inappropriate not to question this decision, as her oncologist thought it wrong. Once the psycho-oncologist focused on Salma's self-criticism and fear of others' compassion, characterized by social disconnection and experiential avoidance, one of her recurrent patterns clearly emerged.

For cancer patients, barriers and blocks in both self-compassion [6] and receiving others' compassion [7] are related to psychological suffering and even to severe forms of psychopathology [8]. Several studies have shown how psychological suffering is typically related to how people detect and respond to threats and losses. Thus, researching how the brain has evolved to detect and respond to threats and losses can help understand and treat this suffering [9,10]. Approaches such as compassion-focused therapy (CFT) are rooted in evolutionary and neurobiological analysis of prosocial motives, such as compassion for self and others and their impact on human affect regulation systems [11]. CFT postulates that the self-soothing system, a mammalian affect regulation system normally triggered by cues of social safeness, is not easily accessible in people whose threat system is hyperactivated by self-criticism, guilt, and shame [12]. Thus, a primary aim of CFT is to increase compassion for one's own suffering as a way to strengthen the ability to generate this self-soothing response. Moreover, CFT hypothesizes that threat responses can be equally, and even concurrently, activated by internal (e.g., shame and self-criticism) and external (e.g., chemotherapy) sources, both of which trigger psychophysiological responses that operate through decreased activity of the vagus nerve and corresponding lower heart rate variability [13].

Once Salma agreed to start a psycho-oncology intervention, the therapist helped her understand how internal and external threats were constantly activating a defense response. They also explored how Salma's most recurrent strategy for steering clear of threat was by hyperfocusing on her job commitments and duties, activating what in CFT is defined as the drive system [11]. Unfortunately, this coping style never allowed Salma to develop and access the compassionate self-soothing skills she deeply needed to face a cancer recurrence, but rather contributed to a demoralization syndrome with several psychosomatic correlates. Consequently, the CFT intervention primarily focused on increasing compassion for herself and seeking the type of compassion she was secretly yearning for from others.

From a clinical psychology point of view, Salma had progressively and maladaptively tried to defend herself from internal and external threats by reducing her range of experiences. She was implicitly assuming a risk-minimizing principle as a way to cope with her tendency to strive for high perfectionistic standards.

CFT, in line with the goals of many other interventions used in psycho-oncology, helps people develop feelings of inner safeness (via increased self-compassion and self-validation) in order to promote the experiential acceptance of how cancer *really* imposes its constraints on their lives. By safely recognizing these constraints, patients can look for internal and external support without wasting their precious resources on trying to change things that cannot be changed, or overly attaching and invalidating the self (a typical defense response in the face of adversities). Depending on the extent to which people experience this acceptance, they can reconnect to their personal and social values and promote healthy self-to-self and self-to-other relationships.

Transcultural and Transreligious Processes

Cultural biases are extremely pervasive and recurrent in counseling and psychotherapy [14]. Despite the adoption of innovative guidelines, cultural competences are difficult to translate into practice. On the one hand, further studies are needed to better understand how to outline effective and culturally unbiased interventions [15]. Such expertise implies exploring both *if* the client is looking for a specific cultural competency and *which* is the least biased therapeutic setting. On the other hand, many scholars support the need for studying, and thus applying, the transcultural and transreligious processes that recur among different clients [16]. Indeed, many factors such as positive and negative values, cognitive and affective aspects, identity formation, and social attitudes are not culturally or religiously specific.

Experimental data and clinical expertise support the transcultural and transreligious reliability of an evolutionarily informed perspective in psychopathology [17,18]. Indeed, evolutionary psychiatry and psychology are rooted in the early studies of primates, indigenous people, and recurrences among different human cultures and races. Evolutionarily informed psychotherapies assume the need for considering mechanisms of onset and treatment of human suffering from an ethological point of view.

Specifically, CFT may turn out to be only a partially biased intervention for two main reasons: it is an evolutionarily informed psychotherapy, and it makes extensive use of experiential techniques. First, the focus of CFT is on strengthening a body-based precognitive emotion regulation system (the soothing system), which has been phylogenetically evolved since the rise of our species, with the function of downregulating the hyperactivity of the threat and the drive system. Compassion for self and others is reputedly an evolved strategy aimed at promoting the reproduction and survival of humankind. The target of CFT is to strengthen an evolutionarily and neurophysiologically based strategy (i.e., the compassionate motive) that has been shown to enable a healthy self-to-self and self-to-other relation [19].

Second, this mind–body vision of psychotherapy is applied through several experiential techniques rooted mainly in contemplative practices. Extensive studies have documented both the physiological underpinnings of caring and compassion [20] and the effect of contemplative practices on compassion and prosociality [21]. At the same time, meditation-based practices report good adaptability across different cultures and contexts [22]. In conclusion, we hypothesize that an intervention targeting the soothing system through experiential techniques may reduce the risk of cultural biases and promote a mind–body adaptative response to either internal or external threats.

Salma, for example, reported a pervasive source of distress: a fracture in her sense of belonging to and connectedness with her cultural and religious heritage; a distress that was specifically targeted by compassion-focused experiential practices. Her experience of being diagnosed with cancer had been complicated by two competing factors, one of which was very common and the other deeply personal. The former refers to the question with which every patient is sooner or later confronted: *Why me?* This question may (and, in Salma's case, did) lead to different kinds of spiritual struggles that, in turn, have almost consistently been associated with poorer health outcomes, especially in the mental health domain [23]. These struggles were worsened by Salma's personal history. About 20 years earlier, she left her home country in North Africa to pursue her career goals. She had become a successful manager but gradually abandoned her cultural roots, partly due to the recurring stereotypes of colleagues and acquaintances and partly due to her desire for emancipation. Although not out-wardly apparent, Salma had painful internal conflicts among her different "selves": a silent but "critical self" that contemptuously reminded her of her father and her for-gotten roots; a "competitive self", constantly oriented to appear as superdiligent in the eyes of colleagues; and a "threatened and disciplined self" that we can consider her manifest self that she presented to the outside world. Rather than negating this multiplicity, CFT promotes an integrative dialogue among the different selves. This integration is achieved by gradually cultivating a compassionate self-identity, charac-terized by the qualities of wisdom, nonjudgment, strength, and desire to help that may support the client's quest for a compassionate, validating relationship with and among all the "selves" [24]. Specifically, after having promoted an accepting, nonjudgmental, and compassionate dialogue among all the selves, the therapist introduced Salma to a widely used contemplative practice: the loving kindness meditation [25]. The goal was to help Salma *retrain* her compassion toward herself, her family, and the people around her.

Clinical Practices and Competencies

A recent meta-analysis supports the idea that CFT is effective in reducing depression, anxiety, and psychological distress while increasing well-being [26]. CFT has been successfully tested with cancer patients as both a specific protocol [27] and an inte-grative component of a wider intervention [28], with promising results. The primary aim in supporting this population is, as usual in CFT, to promote the development of the soothing system via the cultivation of the three flows of compassion (from the other, for the self, and for the other) as a way to help patients manage the internal (e.g., self-criticism) and external (e.g., side effects) threats. As depicted in Salma's case, a patient's journey through cancer is frequently shaped by several, and not always manifest, fears and blocks to compassionately soothe oneself and to be able to ask significant others for care and support. Recent advances in CFT have progressively focused on how to recognize and treat these pervasive inhibitors of compassion [29]. We cope daily with fear-based cognitions such as "compassion is a weakness or self-indulgence" or "others' compassionate efforts will be incompetent or upsetting to the point where I'll have to turn them away from me instead of relying on them for help." Unluckily, the same evolutionary forces that allowed compassion to arise in human history supported the development of competitive motivations that, in turn, may vali-date the idea of caring as a wasteful and risky activity exposing the caregiver to poten-tial threats. At the same time, the more isolated and disconnected persons feel from their social context, the more they will consider it to be risky to ask for help. A therapy such as CFT, focusing on the development of affiliation, caring, and compassion [30], is not intended to disconnect people from other social mentalities or motives, but rather to balance existing human motives and to highlight the need for compas-sionate motives in situations (i.e., cancer) where increased psychophysiological self-regulation is needed. A CFT intervention initially helps the patient understand the evolved nature and difficulties of the human body (an unfortunate predisposition to diseases) and minds (tendencies for negativity bias, negative rumination, shame, and self-criticism). The purpose of this intervention is to help them take an overview of "being human," while depersonalizing one's identification with what is happening to their bodies and within their minds, facilitating a gradual process of de-shaming (from "there is something wrong with me, this is all my fault" to "it is not my fault if humans have tricky brains and tricky bodies, but I can do something to approach all of this in a helpful way"). Patients are then invited to experience how certain practices with a focus on warmth and compassion (soothing rhythmic breathing, compassionate self-stroking and self-talk, visualization of a compassionate place and creature, development of a compassionate self-identity for self and others) stimulate the soothing system with beneficial effects, such as lowering arousal and, in particular, dampening self-criticism.

In order to understand fear and resistance to compassion and to promote a culturally unbiased intervention, a family perspective and competence is also required. An effective psycho-oncology intervention must be contextualized into the patient's family and social narratives [31]. Since the cancer experience, as well as the blocks and resistance to compassion, is expressed through personal, family, and cultural narratives [32], we may consider them as the evolutionary context from where the patient evolved their strategies. As we previously reported, by exploring Salma's life history, we understood and found a way to work with her "inner selves," promoting and balancing the three flows of compassion.

Conclusion

Compassion can be defined as awareness of others' suffering as well as one's own, with the intention to alleviate it. Compassion refers to a distinctive feature of our species that has evolved over millions of years, until the present day. It is not our one and only characteristic, but certainly one of the components that primates and hominids have most refined, allowing them to be competitive despite several manifest weaknesses. Receiving a diagnosis of cancer means suddenly being thrown into a struggle for life, where evolved motives and strategies seem to conflict chaotically. We return to our deeper knowledge and automatisms, often rooted in our early family experiences, of specific cultural, religious, and existential meanings. The more we perceive a discrepancy between our culturally evolved strategies and the way we *currently* deal with the disease, the more we may be at risk of inhibiting our vital search for compassion.

The reported evidence and our clinical experience seemingly support the usefulness of a compassion-focused approach to culture and faith for cancer patients. On the one hand, the evolutionary and neurophysiological foundation of CFT offers a transcultural and transreligious perspective to psychosocial distress. On the other hand, our daily experience with cancer patients suggests that targeting compassion may be extremely useful in hybrid, multicultural contexts, where both the therapist and the client may not necessarily be able or oriented to answer questions that are often unsolvable. Or better, we may assume that cultivating the three flows of compassion as a way of promoting experiential acceptance is the best stance we can offer to our patients to seek for these elusive answers.

References

1. Grassi L, Travado L, Gil F, et al. Hopelessness and related variables among cancer pa- tients in the Southern European Psycho-Oncology Study (SEPOS). *Psychosomatics*. 2010;51(3):201–207. doi:https://doi.org/10.1016/S0033-3182(10)70686-1

2. Robinson S, Kissane DW, Brooker J, Burney S. A systematic review of the demoralization syndrome in individuals with progressive disease and cancer: A decade of research. *J Pain Symptom Manage*. 2015;49(3):595–610. doi:10.1016/j.jpainsymman.2014.07.008

3. Park CL, Pustejovsky JE, Trevino K, et al. Effects of psychosocial interventions on meaning and purpose in adults with cancer: A systematic review and meta-analysis. *Cancer*. 2019;125(14):2383–2393. doi:10.1002/cncr.32078

4. Bobevski I, Kissane DW, Vehling S, McKenzie DP, Glaesmer H, Mehnert A. Latent class analysis differentiation of adjustment disorder and demoralization, more severe depres- sive and anxiety disorders, and somatic symptoms in patients with cancer. *Psychooncology*. 2018;27(11):2623–2630. doi:10.1002/pon.4761

5. Gilbert P. Evolution and depression: Issues and implications. *Psychol Med*. 2006;36(3):287– 297. doi:10.1017/S0033291705006112

6. Pinto-Gouveia J, Duarte C, Matos M, Fráguas S. The protective role of self-compassion in relation to psychopathology symptoms and quality of life in chronic and in cancer patients. *Clin Psychol Psychother*. 2014;21(4):311–323. doi:https://doi.org/10.1002/cpp.1838

7. Trindade IA, Ferreira C, Borrego M, Ponte A, Carvalho C, Pinto-Gouveia J. Going be- yond social support: Fear of receiving compassion from others predicts depression symp- toms in breast cancer patients. *J Psychosoc Oncol*. 2018;36(4):520–528. doi:10.1080/ 07347332.2018.1440275

8. Cheli S, Mancini F. When kindness falls apart: The disrupting effect of dependency, per- fectionism, and narcissism in adjusting to cancer. *Psychooncology*. 2020;29(3):579–581. doi:10.1002/pon.5300

9. Gilbert P. Biopsychosocial approaches and evolutionary theory as aids to integration in clinical psychology and psychotherapy. *Clin Psychol Psychother*. 1995;2(3):135–156. doi:10.1002/cpp.5640020302

10. Gilbert P, Choden. *Mindful Compassion: How the Science of Compassion Can Help You Understand Your Emotions, Live in the Present, and Connect Deeply with Others*.; Oakland, CA: New Harbinger; 2014.

11. Gilbert P. The origins and nature of compassion focused therapy. *Br J Clin Psychol*. 2014;53(1):6–41. doi:10.1111/bjc.12043

12. Gilbert P. Compassion: From Its Evolution to a Psychotherapy. *Front Psychol*. 2020;11:3123. https://www.frontiersin.org/article/10.3389/fpsyg.2020.586161.

13. Petrocchi N, Cheli S. The social brain and heart rate variability: Implications for psycho- therapy. In: *Psychology and Psychotherapy: Theory, Research and Practice*.; 2019;92(2):208– 223. doi:10.1111/papt.12224

14. Pedersen PB. Culturally biased assumptions in counseling psychology. *Couns Psychol*. 2003;31(4):396–403. doi:10.1177/0011000003031004002

15. Sue S, Zane N, Hall GCN, Berger LK. The case for cultural competency in psychother- apeutic interventions. *Annu Rev Psychol*. 2009;60:525–548. doi:10.1146/annurev. psych.60.110707.163651

16. Saroglou V. Trans-cultural/religious constants vs. cross-cultural/religious differences in psychological aspects of religion. *Arch Psychol Relig*. 2003;25(1):71–87. doi:10.1163/ 157361203X00057

17. Fabrega H. Culture and the origins of psychopathology. In: Uwe P. Gielen, Jefferson M. Fish, Juris G. Draguns (eds). *Handbook of Culture, Therapy, and Healing*; London: Routledge; 2012, pp. 15–36. doi:10.4324/9781410610416-9

18. Paris J. Evolutionary Social Science and Transcultural Psychiatry. *Transcult Psychiatr Res Rev.* 1994;31(4):339–367. doi:10.1177/136346159403100401
19. Kim JJ, Parker SL, Doty JR, Cunnington R, Gilbert P, Kirby JN. Neurophysiological and behavioural markers of compassion. *Sci Rep.* 2020;10(1):6789. doi:10.1038/s41598-020-63846-3
20. Porges SW, Furman SA. The early development of the autonomic nervous system provides a neural platform for social behaviour: A polyvagal perspective. *Infant Child Dev.* 2011;20(1):106–118. doi:10.1002/icd.688
21. Luberto CM, Shinday N, Song R, et al. A systematic review and meta-analysis of the effects of meditation on empathy, compassion, and prosocial behaviors. *Mindfulness (N Y).* 2018;9(3):708–724. doi:10.1007/s12671-017-0841-8
22. DeLuca SM, Kelman AR, Waelde LC. a systematic review of ethnoracial representation and cultural adaptation of mindfulness- and meditation-based interventions. *Psychol Stud (Mysore).* 2018;63:117–129. doi:10.1007/s12646-018-0452-z
23. Pargament KI, Koenig HG, Tarakeshwar N, Hahn J. Religious coping methods as predictors of psychological, physical and spiritual outcomes among medically ill elderly patients: A two-year longitudinal study. *J Health Psychol.* 2004;9(6):713–730. doi:10.1177/1359105304045366
24. Bell T, Montague J, Elander J, Gilbert P. "Suddenly you are King Solomon": Multiplicity, transformation and integration in compassion focused therapy chairwork. *J Psychother Integr.* 2021;31(3):223–237. doi:10.1037/int0000240
25. Hofmann SG, Grossman P, Hinton DE. Loving-kindness and compassion meditation: potential for psychological interventions. *Clin Psychol Rev.* 2011;31(7):1126–1132. doi:10.1016/j.cpr.2011.07.003
26. Kirby JN, Tellegen CL, Steindl SR. A meta-analysis of compassion-based interventions: Current state of knowledge and future directions. *Behav Ther.* 2017;48(6):778–792. doi:10.1016/j.beth.2017.06.003
27. Austin J, Drossaert CHC, Schroevers MJ, Sanderman R, Kirby JN, Bohlmeijer ET. Compassion-based interventions for people with long-term physical conditions: A mixed methods systematic review. *Psychol Health.* 2021;36(1):16–42. doi:10.1080/08870446.2019.1699090
28. Cheli S, Caligiani L, Martella F, De Bartolo P, Mancini F, Fioretto L. Mindfulness and metacognition in facing with fear of recurrence: A proof-of-concept study with breast-cancer women. *Psychooncology.* 2019;28(3):600–606. doi:10.1002/pon.4984
29. Gilbert P, Mascaro JS. *Compassion fears, blocks and resistances: An evolutionary investigation.*; 2017.
30. Gilbert P. Explorations into the nature and function of compassion. *Curr Opin Psychol.* 2019;28:108–114. doi:10.1016/j.copsyc.2018.12.002
31. Baider L. Communicating about illness: A family narrative. *Support Care Cancer.* 2008;16(6):607–611. doi:10.1007/s00520-007-0370-4
32. Baider L. Cultural diversity: Family path through terminal illness. In: *Ann Oncol;* 2012;3(23 Suppl):62–65. doi:10.1093/annonc/mds090

14

Enhancing Dignity and Hope in Caring for Cancer Patients through Palliative Care, Italy

Loredana Buonaccorso, Guido Miccinesi, and Carla Ida Ripamonti

Introduction

The care of cancer patients, particularly in the advanced stages and in the terminal phase, requires a global approach to suffering [1]. These patients experience great bodily changes due to both the disease itself and the treatment, feel ashamed and a threat to their dignity, and sometimes experience hopelessness as well. Every patient is not just a physical body on which to intervene to manage symptoms such as pain, fatigue, nausea, loss of appetite, and dyspnea. The physical body has an interconnected history with lived experiences, values, relationships, and social and cultural settings [2,3]. It also expresses emotional experiences that, in turn, are inseparable from the patient's thoughts and meanings [4].

Palliative care has shown that assisting cancer patients with a thorough, personalized approach, considering each one of them as a unique person, improves their quality of life, mitigates the mourning of bereaved families, and reduces the feelings of demoralization, loss of hope and dignity, anxiety and anguish that inevitably occur when someone is confronted with death [1,5,6].

The patient's good is the "heart" of the decision-making process at all stages of a disease, in all care settings. This good is a composite, but it consists mainly in a "personal good" [7]. Therefore, health care professionals (HCPs) try to ensure that the patients, while resetting themselves on the biological and psychosocial level, reach their personal good: being what they deeply want to be.

The doctors, nurses, social workers, pharmacists, psychologists, and hospital chaplains are part of a process that involves, in every step, the dignity and hopes of the patients assisted and of those who take care of them. Beyond HCPs, dignity and hope are important for family members as well [8,9] and for their quality of life [10,11].

Uncontrolled Pain and Symptoms: The First Studies on Dignity and Hope

The cancer patient must endure the clinical symptoms related to the disease, therapies, comorbidities, and diagnostic procedures, all of which are experienced as a disease within the disease [12]. The presence of untreated pain, as well as other symptoms, are causes of lack of dignity and hope for the patient, as well as of psycho-physical suffering. It has been reported that HCPs state loss of dignity as the second leading reason for the request for assisted suicide (in 53% of cases), immediately after the presence of uncontrolled pain (79% of cases) [13,14]. Furthermore, a low sense of dignity is associated with higher levels of psychological and spiritual distress, the loss of positive expectations on life, and living in despair with negative effects within the family [15]. A correlation between the loss of dignity and depression, anxiety, desire for death, hopelessness, feeling as though they are a burden to others, and poor quality of life [16] has also been demonstrated.

Dignity-Conserving Care

Dignity is defined as the "moral nobility that belongs to the nature of man, his skills, and the respect he has for himself and arouses in others because of his condition" [17].

In bioethics, there are three major themes which refer to the concept of dignity [18]:

1. *Attributed dignity*, as the value that human beings receive from other human beings. This involves a choice of what is considered dignified and what is not, and it becomes a value attributed in a conventional way.
2. *Intrinsic dignity*, as the value a person has simply as a human being, and not by virtue or attribution.
3. *Blooming dignity*, as the flowering of the human beings in their life paths, when they implement actions and behaviors that can be considered virtuous and that, therefore, increase the sense of dignity of being in the world. Contrary to the dignity attributed, this does not depend on others but refers to an objective concept of dignity to strive for.

The Universal Declaration of Human Rights of 1948 reported that "the only and sufficient title necessary for the recognition of dignity of an individual is his participation in the common humanity" [19].

The first studies that investigated the patient's dignity examined how it was often associated with a "good death" [13,14]. Emanuel and Emanuel [13] described the dying experience as a process with three critical components: (1) fixed characteristics of the patient, such as the clinical status and the sociodemographic characteristics; (2) modifiable dimensions of the patient's experience, or elements that may respond to events or interventions, such as physical and psychological symptoms, social relationship, economic demands, hope and expectations, and spiritual and existential beliefs; and (3) potential interventions available to family, friends and HCPs, such as the community palliative care services. The overall outcome was determined by the interaction of all those factors. The purpose of such a comprehensive list was to help clinicians systematically evaluate and optimize the care of the dying patient in all areas. Afterward, this framework was used for guiding additional research, for training the HCPs targeted to end-of-life care and dying patients, and for designing health care systems, creating a focus on dignity.

One important study that investigated how to build a model of therapeutic interventions for dignity was conducted by Chochinov and colleagues through a qualitative analysis of 50 interviews with cancer patients at an advanced stage of disease [20].
This eventually resulted in a Model of Dignity for the terminally ill [21], which identifies three main dimensions around which the patients construct a perception of their
dignity and which can be observed, assessed, and appreciated by HCPs: (1) illness-
related concerns; (2) dignity-conserving repertoire; and (3) social dignity inventory.
Within each dimension, some subthemes are identified that can support HCPs to assist patients in enhancing their dignity (see Figure 14.1).

In recent years, starting from this model, other studies have been carried out, expanding parts of it and integrating some new themes into it, according to determined
cultural contexts. A Dignity Care Intervention has been developed in Scotland for
use by nurses caring for persons with palliative care needs [22,23]. This intervention
covers a range of dignity-related concerns, including physical, psychosocial, and existential issues. Community nurses in Scotland and Ireland have found, and patients
have confirmed, that Dignity Care Intervention helps them identify the dignity-related needs of patients and provides a holistic, person-centered care at the end of life
[24,25]. Afterward, Dignity Care Intervention was adapted to a Swedish context, and
a central step was to identify culturally relevant, dignity-conserving care actions, confirming that dignity-conserving care is not just about what is done for the patient, but
also depends on how the patient is viewed by carers [26].

An interesting concept analysis was conducted on "living in the moment," an essential part of dignity-conserving practices in end-of-life care settings [27]. The authors

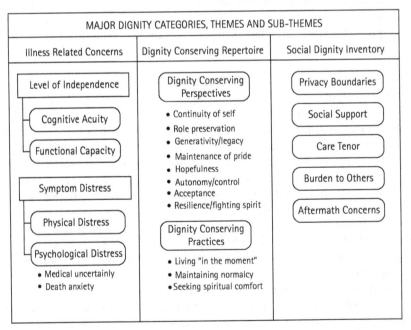

Figure 14.1 The Chochinov Model of Dignity, courtesy of the developer [21]

created a cluster of antecedents, attributes, and consequences frequently associated with this concept, derived from definitions and examples collected in 37 studies. The authors concluded that discussing with the patients the most important things in their lives helps them find meaning in life and to live in the moment, as does talking with them about issues that are nonillness related, encouraging them to partake in various activities, supporting them with carrying out their daily routines, and helping them set realistic goals.

Dignity also concerns the family members. A qualitative descriptive study explored the construct of dignity of the patient–family dyad in hospice palliative care, through semistructured interviews with 34 staff members [28]. The staff members viewed dignity as being reciprocally supported within the patient–family unit, such as respect, comfort, privacy, being informed, and quality family time. The themes solely constituting family dignity included being involved in care, being capable, and being treated fairly.

Another study explored the cancer patients' experiences of the bodily changes in relation to dignity [29]. A hermeneutic qualitative design was conducted by means of individual in-depth interviews with 13 patients with advanced cancer disease, cared for at a hospice inpatient unit. The patients' unpredictable, sick bodies forced them, or gave them the opportunity, to relate to their bodies in an honest way. The data highlights the importance of HCPs having insight into the consequences that bodily changes have for the patient's sense of dignity in order for them to provide good and dignified care [29].

Enhancing Patient Dignity during the Coronavirus Pandemic

Many obstacles to maintaining dignity have been seen during COVID-19, such as having to wear personal protective equipment, which limits opportunities for physical contact and nonverbal communication. Other obstacles include the symptoms related to COVID-19 and its treatment; the *no visitors* policies; patients facing the possibility of their final weeks and days in isolation; and families no longer able to personally offer care, comfort, and support to those they love. The final assault on human dignity is that patients who die from COVID-19 die alone. Table 14.1 shows a contribution that reviewed and implemented ideal practices in conserving dignity, combined with self-awareness, a compassionate presence, and spiritual care [30].

Toolkits for Dignity

Some tools have been developed to support people working in health care as they address dignity [31].

Patient Dignity Question
The Patient Dignity Question (PDQ) is a simple, open-ended question: "*What do I need to know about you as a person to give you the best care possible?*" [32]. After the patient's response, HCPs present a brief summary of the conversation, giving the

Table 14.1 Leaflet for Health Care Providers on Communication and Relation to Enhance Dignity for COVID-19 Patients, courtesy of the developer [30]

COVID-1 issue	Dignity issues	Interventions
Personal Protective Equipment (PPE)	PPE makes communication more challenging; voices may be muffled, eye contact is more difficult to establish, touch is minimal.	Take time to remind yourself who the patient is as a person.
		Eye contact and the *tone of voice* convey important messages and can support difficult communications, even within the limits of PPE.
	Health care providers (HCPs) must be aware of their own anxieties and mindful to balance patients' needs with prudent measures for their own self-protection.	*Tone of care* and *presence* are critical elements of being therapeutic; it lets patients know they are deserving of care and compassion (i.e., not just bodies to be protected from).
Symptoms due to COVID	Shortness of breath can exacerbate/accentuate anxiety.	Aggressive palliation to optimize patient comfort.
	Physical distress will heighten psychological distress; that is, patients will interpret symptoms as a gauge of their illness acuity.	Communicate using simple, accessible language e.g., avoid technical terms; answer all questions honestly, including acknowledging uncertainties regarding COVID-19.
	Needing assistance with personal care can challenge sense of dignity.	Provide patients accurate and clear information, helping them understand what is happening, anticipate what may happen; what is being monitored and what their options are.
	Patient uncertainty about COVID-19 may span from hope for recovery to fear and anticipation of death.	Psychological care includes encouraging expression of emotion and fears; acknowledging distress; normalizing responses to unique circumstances, respecting silence.
		Psychological care for HCPs requires them to be mindful of their own emotional responses, vulnerability and fears.

Isolation/No Visitors	Being cut off from usual sources of support. Feeling out of touch with outside world. Having to rely on health care providers for all medical and supportive (physical and emotional) needs. Health care providers bear the additional responsibility of being the patient's sole point of "in-person" contact.	Help the patient connect with the outside world (phone, video connection, tablet). Availability of television, radio, personal computer (cautioning patients to titrate news exposure, i.e., balance being informed versus frightened or overwhelmed by media reports). Practicing the ABCDs of Dignity Conserving Care (Attitude, Behavior, Compassion, Dialogue) Attitude: be aware that their own attitudes and assumptions can influence the way they deal with patients. Attitude shapes tone of care, presence, and overall emotional stance toward patients Behavior: must be predicated on kindness and respect, validating personhood. Small gestures (adjusting a monitor, giving water, fixing bedclothes, straightening sheets/bedding, adjusting TV settings) take little time to perform but convey caring, support and the idea that they matter. Compassion: being aware of patient suffering and pursuing steps to mitigate their suffering, be it physical, psychological, or spiritual/existential Dialogue: conversations, whether in depth or brief, must acknowledge who they are as persons and the challenges they are facing (e.g., "I can only imagine how hard this must be"; "How are you holding up so far; "What can I do to help you right now"). Ask the Patient Dignity Question: "What do I need to know about you as a person to give you the best care possible"
Death and burial	Patients are dying alone. Family members are denied the opportunity to be with patients in their final days. Traditional burial, funeral, community grieving are postponed or relinquished.	Use communicative technologies to help patients and families stay connected, deliver important final messages (e.g, love, forgiveness, hopes, wishes, goodbyes). A postcard expressing condolences and shared grief was sent to family members after the patient's death. A leaflet for online bereavement support was also sent. Live stream funeral proceedings; virtual memorials

patient the opportunity to correct it as they see fit. If the patient/family wishes, the written summary can be included in the medical file. The PDQ is useful at each stage of care and treatment, such as while carrying out routine physical and diagnostic tests, before providing personal care and/or when discussing arrangements for home care or long-term care.

A scoping review [33] showed that the PDQ promotes patient-centered palliative care, identifying issues and stressors that may be important to consider when planning and delivering someone's care and treatment.

A recent study investigated the feasibility of PDQ screening in palliative care consultation [34]. Data showed that PDQ can be used as a means of eliciting values and perspectives as a component of palliative care consultation. In particular, younger patients were more likely to focus on disease-related concerns; increasing age was associated with preferential discussion of personal perspectives over symptoms.

The Patient Dignity Inventory

The Patient Dignity Inventory (PDI) is designed to measure various sources of dignity-related distress among patients nearing the end of life and serves as a screening tool to assess a broad range of issues that have been reported to influence sense of dignity [35]. It is composed of 25 items, each of which was rated on a five-point scale: 1 – not a problem; 2 – a slight problem; 3 – a problem; 4 – a major problem; 5 – an overwhelming problem. Five-point scales of this nature have been reported as the most reliable on measurements of attitude-judgment, with response categories above five not yielding significant additional discrimination. The PDI has been validated in several languages, such as Italian [36], German [37], Spanish [38], Czech [39], Mandarin [40], and Greek [41].

One study investigated how psychosocial oncology professionals use the PDI during their practice and what utility it might have across the broad spectrum of cancer [42]. Ninety participants used the PDI and submitted a total of 429 feedback questionnaires detailing their experience with individual patients. The benefits of using the PDI in clinical practice were: a screening tool, discovering new issues, reinforcing client-related strengths, tracking client concerns, giving voice to patients, facilitating communication, and promoting insight. Clinicians were more inclined to apply the PDI to patients engaged in active treatment or palliation, rather than those in remission, recently relapsed, or newly diagnosed.

A recent study was conducted on 127 hospice patients with a life expectancy of only a few weeks, assessing the relationship between dignity and patients' other psychosocial and spiritual variables in order to improve patient-centered clinical practices through the use of PDI [43]. Personality traits seem to have an active role in the loss of dignity, whereas spirituality was confirmed to be a positive factor for dignity enhancement.

Dignity Therapy

Dignity Therapy (DT) is a brief psychotherapy targeting depression and suffering in palliative care patients. It was designed to produce a written Generativity Document whereby the patients can tell about their lives and the most significant moments or important thoughts they wish to preserve [44]. Therapy sessions are transcribed and edited, and the resulting Generativity Document is returned to patients who can share it with families, friends, and health care professionals [45]. This psychotherapy protocol begins by giving the patient nine standard questions, which are options for the patients' consideration and reflection about what they want to say. The questions help guide a conversation with a DT-trained health care professional.

A recent systematic review and meta-analysis indicated that, although findings on its efficacy are not consistent, DT has a positive impact on patients and families, particularly for reducing their suffering (anxiety, depression), improving quality of life and the perception of well-being, strengthening the sense of personal dignity, creating the opportunity for patients to talk to their loved ones about important issues, and attending to unfinished business [46].

One study was conducted with 15 advanced colorectal cancer patients who were receiving chemotherapy, showing that DT was a highly feasible, satisfying, and meaningful intervention, resulting in a better understanding of disease and goals of care at the end of life [47].

It has also been reported that an abbreviated DT promotes similar benefits for participants and recipients, making it a promising adaptation warranting further research [48].

A recent online pilot study on DT showed it to be feasible and beneficial, reducing therapist time and clinical cost, and appearing to reach people who would not otherwise receive the therapy [49].

Finally, a recent study explored the meanings emerging in different care setting and stages of cancer through the thematic analysis of two DT questions that are particularly salient to generativity: 'What have you learned about life that you want to pass along to others?'; 'Are the words or perhaps even instructions you would like to offer to your family to help prepare them for the future?' [50]. Generativity is a process whereby patients nearing the end of life invest in those they will soon leave behind. The authors observed that cancer patients, when addressing the topic of legacy, regardless of their disease trajectory, do not tend to focus on death. Providing patients with an opportunity to talk about life lessons (not only those taught by the illness) and share them with love ones appears to be feasible [50].

A novel means of facilitating meaningful conversations for palliative patients and family members, coined Dignity Talk, was designed to prompt end-of-life conversations, adapted from the dignity therapy question framework. The patient–caregiver dyad offers the option to respond only to those questions that are meaningful to them and within their emotional capacity to broach. It is self-administered, and it does not produce a Generativity Document. No therapist is needed, although ideally one would be available before or after Dignity Talk for added support [51].

Fostering Hope in Care

Hope has been defined as "a multidimensional dynamic life force characterized by a confident, yet uncertain, expectation of achieving a future good which, to the hopeful person, is realistically possible and personally significant" [52,53]. Many qualitative, nonexperimental, and quasi-experimental studies were conducted on cancer patients at every stage to investigate the relationship between hope and physical or social characteristics and quality of life, as well as to understand the factors associated with variations of hope in time, and to take any necessary action [52–54]. Hope has been confirmed to be important in palliative care for both cancer patients and their families. The presence of hope has been shown to be an essential factor contributing to increased family well-being. Furthermore, many people with cancer receiving palliative care require hope in order to maintain their dignity and enhance their quality of life [55].

Olsman et al. [56] revealed that cancer patients and their families may emphasize different dimensions within hope: a patient may emphasize the hope to continue living as long as possible, while the family member may emphasize the suffering from symptoms, which was not worth the hope.

In a study conducted by Johnson, attributes of hope were outlined for a sample of terminally ill patients [57]. The study suggested that the strategies that patients most commonly implement are: religion and prayer; to live for the day; relationships with others; symptom control; control of the situation; thinking positively and focusing on positive memories. Those attributes seem congruent with the results of another qualitative study that examined patients' coping strategies for maintaining hope despite the advanced stage, conducted by Herth [58]. He showed the main elements that can help patients hope, such as feeling loved, giving love, and having goals in the short and long term, as well as those that can obstruct the construction of hope, such as abandonment, isolation, uncontrolled pain, and internal suffering.

The family members' hope plays a role in maintaining the patient's hope as well, suggesting that interventions to increase family members' hope will also have a positive effect on the patient's hope [59]. The HCPs can use knowledge of the attributes of hope to build a relationship aimed at maintaining and supporting hope in cancer patients. For example, reasons of hopelessness can be related to fear of painful death and inadequate symptom management. In this case, supporting hope means ensuring adequate pain therapy and symptom control with routine symptom assessments.

Spirituality is an important component of hope, and the Institute of Medicine (IOM) identifies spiritual well-being as an important area of supportive care for advanced-stage patients. Pain and spiritual suffering affect the social and psychological integrity of the patient and can manifest themselves as physical symptoms, psychological stress, crisis of faith, or destruction of social relationships. Interventions aimed at mitigating this spiritual suffering and existential distress support the patient's hope and have a potentially positive effect on various aspects of the disease experience [52,57,60].

We propose a summary table that reports the major contributions to the qualitative studies on fostering or hindering hope in palliative care cancer patients and their family members, and the intervention to foster personalized assistance [30,57,58]. The elements also intersect with the themes and subthemes of dignity-conserving care [61] (See Table 14.2).

Evaluating Hope

Based on the identified factors, a survey instrument of hope in cancer patients has been developed: the Herth Hope Index (HHI) [62], consisting of 12 items on the Likert Scale. A high score in the HHI indicates a greater presence of hope in the patient.

Table 14.2 Elements that promote and hinder hope in palliative care patients

	Promote hope	Hinder hope	Interventions [30]
Patient	- **Emotional experience**: to feel loved and give love, especially within the family - **Positive expectations**: a positive forecast with hope for a better tomorrow, despite the poor prognosis - **Personal qualities**: an inner strength, an approach to life aimed at solving problems and achieving important goals - **Humor**: a good dose of humor as the ability to defuse difficult situations - **Spirituality and faith**: faith in a superior being/God; hope of a life after death where they can meet loved ones again by finding a purpose to live what remains of life - **Goals**: setting and achieving short- and long-term goals, maintaining as much autonomy as possible (both physical and mental, such as being involved in the process of care and daily decision making) - **Comfort**: being pain-free and comfortable - **Assistance**: the behavior of others for physical contacts, attention to mood and giving honest information; feel supported by the HCPs and have a good relationship with them (good communication, feeling in a position to express doubts and fears that may be contained) - **Interpersonal relationships**: loving relationships with friends and family, honest relationships with carers - **Control**: possibility to decide on own care - **Legacy**: leaving something of value to others - **Memories and review of one's life**: recognizing the goals achieved and contributions made to improve the lives of others in order to keep them pleasant; memories one can share with family members to retrace the most important phases of one's life	- **Abandonment and isolation**: inadequate communication within the family about the disease, dying and death - **Uncontrolled symptoms**: pain and internal suffering, such as anxiety and depression - **Depersonalization**	- **Take time to remind yourself who the patient is as a person** - **Aggressive palliation** to optimize patient comfort - Provide patients accurate and **clear information**, helping them understand what is happening, anticipate what may happen; what is being monitored and what their options are - **Psychological care** includes encouraging expression of emotion and fears; acknowledging distress; normalizing responses to unique circumstances; respecting silence - Psychological care for HCPs requires them to **be mindful of their own emotional responses, vulnerability, and fears** - Practicing the **ABCDs of Dignity Conserving Care** (Attitude, Behavior, Compassion, Dialogue [61]) - Attitude: be aware that their own attitudes and assumptions can influence the way they deal with patients - Behavior: must be predicated on kindness and respect, validating personhood - Compassion: being aware of patient suffering and pursuing steps to mitigate their suffering - Dialogue: conversations, whether in depth or brief, must acknowledge who they are as persons and the challenges they are facing - **Personalized approach**: use the Patient Dignity Question [32] - Focus on the legacy of the patient: use dignity therapy [44,51]

Continued

Table 14.2 Continued

	Promote hope	Hinder hope	Interventions [30]
Family members	- Interpersonal relationship: involvement in relationships with patient and HCPs perceived as warm and nourishing - Personal qualities: a conscious reframing of perceived threats in a more positive context, talking to oneself and using meditation - Living in the moment: live for the day, supported in unexpected changes - "Being with": having realistic expectations and focus on the sense of "being with" as opposed to "doing" when death approaches - Spirituality and faith: practice spiritual faith and manage available energies	- Abandonment and isolation: the sense of isolation - Recent and past experiences: feeling overwhelmed by other losses, especially recent experiences - Uncontrolled symptoms: the patient's symptoms are not adequately controlled - Communication with the clinicians: to have difficulties gives a feeling of loss of personality and of receiving negative messages	- Global assistance: the care intervention is dedicated to the patient/family dyad - Provide family members accurate and clear information, helping them understand what is happening, anticipate what may happen; what is being monitored, and what their options are - Psychological care includes encouraging expression of emotion and fears - Personalized approach to the dyad: use the Dignity Talk [50]

A recent systematic review showed that the HHI has been translated and psychometrically tested in many languages across numerous countries [63]. The reliability of the HHI was reported as making it acceptable in all of the studies.

Conclusion

Introducing a biopsychosocial-spiritual model of care across the cancer trajectory would most likely improve the care of patients [64]. This model sustains the integration of the spiritual dimension, in addition to the physical, emotional, and social aspects, into the assessment of cancer patients regardless of the stage of the disease, in order to offer a comprehensive needs-tailored intervention, which includes dignity and hope.

The HCPs can use standardized questionnaires to assess the dignity-related distress and the sense of hope in cancer patients during all phases of the disease. No cutoff is indicated for the correct use of these questionnaires. The aim of the questions is more to open a dialogue with the patient and to make them feel safe and trust the HCPs who better know what is really important for them. Indeed, critical passages in the course of the disease can be better dealt with if this dialogue on important personal preferences and values has already been opened.

The multidimensional assessment of cancer patients on physical, psychological, social, and spiritual (including hope and dignity) dimensions, in any phase of the disease, made by well-trained HCPs, offers them a better understanding of the dynamic process of coping with the disease, and finding out which paths are still viable for well-being, even in the presence of a life-threatening disease. Some studies showed that cancer patients who are involved in decision-making processes on their own care have a higher compliance rate with suggested treatments and cope better with the disease, resulting in a higher level of well-being [64].

The HCPs should consider expanding their role and involving themselves more in the holistic aspects of care. It is possible to help cancer patients to cope with feelings of isolation and hopelessness. To act on hope, one must act on the needs (especially on the psychoemotional needs), the symptoms, and the spiritual dimension: they all have a specific and independent effect on hope. From a supportive care perspective, issues such as hope, meaning, and dignity are to be dealt with from the very beginning of any serious disease.

References

1. Bruera E, Hui D. Integrating supportive and palliative care in the trajectory of cancer: Establishing goals and models of care. *J Clin Oncol.* 2010;28:4013–4017. https://doi.org/10.1200/jco.2010.29.5618
2. Pask S, Pinto C, Bristowe K, et al. A framework for complexity in palliative care: A qualitative study with patients, family carers and professionals. *Palliat Med.* 2018;32:1078–1090. https://doi.org/10.1177/0269216318757622
3. Grassi L, Caruso R, Sabato S, et al. The UniFe Psychiatry Working Group Coauthors, Psychosocial screening and assessment in oncology and palliative care settings. *Front Psychol.* 2015;7;5:1485. doi: 10.3389/fpsyg.2014.01485. eCollection 2014

4. Winger JG, Ramos K, Steinhauser KE, et al. Enhancing meaning in the face of advanced cancer and pain: Qualitative evaluation of a meaning-centered psychosocial pain management intervention. *Palliat Support Care*. 2020;18(3):263–270. doi:10.1017/S1478951520000115

5. Jordan K, Aapro M, Kaasa S, et al. Supportive and palliative care: It's all about the patient. European Society for Medical Oncology ESMO position paper. *Ann Oncol*. 2018;29(1):36–43.

6. Vehling S, Lehmann C, Oechsle K, et al. Global meaning and meaning-related life attitudes: Exploring their role in predicting depression, anxiety, and demoralization in cancer patients. *Support Care Cancer*. 2011;19:513–520. doi:10.1007/s00520-010-0845-6

7. Pellegrino D, Thomasma DC. *For the Patient's Good*. Oxford: Oxford University Press; 1988.

8. Balboni TA, Balboni MJ. The spiritual event of serious illness. *J Pain Symptom Manage* .2018;56(5):816–822.

9. Delgado-Guay MO, Chisholm G, Williams J, et al. Frequency, intensity, and correlates of spiritual pain in advanced cancer patients assessed in a supportive/palliative care clinic. *Palliat Support Care*. 2016;14(4):341–348. [PubMed: 26481034]

10. McClement SE, Chochinov HM, Hack TF, et al. Dignity-conserving care: application of research findings to practice. *Int J Palliat Nurs*. 2004;10(4):173–179.

11. McClement SE, Chochinov HM. Hope in advanced cancer patients. *Eur J Cancer*. 2008;44(8):1169–1174.

12. Ripamonti CI, Bossi P, Santini D, Fallon M. Pain related to cancer treatments and diagnostic procedures: a no man's land? *Ann Oncol*. 2014;25(6):1097–1106. doi: 10.1093/annonc/mdu011. Epub 2014 Mar 13

13. Emanuel EJ, Emanuel LL. The promise a good death. *Lancet*. 1998;351 (Suppl 2):S1121–S1129.

14. Van der Maas PJ, van der Wal G, Haverkate I, et al. Euthanasia, physician-assisted suicide, and other medical practices involving the end of life in the Netherlands, 1990–1995. *N Engl J Med*. 1996;335:1699–1705.

15. Chochinov HM, Wilson KG, Enns M, Lander S. Depression, hopelessness, and suicidal ideation in the terminally ill. *Psychosomatics*. 1998;39:66–370.

16. Guerrero-Torrelles M, Monforte-Royo C, Tomás-Sábado J, et al. Meaning in life as a mediator between physical impairment and the wish to hasten death in patients with advanced cancer. *J Pain Symptom Manage*. 2017;54(6):826–834.

17. Debes R (ed). *Dignity: A History*. New York: Oxford University Press; 2017.

18. Lanigan (ed). *Human Dignity and Bioethics*. New York: Nova Science Publisher; 2008.

19. Universal Declaration of Human Rights, December 10, 1948, art.1. www.ohchr.org/EN/UDHR/Pages/SearchByLang.aspx

20. Chochinov HM, Hack T, Hassard T, et al. Dignity in the terminal ill: A cross sectional, cohort study. *Lancet*. 2002;360:2026–2030.

21. Chochinov HM, Hack T, McClement S, Kristjanson L, Harlos M. Dignity in the terminally ill: A developing empirical model. *Soc Sci Med*. 2002;54:433–443.

22. Brown H, Johnston B, Östlund U. Identifying care actions to conserve dignity in end-of-life care. *Br J Community Nurs*. 2011;16:238–245.

23. Johnston B, Östlund U, Brown H. Evaluation of the dignity care pathway for community nurses caring for people at the end of life. *Int J Palliat Nurs*. 2012;18:483–439.

24. McIlfatrick S, Connolly M, Collins R, et al. Evaluating a dignity care intervention for palliative care in the community setting: Community nurses' perspectives. *J Clin Nurs*. 2017;26:4300–4312.

25. Johnston B, Papadopoulou C, Östlund U, Hunter K, Andrew J, Buchanan D. What's dignity got to do with it? Patients experience of the dignity care intervention: A qualitative evaluation study. *SAGE Open Nurs*. 2017;3:1–12.26.

26. Östlund U, Blomberg K, Annika Söderman A, Werkander Harstäde C. How to conserve dignity in palliative care: Suggestions from older patients, significant others, and health-care professionals in Swedish municipal care. *BMC Palliat Care*. 2019;18:10. https://doi.org/10.1186/s12904-019-0393-x

27. Donmez ÇF, Johnston B. Living in the moment for people approaching the end of life: A concept analysis. *Int J Nurs Stud Adv*. 2020;108:103584. doi: 10.1016/j.ijnurstu.2020.103584 (PMID:32450405)

28. Guo Q, Zheng R, Jacelon CS, McClement S, Thompson G, Chochinov H. Dignity of the patient-family unit: further understanding in hospice palliative care. *BMJ Support Palliat Care*. July 14, 2019:bmjspcare-2019-001834. doi: 10.1136/bmjspcare-2019-001834

29. Lorensten VB, Nåden D, Sæteren B. The meaning of dignity when the patients' bodies are falling apart. *Nurs Open*. May 22, 2019;22;6(3):1163–1170. doi: 10.1002/nop2.301

30. Tanzi S, Buonaccorso L. Enhancing patient dignity: Opportunities addressed by a specialized palliative care unit during the coronavirus pandemic. *J Palliat Med*. 2021 Mar;24(3):324–326. doi: 10.1089/jpm.2020.0661

31. https://www.dignityincare.ca/en/toolkit.html#top

32. Chochinov HM, McClement S, Hack T, Thompson G, Dufault B, Harlos M. Eliciting personhood within clinical practice: Effects on patients, families and health care providers. *J Pain Symptom Manage*. 2015;49(6):974–980.e2. doi: 10.1016/j.jpainsymman.2014.11.291

33. Arantzamendi M, Belar A, Martinez M. Promoting patient-centred palliative care: A scoping review of the Patient Dignity Question. *Curr Opin Support Palliat Care*. 2016 Dec;10(4):324–329.

34. Hadler R, Goldshore M, Nelson J. The Patient Dignity Question in routine palliative care consultation: Implementation and implications (TH322D). *J Pain Symptom Manage*. 2020;59(2):419–420.

35. Chochinov HM, Hassard T, McClement S, et al. The Patient Dignity Inventory: A novel way of measuring dignity-related distress in palliative care. *J Pain Symptom Manage*. 2008;36:559–571.

36. Ripamonti CI, Buonaccorso L, Maruelli A, et al. Patient Dignity Inventory (PDI) questionnaire: The validation study in Italian patients with solid and hematological cancers on active oncological treatments. *Tumori*. 2012;98:491–500.

37. Sautier LP, Vehling S, Mehnert A. Assessment of patients' dignity in cancer care: Preliminary psychometrics of the German version of the Patient Dignity Inventory (PDI-G). *J Pain Symptom Manage*. 2014;47(1):181–188. doi: 10.1016/j.jpainsymman.2013.02.023. Epub 2013 Jul 3

38. Rullán M, Carvajal A, Núñez-Córdoba JM, et al. Spanish version of the Patient Dignity Inventory: Translation and validation in patients with advanced cancer. *J Pain Symptom Manage*. December 2015;50(6):874–881.e1. doi: 10.1016/j.jpainsymman.2015.07.016

39. Kisvetrová H, Školoudík D, Danielová L, et al. Czech version of the Patient Dignity Inventory: Translation and validation in incurable patients. *J Pain Symptom Manage*. 2018;55(2):444–450. doi: 10.1016/j.jpainsymman.2017.10.008. Epub

40. Li YC, Wang HH, Ho CH. Validity and reliability of the Mandarin version of Patient Dignity Inventory (PDI-MV) in cancer patients. *PLoS One*. 2018;13(9):e0203111. doi: 10.1371/journal.pone.0203111. eCollection 2018

41. Parpa E, Kostopoulou S, Tsilika E, Galanos A, Katsaragakis S, Mystakidou K. Psychometric properties of the Greek version of the Patient Dignity Inventory in advanced cancer patients. *J Pain Symptom Manage*. 2017;54(3):376–382. doi: 10.1016/j.jpainsymman.2017.07.002. Epub 2017 Jul 13. PMID: 28711753

42. Chochinov HM, McClement SE, Hack TF, et al. The Patient Dignity Inventory: Applications in the oncology setting. *J Palliat Med*. 2012;15(9):998–1005. doi: 10.1089/jpm.2012.0066

43. Bovero A, Sedghi NA, Botto R, Tosi C, Ieraci V, Torta R. Dignity in cancer patients with a life expectancy of a few weeks. Implementation of the factor structure of the Patient Dignity Inventory and dignity assessment for a patient-centered clinical intervention: A cross-sectional study. *Palliat Support Care* 2018;16(6):648–655. doi: 10.1017/S147895151700102X

44. Chochinov HM, Hack T, Hassard T, et al. Dignity therapy: A novel psychotherapeutic intervention for patients near the end of life. *J Clin Oncol.* 2005;23:5520–5525.

45. McClement S, Chochinov HM, Hack T, Hassard T, Kristjanson LJ, Harlos M. Dignity therapy: Family member perspectives. *J Palliat Med.* 2007;10:1076–1082. https://doi.org/10.1089/jpm.2007.0002

46. Xiao J, Chow KM, Liu Y, Chan C WH. Effects of dignity therapy on dignity, psychological well-being, and quality of life among palliative care cancer patients: A systematic review and meta-analysis. *Psychooncology.* 2019;28(9):1791–1802.

47. Vergo MT, Nimeiri H, Mulcahy M, Benson A, Emanuel LA. Feasibility study of dignity therapy in patients with stage IV colorectal cancer actively receiving second-line chemotherapy. *J Commun Support Oncol Actions.* 2014;12(12):446–453. doi: 10.12788/jcso.0096

48. Beck A, Cottingham AH, Stutz PV, et al. Abbreviated dignity therapy for adults with advanced-stage cancer and their family caregivers: Qualitative analysis of a pilot study. *Palliat Support Care.* June 2019;17(3):262–268. doi:10.1017/S1478951518000482

49. Bentley B, O'Connor M, Williams A, Breen LJ. Dignity therapy online: Piloting an online psychosocial intervention for people with terminal illness. *Digit Health.* 2020;6:2055207620958527. doi: 10.1177/2055207620958527

50. Buonaccorso L, Tanzi S, De Panfilis L, et al. Meaning emergin from dignity therapy among cancer patients. *J Pain Symptom Manage.* 2021 Oct;62(4):730–737. doi: 10.1016/j.jpainsymman.2021.02.028. Epub 2021 Feb 20.

51. Guo Q, Chochinov HM, McClement S, Thompson G, Hack T. Development and evaluation of the Dignity Talk question framework for palliative patients and their families: A mixed-methods study. *Palliat Med.* 2018;32(1):195–205. doi: 10.1177/0269216317734696. Epub 2017 Nov 13

52. Dufault K, Marmocchio BC. Symposium on compassionate care and the dying experience. Hope: Its spheres and dimensions. *Nurs Clin North Am.* 1985;20:379–391.

53. Butt CM. Hope in adults with cancer: State of the science. *Oncol Nurs Forum.* 2011;38/5:E341–E350.

54. Chi GC. The role of hope in patients with cancer. *Oncol Nurs Forum.* 2007;34:415–424.

55. Olsson L, Ostlund G, Strang P, et al. The glimmering embers: experiences of hope among cancer patients in palliative home care. *Palliat Supp Care* 2011;9(1):43–54.

56. Olsman E, Willems D, Leget C. Solicitude: Balancing compassion and empowerment in a relational ethics of hope-an empirical-ethical study in palliative care. *Med Health Care Philos.* 2016;19(1):11–20.

57. Johnson S. Hope in terminal illness: An evolutionary concept analysis. *Int J Palliat Nurs.* 2007;13:451–459.

58. Herth K. Fostering hope in terminally ill people. *J Advanced Nurs.* 1990;15:250–1259.

59. Fu F, Chen YY, Li Q, Zhu F. Varieties of hope among family caregivers of patients with lymphoma. *Qual Health Res.* 2018;28(13):2048–2058. doi: 10.1177/1049732318779051. Epub 2018 Jun 11

60. Wang YC, Lin CC. Spiritual well being may reduce the negative impacts of cancer symptoms on the quality of life and the desire for hastened death in terminally ill cancer patients. *Cancer Nurs.* 2016;39:E43–E60.

61. Chochinov HM. Dignity and the essence of medicine: The A, B, C, and D of dignity conserving care. *BMJ.* 2007;335:184–187.

62. Herth K. Abbreviated instrument to measure hope: Development and psychometric evaluation. *J Adv Nurs.* 1992;17:1251–1259.
63. Nayeri ND, Goudarzian AH, Hert K, et al. Construct validity of the Herth Hope Index: A systematic review. *Rev Int J Health Sci.* 2020;14(5):50–57.
64. Ripamonti CI, Giuntoli F, Gonella S, Miccinesi G. Spiritual care in cancer patients: A need or an option? *Curr Opin Oncol.* 2018;30(4):212–218.

15

Meaning-Making in Coping with Cancer

The Impact of Spirituality and Culture among Cancer Patients in the Philippines

Maria Minerva P. Calimag

The Global Cancer Burden

The global cancer burden rose to an estimated 18.1 million new cases and 9.6 million deaths in 2018, up from the estimated 12.7 million new cancer cases and 7.6 million cancer deaths recorded in 2008. Globally, the combined statistics for both men and women show that nearly half of the new cases and more than half of the cancer deaths worldwide in 2018 were estimated to occur in Asia, mainly because Asia accounts for nearly 60% of world population. Asia shows a higher proportion of cancer deaths (57.3%) than the proportion of incident cases (48.4%) as compared to other world regions. Many families have had at least one family member who has been afflicted with or has died from cancer. Asia is largely beleaguered by limited access to timely diagnosis and treatment, and by a higher frequency of certain types of cancer associated with poorer prognosis and higher mortality rates. At least one in five men and one in six women develop cancer throughout their lives, and one in eight men and one in eleven women die from the condition [1].

Respecting cultural differences and beliefs is key in cancer care. Our ultimate goal in the practice of cancer care is to remember that we are not just treating diseases. We are caring for people who are living with cancer. Unfortunately, many of these patients living in low- and middle-income countries will die of this disease. The total number of people living within five years of a cancer diagnosis, called the five-year prevalence, is estimated to be 43.8 million. It is to these cancer survivors that the adequate management of cancer and the accompanying pain matter most, as it impacts their quality of life.

Cancer is the third leading cause of morbidity and mortality in the Philippines [2]. It is one of the four epidemic noncommunicable diseases (NCDs) or lifestyle-related diseases (LRDs), which include cardiovascular diseases, diabetes mellitus, and chronic respiratory diseases [3]. The Philippine population of 109.58 million, equivalent to 1.41% of the total world population (Worldometer), is made up of ethnic groups with diverse cultural ethnicities: Tagalog 28.1%, Cebuano 13.1%, Ilocano 9%, Bisaya/Binisaya 7.6%, Hiligaynon Ilonggo 7.5%, Bikol 6%, Waray 3.4%, other 25.3% (2000 census). The Philippines has two official languages: Filipino (based on Tagalog) and English, and it has eight major ethnolinguistic strands: Tagalog, Cebuano, Ilocano, Hiligaynon or Ilonggo, Bicol, Waray, Pampango, and Pangasinan [4].

Meaning-making in Oncology

Searching for meaning has sometimes been shown to be adaptive [5], leading to resilience and recovery, but at other times it has been found to be related to higher levels of distress and dysfunction [6]. The process of meaning-making coping involves efforts to understand a stressor (appraised meaning) and to incorporate that understanding into one's global meaning system [7]. Individuals maintain equilibrium and a sense of coherence when they view their lives as comprehensible, manageable, and meaningful [8,9]. The occurrence of cancer often violates individuals' beliefs in these areas because a negative life event threatens one's perceptions about meaning in life, especially one's sense of harmony and peace [10,11].

To relieve the anxiety brought about by cancer, survivors' meaning-making following cancer entails attempts to reduce the discrepancy between their situational meaning (appraisals, meaning making, and meanings made) versus their global meaning (global beliefs and goals) of the cancer [7,12]. Meaning-making is very common in cancer survivors [13,14] and is believed to be important in their psychological adjustment [15]. Although this process is considered to be initially adaptive, it can devolve into maladaptive brooding or depressive rumination if satisfactory meanings cannot be constructed [16]. Eventually, their psychological adjustment depends on the cancer survivors' efforts at meaning-making, which may influence the extent to which they successfully make meaning from their experience and the meanings arrived at after the experience, that is, posttraumatic growth, meaningful life, and restored beliefs in a just world.

Culture and Care in Health and Disease

Culture is a complex concept that consists of integrated patterns of traditions, beliefs, values, norms, symbols, and meanings that are shared, to varying degrees, by members of a community. It refers to shared realities and norms that constitute the learned systems of meaning for a particular community [17], including thresholds for pain [18] and other forms of suffering and affliction that are shaped by culture [19,20,21,22]. Culture influences the perceived scope and significance of obligations, duties, and interdependence with family; the perceived role of the patient in the decision-making process relative to that of other stakeholders in medical decision making; and the perceived likelihood that harm will arise from patient involvement in the decision-making process [17].

Culture shapes how people respond to disease. The concept of "care" is likewise strongly related to the cultural and historical roots of a society so that it is differently interpreted and applied in a diverse sociocultural context [23]. Culture also influences how the sick interpret symptoms, label them, understand them, communicate with others about them, and give meaning to them. As culture shapes the explanation and meaning one has for a disease, it also determines how one believes that disease is to be medically treated and cared for psychosocially. Kleinman [24] posited a model whereby health, illness, and health care-related aspects of societies are articulated as cultural systems. He further observed that while professional practitioners typically focus on the disease itself, the patient and the patient's family address the disease as an experience (i.e., illness) in its social and spiritual contexts.

Cultural competence in medicine is a complex multilayered accomplishment, requiring knowledge, skills, and attitudes whose acquisition is needed for effective cross-cultural negotiation in the clinical setting leading to improved therapeutic outcomes and decreased disparities in care. Effective cultural competence is based on knowledge of the notion of culture; on awareness of possible biases and prejudices related to stereotyping, racism, classism, sexism; on nurturing appreciation for differences in health care values; and on fostering the attitudes of humility, empathy, curiosity, respect, sensitivity, and awareness.

In clinical practice, the culturally competent oncologist must be aware of his own cultural beliefs and values and be able to communicate with cancer patients in culturally sensitive ways. He should develop a sense of appreciation for differences in health care values, based on the recognition that no culture can claim dominance over others and that cultures are evolving under their reciprocal influence on each other. Medical schools and oncology training must teach communication skills and cultural competence, while fostering in all students and young physicians those attitudes of humility, empathy, curiosity, respect, sensitivity, and awareness that are needed to deliver effective and culturally sensitive cancer care [25].

The world can be divided into two ethical cultures that are either autonomy-based (found mainly in North America, Northern Europe, and Australasia) or family-centered (the dominant type in Mediterranean, Eastern European, Asian, and traditional societies) [26,27]. This brings to fore the concept of cultural sensitivity. Cultural sensitivity is based on the recognition of cultural diversity and on the avoidance of stereotyping, but also common universal similarities beyond cultural differences [25,28]. Autonomy-based ethical cultures strongly focus on the individual patient's decision making and full disclosure to facilitate informed decision making. In contrast, family-centered ethical cultures are characterized as protecting patients from bad news in difficult situations. Cultural differences between patients and health care professionals often give rise to some common bedside misunderstandings and conflicts with respect to truth-telling, end-of-life choices, prevention and screening, and involvement in clinical trials. An example of the importance of cultural sensitivity in cancer care is the notion of "offering the truth" and truth-telling when breaking bad news to cancer patients [29,30,31]. This notion, based on allowing individual patients to choose their own paths and rhythm, was proposed as an effective means to respecting patients' autonomy to follow their own cultural norms. Simultaneous research in different countries was undertaken in the 1990s, and Ngelangel et al. [32] contributed their share when they expounded on the process of disclosure in Philippine oncological practice, emphasizing that different cultural reasons in every country and region support its degree of commitment to truth-telling.

Religiosity and Spirituality in Philippine Culture

Religion holds a central place in the life and culture of Filipinos [33]. Ninety-three percent of the population are Christians (mostly Roman Catholics), 5% are Muslim, and 2% are unspecified [4]. Religion is integrated into the country's public life, social networks, and personal spirituality and figures prominently in their corporate and personal sense of identity. Among the Christian community, the Catholic Church has established a strong relationship between Christian doctrine and the pattern of family and community life. Filipinos express strongly held beliefs in a host of experiences, ceremonies, rituals, novenas, and devotions. These patterns of behavior provide continuity in life, cohesion in the community, and, more importantly, a moral compass that is the essence of Filipino life. In this context, human mortality is viewed in a broader context, informed by belief, and surrounded by mystery [34].

Key concepts to consider in understanding the Filipino perspective on death and dying include cultural values and beliefs related to religion, family, and interpersonal harmony. Miranda and colleagues (cited in Doorenbos et al) [35] found that deeply religious Filipinos tended to attribute illness to reasons of God or a higher power. The predominant belief in the causes of disease and death were the "will of God," even though individuals also believed in personal responsibility [36]. As a nation, and individually as well, Filipinos are known for their grit and resilience [37]. The Filipino's spiritual richness—their great faith and hope in God's plan for their lives, their attitude toward God's providence, their often fatalistic and deterministic attitude toward life—all have given substance to the physical pain and the feelings of emptiness brought about by their diseased status. Overall, however, Filipino cancer patients are able to maintain a moderate to high quality of life. A significant factor contributing to rather good quality of life among Filipino cancer patients is their seemingly strong tendency to find meaning in their suffering. They can metamorphose themselves from an existentially sick person to an existentially well person [38]. This same spiritual affluence has led the patients to have a strong sense of hope, either imagined or real. Anchored on Snyder's hope theory [39], Calimag, Gonzales et al. (unpublished) [40], in their study entitled "Images of Hope: Photography as Therapy among Filipino Adolescents with Cancer," explored how Filipino adolescent cancer patients, instilled with a sense of hope, helped themselves go through the initial stages of anger, denial, and grief until they finally learned to accept their health status. Hope is "goal-directed thinking, in which people appraise their capability to produce workable routes to goals (pathway thinking), along with their potential to initiate and sustain movement via a pathway (agency thinking)" and when people hope, they hope for something, that is, a goal [39,41].

Doorenbos et al. [36] described 4 of the top 20 most important interventions designed to promote dignified dying in the Philippines as spiritual comfort interventions: to "encourage patient to express spiritual concerns," "protect religious beliefs," "provide spiritual support," and "provide privacy for spiritual behaviour." These interventions to promote dignified dying are consistent with Periyakoil et al.'s [42] study of Filipino Americans, which reported that finding meaning in one's existence and death was one of the factors influential in preserving dignity at the end of life, as well as with Yanez et al.'s [43] study on the facets of spirituality as predictors of adjustment to cancer.

Within Filipino hospice programs, this blending of belief and care may be seen as a motivating factor that draws volunteers toward the dying: in effect, they frame the nature of the interaction and provide succor for both patient and caregiver. From the website of the Madre de Amor Hospice Foundation [44] volunteers speak readily and clearly about their commitment as:

End of Life: Hard but Beautiful: *"During the pandemic, I still get to meet and chat with my hospice patient online. I delight in listening to her and hearing her stories."* (Fiona C. Vasallo, July 19, 2021)

Cruising in the Life of Angels: *"When I joined Madre de Amor Hospice Foundation six years ago, I had no inkling that it would be the realization of my youthful dream, I call it cruising in the life of angels."* (Jenelyn A. Rualo, RN April 3, 2019)

My Journey as a Hospice Doctor: *"I find the process of addressing the concerns of the patient and the family to be something of a reward in itself."* (Jeromel Lapitan, MD, March 20, 2019)

There is a need to recognize and address social and cultural beliefs that may be impeding efforts to improve cancer care, as well as to develop local cancer care expertise among community members who are familiar with cultural attitudes and beliefs [45]. There is also a need to support coping by giving hope, while a person's spirituality is impacted by chronic illness as well, with 80–93% of people reporting that spirituality helps them cope with serious illness and 50% reporting they became more spiritual after diagnosis of a serious condition [46].

The Filipino Family and Coping with Cancer

The family is the basic social and economic unit of Filipino kinship. Although family is important in many cultures, its central role in the lives of its members in the Philippines is unusually significant, with family being rated the most important source of happiness [47]. In times of illness, the extended family provides support and assistance [33]. Important values that might affect interactions between providers and patients and families in the context of terminal illness include a strong respect for elders, a strong reliance on family as decision makers in case of illness, and strong expectations of care by the family.

Lagman et al. [48] expound on this concept of "Leaving it to God" as a distinctly Filipino trait. Calimag, Mabanta et al. (unpublished) [49], in a study of coping among Filipino families of children with leukemia, has developed the following Shield of Resilience themes: core-based strategies ("Ako and Bahala," *"I am in charge"*); relationship-based strategies ("Tayo ang Bahala," *"We can do it together"*); culture-based strategies ("Bahala na," *"Just let go and we will overcome this no matter what"*); and faith-based strategies "Bathala na," *"It is all up to the Supreme Being," "Leaving it to God," "Trusting in the Lord"*), emphasizing a faith-based family-centered approach to cancer care [50]. Filipino values refer to the set of values that a majority of the Filipinos have historically held important in their lives. This Philippine values system includes their own unique assemblage of consistent ideologies, moral codes, ethical practices, etiquette, and cultural and personal values that are promoted by their society. As with any society, however, the values that individuals hold sacred can differ based on religion, upbringing, and other factors. As a general description, the distinct value system of Filipinos is rooted primarily in personal alliance systems, especially those based in kinship, obligation, friendship, religion (particularly Christianity), and business relationships [51]. The anthropologist Mercado [51] avers that the Filipino worldview is basically "nondualistic." Based on his linguistic analyses of Filipino value terms like *loob* (Cebuano *buot*), Mercado concludes that Filipinos desire harmony, not only in interpersonal relationships, but also with nature and religion, while remaining nondichotomous. One can note how *Hiya* (propriety/dignity), *Pakikisama* (companionship/esteem), and *Utang na loob* (gratitude/solidarity), are merely *surface values*—readily seen and observed values exhibited and esteemed by many Filipinos. These three values are considered branches from a single origin—the actual *core value* of the Filipino personality—*Kapwa*, which means "togetherness" and refers to community or not doing things alone. *Kapwa* is divided into two categories: *Ibang Tao* (other people) and *Hindi Ibang Tao* (akin to oneself). The surface values spin off of the core values through the pivotal aspect of *Pakikiramdam*, or shared inner perception (feeling for another) or *Pakikiramay* (empathy).

In her article "Filipino Attitude towards Pain Medication," Galanti [52] mentioned the fact that "Filipino nurses tend to undermedicate their patients ... because stoicism is highly valued and, for Catholic Filipinos, suffering is an opportunity to demonstrate virtue." Calimag [53], in a Q-Methodology analysis of perceptions of chronic pain among Filipino patients, found that the participants developed consensus around the statement, "My spiritual direction has allowed me to bear the pain silently," yet carried on with their activities of daily living. Thus, they lived through their chronic pain experience while fostering a balance between hope and resignation.

Patients use several cognitive and behavioral strategies to cope with their pain, including religious/spiritual factors such as prayers, and spiritual support to manage their pain. Tan [54] opines about how "Filipino pathos and algos are shaped by two important forces: religion and feudalism." Narratives about how Filipinos cope with pain are profuse using the concept of redemptive pain. According to Galanti [55], to stereotype is to reach an ending point whereby no effort is made to ascertain whether it is appropriate to apply it to the person in question; a generalization, on the other hand, serves as a starting point. "Knowledge of cultural customs can help avoid misunderstanding and enable practitioners to provide better care" [56].

A study by Calimag, Clutario et al. (unpublished) [57] entitled "Pain Things: The Lived Experience of Gynecologic Cancer Pain in Filipino Women" shows that the pain suffered by cancer patients is multidimensional. Anchored on the Roy Adaptation Model [58], the themes evolved included the following: dis-ease and dysfunction as pain of the physical wounds of cancer encompassing the pain from cancer; pain from the side effects of their treatment as well as pain from the different procedures; denial and deprivation as pain of the emotional wounds in cancer encompassing the feelings of denial about their present condition and the deprivation brought about by feelings of insecurities about the disease progression; fear of the unknown and the deprivation of fulfilling the spouse's needs due to dyspareunia and the loss of purpose due to the loss of the ability to procreate; division and desolation as pain of the social wounds in cancer encompassing their inability to fulfill their role in the family, and the limitation of participation in family functions, as well as the inability to work and participate in activities of daily living; detachment and destitution as the financial wounds of cancer that encompasses the times of reversals owing to the financial resources needed for treatment; and despair and devastation as the pain of spiritual wounds stemming from thoughts of impending and/ or untimely death and feelings of being neglected by a Higher Being. Other notable key elements or motivations are optimism about the future; pessimism regarding present situations and events; concern and care for other people, especially within the context of the Filipino family; the existence of friendship and friendliness; the habit of being hospitable; religious nature; respectfulness to self and others; respect for the female members of society; and the fear of God. It behooves the culturally competent oncologist to know the impact of social-emotional-financial contexts in chronic cancer pain in order to provide holistic care for the patient [59,60].

The importance of spousal caregiving and dyadic coping was explored in yet another paper by Calimag, Siongco et al. (unpublished) [61] entitled "Faces and Paces: The Phenomenology of Filipino Males with Cancer-Stricken Wives." The study answers the central question: "What typifies Filipino male spouses' portrayal of their coping strategies as caregivers of their cancer-stricken wives?"

Evidence indicates that responses within the couple that inhibit open communication between partner and patient are likely to have an adverse impact on psychosocial outcomes. Models that incorporate the interdependence of emotional responses and coping behaviors within couples have an emerging evidence base in psycho-oncology and may have the greatest validity and clinical utility in this setting [62,63]. The study is based on the social network theory [64], and the relational cultural theory [65]. The social network theory posits that the health-related outcomes of cancer patients are the result of interactions among types of informal caregivers, the nature of the caregiving relationship, caregiving as a function of such relationships, and the internal processes of the care recipient. The relational cultural theory, on the other hand, focuses on the unique social concerns that cancer survivors may face in maintaining authentic and mutual relationships, including relationships with a caregiver who may happen to be the spouse. The theory offers a complex integration of interpersonal and cultural dynamics to address cancer survivors' risks for disconnection, isolation, and social stigma, the context of which is highlighted in the De Laurentis et al. [59] study.

Although the consensus of researchers on caregiving and culture is that the caregiving experience differs significantly among cultural/ethnic groups, the question remains as to how cultural values and norms influence the caregiver experience [66]. Caregiving spouses want consolation too and must overcome their solitude by articulating experiences, being listened to, and, in this way, re-creating and strengthening their identity. As the head of the family, Filipino males are expected to be firm and in control, and yet resilient in every situation that the family encounters. As spouses of sick individuals, husbands of cancer-stricken wives often portray a positive attitude of "fighting" the disease beside their loved ones. Filipino males embrace a "macho" image [67,68]; thus, their emotional and psychological well-being as caregiving spouses may be inadvertently overlooked.

The coping themes evolved from the participants' narratives were clustered around five themes: Face Down, Face Away, Face It, Face With, and Face Up. The face is an apt metaphor, for it is something that is emotionally invested, thereby mirroring the vulnerability of the person's psyche. *Face Down* typifies the spouse's shock and fear upon learning of their wife's cancer diagnosis; *Face Away* reflects the isolation and grief about the whole situation; *Face It* reveals the positive coping stance of steadfastness despite knowledge of the wife's diagnosis and the courage to confront the problem head on; *Face With* entails coping and drawing strength from wife, children, and other relatives typical of the family-oriented approach to illness among Filipinos; and *Face Up* signifies the reliance on and supplication to a Supreme Being who is in control. Having cancer is a life-changing experience for most people. It is not uncommon for people to face down while experiencing anxiety, terror, shock, and upset, as well as emotional numbness and personal or social disconnection [69]. It is natural for anyone to feel sadness, fear, and uncertainty. It shows that the person has at least begun to accept the reality based on the Grief Cycle model first published in Kübler-Ross's classic work, *On Death and Dying* [70].

People have different reactions to life events. Deeply upset and agitated, husbands may *face down* after learning about the condition of their wives, which results from their lack of drive to accomplish other priorities. They tend to isolate themselves, fail to verbalize feelings, avoid interaction with peers, and cry to self—*Face Away* strategies that are unsupportive; negative effects may have a profound impact on the partner's mental and physical health, sometimes outweighing the positive impact of supportive exchanges [71]. These men keep their problems and struggles regarding the event to themselves, believing that as husbands, and men specifically, they should be strong and brave. For these men, airing out feelings and emotions is not an action they feel they should take. Men are traditionally thought of as being less emotional than women, but the evidence points more to a situation where men tend to show emotions that are bad for themselves and the people around them. There is substantial evidence that men have more difficulty showing their emotions and exert greater control over the expression of emotions. Some men tend to have a hard time enjoying the company of friends for a couple of reasons: first, because they cannot enjoy life as much as their friends do; and second, because their priorities are now differently set. Most of the respondents found it difficult to adjust and just blend in when they felt that they had more complicated problems than their friends. Several studies have shown that caregivers suffer physical and psychological ailments when they do not accept help [72,73,74].

Some husbands eventually turn their gaze toward the home. Filipino men with cancer-stricken wives then develop a positive outlook in life amidst their struggle for acceptance and adjustments and take responsibility for their lives and family as well. In these *Face It* strategies, these men realize that they are not only spouses to their cancer-stricken wives but also fathers to their children. *Face It* and *Face With* strategies are congruent with studies that propose better outcomes for the well-being of a relationship when partners view the illness as a relationship issue rather than an individual issue. This concept is known as dyadic coping [75]. Most of the caregiving Filipino husbands considered their family, especially their children, as a reason to keep their lives intact amidst an event beyond their control. Now that their wives are facing an unfortunate fate, they are left with what they consider as both a burden and a blessing to be the sole provider and caregiver for their wives and children. In families of cancer patients, poor family functioning has been associated with increased risk of depression and anxiety. The courage shown by these men is made possible through the value they put into their family and how Filipinos deal with crises as a family. This can be seen in supportive family types [76].

These findings among Filipino males are contrary to the findings of a study conducted by the University of Michigan Health System [77] which showed that spouses of cancer patients solely carried the load and were left alone without any information to deal with the problems in such situations. Spouses in this study were also reported to have less confidence than the patients in their ability to manage the illness, showed more uncertainty about the illness, and managed with less social support than the patient. Lewis and Deal [78] proposed that surviving strategies include learning to live with the condition, talking about the children, and being in control. Healing strategies include making progress and moving on, maintaining optimism, and trying to keep stress to a minimum.

Some of the respondents developed stronger relationships with their friends. In these *Face With* strategies, husbands found solace in the company of friends and recognized their sincere concern. Friends either allowed them to wind down after a long day or helped out with errands that must be accomplished. They claimed that friends provided perspective, gave them another view of reality, and gave honest feedback on their skewed version of that same reality. Trusted friends provided nuggets of advice, strength, and huge encouragement. Friends also provided financial support in paying bills related to hospital expenses and their everyday needs. Barriers to help-seeking behaviors should be explored and addressed [79], and health care professionals should encourage caregivers to reach out for help, and request and receive assistance from caregiving external supports from family, friends, and formal caregivers in order to promote caregiver resilience [80,81,82].

Facing Up, Filipino males pray to God for strength to accept their situation. Filipinos find inner strength and purpose during contemplation in a Supreme Being, especially whenever an unfortunate event happens. The verbalizations of the participants support the Filipinos' strong belief in a Supreme Being and show that their faith is intensified with suffering. Most of the respondents realized that they have no right to question God about their circumstances. Instead, they put their faith in the will of God. Vitaliano et al. [83] observed that "for Filipinos, God is the hope of the world." Religion may assist individuals in crises to salvage a sense of control or stability by giving some meaning to negative, chaotic events [84]. Belief in a Supreme Being is one of the Filipino values that husbands utilize as a means of coping, and it helps them wholeheartedly accept their caregiver role.

For many cancer patients, religion and spirituality play a strong role in coping with illness. They also play an important role in the management of older cancer patients, as with aging there is an increased interest in the meaning of life and in spiritual accomplishments (gerotranscendence) [85]. Several studies have documented a relationship between public religiousness (e.g., church attendance) and mortality [86]. Levin [87] has also presented strong evidence that religiousness is an important resource. Religiosity as a cultural resource can also be found in other cultural contexts [88,89].

Caregiving is a dynamic relationship that evolves over time. As the number of caregiving tasks increase, so does stress on the caregiver. A caregiver and their loved one will manage this challenge successfully if each person is able to express directly what they need, want. or can do. A relationship that allows for and respects boundaries and individual limitations can expand to include other caregivers without the risk of lessening the importance of the primary relationship that sustains the cared-for in the caring process. Filipino spouses of cancer-stricken wives view their situation as a fearful, stressful life-changing event, but their life experience of adjusting to their situation reflects Filipino historical, social, and cultural influences. The negative stigma of cancer, the role of the man in Filipino families as the breadwinner, and the embedded role of religion in Filipino society are the bases for the differences in the coping strategies of Filipino men as compared to men from other cultures.

Conclusion

To be culturally competent and supportive of culturally diverse patients' spiritual beliefs and practices, a health care professional must assume an attitude of receptivity to learning about other beliefs and maintain an attitude of acceptance toward every patient who is, inevitably, different. They should respond to patients in ways that allow them to integrate their spiritual experience rather than repress it. A health care professional engaged in oncology who fails to appreciate such spiritual-cultural values, beliefs, and behaviors will likely encounter some conflicts between the carer and the cared-for.

Health care professionals should also develop an attitude of sensitivity toward patients who make religious requests that are counter to medical traditions and institutional policies and use creativity and critical thinking to resolve the problems such requests might stir. When an impasse occurs, a spiritual care expert from the patient's culture or religion can be invited to participate. A religious leader often can provide a client with an alternative approach to religious observance that is compatible with Western health care practices.

In the Philippines, hospice and palliative care development, albeit with some challenges [90], is making progress after a checkered history that began with a groundswell of enthusiasm and the unequivocal support of the government: a factor that later waned, leading to a loss of momentum and a reduction in services. In a country that has insufficient investment in health services, a weak primary care system, high migration rates among health professionals, and widespread poverty—particularly among the indigenous population—such support is crucial if quality service is to become available to the Filipino needy at the end of life. There are some encouraging signs. Public awareness of hospice-palliative care is increasing. The number of service providers has risen to its highest level. Individuals are supplementing their initial training by enrolling in palliative courses. Highly motivated volunteers, both young and not-so-young, provide psychosocial support to patients and their family, or perform other tasks that support the delivery of care. The national organizations have become invigorated, exploring new ways of supporting its members, engaging with government, and seeking the means to encompass culturally competent palliative care within the public health system.

References

1. Ferlay J, Colombet M, Soerjomataram I, et al. Estimating the global cancer incidence and mortality in 2018: GLOBOCAN sources and methods. *Int J Cancer.* 2019;144(8):1941–1953.
2. The Philippine Cancer Control Program, Department of Health, 2020. Available from https://www.doh.gov.ph/philippine-cancer-control-program accessed March 15, 2020
3. Mery L, Bray F. Population-based cancer registries: a gateway to improved surveillance of non-communicable diseases. *ecancermedicalscience.* 2020 Jan1;14:1–4. DOI:10.3332/ecancer.2020.ed95
4. Central Intelligence Agency. *World Factbook 2018.* Available from https://www.cia.gov/library/publications/download/download-2018/index.html accessed March 15, 2020.
5. Park CL, Blake, EC. Resilience and recovery following disasters: The meaning making model. In SE Schulenberg (Ed.), *Disaster mental health and positive psychology.* Cham, Switzerland: Springer International; 2020:9–25. https://doi.org/10.1007/978-3-030-32007-2_2
6. Bonanno GA, Papa A, Lalande K, Zhang N, Noll JG. Grief processing and deliberate grief avoidance: a prospective comparison of bereaved spouses and parents in the United States and the People's Republic of China. *J Consult Clin Psychol.* 2005;73(1):86.
7. Park CL, Folkman S. Meaning in the context of stress and coping. *Rev Gen Psychol.* 1997;1(2):115–144.
8. Antonovsky A. *Unraveling the Mystery of Health—How People Manage Stress and Stay Well.* San Francisco: Jossey-Bass; 1987
9. Antonovsky A. Studying health vs. studying disease. Lecture at the Congress for Clinical Psychology and Psychotherapy, Berlin, February 19. 1990. Available online from the Universidade Nova de Lisboa.
10. Holland JC, Reznik I. Pathways for psychosocial care of cancer survivors. *Cancer: Interdisc Int J ACS.* 2005;104(S11):2624–2637.
11. Jim HS., Richardson SA, Golden-Kreutz DM, Andersen BL. Strategies used in coping with a cancer diagnosis predict meaning in life for survivors. *Health Psychol,* 2006; 25(6):753.
12. Horowitz MJ. Stress Response Syndromes: PTSD, Grief, Adjustment and Dissociative Disorders. Jason Aronson, Incorporated; 2011 Sep 16.
13. Vachon ML. Meaning, spirituality and wellness in cancer survivors. *Seminars Oncol Nurs,* 2008;24(3):218–225. WB Saunders. https://doi.org/10.1016/j.soncn.2008.05.010
14. van der Spek N, Vos J, van Uden-Kraan, CF, et al. Meaning making in cancer survivors: A focus group study. *PloS one.* 2013 Sep 26;8(9):e76089.
15. Park, CL, Edmondson D, Fenster JR, Blank TO. Meaning making and psychological adjustment following cancer: The mediating roles of growth, life meaning and restored just-world beliefs. *J Consult Clin Psychol.* 2008;76(5):863.
16. Pearson KA, Watkins ER, Kuyken W, Mullan EG. The psychosocial context of depressive rumination: Ruminative brooding predicts diminished relationship satisfaction in individuals with a history of past major depression. *Br J Clin Psychol.* 2020;49(2):275–280.
17. Ting-Toomey S, Chung LC. What are the essential cultural value patterns? In: Ting-Toomey S Chung LC. *Understanding Intercultural Communication.* Oxford University Press; 2007: 51–82.
18. Zatzick DF, Dimsdale, JE. Cultural variations in response to painful stimuli. *Psychosom Med.* 1990;52 (5):544–557.
19. Kirmayer LJ. Cultural variations in the response to psychiatric disorders and emotional distress. *Soc Sci Med.* 1989; 29(3): 327–339.
20. Kirmayer LJ, Young A. sulture and Somatization: Clinical, epidemiological, and ethnographic perspectives. *Psychosom Med.* 1998;60 (4):420–430.

21. Kirmayer LJ. Re-visioning psychiatry: Toward an ecology of mind in health and illness. In Laurence J, Kirmayer R (eds), *Cultural phenomenology, Critical Neuroscience and Global Mental Health*, 2015.

22. Kirmayer LJ., Gomez-Carrillo A, Veissière SPL. Culture and depression in global mental health: An ecosocial approach to the phenomenology of psychiatric disorders." *Soc Sci Med.* 2017;183:163–168.

23. Olarte JN. Cultural difference and palliative care. In Munroe, B, Oliviere D. (eds). *Patient Participation in Palliative Care: A Voice for the Voiceless.* Oxford: Oxford University Press; 2003:74–87. DOI:10.1093/acprof:oso/9780198515814.003.0006

24. Kleinman A. Concepts and a model for the comparison of medical systems as cultural systems. In Stewart R (ed) *Management of Health Care* Routledge; 2019 Oct 8. pp3–11.

25. Surbone A. Cultural aspects of communication in cancer care. *Support Care Cancer.* 2008;16(3):235–240.

26. Pellegrino ED. Is truth telling to the patient a cultural artifact? *JAMA.* 1997;268:1734–1735.

27. Cherny NI. Controversies in oncologist-patient communication: A nuanced approach to autonomy, culture and paternalism. *Practice.* 2012;26(1):37–43.

28. Bakan AB, Yıldız M. An investigation of the relationship between intercultural sensitivity and religious orientation among nurses. *J Relig Health.* 2021;60(1):178–187.

29. Yao T, Metzler T, Gorrell B. Truth-telling or Not: A dilemma for health care providers regarding disclosure of cancer in China. *J Law Med.* 2019;27(2):316.

30. Hahne J, Liang T, Khoshnood K, Wang X, Li X. Breaking bad news about cancer in China: Concerns and conflicts faced by doctors deciding whether to inform patients. *Patient education and counseling.* 2020;103(2):286–291.

31. Akanuwe JN, Black S, Owen S, Siriwardena AN. Communicating cancer risk in the primary care consultation when using a cancer risk assessment tool: Qualitative study with service users and practitioners. *Health Expectations.* 2020 Apr;23(2):509–518.

32. Ngelangel CA, Ramiro LS, Perez E, et al. Process of disclosure in Philippine oncological practice. *Phil J Oncol.*1996;2(1):13–27.

33. Wright M, Hamzah E, Phungrassami T, Bausa-Claudio A. *Hospice and Palliative Care in Southeast Asia: A Review of Developments and Challenges in Malaysia, Thailand and the Philippines.* Oxford: Oxford University Press; 2010.

34. Donlan RE (ed). Philippines: A country study. Washington, DC: GPO for the Library of Congress; 1991. http://countrystudies.us/philippines/45.htm Accessed 6 April 2008.

35. Doorenbos AZ, Perrin ME, Eaton L, et al. Supporting dignified dying in the Philippines. *International journal of palliative nursing.* 2011;17(3):125–130.

36. Clark S. Death and loss in the Philippines; 1998. Available in https://aboutphilippines.org/files/Death-and-Loss-in-the-Philippines.pdf. accessed March 7, 2020

37. Quismundo T. No doubting Thomas when it comes to Filipino grit. *The Philippine Daily Inquirer* inquirer.net [newspaper online] 2012 Aug 17 [cited 2021 Nov 15]. Available from https://globalnation.inquirer.net/47364/no-doubting-thomas-when-it-comes-to-filipino-grit

38. Ngelangel CA. Quality of life of Filipino cancer patients. *Can J Psychiatry.* 1994;39(10):617.

39. Snyder CR, Rand KL, Sigmon DR. Hope theory: A member of the positive psychology family. In: Gallagher MW, Lopez SJ, editors. 2017 The Oxford Handbook of Hope: Oxford University Press. Available from psycnet.apa.org accessed March 7, 2020.

40. Calimag MMP; Gonzales, MLJ; Gonzalez JMI, et al. Images of hope: Photography as therapy among Filipino adolescents with cancer. (Unpublished).

41. Cheavens JS, Feldman DB, Gum A, Michael ST, Snyder CR. Hope therapy in a community sample: A pilot investigation. *Soc Indic Res.* 2006;77:61–78.

42. Periyakoil VS, Noda AM, Chmura Kraemer H. Assessment of factors influencing preservation of dignity at life's end: Creation and the cross-cultural validation of the preservation of dignity card-sort tool. *J Palliat Med.* 2020;13(5):495–500.

43. Yanez B., Edmondson D., Stanton AL et al. Facets of spirituality as predictors of adjustment to cancer: relative contributions of having faith and finding meaning. *J Consult Clin Psychol.* 2009;77(4):730.

44. Madre de Amor Hospice Foundation.2021 [cited 2021 Nov15] Available from http://www.hospice.org.ph

45. Seow H, Bainbridge D, Brouwers M, Bryant D, Toyofuku ST, Kelley ML. Common care practices among effective community-based specialist palliative care teams: a qualitative study. *BMJ Support Palliat Care.* 2020;10(1):e3–e3.

46. Friebohle C. Taking care of the forgotten: A pastoral response to the hospice care professional. 2020, 1–40. DigitalCommons@CSB/SJU [cited 2020 Mar 15] Available from https://digitalcommons.csbsju.edu/sot_papers/1928/

47. Virola RA, Encarnacion JO, Pascasio MC. Improving the way we measure progress of society: The Philippine happiness index among the poor and the unhappy. Published by the International Statistical Institute, The Hague, The Netherlands, December 2012. In *Proc. 58th World Statistics Congress, International Statistical Institute, Dublin, Ireland, 2011,* 4985–4990. Available from http://www.2011.isiproceedings.org/papers/950161.pdf

48. Lagman RA, Yoo GJ, Levine EG, Donnell KA, Lim HR. "Leaving it to God" religion and spirituality among Filipina immigrant breast cancer survivors. *J Relig Health.* 2014;53(2):449–460.

49. Calimag MMP, Mabanta ELD, Macarubbo NA, Madrona VAC, Magadia JKS. The shield of resilience: The lived experience of Filipino families of children with leukemia. (Unpublished).

50. Mooney-Doyle K, dos Santos MR, Woodgate RL. Family-centered care in pediatric cncology. In *Pediatric Oncology Nursing* (pp. 7–19). Cham, Switzerland: Springer;2020:7–19.

51. Mercado L. *Elements of Filipino Philosophy.* 1993 Divine Word University Publications, Tacloban City.

52. Galanti GA. An introduction to cultural differences. *West J Med.* 2000;172(5):335.

53. Calimag, MMP. The P-A-I-N-S typology of health literacy perspectives among Filipino chronic non-malignant pain sufferers: A Q methodology study. *J Med Univ Santo Tomas.* 2020;4(1):394–406. doi: 10.35460/2546-1621.2020-0008

54. Tan, M. Filipino Pain. *Philippine Daily Inquirer* inquirer.net [newspaper online] 2013 Jul 16. [cited 2019 Dec 30] Available from https://opinion.inquirer.net/56715/filipino-pain

55. Galanti GA. Filipino attitudes toward pain medication. A lesson in cross-cultural care. *West J Med.* 2000;173(4):278–279.

56. Galanti G. *Caring for Patients from Different Cultures.* 2nd ed. Philadelphia: University of Pennsylvania Press; 1997.

57. Calimag MMP, Clutario JD; Co, C; Co, IDK; Co, JJ; Co, LK. Pain things: The lived experience of gynecologic cancer pain in Filipino women (Unpublished).

58. Hanna DR, Roy C. Roy adaptation model and perspectives on the family. *Nurs. Sci. Q.* 2001 Jan;14(1):10–13.

59. De Laurentis M, Rossana B, Andrea B, Riccardo T, Valentina I. The impact of social-emotional context in chronic cancer pain: Patient-caregiver reverberations. *Support Care Cancer.* 2019;27(2), 705–713.

60. Graboyes EM, Gupta A, Sterba KR. Financial impact of cancer treatment. In Fundakowski CE (ed). *Head and neck cancer.* Cham, Switzerland: Springer; 2020:173–186.

61. Calimag MMP, Singson AS, Siongco PRL, Sisante LC, DR, Sison, KM. So, JM. Faces and paces: The phenomenology of Filipino males with cancer-stricken wives (Unpublished).

62. Kim Y, Kashy DA., Wellisch DK, et al. Quality of life of couples dealing with cancer: dyadic and individual adjustment among breast and prostate cancer survivors and their spousal caregivers. *Ann Behav Med*. 2008; 35(2):230–238.

63. Regan TW, Lambert SD, Kelly B, Falconier M, Kissane D, Levesque JV. Couples coping with cancer: exploration of theoretical frameworks from dyadic studies. *Psychooncology*. 2015;24(12):1605–1617.

64. Segrin C, Badger TA. Psychological distress in different social network members of breast and prostate cancer survivors. *Res Nurs Health*. 2010;33(5):450–464.

65. Raque-Bogdan TL. Relational cultural theory and cancer: Addressing the social well-being of a growing population. *Pract Innov*. 2019 Jun;4(2):99–111.

66. Pharr JR, Dodge Francis C, Terry C., Clark MC. Culture, caregiving, and health: exploring the influence of culture on family caregiver experiences. *ISRN Public Health*, 2014;1–8. DOI:http://dx.doi.org/10.1155/2014/689826

67. Angeles LC. The Filipino male as "macho-machunurin": Bringing men and masculinities in gender and development studies. *Kasarinlan J Third World Issues*. 2001;16(1):9–30. Third World Studies Centre, University of the Philippines

68. Modequillo A. The "Macho" Image. The Freeman Cebu Lifestyle under the banner of *The Philippine Star*, June 5, 2016.

69. Najjar N, Davis LW, Beck-Coon K, Carney Doebbeling C. Compassion fatigue: A review of the research to date and relevance to cancer-care providers. *J Health Psychol*. 2009;14(2):267–277.

70. Kübler-Ross E. *On death and dying*. London: Routledge; 1973.

71. Mokuau N, Braun KL, Daniggelis E. Building family capacity for Native Hawaiian women with breast cancer. Health & Social Work. 2012 Nov 1;37(4):216–224.

72. Bernard LL, Guarnaccia CA. Two models of caregiver strain and bereavement adjustment: A comparison of husband and daughter caregivers of breast cancer hospice patients. *The Gerontologist*. 2003;43(6):808–816.

73. Clukey L. "Just be there": Hospice caregivers' anticipatory mourning experience. *J Hospice Palliat Nurs*. 2007;9(3):150–158.

74. Kris AE, Cherlin EJ, Prigerson H, et al. Length of hospice enrollment and subsequent depression in family caregivers: 13-month follow-up study. *Am J Geriatr Psychiatry*. 2006;14(3), 264–269.

75. Acitelli LK, Badr HJ. My illness or our illness? Attending to the relationship when one partner is ill. In: Revenson TA, Kayser K, Bodenmann G (eds). *Couples coping with stress: Emerging perspectives on dyadic coping*. Washington, DC: American Psychological Association, 2005: 121–136. https://doi.org/10.1037/11031-006.

76. Nissen KG, Trevino K, Lange T, Prigerson HG. Family relationships and psychosocial dysfunction among family caregivers of patients with advanced cancer. Journal of pain and symptom management. 2016 Dec 1;52(6):841–849.

77. University of Michigan Health System. "Cancer patients, spouses report similar emotional distress." *Science Daily*. [newspaper online] 2007 Sep 21 Available from http://www.sciencedaily.com/releases/2007/09/070920111419.htm

78. Lewis F, Deal L. Balancing our lives: A study of the married couple's experience with breast cancer recurrence. *Oncol Nurs Forum*. 1995;22(6):943–953.

79. Mansfield AK, Addis ME, Courtenay W. Measurement of Men's Help Seeking: Development and Evaluation of the Barriers to Help Seeking Scale. *Psych Men Masculinity*. 2005;6(2):95.

80. Northfield S, Nebauer M. The Caregiving Journey for Family Members of Relatives With Cancer. How do the cope? *Clin J Oncol Nursg*. 2010;14(5):567–577.

81. Litzelman K, Reblin M, McDowell HE, DuBenske LL. Trajectories of social resource use among informal lung cancer caregivers. *Cancer*. 2020;126(2):425–431.

82. Shin JY, Choi SW. Interventions to promote caregiver resilience. *Curr Opin Support Palliat Care*. 2020;14(1):60.

83. Vitaliano PP, Zhang J, Scanlan JM. Is caregiving hazardous to one's physical health? A meta-analysis. Psychological bulletin. 2003 Nov;129(6):946.

84. Szałachowski RR, Tuszyńska-Bogucka W. "Yes, in Crisis We Pray." The Role of Prayer in Coping with Pandemic Fears. Religions. 2021 Oct;12(10):824 Springer, Cham.

85. Balducci L. The older cancer patient: Religious and spiritual dimensions. In Extermann M (eds) *Geriatr Oncol.* 2020:1015–1027. DOI: https://doi.org/10.1007/978-3-319-57415-8_19.

86. Page RL, Peltzer JN, Burdette AM, Hill TD. Religiosity and health: a holistic biopsychosocial perspective. *Journal of Holistic Nursing.* 2020 Mar;38(1):89–101.

87. Levin JS. Religion and health: Is there an association, is it valid, and is it causal?. *Social Science & Medicine.* 1994 Jun 1;38(11):1475–1482. https://doi.org/10.1016/0277-9536(94)90109-0.

88. Oman D, Syme SL. Weighing the evidence: What is revealed by 100+ meta-analyses and systematic reviews of religion/spirituality and health?. Why religion and spirituality matter for public health. 2018:261–281.

89. Almuhtaseb MI, Alby F, Zucchermaglio C, Fatigante M. Religiosity as a cultural resource for Arab-Palestinian women's coping with cancer. *SAGE Open.* 2020;10(1):2158244019898730.

90. Calimag MP, Silbermann M. Current challenges and evolving strategies in implementing cancer and palliative care services in the Philippines. *Br J Cancer Res.* 2019;2(2):257–263. doi: 10.31488/bjcr.127

16

Spiritual and Religious Impacts on Advanced Cancer Care in Australia

Clare O'Callaghan, Natasha Michael, and David Kissane

A holistic approach to care is vital to truly support patients with advanced cancer as they adapt to physical and functional decline and deal with psychoexistential concerns [1]. Equally, family caregivers require attention as they undertake the sometimes rewarding but isolating and overwhelming role of caregiving that, when unsupported, leads to misdirected anger and distress that can negatively impact patient care [2,3]. Central to a holistic approach to care of the cancer patient is the provision of spiritual care. Beliefs held by the patients and caregivers, whether religious or more broadly spiritual, are entwined within their sociocultural backgrounds and can shape how they come to terms with a diagnosis of cancer [4]. Although many patients come to accept their mortality, some experience intense angst and spiritual despair [5].

While debates about definitions of spirituality continue [6], one international consensus team described spirituality as the means through which "persons seek ultimate meaning, purpose, transcendence, and experience relationship to self, family, others, community, society, nature, and the significant or sacred" [7, p. 887]. Many turn to spirituality in their efforts to cope with advanced cancer [8,9], and care guidelines recommend access to spiritual care from specialist (chaplains, pastoral carers) and generalist health workers [10,11]. Religion can be a part of spirituality and is associated with organised beliefs, practices, and closeness with the transcendent [12].

Oversight of this landscape leaves little doubt about the importance of attention to matters spiritual within the health and sociocultural context and the need for routine inquiry into the spiritual concerns of those suffering from advanced illness. Religious beliefs can affect treatment decisions [13], and spiritual well-being can protect patients against psychological distress [14], anxiety, and depression [15]. Religiousness can also help caregivers to experience peace, comfort, strength [16], and more adaptive bereavement [17]. Hospital-based spiritual support is also associated with higher hospice usage, and lower aggressive interventions, death in the intensive care unit, and end-of-life care costs [13]. Unaddressed spiritual issues can contribute to increased spiritual pain [18,19] and reduced quality of life [20], coping [9], care satisfaction, and perception of care quality [21]. Conversely, negative religious coping framed by deeply held cultural or religious beliefs such as belief in divine punishment, can lead to suicidal ideation [22], while religious guilt and feeling abandoned by God can mitigate the use of religious resources [23,24].

Thus, in striving to meet spiritual needs [25], we aim to ameliorate suffering related to existential, religious, or other concerns. Despite patients and caregivers attesting to the helpfulness of spiritual care in the hospital setting [3] and articulating that their doctors should inquire about spiritual needs and sources of support [26], there has been sparse research and implementation of this domain in the Australian setting [27,28]. To optimize spiritual care in advanced illness, further understanding of patients' and caregivers' views about spirituality, religion, and spiritual care is needed. In this chapter, we report on a series of studies conducted in Australia examining spiritual needs, concerns, and care provision.

A Multisite Project: Australian Patients' and Caregivers' Spiritual Well-being and Views

Across the years 2016–2019, we conducted a range of studies at three Christian, faith-based hospitals in Melbourne and Sydney, Australia. Using mixed methods and qualitative designs in cross-sectional and observational studies, we examined spirituality among 370 patients and caregivers affected by advanced illnesses.

Our overarching research question was: What are the spiritual encounters (experiences) and requirements of adult patients and caregivers affected by advanced, serious illness including cancer, and what are their implications for service provision?

The vast majority of participants had been ill with advanced cancer for some years; one-quarter were nonreligious and one-third were born overseas. A Judaeo-Christian orientation was prominent among those who were religiously affiliated. We used the well-known Functional Assessment of Chronic Illness Therapy-Spiritual Scale-12 (FACIT-SP-12) [29] and explored their views about the roles of spirituality, religion, and spiritual care using questions derived primarily from Balboni and colleague's 2007 study [30] of religious and spiritual support. We also developed a screening tool to identify unrecognized needs, the Spiritual Concerns Checklist (SCC) [31], and assessed how well our services delivered spiritual care. A subgroup of participants self-nominated for a qualitative interview to examine views about spiritual care more specifically. About half of those invited to participate in these studies did so. A synthesis of our findings follows, together with their implications for spiritual care. Further study details, including sociodemographic and clinical characteristics of participants, can also be found in published manuscripts [31–34].

The Importance of Spirituality/Religion

Around 60% of our participants were Christian, about one-quarter had no religious affiliation, 7% were Jewish, and 3% were Buddhist. The predominance of participants with Judaeo-Christian beliefs reflected the catchments of our collaborating hospitals. By way of comparison, Australian census data reveals the following affiliations: 52% are Christian, 30% no religion, 2.6% Buddhism, and 0.4% Judaism [35]. In our studies, approximately two-thirds of patients and their caregivers reported that spirituality and religion were important. Many described how spirituality inspired their individual, communal, and aesthetic lives, as well as their belief systems. After the initial cancer diagnosis, half of the patients and one-third of their caregivers prayed more than once a week, compared with one-third or less before diagnosis. Moreover, nearly half of the patients and one-third of caregivers meditated more than once a week compared with only one-quarter beforehand. These spiritual/religious activities helped them to cope, but, as illness advanced, attendance at church or synagogue services declined because of health needs.

In contrast to this group embracing spiritual/religious practice, one-third described spirituality or religion as not important and one-quarter reported that both were unimportant. Some spoke of humanitarian values or the wonders of science, while others referred to church-related disgraces exemplified by sexual abuse.

Spiritual Well-being and Associations with Religious Affiliation and Spiritual Support

Participants' overall FACIT-Sp-12 scores are found in Table 16.1. For both patients and caregivers, patients with Christian or Buddhist affiliations, and caregivers with any affiliation, there were higher faith subscale scores on the FACIT-Sp-12 (suggesting higher spiritual well-being) than those who reported no religious affiliation. There were no associations between the FACIT-Sp-12 meaning and peace subscale and religious affiliations.

Religious/faith communities away from hospitals were supporting one-third of patients and a quarter of caregivers. Those who received at least some (patients) or moderate (caregivers) spiritual support had higher Total FACIT-SP-12 well-being scores compared to those whose needs were less met by their communities. For the 27% of patients who had at least moderate spiritual support needs met by the hospital, the total FACIT-SP-12 score was significantly higher than those whose needs were less met. Among caregivers, 19% had spiritual needs met by hospitals to at least a moderate extent, but their spiritual well-being did not differ from that of people whose needs were unmet by hospitals.

Spiritual Requirements and Concerns

One-third of patients and 40% of caregivers reported that they did not have spiritual requirements, and just under half of the patients (45%) and caregivers (44%) reported no religious requirements. However, while only 15% of patients directly sought spiritual care, nearly 62% of all patients reported at least one spiritual concern on the SCC

Table 16.1 FACIT Sp-12 Well-being Scores [mean (SD)]

	Patients N = 261	Caregivers N = 109
Meaning/Peace (0–32)	23.3 (5.8)	22.8 (5.4)
Faith (0–16)	8.7 (5.0)	8.0 (4.5)
Total score (0–48)	31.9 (8.6)	30.5 (8.4)

[25]. Most commonly reported were existential concerns, exemplified by fear of the dying process (32% of patients) and loss of control (31% of patients). Additionally, patients reported religious and emotional concerns of regret (20%) and guilt (13%) about past behaviors, self-forgiveness (17%) and need to forgive others (14%), loss of meaning (15%), and loss of hope (13%).

Among caregivers, 52% reported at least one spiritual concern, with the highest ranking concerns including guilt over past behaviors (25%), losing control (21%), loss of hope (17%), and fear of death (13%). Among those patients who were religiously oriented, the median number of concerns was two, while one-quarter of the patient cohort expressed more than four concerns. Psychometric appraisal of the SCC revealed a single factor, with a satisfactory Cronbach's alpha of 0.82. Concurrent validity was demonstrated with the FACIT-Sp-12 and indicated that having unaddressed spiritual concerns was negatively associated with a sense of meaning and peace about life. Though the preliminary psychometric analysis of the SCC suggests the need for further refinement and validation, these data point to the benefit of screening to better recognize and support people with spiritual concerns.

Pastoral Care (Chaplain) Experiences

Among patients, two-thirds were offered, and one-third received, pastoral care visits. The visit content included shared prayer, receipt of sacraments, existential or general discussions, and informational support. Two respondents described how visits helped them to reconnect with their spiritual lives. Some individuals described how visits offered understanding, relieved concerns, reassured, and/or elicited peace. Among caregivers, pastoral care visits were offered to two-fifths and were received by one-third. Many also reported that they were calming, comforting, and/or encouraged faith. However, care in interpretation is always needed as five caregivers experienced discomfort with such visits. One, for example, erroneously interpreted that the visit indicated that a patient's recent treatment was unsuccessful.

The Role of Hospitals in Supporting Spiritual/Religious Requirements

When asked if Australian hospitals should support patients' and caregivers' spiritual requirements when affected by advanced illnesses, 75% of patients and 80% caregivers agreed; small numbers (around 1 in 20) disagreed. Patients who agreed explained that spiritual care, when desired, addressed the whole person and that many with advanced illnesses needed psychoexistential support for demoralization, fear, suffering, feeling of burden, and existential issues. Some noted that spiritual support could strengthen, comfort, help faith, and promote acceptance, coping, and/or motivation "to battle on." A few believed that God could help to lengthen lives and one wrote, "Physical and spiritual release are essential for closure."

Caregivers who agreed that hospitals should support spiritual requirements noted that caregivers can be stressed and potentially have spiritual questions while watching a loved one suffer. They could therefore benefit from support and comfort. Many patients and caregivers wrote that spiritual care could help others but not themselves, while only a small group considered it inappropriate, explaining that hospitals should be secular; that community and family/friend spiritual support were enough; that beliefs were personal; and/or that staff kindness and positive aesthetics were sufficient:

> ... kindness and understanding of staff members ... very important. The ambience of the hospital is also important—e.g. peace, lovely gardens, lack of sterility.... A kind word, a gentle approach (not necessary efficiency) a little time can mean everything to a person who is stressed in the hospital environment.

In added comments related to how hospitals could extend spiritual support, some patients and caregivers emphasized the importance of staff compassion and the availability of quiet, reflective, and private spaces. Gratitude was expressed when a staff member found a private room for family when they were "overwhelmed and upset."

Qualitative Interview Findings from Patients and Caregivers

We interviewed 40 participants and 10 caregivers and invited them to describe health care experiences that connected them with what they considered to be sacred or important to their well-being [34]. The thematic analysis revealed three themes: (1) participants held contested and varied beliefs about spiritual care; (2) they valued staff affirming their worth and dignity; and (3) they recognized how the hospital's organizational and environmental ethos impacted their holistic well-being. Strikingly, views about spirituality and spiritual care were disparate, reflecting norms in society. Spirituality and religion could be conflated, that is, considered as "one and the same," or they could be completely independent. Examples of these discordant views included that it was only the province of pastoral care; any quality care is spiritual; staff care couldn't be spiritual; and clinicians ought not to be distracted by cultural or spiritual beliefs. Some participants considered spiritual terms to be nebulous or disrespectful of the atheist. This highlighted the practical challenges in delivering spiritually oriented care.

In summary, while *some* participants resonated with the term *spiritual care* referring to helping individuals to find peace, deal with fear of death and other existential issues, *all* participants valued concepts within the spiritual care definition. They welcomed respectful care that valued patients and families, as well as religious affiliations, and/or improved the quality of their lives. Importantly, participants emphasized how the hospital's policies, services, and environmental features helped their sense of well-being. No one was offended by the presence of religious icons, including participants without religious or Christian affiliations. One summed it up as care that helped them to "want to live life to live rather than live life to die." The kindness found in humanistic and compassionate care was deeply appreciated. Those who experienced pastoral care valued connections made and shared prayers, sacraments, and rituals.

Discussion, with Implications for Spiritual Care

These Australian studies highlight that most patients and caregivers affected by advanced cancer regard spirituality and religion as important. Indeed, they held spiritual concerns and believed that spiritual care should be available for those who needed it. This confirmed international findings regarding the importance of spirituality and addressing spiritual concerns in patients with advanced illness [3,6]. The word "spirituality" is better understood in the community than "existential," but regrettable confusion still exists about its meaning [36]. Many participants engaged in more prayer and meditation following diagnoses but because of declining health attended fewer religious services. Similar findings have been described in a study of American cancer patients [30]. As a more secular society, Australians, however, attended substantially fewer services than those patients in the United States (pre- to postdiagnosis: 56–44% in the United States versus 15–7% in Australia) [30,31].

Cultural differences likely influence findings in spiritualty studies in complex ways [4]. For example, while our participants' Christian and nonreligious affiliations were comparable to the general Australian (52% Christian; 25% no religion) and U.S. (65% Christian; 26% nonreligious) populations, there were differences across countries regarding the importance of religion. In the United States, 88% of patients consider it important [30], compared to 61% in our study [31]. Cultural variations are also apparent in FACIT Sp-12 spiritual well-being scores. Australia's FACIT Sp-12 scores are lower than those scores in the United States [37], but comparable to ratings in Singapore [38], South Korea [39], and Switzerland [40].

One cultural consideration is the meaning attributed to the word "spiritual" in the United States, where 98% of patients considered themselves spiritual [18] and recorded higher spiritual well-being scores than the Australians [37]. The interpretation of the FACIT Sp-12 scale as a measure of spiritual well-being, in terms of both baseline population variations and responsiveness, is worth further examination, including how the measure aligns with diverse perspectives.

For a secular society with falling rates of religious affiliation, the nature of ritual that supports adaptation to loss and mourning emerges as a new challenge. Sociology has long recognized the contribution of religious ritual to coping and adaptation. Some see the therapist's couch taking the place of the chaplain's prayerbook. Others see the celebratory dinner with speeches of gratitude replacing the celebrant's homily; the biography and life review aided by a volunteer creating a legacy for the family; and music aided by a therapist replacing the sacred chant. Thus, caution may be needed in endorsing perceptions that facing one's mortality is a spiritual event [41] or theorizing health care as a spiritual act [42]. Great care is needed that health care providers respect patients' and caregivers' views, whether these are faith-based, spiritual, or secular in nature.

The broad meaning of spirituality has been considered both a weakness, given how it can be misunderstood, and a strength, for allowing pluralist views [36]. Breitbart associates "spirituality" with the uniquely human capacity for self-contemplation and creativity beyond biological limitations [43], and many respondents in our studies affirmed the value of spirituality for guidance, self-discovery, meaning, strength, and hope. However, some Australians struggle with the term, and this is likely to continue as Australia becomes increasingly multicultural and secularized, with greater than one-quarter of residents now overseas-born [35]. Hence, additional, relatable term/s are needed to communicate each hospital's endeavors to support patients' and caregivers' holistic well-being. Terms could include *values-based care* [44], which refers to care that people regard as significant; *humanistic medicine* [45–47] embracing narratives, the shared human experience and pursuit of the good for the patient; and *hospitality*, a term derived from medieval hospice shelters that described the gracious disposition toward travelers [48].

Our participants offered valuable suggestions for how the health services could reinforce and extend their personhood as they experienced challenges associated with patients' advancing illnesses. These included faith-based hope and/or meaning-focused practices, and chapels, religious leaders, texts, and icons traditionally associated with spiritual care. They also included welcoming, considerate behaviors, and organizational and environmental characteristics with more supportive and "home-like" associations, such as information, family meeting areas, and gardens. Appreciation of being helped to "live in the moment," sensory experiences, and so-called "small things in life" have also been highlighted by patients in spirituality research elsewhere [49]. Many of these qualities resonate with hospitality theory, which focuses on the nature of host communities and guests [50]: Hospitality values all diverse and unique individuals needing care [51], is concerned for another's comfort, goes beyond what is generally expected, and communicates friendliness, kindness, availability, and "something of oneself" [52,53]. Hospitality supports holistic well-being through providing a welcoming human presence and home-like context where patients and families can flourish. It reaches to the essence of humanistic medicine taught by so many for the secular world.

Specialist (chaplains, pastoral carers) and generalist health workers are well placed to offer hospitality alongside humanistic or spiritual care. Importantly, health workers need to ask patients and caregivers affected by advanced cancer of their spiritual concerns and offer support when needed. Our studies found that spiritual and religious needs will be sufficiently met by external faith-based communities for some we meet. Additionally, health workers need to inquire about what helps patients and caregivers to feel welcome and valued; "what really matters" [36] at human relationship, organizational, and environmental levels, and appropriately respond as much as possible. Such inquiry can be in formal assessments and/or embedded in daily clinical care [54].

Conclusion

A single definition of spirituality will not likely accommodate the multitude of views on life, death, cosmology, ethics, and human destiny. Research findings on spirituality will also likely remain contextually relevant and logically generalizable. As such, seeking terminology and constructs, such as hospitality, that are universally understood and esteemed across traditions may prove to resonate more significantly across cultures. Hospitality alongside spiritual care provides opportunities for patients and caregivers to create goals, experience what is valued, articulate the existential and meaningfully live until death, and yield memories that may sustain the bereaved. We suggest that providing hospitality alongside spiritual care could respectfully convey person-centered care that is humanistic in its nature and suited to pluralist palliative care communities as found in Australia. Humbly respecting the other, finding common ground, accompanying and listening with empathy and compassion, we can bring excellent diagnostic and clinical skills together in a value-driven pathway that will improve holistic advanced cancer care.

Acknowledgment: We thank our collaborators, including Drs. I. Bobevski, J. M. Clayton, E. Georgousopoulou, and D. Seah, for their assistance with these studies. We also thank our funders, Cabrini Foundation Sambor Family Clinical Research Grant, St Vincent's Curran Foundation Grant, and the University of Notre Dame Australia SoMS Research Support Grant.

References

1. Chochinov HM, Hassard T, McClement S, et al. The landscape of distress in the terminally ill. *J Pain Symptom Manage.* 2009;38(5):641–649.
2. Henriksson A, Carlander I, Arestedt K. Factors associated with feelings of reward during ongoing family palliative caregiving. *Palliat Support Care.* 2015;13:505–512.
3. Selman LE, Brighton LJ, Sinclair S, et al. Patients' and caregivers' needs, experiences, preferences and research priorities in spiritual care: A focus group study across nine countries. *Palliat Med.* 2018;32:216–230.
4. Speck P. Culture and spirituality: essential components of palliative care. *Postgrad Med J.* 2016;92:341–345.
5. Kissane DW. The relief of existential suffering. *Arch Intern Med.* 2012;172:1501–1505.
6. European Association for Palliative Care. EAPC taskforce on spiritual care in palliative care. 2010. Available at: http://www.eapcnet.eu/themes/clinicalcare/spiritualcareinpalliat ivecare.aspx Accessed April 15, 2016. 2010.
7. Puchalski C, Ferrell B, Virani R, et al. Improving the quality of spiritual care as a dimension of palliative care: The report of the Consensus Conference. *J Palliat Med.* 2009;12:885–904.
8. Piderman KM, Kung S, Jenkins SM, et al. Respecting the spiritual side of advanced cancer care: A systematic review. *Curr Oncol Rep.* 2015;17:1–9. Doi 10.1007/s11912-014-0429-6
9. Vallurupalli M, Lauderdale K, Balboni MJ, et al. The role of spirituality and religious coping in the quality of life of patients with advanced cancer receiving palliative radiation therapy. *J Support Oncol.* 2012;10:81–87.
10. Handzo G, Bowden J. A response to Geriatric Oncology, Spirituality, and Palliative Care by Dr. Lodovicio Balducci. *J Pain Symptom Manage.* 2019;58:e1–e2.
11. National Consensus Project for Quality Palliative Care. Clinical practice guidelines for quality palliative care, 4th ed. 2018. Richmond, VA: National Coalition for Hospice and Palliative Care. Available from https://www.nationalcoalitionhpc.org/ ncp. Accessed March 1, 2019.
12. Koenig HG, King DE, Carson VB. *Handbook of Religion and Health.* 2nd ed. Oxford: Oxford University Press; 2012.
13. Balboni TA, Balboni M, Enzinger AC, et al. Provision of spiritual support to patients with advanced cancer by religious communities and associations with medical care at the end of life. *JAMA Intern Med.* 2013;173:1109–1117.
14. Bernard M, Strasser F, Gamondi C, et al. Relationship between spirituality, meaning in life, psychological distress, wish for hastened death, and their influence on quality of life in palliative care patients. *J Pain Symptom Manage.* 2017;54:514–522.

15. Johnson KS, Tulsky JA, Hays JC, et al. Which domains of spirituality are associated with anxiety and depression in patients with advanced illness? *J Gen Intern Med.* 2011;26:751–758.

16. Paiva BS, Carvalho AL, Lucchetti G, Barroso EM, Paiva CE. "Oh, yeah, I'm getting closer to God": Spirituality and religiousness of family caregivers of cancer patients undergoing palliative care. *Support Care Cancer.* 2015;23:2383–2389.

17. Fenix JB, Cherlin JB, Prigerson HG. Religiousness and major depression among bereaved family caregivers: A 13-month follow-up study. *J Palliat Care.* 2006;22:286–292.

18. Delgado-Guay MO, Hui D, Parsons HA, et al. Spirituality, religiosity, and spiritual pain in advanced cancer patients. *J Pain Symptom Manage.* 2011;41:986–994.

19. Mako C, Galek K, Poppito SR. Spiritual pain among patients with advanced cancer in palliative care. *J Palliat Med.* 2006;9:1106–1113.

20. Perez-Cruz PE, Langer P, Carrasco C, et al. Spiritual pain is associated with decreased quality of life in advanced cancer patients in palliative care: An exploratory study. *J Palliat Med.* 2019;22:663–669.

21. Astrow AB, Kwok G, Sharma RK, Fromer N, Sulmasy DP. Spiritual needs and perception of quality of care and satisfaction with care in hematology/medical oncology patients: A multicultural assessment. *J Pain Symptom Manage.* 2018;55:56–64 e51.

22. Trevino KM, Balboni M, Zollfrank A, Balboni T, Prigerson HG. Negative religious coping as a correlate of suicidal ideation in patients with advanced cancer. *Psychooncology.* 2014;23:936–945.

23. Winkelman WD, Lauderdale K, Balboni MJ, et al. The relationship of spiritual concerns to the quality of life of advanced cancer patients: preliminary findings. *J Palliat Med.* 2011;14:1022–1028.

24. Zarzycka B, Sliwak J, Krok D, Ciszek P. Religious comfort and anxiety in women with cancer: The mediating role of hope and moderating role of religious struggle. *Psychooncology.* 2019;28:1829–1835.

25. Pearce MJ, Coan AD, Herndon JE, 2nd, Koenig HG, Abernethy AP. Unmet spiritual care needs impact emotional and spiritual well-being in advanced cancer patients. *Support Care Cancer.* 2012;20:2269–2276.

26. Best M, Butow P, Olver I. Spiritual support of cancer patients and the role of the doctor. *Support Care Cancer.* 2014;22:1333–1339.

27. Penman J, Ellis B. Palliative care clients' and caregivers' notion of fear and their strategies for overcoming it. *Palliat Support Care.* 2015;13:777–785.

28. Tan HM, Wilson A, Olver I, Barton C. The experience of palliative patients and their families of a family meeting utilised as an instrument for spiritual and psychosocial care: A qualitative study. *BMC Palliat Care.* 2011;10:7.

29. Peterman AH, Fitchett G, Brady MJ, Hernandez L, Cella D. Measuring spiritual well-being in people with cancer: The functional assessment of chronic illness therapy--Spiritual Well-being Scale (FACIT-Sp). *Ann Behav Med.* 2002;24:49–58.

30. Balboni TA, Vanderwerker LC, Block SD, et al. Religiousness and spiritual support among advanced cancer patients and associations with end-of-life treatment preferences and quality of life. *J Clin Oncol.* 2007;25:555–560.

31. O'Callaghan CC, Georgousopoulou E, Seah D, Clayton JM, Kissane D, Michael N. Spirituality and religiosity in a palliative medicine population: mixed-methods study. *BMJ Support Palliat Care.* 2020. Epub ahead of print. Doi:10.1136/bmjspcare-2020-002261

32. Michael NG, Bobevski I, Georgousopoulou EN, et al. Unmet spiritual needs in palliative care: psychometrics of a screening checklist. *BMJ Support Palliat Care.* 2020. Epub ahead of print. Doi:10.1136/bmjspcare-2020-002636

33. O'Callaghan C, Seah D, Clayton JM, et al. Palliative caregivers' spirituality, views about spiritual care, and associations with spiritual well-being: A mixed methods study. *Am J Hosp Palliat Med*. 2020;37:305–313.

34. O'Callaghan C, Brooker J, de Silva W, et al. Patients' and caregivers' contested perspectives on spiritual care for those affected by advanced illnesses: A qualitative descriptive study. *J Pain Symptom Manage*. 2019;58:977–988.

35. Australian Bureau of Statistics. Census. 2016. Available online at www.abs.gov.au (accessed 22th August, 2020).

36. Egan R, Maclead R, Jaye C, et al. What is spirituality? Evidence from a New Zealand hospice study. *Mortality*. 2011;16:307–324.

37. Piderman KM, Radecki Breitkopf C, Jenkins SM, et al. Hearing and heeding the voices of those with advanced illnesses. *J Palliat Care*. 2020;35:248–255.

38. Yang GM, Tan YY, Cheung YB, et al. Effect of a spiritual care training program for staff on patient outcomes. *Palliat Support Care*. 2017;15:434–443.

39. Shin DW, Suh SY, Kim SH, et al. Is spirituality related to survival in advanced cancer in-patients in Korea? *Palliat Support Care*. 2018;16:669–676.

40. Pautex S, Gamondi C, Philippin Y, et al. Advance directives and end-of-life decisions in Switzerland: Role of patients, relatives and health professionals. *BMJ Support Palliat Care*. 2018;8:475–484.

41. Balboni TA, Balboni MJ. The spiritual event of serious illness. *J Pain Symptom Manage*. 2018;56:816–822.

42. Davis CS. Hospitality happens: dialogic ethics of care. *Sociology*. 2019;56:130–134.

43. Breitbart W. Special issue on spirituality in palliative and supportive care: who are we talking to when we are talking to ourselves? *Palliat Support Care*. 2015;13:1–2.

44. Lewis S. Value-based healthcare - meeting the evolving needs of our population. *Aust Health Rev*. 2019;43:485.

45. Weissmann PF, Branch WT, Gracey CF, Haidet P, Frankel RM. Role modeling humanistic behavior: learning bedside manner from the experts. *Acad Med*. 2006;81:661–667.

46. Ferry-Danini J. A new path for humanistic medicine. *Theor Med Bioeth*. 2018;39:57–77.

47. Lee Roze des Ordons A, de Groot JM, Rosenal T, Viceer N, Nixon L. How clinicians integrate humanism in their clinical workplace—"Just trying to put myself in their human being shoes." *Perspect Med Educ*. 2018;7:318–324.

48. Balboni MJ, Balboni TA. *Hostility to Hospitality: Spirituality and Professional Socialization within Medicine*. New York: Oxford University Press; 2019.

49. Selby D, Seccaraccia D, Huth J, Kurppa K, Fitch M. Patient versus health care provider perspectives on spirituality and spiritual care: the potential to miss the moment. *Ann Palliat Med*. 2017;6:143–152.

50. Lashley C, Morrison A (eds). *In Search of Hospitality: Theoretical Perspectives and Debates*. Oxford: Butterworth-Heinemann; 2000.

51. Gula RM. *The good life: Where Morality and Spirituality Converge*. New York: Paulist Press; 1999.

52. Telfer E. The philosophy of hospitableness. In: Lashley C (ed). *The Routledge Handbook of Hospitality Studies*. New York: Routledge; 2016, 38–55.

53. Marcel G. *Creative Fidelity*. Robert Rosthal (trans). New York: Fordham University Press; 2002.

54. Rohde G, Kersten C, Vistad I, Mesel T. Spiritual well-being in patients with metastatic colorectal cancer receiving noncurative chemotherapy: A qualitative study. *Cancer Nurs*. 2017;40:209–216.

17

The Influence of Spirituality on Quality of Life during Cancer, United States

Jeannine M. Brant and Annette Brant Isozaki

Introduction

Traditional medical models have focused on physical health and management of physical symptoms, and yet new paradigms have shifted this focus to a more holistic approach. In the late 1970s, Dame Cicely Saunders, a nurse, social worker, physician, and palliative care pioneer, was one of the first health care professionals to promote this paradigm shift in her recognition of pain and suffering that extends beyond the physical realm [1]. She coined the term *total pain* to recognize that not only physical symptoms, but accompanying psychological, social, and spiritual suffering exists and composes the whole person (Figure 17.1). Clinicians should be reminded that if suffering includes all realms, then quality cancer care must also address all realms as well.

Spirituality lies at the core of whole-person health. Dame Saunders specifically addressed spirituality, noting: "Where a desolate sense of meaninglessness is encountered by the person at the end of life, one finds the essence of 'spiritual pain'" [2]. While spiritual pain tends to peak during the end of life, it can surface at any point during the cancer trajectory.

Within the mythos of spirituality, deeply mysterious questions can emerge from patients with cancer, ones that philosophers and religions have sought to answer for ages [3]. The questions often pondered include: (1) what is the meaning of my life, (2) how does one define joy, (3) has my life made a difference, (4) can physical suffering have a purpose, (5) what is the meaning of good and evil in the world, and (6) where will one spend eternity, and does it exist? With these deep-seeded questions and spiritual pain comes a significant responsibility for clinicians to address spirituality and spiritual pain. And yet, studies reveal that spirituality is one of the most underassessed and underrecognized aspects of whole-person care. Even within the palliative care environment, where there is greater recognition of spirituality, one study found that spirituality was only addressed in half of the consultations [4]. This chapter will focus on assessment and management of spirituality in cancer care and the positive outcomes of spiritual well-being. A case study will highlight the impact that clinicians have by assessing spirituality and addressing spiritual concerns.

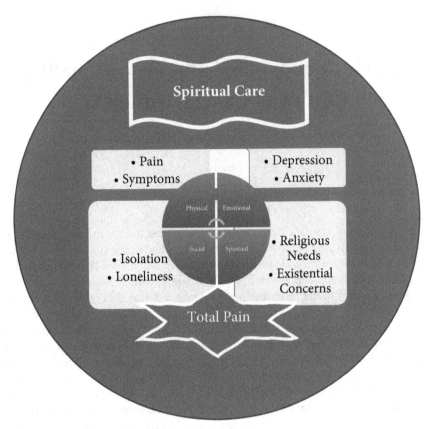

Figure 17.1 Spiritual Care for Total Pain

Definitions

Understanding definitions and terms surrounding religion and spirituality are foundational to addressing spiritual pain. Some terms can be used incorrectly, and definitions have also evolved over time. The goal of standardizing definitions is to promote nonjudgmental conversations, honor individual beliefs, capture the breadth and diversity of experiences of persons with cancer, and recognize similarities and crosscutting themes [5]. Clarity of definitions is also needed for research, so that variables can be standardized and captured in a similar framework. Some common terms with definitions are included in Table 17.1 [5–8].

Within these standard definitions, it is also important to recognize cultural differences that exist. For example, Native Americans may find it difficult to separate spiritual pain from emotional and physical pain [9–10]. Their worldviews include a medicine wheel that intertwines the physical, emotional, mental, and spiritual realms, thereby blurring these concepts as distinct entities.

Table 17.1 Definitions

Term	Definition
Chaplain (health care)	• A professionally trained person or clergy member who supports patients and staff with spiritual and religious concerns to help navigate the health care experience
Faith	• Complete trust or confidence in something or someone
Religion	• That which "binds together" • Connections to deity—includes shared beliefs and customs • An organized system to facilitate the relationship and responsibility with others in a given community
Religious Affiliation	• Religious community in which the individual associates and participates
Sacred	• That which is set apart from the ordinary
Spirituality	• Spiritual or religious beliefs that transcend meaning or life purpose • A search for that which is sacred to the individual
Spiritual Pain	• A struggle to find sources of meaning, hope, love, peace, comfort, strength, and connection in one's life
Spiritual Well-being	• Meaning, value, transcendence, connecting with a higher power, and growth in life
Suffering	• Undergoing pain, distress, or hardship
Transcendence	• To experience or exist beyond the normal physical realm

Data from [5–7]

Assessment

Assessment of spirituality is foundational to understanding each person's lens of their spiritual journey. Without assessing spirituality, spiritual distress and pain cannot be recognized and can easily be forgotten in lieu of the physical and emotional care of the patient. Spiritual discussions and assessments may be more common in palliative care as the definition of palliative care in itself includes spirituality: "palliative care integrates the psychological and spiritual aspects of care" [11]. And yet spirituality is not always consistently addressed in palliative care and even more often, not addressed throughout the cancer trajectory. One study found it addressed in only half of palliative care consultations. Providing patients with a prompt list has been shown to increase spiritual discussions, allowing patients to ask questions that they may not have considered [4]. All clinicians should take part in recognizing spiritual pain and in uncovering distress so that appropriate referrals and interventions can ensue.

Inquiring about spirituality and religion falls into three major categories: screening, history-taking, and assessment [12]. A variety of tools for each category are included in Table 17.2. First, all clinicians should conduct a brief screen to identify patients in need of a spiritual care referral. These tools often contain a single item that can identify spiritual or religious distress, depression, and worse quality of life. Screening should occur at least at an initial visit, but the timing of follow-up screening is not well established. Second, a clinical nurse or provider can further obtain a spiritual history

Table 17.2 Spiritual Assessment

Tool or Model	Item(s)	Comments
Spiritual Screening		
Mako's tool [32]	Do you have spiritual pain?	Can indicate depression as well
Rush Spiritual Screening Protocol [33]	Is religion or spirituality important to you as you cope with your illness?	Protocol uses a series of questions based on yes/no to the foundational question; assumes that patients may not report in brief history-taking and an indirect approach needed
Steinhauser tool [34]	Are you at peace?	Associated with emotional and spiritual well-being
History-Taking		
FICA [35]	F – What is your faith or beliefs? I – Is it important in your life? C – Are you part of a spiritual or religious community? A – How should we address these issues in your care?	Research supports feasibility and concurrent validity
HOPE [36]	H – Sources of hope O – Organized religion P – Personal spirituality and practices E – Effects on medical care and end-of-life issues	Originally developed as a teaching tool to help medical students, residents, and physicians incorporate spiritual assessment into practice
SPIR [37]	S – Describe self as a believing or spiritual person? P – Place of spirituality in life I – Integrated into a spiritual community R – Role you would like to assign your care team in providing spiritual care	Authors suggest that several follow-up questions can be asked under each of the major categories
SPIRIT [38]	S – Spiritual belief system P – Personal spirituality I – Integration with a spiritual community R – Rituals I – Implications of spirituality T – Terminal event planning	Based on the belief that spiritualty impacts medical problems; developed to aid physicians in spiritual history-taking

Table 17.2 Contined

Tool or Model	Item(s)	Comments
Spiritual Assessment		
7x7 Spiritual Assessment Model [39]	Holistic 7 assessment: medical, psychological, family systems, psychosocial, ethnic/racial/ cultural, social, spiritual Spiritual 7 assessment: belief/ meaning, vocation/obligations, experience/emotions, doubt/ growth, ritual/practice, community, authority/guidance	Includes 7 holistic and 7 spiritual assessment parameters to be considered in a comprehensive assessment
Discipline for Pastoral Care Giving [40]	Includes concepts about meaning, hope, and holiness Integrates faith community	Based on a disciple-oriented model for chaplains that is focused on outcomes and deepened relationships with patients
MD Anderson Spiritual Assessment Tool and Model [41]	Despair versus Hopeful Broken versus Whole Dread versus courage Alienated versus connected Meaningless versus meaningful Guilt/shame versus accepted Helpless versus Empowered	Combines physical assessment and spiritual assessment to examine spiritual distress and other symptom correlates Items are compared on a 7-item scale
National Institutes of Health Healing Experience of All Life Stressors (HEALS) [42]	3 subscales: Connection, Introspection & Reflection, and Trust & Acceptance	Includes 42 items Assesses an individual's psycho-social-spiritual mechanisms for coping during life's difficult situations Established validity and reliability
Spiritual AIM [15]	Diagnosis of unmet spiritual needs Devise and implement a plan to address needs Evaluate the outcome of the intervention	One of the few models that offers spiritual intervention
Spiritual Distress Assessment Tool (SDAT) and Model [43]	Need for life balance Need for connection Need for values and acknowledgment Need to maintain control Need to maintain identity	Includes 4 dimensions: meaning, transcendence, values, and psychosocial identity SDAT is one component of the model

by asking open-ended questions about whether the patient has a faith community and how they hope to see spiritual needs met throughout their care trajectory. And finally, a spiritual assessment is more in depth and provides a framework for the development of a spiritual care plan. A trained professional such as a board-certified chaplain or other individual with spiritual training should conduct this assessment.

Assessing spirituality can also involve many domains. A recent systematic review of 58 measures revealed the following tools that measured suffering ($n = 2$), hopelessness/demoralization ($n = 7$), hope ($n = 5$), meaning ($n = 20$), spiritual well-being ($n = 11$), multidimensional quality of life (QOL; $n = 9$), spiritual distress ($n = 2$), and distress in palliative care ($n = 2$) [13]. These tools can be used to further identify specific distress areas.

While a variety of tools are available to screen, take a history, and fully assess spirituality, some significant gaps exist. Not all have established validity and reliability. And most have been used in the cancer and/or palliative care setting and may not be applicable to other patient populations. Tools have also not been tested in other cultures, and some of the questions may pose challenges for some groups of individuals. More research is needed in this area to test these tools, translate them to other languages, and explore their use with diverse populations [12].

Spiritual Interventions

Spiritual interventions are integral to the holistic care of the patient. Once spiritual distress is assessed, clinicians should determine the best intervention for the patient and family. While clinicians and direct caregivers can deliver some of the necessary spiritual interventions, lack of time and lack of spiritual training and competence often limit their depth and types of interventions that they can employ. Because of these challenges, the clinician can refer the patient and/or family to a spiritual counselor or chaplain trained in spiritual care who can deliver the appropriate interventions. Referring the patient and family to the trusted spiritual care resource is essential in incorporating spiritual care into the patient's individualized plan of care.

Chaplains play an important role on the health care team and are commonly employed in most hospitals and hospices in the United States and Western world. Globally, they are becoming increasingly recognized, and training programs are emerging in many parts of the world such as the Middle East [14]. Referring a patient or family to a chaplain can be for several reasons that reach beyond religion. Chaplaincy theories indicate goals of care, include integrating theology into care, recognizing interpersonal dynamics within the person and family, having cultural humility and competence with care, providing ethical care, and recognizing and incorporating theories of human development into care [15]. Therefore, struggles with religion, total pain (including physical pain), interpersonal and family conflict, ethical dilemmas, questions about end-of-life goals, and existential suffering are all challenges presented by both patients and families, in which a chaplain referral may be indicated and beneficial.

While in Western health care systems, anyone can make a referral to a chaplain, one study found that nurses are the most likely team member to refer to chaplains, and the most common reason was for patient-related emotional distress. Physicians also are likely to refer to chaplains for emotional care but also for end-of-life issues. Patients and families, on the other hand, request a chaplain visit most often for spiritual or religious needs. Chaplains serve in all of these roles, and it is likely that patients and families don't understand the full role of the chaplain; therefore, it is important that clinicians clarify their role to patients and families [16].

Table 17.3 Spiritual Care Interventions

Spiritual intervention	Description
Chaplain Care	Clinicians can refer patients to a chaplain who can provide spiritual assessment and interventions as needed
Life Review	Interventions that engage the patient to discuss life experiences to preserve dignity; examples include dignity therapy and outlook life review
Mind-Body Interventions	Interventions provided to comfort the body and the mind, such as meditation, massage, reiki therapy, and mindfulness
Music Therapy	Music listening and playing according to the patient and family's desired genre
Prayer	Praying for the patient or providing intercessory prayer; can be performed by clinicians, family members, friends, and trained spiritual care providers
Religious Rituals	Some patients use rituals to integrate religion into their care; examples include providing holy communion to Christian and Catholic patients and the use of ceremonial smoke in Native American culture
Scripture	Reading, meditating on, or listening to scripture from a religious book such as the Bible, Quran, or other spiritual guide
Traditional Ceremonies	Specific to a culture
	Examples include ceremonial dancing, community gatherings, and celebration with food

Data from [9,17,19–22].

As noted, clinicians lack the training and skill to deliver many spiritual interventions. However, they can incorporate some interventions into daily care such as prayer, therapeutic touch, and empathic listening. Some clinicians choose to receive additional training in spiritual care and can then engage in other in-depth interventions such as life review, dignity therapy, and meditation if time allows. A list of spiritual interventions is included in Table 17.3 [12,17–22].

Spirituality Outcomes

Spiritual screening, assessment, and interventions are important to incorporate into cancer care, but the most important reasons for integration lie in the evidence-based outcomes attained when both patient and family are spiritually well. And reaching spiritual wellness means that the individual is at peace, has found meaning in the cancer and suffering, and finds purpose in life in the midst of the crisis. Because total pain and suffering encompasses all components, spiritual wellness involves improving outcomes in all care realms, including physical, emotional, social, and spiritual well-being. Often, relieving suffering in one area can relieve suffering in another. For example, relief of emotional pain can often relieve physical pain [23]. It is the interconnection of the body, mind, and spirit that makes us uniquely human beings, representing all of the various races, cultures, and religions of the world. And care for our interconnected beings is what institutes the art of palliative and cancer care [24].

According to the evidence-based literature, religious and spiritual well-being have many benefits. In a meta-analysis of 32,000 adult cancer patients representing 101 unique samples, physical well-being and symptoms ($p < .001$), functional well-being ($p < .01$), and cognitive well-being ($p < .05$), all demonstrated a significant benefit when compared to patients without religious and/or spiritual well-being [25].

Quality of Life

Another systematic review of 36 studies found a positive association between overall spiritual well-being and overall QOL. Effect sizes ranged from 0.36 to 0.70, indicating a moderate to large size, with emotional and affective factors such as meaning and peace showing a stronger effect and physical health a lower effect, which was similar to the findings by Jim et al. [26]. These studies underscore the importance of addressing spiritual health. Each of the QOL domains (physical, emotional, and social) is more carefully examined below in examining their relationship with spirituality.

Physical Distress

Physical symptoms such as pain, dyspnea, nausea, vomiting, and fatigue are common among patients with cancer due to the disease itself, cancer treatment, or comorbid conditions. Treatment for these conditions often includes opioids, antiemetics, and other pharmacologic modalities. And yet studies reveal that spiritual wellness can also improve symptoms, as spiritual distress can disrupt symptom tolerance. One large meta-analysis of 44,000 patients found a significant relationship between physical well-being and religion/spirituality, with effect sizes estimated at 0.15. One of the challenges with this research is that concepts overlap. For example, affective or emotional wellness is also related to symptom relief, with effect sizes estimated at 0.26. But regardless, improvement in spiritual wellness and emotional wellness may improve symptom intensity and distress in patients with cancer [27].

Emotional Distress

Emotional health, another QOL domain, has been shown to be significantly impacted by spiritual wellness. Emotional health includes many concepts such as mental health, depression, anxiety, hopelessness, and others. According to the same meta-analysis of 44,000 patients, emotional health demonstrated the largest effect size of 0.19 in relation to spiritual wellness [27]. Another study that focused specifically on the relationships between anxiety, depression, and spirituality found a significant negative correlation between spiritual well-being and anxiety and depression scores ($p < .0001$), indicating that those with greater spiritual wellness suffered from less anxiety and depression. Interestingly, religion did not demonstrate this same relationship, indicating once again that religion and spirituality are separate concepts [28]. Another study had similar findings, with a significant relationship between the Hamilton Depression Scale and the Functional Assessment of Cancer Treatment Scale (FACIT), but religion also was not significant [29].

Another study examined 160 patients with cancer and a limited life expectancy regarding emotional issues and spirituality. Findings revealed that those with higher spiritual well-being had a significantly higher desire for hastened death ($r = -0.51$) and lower hopelessness ($r = -0.68$) and suicidal ideation ($r = -0.41$). The authors concluded that spiritual well-being may protect against despair at the end of life [30]. Other implications could exist for advanced care planning as those patients who are more spiritually well may also not be as likely to ask for life-sustaining treatment and futile care at the end of life. But more research is needed in this area.

Social Distress

Regarding social well-being, one large meta-analysis of 178 independent samples encompassing 14,277 patients found social health significantly associated with overall religion/spirituality (Fisher z effect size = .20; $p < .001$). The authors defined social health as the extent of involvement in social roles, relationships, or activities, and the perceived quality of that involvement. Social well-being, social distress, and social support were all embedded within the context of social health. The authors concluded that social health is related to involvement in religion/spirituality and that the effect is moderate [31].

Research Considerations

When examining this combined evidence, limitations exist with many of the studies, including methodologic and conceptual concerns. First, outcomes in the studies varied, as did the measures and their quality. Some had sound psychometric properties, whereas other measures were not as well defined. Second, most of the research was cross-sectional, and so whether the effects stay stable over time is unknown. Third, studies lacked a heterogeneous sample. Most participants were Caucasian and had a Christian faith background; therefore, generalizability of the studies may be limited. Finally, confounding factors may exist, especially socioeconomic status, which is highly correlated with religion/spiritual well-being. Further studies should be mindful of these challenges in this body of research [27].

One of the biggest recommendations for research is to employ more intervention studies to answer several questions. For example, which interventions work best in which populations? Are interventions generalizable to individuals from various religious backgrounds? Additionally, what is the best timing of the interventions, and how often should interventions be delivered? Opportunity exists for this area of research, especially in diverse populations and in low- to middle-income countries.

Case Studies

Integrating spiritual screening, assessment, and interventions into cancer care is therefore an essential component of holistic care. The two case studies presented here exemplify how clinicians can incorporate some of these principles into practice.

Case Study 1

Carolee (C.M.) is a 48-year-old female recently diagnosed with aplastic anemia. She was admitted for a stem cell transplant with anti-thymocyte globulin conditioning prior to treatment. It was C.M.'s first night in a hospital. She had three young children at home and was feeling very distressed. When the night nurse came onto shift, the patient expressed anxiety and uncertainty with the unknown factors regarding her treatment. She feared death and leaving her three children behind. The nurse identified that fear of the unknown was driving the patient's anxiety. She explained the patient's conditioning regimen and expectations for treatment. The patient's anxiety seemed to subside.

Later that night, close to midnight, the patient lay wide awake. When the nurse went into the room, she identified a devotional book lying at the patient's side. Recognizing emotional and potentially spiritual distress, the nurse also used the FICA tool to better understand how Carolee might like spirituality issues addressed in her care. Carolee identified herself as a Christian and indicated that faith was very important to her. She indicated that she belonged to a nondenominational evangelical church, and she felt that she would appreciate visits from the pastor at her church. She also stated that prayer is important to her. The patient reported that she had been feeling anxious again about her disease and treatment. She said that her devotional book and prayer brought her comfort, but she still felt very anxious. The nurse offered to pray for her, and the patient agreed. The nurse prayed for peace and for the patient's anxiety to be alleviated. Almost as soon as the prayer finished and the nurse left the room, the patient lay fast asleep for the rest of the night. This case highlights the role of a clinician (nurse) in taking a spiritual history and providing spiritual care. Listening, therapeutic touch, and prayer were used to allay a patient's anxiety and distress.

Case Study 2

Manuel is a 75-year-old male diagnosed with multiple myeloma (MM) 14 years prior. His myeloma remained under control with a previous autologous stem cell transplant and chemotherapy. Eight months ago, his disease began to rapidly progress, and he was started on a clinical trial. Initially, he had a good response to treatment but was later readmitted for elevated creatinine, confusion, and electrolyte imbalance. Upon further evaluation, the team determined that the patient's current symptoms were treatment-related and not disease induced. As such, the physician determined that the patient would not be eligible for further treatment on the current clinical trial due to the toxicities experienced. No other clinical research studies could be identified for the patient given his current condition. At this time, the physician determined that it was time to withdraw treatment and allow for natural death as there were no more curative or disease control options of treatment for the patient. The palliative care team was consulted for a family meeting to discuss the patient's prognosis.

The social worker, case manager, chaplain, palliative care specialist, nurse practitioner, physician, nurse, wife, and patient agreed on a time that was conducive for a family meeting. Given the COVID-19 pandemic, the patient's family member was contacted via video chat for the meeting. The social worker made sure that all members were present on screen and that voices were audible prior to the start of the meeting. Once technological issues were addressed, the palliative care specialist introduced the team and began the meeting with identifying the wife's and patient's current understanding of Manuel's disease process and treatment. The palliative care specialist then asked the physician what his interpretation of the patient's current response to treatment was. Through this process, the team was able to identify gaps in the patient and wife's interpretation of the illness and contrast it to reality. Once the patient and his wife had no other questions, the palliative care specialist asked the family and patient to repeat their understanding of the patient's current prognosis given the information they had just received. Since the interpretations of prognosis matched, the team concluded that the family and patient had a realistic understanding of Manuel's prognosis. The palliative care specialist allowed time for the family to ask any questions necessary before ending the meeting. The patient was made Do Not Resuscitate (DNR) with plans to be discharged home once the renal function resolved.

Once the meeting had ended, the palliative care chaplain assisted the patient with calling his wife so that they could have time to grieve the conversation and his terminal prognosis together. After the wife and husband's conversation had ended, the chaplain provided empathetic listening and space for the patient to share his response to his prognosis. Following the phone call, the chaplain conducted a spiritual history and assessment of the patient to identify any potential spiritual distress and to better incorporate spirituality into the patient's care. Manuel noted that his biggest regret in life was not telling his wife how precious she was to him. The chaplain sat with the patient as Manuel reminisced about his life. He told stories of his childhood and expressed distress with leaving his wife. The chaplain sat and listened to the patient to allow him to process and grieve things that he felt he could not tell his wife. After listening to the patient's stories, life successes and challenges, and grief about leaving his good life, the chaplain offered the patient a dignity therapy intervention. This therapy offered Manuel an opportunity to reflect on his life and transmit messages that he wanted to be relayed to his wife and family.

Over the next week, the chaplain visited the patient for 30 minutes daily, interviewing the patient and recording his responses and messages. The patient shared with the clinician that he felt like a load was lifted from his chest by sharing his story. A copy of the transcript was then given to Manuel who could provide it to his wife and family as desired. The patient was discharged home the following week and died two months later. Following the patient's death, the chaplain followed up with Manuel's wife, who reported that Manuel left her a packet that he requested she open after he died. She revealed that the messages shared by Manuel would be treasured forever by her and her family and that somehow these messages gave her comfort as she coped with his loss. This case involves a more detailed spiritual care intervention delivered by a trained spiritual person and illustrates the potential impact on patient and family outcomes.

Conclusion

Spirituality is an important domain within quality of life that plays a significant role in holistic health and well-being. Spirituality is one of the most underrecognized aspects of care, and this chapter reinforces the importance of incorporating spirituality more consistently into cancer care to improve patient and family outcomes, including physical, emotional, and social distress. To do so, all clinicians should incorporate spiritual screening into daily care, at each clinic visit and with each admission to the hospital or a hospice setting. Once spiritual distress is detected, a more comprehensive spiritual assessment should ensue by a chaplain or clinician trained in spiritual assessment. The spiritual assessment should then drive the spiritual care interventions. While clinicians may be able to readily incorporate some interventions into care such as prayer, therapeutic touch, and empathetic listening, other interventions require more time and expertise beyond most clinicians' scope of practice. Therefore, again, having a chaplain or spiritual expert as part of the interdisciplinary team is essential in providing holistic cancer care. Total suffering involves all aspects of care, and holistic healing must involve the same.

References

1. Saunders CM. *The Management of Terminal Malignant Disease*. London: Edward Arnold; 1978.
2. Saunders C. Spiritual pain. *J Palliat Care*. 1988(4):29–32.
3. Sulmasy DP. Ethos, mythos, and thanatos: Spirituality and ethics at the end of life. *J Pain Symptom Manage*. 2013;46(3):447–451.
4. Best M, McArdle MB, Huang YJ, Clayton J, Butow P. How and how much is spirituality discussed in palliative care consultations for advanced cancer patients with and without a question prompt list? *Patient Educ Couns*. 2019;102(12):2208–2213.
5. Steinhauser KE, Fitchett G, Handzo GF, et al. State of the science of spirituality and palliative care research. Part I: Definitions, measurement, and outcomes. *J Pain Symptom Manage*. 2017;54(3):428–440.
6. Fisher JW, Francis LJ, Johnson P. Assessing spiritual health via four domains of spiritual wellbeing: The SH4DI. *Pastoral Psychol*. 2000;49(2):133–145.
7. Koenig HG. Religion and medicine IV: Religion, physical health, and clinical implications. *Int J Psychiatry Med*. 2001;31(3):321–336.
8. Koenig HG. Religion, spirituality, and medicine: How are they related and what does it mean? *Mayo Clin Proc*. 2001;76(12):1189–1191.
9. Haozous EA, Knobf MT. "All my tears were gone": Suffering and cancer pain in Southwest American Indians. *J Pain Symptom Manage*. 2013;45(6):1050–1060.
10. Haozous EA, Knobf MT, Brant JM. Understanding the cancer pain experience in American Indians of the Northern Plains. *Psychooncology*. 2011;20(4):404–410.
11. World Health Organization. Integrating palliative care and symptom relief into primary health care: A WHO guide for planners, implementers and managers. World Health Organization. 2018. Accessed December 2, 2018.
12. Balboni TA, Fitchett G, Handzo GF, et al. State of the science of spirituality and palliative care research. Part II: Screening, assessment, and interventions. *J Pain Symptom Manage*. 2017;54(3):441–453.

13. Best M, Aldridge L, Butow P, Olver I, Price M, Webster F. Assessment of spiritual suffering in the cancer context: A systematic literature review. *Palliat Support Care.* 2015;13(5):1335–1361.

14. Silbermann M, Pitsillides B, Al-Alfi N, et al. Multidisciplinary care team for cancer patients and its implementation in several Middle Eastern countries. *Ann Oncol.* 2013;24 (Suppl 7):vii, 41–47.

15. Shields M, Kestenbaum A, Dunn LB. Spiritual AIM and the work of the chaplain: A model for assessing spiritual needs and outcomes in relationship. *Palliat Support Care.* 2015;13(1):75–89.

16. Galek K, Vanderwerker LC, Flannelly KJ, et al. Topography of referrals to chaplains in the Metropolitan Chaplaincy Study. *J Pastoral Care Couns.* 2009;63(1-2): 1–13.

17. Tsai HF, Chen YR, Chung MH, et al. Effectiveness of music intervention in ameliorating cancer patients' anxiety, depression, pain, and fatigue: A meta-analysis. *Cancer Nurs.* 2014; 37(6) E35–50.

18. Best M, Aldridge L, Butow P, Olver I, Price MA, Webster F. Treatment of holistic suffering in cancer: A systematic literature review. *Palliat Med.* 2015;29(10):885–898.

19. Martínez M, Arantzamendi M, Belar A, et al. 'Dignity therapy', a promising intervention in palliative care: A comprehensive systematic literature review. *Palliat Med.* 2017;31(6):492–509.

20. Miranda TPS, Caldeira S, de Oliveira HF, et al. Intercessory prayer on spiritual distress, spiritual coping, anxiety, depression and salivary amylase in breast cancer patients during radiotherapy: Randomized clinical trial. *J Relig Health.* 2020;59(1):365–380.

21. Oh PJ, Kim SH. The effects of spiritual interventions in patients with cancer: A meta-analysis. *Oncol Nurs Forum.* 2014;41(5):E290–301.

22. Xing L, Guo X, Bai L, Qian J, Chen J. Are spiritual interventions beneficial to patients with cancer?: A meta-analysis of randomized controlled trials following PRISMA. *Medicine.* 2018;97(35):e11948.

23. Brant JM. Holistic total pain management in palliative care: Cultural and global considerations. *Palliat Med Hospice Care.* 2017:S32–S38.

24. Brant JM. The art of palliative care: living with hope, dying with dignity. *Oncol Nurs Forum.* 1998;25(6):995–1004.

25. Jim HS, Pustejovsky JE, Park CL, et al. Religion, spirituality, and physical health in cancer patients: A meta-analysis. *Cancer.* 2015;121(21):3760–3768.

26. Bai M, Lazenby M. A systematic review of associations between spiritual well-being and quality of life at the scale and factor levels in studies among patients with cancer. *J Palliat Med.* 2015;18(3):286–298.

27. Park CL, Sherman AC, Jim HS, Salsman JM. Religion/spirituality and health in the context of cancer: Cross-domain integration, unresolved issues, and future directions. *Cancer.* 2015;121(21):3789–3794.

28. McCoubrie RC, Davies AN. Is there a correlation between spirituality and anxiety and depression in patients with advanced cancer? *Support Care Cancer.* 2006;14(4):379–385.

29. Nelson CJ, Rosenfeld B, Breitbart W, Galietta M. Spirituality, religion, and depression in the terminally ill. *Psychosomatics.* 2002;43(3):213–220.

30. McClain CS, Rosenfeld B, Breitbart W. Effect of spiritual well-being on end-of-life despair in terminally-ill cancer patients. *The Lancet.* 2003;361(9369):1603–1607.

31. Sherman AC, Merluzzi TV, Pustejovsky JE, et al. A meta-analytic review of religious or spiritual involvement and social health among cancer patients. *Cancer.* 2015;121(21):3779–3788.

32. Mako C, Galek K, Poppito SR. Spiritual pain among patients with advanced cancer in palliative care. *J Palliat Med.* 2006;9(5):1106–1113.

33. Fitchett G, Risk JL. Screening for spiritual struggle. *J Pastoral Care Couns.* 2009;63(1-2): 1–12.
34. Steinhauser KE, Voils CI, Clipp EC, Bosworth HB, Christakis NA, Tulsky JA. "Are you at peace?": One item to probe spiritual concerns at the end of life. *Arch Int Med.* 2006;166(1):101–105.
35. Puchalski CM. Formal and informal spiritual assessment. *Asian Pac J Cancer Prev.* 2010;11(Suppl 1):51–57.
36. Anandarajah G, Hight E. Spirituality and medical practice: Using the HOPE questions as a practical tool for spiritual assessment. *Am Fam Phys.* 2001;63:81–88.
37. Frick E, Riedner C, Fegg MJ, Hauf S, Borasio GD. A clinical interview assessing cancer patients' spiritual needs and preferences. *Eur J Cancer Care (Engl).* 2006;15(3):238–243.
38. Maugans TA. The SPIRITual history. *Arch Fam Med.* 1996;5(1):11–16.
39. Fitchett G. *Assessing Spiritual Needs: A Guide for Caregivers. 2nd ed.* Augsburg: Academic Renewal Press; 2002.
40. Lucas AM. Introduction to the discipline for pastoral care giving. *J Health Care c\ Chaplaincy.* 2001;10(2):1–33.
41. Hui D, de la Cruz M, Thorney S, Parsons HA, Delgado-Guay M, Bruera E. The frequency and correlates of spiritual distress among patients with advanced cancer admitted to an acute palliative care unit. *Am J Hosp Palliat Care.* 2011;28(4):264–270.
42. Ameli R, Sinaii N, Luna MJ, Cheringal J, Gril B, Berger A. The National Institutes of Health measure of healing experience of all life stressors (NIH-HEALS): Factor analysis and validation. *PloS one.* 2018;13(12):e0207820–e0207820.
43. Monod SM, Rochat E, Bula CJ, Jobin G, Martin E, Spencer B. The spiritual distress assessment tool: An instrument to assess spiritual distress in hospitalised elderly persons. *BMC Geriatr.* 2010;10:88.

18

Suffering and Compassion

The Role of Faith in the United States

Lodovico Balducci

The Middle East Cancer Consortium (MECC) [1] is an organization, a movement, and a personal adventure. Any attempt to dissect these aspects in a list of goals and results shortchanges the wholeness of MECC where these dimensions are complementary, much as the two chains of the DNA are to each other. The organization could not subsist without common beliefs born out of a personal adventure.

Asked to unravel the meaning of MECC, I face the arduous task of describing how the vision of a man arrived, to be shared by a community of individuals from diverse and often mutually hostile cultures, and how this vision empowered the movement and succeeded in influencing the medical, cultural, political, and social structures of the war-torn Middle East. For this purpose, I ask the reader to accompany my travel through MECC. I find an on-site journey more instructive and persuasive than a pedantic analysis.

A "Eureka" Moment

Two important messages emerged from an ASCO-MECC (Middle Eastern Cancer Consortium) [1] palliative care program for health professionals in a republic of Central Asia:

First, the age-old tendency to blame a person for causing their disease is sometimes reinforced rather than squelched in the culture of contemporary medicine. This tendency can create misunderstandings between practitioner and patients and hinder delivery of palliative care.

Second, compassion is a universal language that transcends differences in geography, ethnicity, culture, politics, and language.

These are some of the messages that MECC endeavored to broadcast since its beginning: the management of pain and suffering is born out of basic human decency and should never be judgmental. The commitment to palliative care is inspired by compassion and nurtures compassion. In turn, compassion nurtures peace.

As a physician, I had a Eureka! moment during a role-playing exercise, relearning a lesson I've witnessed over and over in my decades of practice: guilt and disease are intertwined. Enlightened as we supposedly are, the roots of this commingling date at least as far back to the Bible. More about the story of Job and how it fits in will be covered later, but first, more about the role playing.

I took on the persona of a cancer-stricken man. He had sired a child out of wedlock and abandoned the mother and child. He endured his disease as punishment for these callous acts. Playing the doctor: a local provider.

He took my hand. In a firm yet warm and empathetic voice, he told me, "Nobody deserves to suffer that much."

The young nurse taking part in the scene broke down. She was no longer acting, and the whole room knew it. Silence fell.

"I wish the doctor had been so compassionate when my father ...." she began. She was unable to continue.

The silence was compelling because the auditorium was filled with scores of usually rowdy conference attendees. Only occasional sobs could be heard as the playacting awkwardly ground to a halt. For me—and I hope for other medical professionals—insights emerged as emotions became acute [2].

Overwhelmed by emotional pain, the nurse could say no more. At least not in public.

I pursued her during the coffee break. She agreed to elaborate.

Her father had developed hepatocellular carcinoma at age 31. A few months earlier, he had come home to his family after a seven-year absence in a distant oilfield. With the money he had earned, thanks to hard work and thrifty saving, he had planned to ensure his family's livelihood. His assets included a small house and a family-owned enterprise. He had come home animated by hope, ready to reap the fruits of his own and his family's sacrifices.

At bedside, the family heard a blunt message from the oncologist: The cancer resulted from work-related exposure to toxic components of oil refinement; the patient had asked for medical attention too late; there was nothing the physician could do! Even terminal-pain management failed to take place effectively, impeded by strict rules controlling the administration of opioids. Only parenteral morphine was available, and the dose was not to exceed 50 mg daily.

Reliving her role as distressed daughter, the nurse broke into tears several times as she recounted the story. She brought to life the tragedy of a healthy and hopeful young man who laid down a love-inspired blueprint for his family's future, only to see his plans shattered. Over a few months, disease had sapped his energies, consumed his muscles, and transformed him into a skeleton-like form contorted by pain. All other designs dissipated; an early death was the only hope for him.

Of course, the doctor's callousness only added more discomfort and extra pain. She told me that more than once the physician refused the family's invitations to visit the dying man. The doctor's claims: He was too busy, there was nothing he could do, and in any event the patient had only himself to blame for his work in the oilfields, the vodka he had sipped during his solitary weekends, and his lack of attention to the initial symptoms of cancer.

Amazingly, almost none of the attendees, including the one playing the compassionate doctor, spoke English. We had communicated through interpreters throughout the performance, yet no word seemed to have gotten lost. The universal language of compassion provided a connection much stronger than a shared parlance.

From the Latin *cum pati* (to suffer together), the word "compassion" implies that human suffering pertains to all members of humanity. The comedian John Cleese crystallized this concept when he said, "Life is a terminal disease and is sexually trans-mitted." If death is the ultimate enemy of our profession, we are set up for defeat. This awareness of a common destiny is the basis of compassion and of our ability to share other people's suffering, and compassion is the inspiration to defeat death by man-aging the pain that precedes and accompanies the experience of death. So, too, we help patients to discover the ultimate meaning of life in their personal histories.

Medical resources vary greatly from one country to another. In some countries, the availability of opioid and other pain medications is restricted, but the provider presence, encouragement, and care are available even in the direst economic circum-stance [3].

It was rewarding to witness such profound understanding despite the different lan-guages spoken during the ASCO-MECC conference. Compassion proved to be a uni-versal language in which authentic human experience trumped and transcended the spoken word.

For more than 20 years the MECC, which supported this conference, has relent-lessly promoted palliative care of cancer throughout a war-torn Middle East on the assumption that compassion may overcome the Babel of languages via the aware-ness of our common destiny. For me MECC has represented a living laboratory of compassion.

During annual member conferences, I have witnessed astounding acts: a Palestinian nurse comforting an Israeli doctor, for instance, and a rabbi ministering to an Arab patient from war-torn Syria. The commitment of people from countries at war, working together to defeat the suffering caused by cancer with whatever means were available, is beyond inspiring.

MECC has allowed me to reflect on the richness of the English language, which dif-ferentiates between "curing" and "healing." We may not be able to cure cancer, but we can always invoke the powerfully healing nature of compassion [4].

A Common Language

Human cohesion is founded on a common language. According to the Bible, the loss of a common language began with the attempt to build the Babel tower in present-day Iraq. It certainly became more widespread with the emergence of different beliefs and rituals and thereafter with the division of the earth into major imperial blocks, and it was accelerated in recent years by globalization. While in recent past the regions of the world might have built a common language over a common culture, the communality of culture all but waned when even small country towns started hosting representa-tives of unrelated cultures.

It is well known that a language involves much more than the spoken word. Indeed, we are all familiar with situations in which facial expressions and general behavior ex-press a message opposite from the one emerging from the mouth. And expressions are often more comprehensive than the spoken words that define an idea with little room for variables or nuances. In his fourth eclogue, the Latin poet Virgil described how comprehensive may be the smile of a little child who learns for the first time to recog-nize the mother (*Incipe parve puer risu conoscere matrem*).

In other words, to use a common language means to partake of each other's emotion. In this respect, MECC is a training camp in a common language for different players. The focus of MECC is the relief of suffering caused by cancer, with the understanding that cancer is just a component of the suffering experience. To relieve human suffering requires understanding of the components of suffering, understanding and participation of the emotional and spiritual domains involved in suffering. It involves the ability to express understanding and allegiance with proper comments, with open questions, with reflexive listening, and mainly with proper demeanor. For sensory-deprived older individuals, touch may be much more communicative than any words or facial expression. A common language is more comprehensive than a common idiom! All members of MECC master English, but that is only the beginning of the search; it is an instrument to share ongoing discoveries. The reason is that central to the MECC encounters are sessions where people learn from each other how to communicate pain and how to signify understanding.

Equally important as a common language, MECC coopted the religious hypothesis, which involved the belief in a transcendency capable of giving meaning to human suffering. The modern culture spawned from the illuminism has enshrined human reason, and later science and technology, as the modern deity. The underlying belief is that humankind is self-sufficient. This belief involves a perennial escape from the thought of death and the blind faith that all human sufferings may be explained by reason and cared for by science. More than refusing the religious hypothesis, the secular culture disregards it as an instrument of the past, as a wooden stove at the time of electrical heating. The disregard of the religious hypothesis restrains human interventions within the boundary of earthly life and impedes the discovery of the meaning of suffering. Without endorsing any particular religion, MECC encourages its members to utilize beliefs, values, and prayer as a nonrenounceable approach to suffering. It may be poetic justice that the world may obtain a common language in the very Middle East where the Bible says the common language was first lost.

Sadly, the doctor who had abandoned the patient after diagnosing incurable liver cancer had refused to partake of the common language of compassion. Armed with scientific presumption, he failed to recognize his role as a healer. As is true of most current practitioners of medicine, he had chosen to live in a desert where human interactions were impersonal and unhelpful. Paradoxically, he provided an example of how the MECC vision and training were wanted beyond the Middle East and beyond the realm of medicine.

MECC and Job

The tale of the young woman sparked flashes of heartbreaking déjà vu. A childhood friend of mine was told that he was responsible for his lifelong tetraplegia because he had engaged his new motorcycle in a race with a sports car.

And here are two stories from my student days and from my practice that could be developed into case studies to illustrate any number of points:

A young black woman discharged 212 times in a year from a town's emergency rooms with the diagnosis of pelvic inflammatory disease (PID) kept cycling through hospitals until a compassionate physician, interested enough to take a patient history, offered a diagnosis of Crohn's disease. The diagnosis of PID was based on social prejudices: she was black and poor and came from a Southern state of the United States. The failure to soothe her pain spawned from the persuasion that she herself had been responsible for her disease, even if she had not had any sexual encounter during the full year.

A young woman dying of postpartum breast cancer felt responsible for her imminent death; her passing would leave her newborn deprived of a mother. What overwhelmed her with guilt? She had heard the American Cancer Society claiming that women can conquer breast cancer if they do everything right—or so she thought the message was.

How strange that we should still think this way, given our scientific bent and given that we can point to evidence that the connection between guilt and disease was found void in biblical times. Earlier I mentioned the Book of Job. Here is a summary for those who may be unfamiliar with this story in the Old Testament:

Because the devout and wealthy Job, a leader in his community, was a favorite of God's, the devil (from the Greek δίϐβολος, which means "lawyer") stepped in. The devil claimed he could turn Job against God by depriving him of his good life on the grounds that Job's privileged status was the only basis for his love of God. God agreed to the challenge. Job soon lost everything: In a matter of a few days he found himself childless, destitute, affected by a painful disease that ulcerated his skin, and scorned by people who once revered him. Lying on a heap of rubbish at the edge of town, he tried to ease his pain by scratching his skin with potsherds or inviting dogs to lick his wounds.

Three well-meaning friends visited Job and encouraged him to acknowledge that his suffering was God-inflicted punishment for a hidden sin. Once he had avowed his guilt and repented, God would then certainly restore him to health and wealth!

Job rejected this assertion and refused the advice. The friends denounced his stubbornness and identified his denial as the cause of his disgrace and affliction.

God (the *deus ex machina* [5] of the ancient Greek tragedies) appears at the climactic moment. Praising Job's sincerity, God rebukes the friends for their arrogance in claiming authority to interpret God's designs. Ultimately, God sides with Job and rejects any casual connection between guilt and disease or, in fact, any form of human misfortune.

Almost 3,000 years after Job, we still seem unable to accept that "bad things happen to good people" through no fault of their own, and we try to make the sick guilty of bringing on their diseases. Perhaps it is a basic human need to look for an explanation of human suffering, a way to reassure ourselves that good and healthy behaviors will preserve us from the ills that beset others. This need is even more urgent in a secular culture than in a religious one, which may rely on God's will as the default explanation of all human events.

Increasingly, however, scientific evidence seems to support the claim that people may bear at least some responsibility for their own health. We know that cancer as well as other diseases may be triggered by habits such as drinking, smoking, and consuming certain types of food. We also have numbers to prove that some screening mechanisms may prevent deaths—but only if people avail themselves of the screenings.

Mental illness—in at least some forms—also provides rich fodder for a discussion of patient responsibility. David Burns, MD, an expert on depression whose book *Feeling Good: The New Mood Therapy* has sold more than four million copies, spends much time attempting to signal to patients the import of the thoughts they think. Thoughts (over which the patient may exercise control) come first, he points out; emotions follow; and then biochemical changes occur in brain and body. While he prescribes drugs to his patients in some cases, he tries to educate them to the powerful triggering mechanisms of their own downward-spiraling thoughts.

Much has been written in the media about the connection between stress and wellness, not to mention diet and exercise. All this is to say that while tying disease to sin—as happened in Job's time and still happens in our own—is preposterous, it's not the same as rejecting evidence that human behavior can and does play a role in sickness.

Such evidence is the basis of public health discussions about whether taxpayers should bear the costs of smoking-related diseases or of brain traumas in people who refuse to wear helmets when riding motorcycles. These debates are legitimate and necessary. Yet physicians heeding the cry of the young woman—"I wish the doctor had been so compassionate when my father...."—should stay clear of them. That young woman highlighted through the power of her experience that compassion is the first duty of a provider and the first expectation of a patient. And compassion is incompatible with judgment.

Job's friends are alive and well today, comforted by science and technology, the deity of our times. Of course it is convenient to hold people responsible for their own suffering, for a two-fold reason. Their responsibility absolves everybody else from getting involved in their problems. Their responsibility represents a form of insurance that prevents other people from undergoing the same ordeal. In the case presented, the physician felt he could wash his hands of the pain of a terminal patient because the liver cancer was his fault. I also described how the well-meaning recommendations for breast cancer screening made a young woman guilty of her own death.

Even more lacking in compassion has been the approach to patients affected by a disease spawned from their behavior, such as lung cancer or AIDS. I remember very well how at the beginning of the AIDS epidemics many physicians were reluctant to take care of AIDS patients, and they provided multiple reasons such as the fact that these patients' disease had been caused by their sinful behavior, and besides, their care would have increased the cost of health care for the whole population. I remember a self-righteous medical student begrudging a shot of whisky the chaplain had offered for Christmas to a veteran dying of lung cancer as an "unnecessary medical expense."

In an area ravaged by millennial enmities such as the Middle East, it is easy to ascribe the suffering of millions to political choices, such as the Intifada or the Arab Spring.

MECC takes to task Job's friends as it realizes the fallacy of the assumption that suffering is ever deserved and ever proportioned to the individual's faults. MECC principles involve three corollaries of the Book of Job:

1. Suffering concerns everybody because everybody has the ability to relieve or to worsen other people's suffering. When it comes to suffering, there is no such thing as a neutral bystander. Despite their good intentions, Job's friends added

insult to injury by making him responsible for his misfortune, and they lost the opportunity to console him. Prisoners of their religious prejudices, they could not develop compassion, which is the basis of lasting human relationships. They refused the opportunity that the Indian Siddhartha accepted. Siddhartha was a rich prince who lived within the walls of his domains and knew only privilege. Once he walked out of the city walls, he met people suffering all types of physical, emotional, and spiritual ills. Instead of withdrawing, as Job's friends would have done, he decided to live with them, and out of this experience he developed a wisdom founded on compassion and more valuable than any material privilege. Now Siddhartha is known to the world as Buddha.

2. As the deity made very clear in the Book of Job, nobody is exempt from human suffering. The development of compassion is a most important coping mechanism to deal with one's own disgraces, as well as an occasion to build allegiance based on common suffering. Again the Bible highlights the foolishness of self-righteousness in Psalm 130: "if you keep a record of sin, God, who will stand?"

3. Desperate people may become rebellious and dangerous when they have nothing to lose. The Russian Revolution was born out of desperation, and so was the French Revolution. In other words, evil begets evil results.

In conclusion, MECC holds that any suffering experience belongs to and affects the whole of humanity, and at the time we allay other people's suffering, we do rescue ourselves.

We Are All in It Together

No man is an island,
Entire of itself,
Every man is a piece of the continent,
A part of the main.
If a clod be washed away by the sea,
Europe is the less.
As well as if a promontory were.
As well as if a manor of thy friend's
Or of thine own were:
Any man's death diminishes me,
Because I am involved in mankind,
And therefore never send to know for whom the bell tolls.
It tolls for thee.

This poem, "No Man Is an Island," by John Donne collapses in crystal-clear terms the mission of MECC: "it is everybody's responsibility to rebuild a city or a country from the devastation of war or of a natural cataclysm."

Written in 1623 as part of a collection of poems titled *Devotions*, "No Man Is an Island" was inspired by the human solidarity promoted by the Judeo-Christian vision and embraced by Islam as well. All children of the same God are part of a design, and each human action enhances or jeopardizes the divine project. This vision has also been subscribed to by atheists or agnostics desperate to find meaning in human suffering. Think of the philosopher Arthur Schopenhauer, of the Nobel Prize winners Ernest Hemingway and Albert Camus, the Italian Poet Giacomo Leopardi, and many, many more that there is not enough space to quote. Though they could not be comforted by a religious faith, these generous individuals refused to accept the absurdity of human life.

One may say that human solidarity is foreign to a Western culture focused on individual achievements and individual rights, a culture that holds each person responsible for their successes or failures and disregards as inconsequential noises any environmental and societal contribution. Yet, the recent COVID-19 pandemic refuted in no middle terms Western individualistic tenets. The closure of a meat plant in South Dakota caused food shortages in California; the closure of restaurants in New York caused the bankruptcy of some agricultural enterprises in Iowa; the travel of grandparents from Asia or Europe to celebrate the graduation of a grandchild caused tens of thousands of deaths in the United States and the economic decline of the richest country in the world.

MECC chose as its field of intervention the Middle East, arguably the most restless region of the world, ravaged by wars since the beginning of history. This choice was inspired by a twofold motive. The Middle East, more than any other area of the world, is in want of peace, and the approach of MECC would have been best vindicated if it could unravel the knot of tribal conflicts that underlie the perennial Middle East War.

MECC involves health care professionals whose vocation and training are to heal [5]—to heal and not necessarily to cure. Cure involves the care of the disease: healing the care of the suffering. Even if the disease is not curable, even when it is lethal, healing is always possible and it occurs with the control of physical, emotional, and spiritual suffering—in other words when a person can come to terms with their suffering and with their death.

The Middle East comprehends some of the richest and some of the neediest countries in the world as well as a hodgepodge of beliefs, prejudices, and tribal feuds. The first task of MECC was to identify a common ground for action suitable to health professionals. Palliative care of cancer, a disease endemic in the region, appeared immediately as an appropriate goal, as suffering knows no religious, ideological, or ethnical bindings. Indeed, the same diversity responsible for the political unrest may become a unique resource to allay suffering and to promote peace. Different cultural approaches to suffering may blend into a holistic management as well as a mutual understanding fostered by the common goal. Professionals used to very expensive technological approaches to pain may be surprised by how far human contact and prayer may be effective in countries so poor of resources that they cannot even access opioids [2].

As important is the point that the only way to appreciate the benefits of human solidarity involves its practice. Only after they have overcome the initial reluctance to make the effort and engage in a long climb can the hiker appreciate the beauty of a mountain and remain enamored of it.

MECC and Fulfilling a Destiny

One may think of MECC as the accomplishment of a destiny. Arguably, human history began in the Fertile Crescent where nomadic people of different origins found favorable conditions for setting up a permanent residence. From Egypt to Babylon, the Middle East oversaw the most important cultural developments, including scripture, calculus, and observation of the stars. And the Middle East was the cradle of the first monotheistic religion, whose outgrowths, Christianity and Islam, account for the religion of more than half the world population.

In the process of enriching the world, the Middle East impoverished itself through a succession of mutual destructions that persists into our time. The destiny of the Middle East was never accomplished "on location." No matter how well intentioned, peace initiatives are bound to fail as long as they involve the overpowering of one culture by another culture.

Health care professionals are best positioned to promote a peace based on a common want, as diseases do not recognize geographic, cultural, or religious boundaries. Hostile tribes may be involved in the same suffering and may need each other's cooperation to overcome the common pain. Even more important, that common pain may become a shared language. One may be reluctant to save the life of a wounded enemy, but very few people would refuse to relieve the pain of a dying enemy, an experience of mutual healing.

To embrace the MECC mission to allay the suffering caused by cancer throughout the Middle East, one has to recognize that suffering is a common problem and that management of suffering is a human call that defines our humanity, that it is a call to be human, to discover the unsuspected richness of our humanity; to discover the power of science and in the meantime the power of compassion expressed in words, touches, looks.

Miguel de Unamuno opens his essay "Agony of Christianity" with a description of the relation between King David and Abishai the Sunamite. David was a notorious philanderer with God's blessing, and Abishai was a very attractive virgin who at other times would have excited the king's covetousness. Yet the old king did not know Abishai but used her body to keep warm. His sexual impotence represented for David an opportunity to establish an even more binding relation, as he needed Abishai more than he had needed the many women he had used and discarded, to start with the poor Michal, daughter of Saul.

Likewise, suffering is a unique opportunity to recognize the riches of our own humanity and of the people we serve. The suffering that aborted the development of the Middle East more than 3,000 years ago becomes through MECC the means to share each other's richness, to accomplish the promises of history.

Arrival

What have we learned from this brief journey through MECC? I feel myself anchored to MECC by these inspirations that inform my daily life:

- Every human experience is an opportunity to visit and develop our humanity. The avoidance of pain, suffering, and death represents an escape from our own humanity; compels us to a perpetual exile from ourselves. The biblical metaphor of this situation is Cain, as incapable of living as he is incapable of dying.
- Pain and suffering are universal. The relief of pain and suffering is a universal task in want of a universal language. This language is compassion.
- Compassion may be learned and nurtured at the moment we exercise it. MECC is mostly a laboratory and a training camp of compassion and accordingly of a universal language, and it is made of living more than of spoken words. Through MECC initiatives, its members learn to understand and support each other even when they partake of cultures that are diverse and hostile to each other.
- The main obstacles to compassion include fear of pain and self-righteousness. The members of MECC have learned the difference between the pain caused by an abscess and the pain necessary to drain the abscess. They learn not to fear the pain necessary to prevent and relieve more pain. Likewise, the members of MECC know that their first task is to help the wounded and succor the homeless when they are faced with the destruction of war, rather than pursue the culprits of the destruction. They are aware that each death involves all of us. Every time the bell tolls it tolls for all of us.
- Science and technology may represent an obstacle to compassion. Through MECC, representatives of a so-called developed country may learn how to manage suffering when technology is scarce.
- The war-torn Middle East provides a most promising ground to test the message of MECC, but the message is universal; it is a prescription for an increasingly war-weary world.

References

1. Silbermann M, Fink RM, Min SJ, et al: Evaluating palliative care in Middle Eastern countries. *J Pall Med.* 2015;18:18–25.
2. Schapira L: Communication skill training in clinical oncology: The ASCO position review and an optimistic personal perspective. *Crit Rev Oncol Hematol.* 2003;46:25–31.
3. Silbermann M, Dweib Khleif A, Balducci L: Healed by cancer. *J Clin Oncol.* 2010;28:1436–1437.
4. "Deus ex machina." https://www.britannica.com/art/deus-ex-machina
5. Byock I: The meaning and value of death. *J Palliat Med.* 2002;5:279–288.

19

The Role of Spirituality among Palliative Care Patients in Poland, Poland

Jakub Pawlikowski, Małgorzata Krajnik, and
Aleksandra Kotlińska-Lemieszek

Introduction

All patients have their own sense of spirituality with personal value and belief systems. Person-centered and culturally sensitive health care, particularly at the end of life (EOL), should consider these needs [1]. Spiritual care is an intrinsic and essential component of palliative care (PC), central to the founder of the modern hospice movement, Cicely Saunders, and has been included in the World Health Organization definition of PC for almost 20 years [2]. High-quality spiritual care for cancer patients may influence the use of aggressive treatment, length of hospitalization, and frequency of dying in hospitals, and should be a key component of EOL care guidelines [3,4].

The Polish population provides an interesting background for analysis of the development of holistic care with spiritual support for people with cancer. On one side, Poland is among the many countries reporting a high mortality rate from cancer. On the other side, Poland is one of the most religious countries in the world, as measured either by church attendance, religiosity, or the percentage of the population that declares a belief in God [5,6]. Over the past 30 years, Poland has been undergoing a process of transformation from a communist to a democratic state. Religiousness and the Solidarity movement have influenced the development of PC in Poland [7]. However, in recent years, the Polish population, especially the youth, has become more secular, and regular Sunday Mass attendance has declined, from 51% in 1980 to 41% in 2010 and 38% in 2018 [8,9]. At the same time, the process of medicalizing death is progressing, and most Poles die in hospitals. This brings new challenges to providing spiritual care for patients (which should not be reduced to just pastoral care). Members of medical staff should recognize these needs and provide basic spiritual support at all settings where patients are cared for during the last days of their lives.

Hospice Movement and Palliative Care in Poland

The origin of hospice and PC goes back to 1970 and the early 1980s when groups of medical and nonmedical volunteers started congregating at local Roman Catholic parish churches with the aim of caring for people with incurable advanced diseases living in nearby neighborhoods [7,10]. Spiritual care, as an important component of the holistic approach, has since then been deeply grounded in PC [7]. These initially local initiatives greatly expanded in the 1980s during the time of martial law, when most forms of social activity were prohibited, as well as during subsequent years of social and political transformation in Poland (from 1981 to 1983 until the 1990s) [10]. The goal of these hospice teams, composed of volunteers, was to provide care for people near the EOL whose needs were not being addressed by the public health care system at that time, reflecting the peoples' will for solidarity and a protest against political restrictions. As soon as the late 1980s, the first inpatient and home care units within the public health care system were established, followed in the early 1990s by the establishment of PC departments at medical universities (Poznan, Gdansk, Bydgoszcz, and others). Specializations in palliative medicine for physicians and in PC for nurses were introduced in 1998–1999 (Poland was the third country in the world to offer a diploma for specialization in PM for physicians). Thanks to the assistance of Dr. Robert Twycross, a WHO expert and the head of the Sir Michael Sobell House in Oxford, as well as the support of the Polish Hospice Fund and other foundations in the late 1990s and early 2000s, for over 10 years Poland was a center of education in PC for medical and nonmedical professionals from Eastern/Middle European countries [10,11]. Each year, 80–100 of them attended advanced courses chaired by Dr. Twycross and Prof. Jacek Łuczak, the pioneer and first national consultant in PC in Poland. Since the year 2000, PC has developed rapidly within the national health care system, with the creation of many hospices and home hospice care programs, as well as the implementation of PC educational and training programs for pre- and postgraduates of medicine [10].

At present, PC in Poland is a well-developed system integrated with the national public health care system, including almost 200 hospices and PC inpatient units and above 400 home care services operating throughout the country. However, until now, PC has been focused mostly on the care of patients with cancer. Patients with other diseases constitute only 10–20% of patients under care, and their access to specialized PC is still limited due to criteria for admission formulated in law. Paradoxically, the access to PC is also markedly limited for hospitalized patients (of Poles who die a year in Poland about 52% die in hospital wards). PC specialist consultations are not available in most of these institutions. Aside from the units specified for adult patients, a separate PC system exists for children; in addition, in recent years, prenatal PC teams have been funded in some maternity wards. Although the vast majority of PC units and hospices are run by public health care, some hospices are funded by social and religious (mainly Catholic) charities.

The Act on Healthcare Services Financed from Public Funds (2004) and the Regulation of the Minister of Health on guaranteed services in PC (2009) ensure public financing for hospices operating in public, as well as nonprofit and private sectors.

The Role of Chaplains in Spiritual Care

Patients in Poland have been legally guaranteed the right to pastoral care, which includes enabling the participation of religious ceremonies in health care entities; in addition, chaplains are financed from public funds [12]. When the disease causes severe deterioration in the patient's health and becomes life threatening, the hospital facilitates contact with the clergy of their denomination, upon request of patients and/or their caregivers [12]. A list of phone numbers and addresses for each particular denomination should be available in every ward. The main religion in Poland is Catholicism (86%), followed by Orthodoxy (1.5%) and various Protestant factions (1%). It is estimated that the number of priests employed or working as volunteers in Poland amounts to approximately 900, including 700 hospital chaplains, which roughly corresponds to the number of hospitals. About 11% of nuns work in health care units as nurses and doctors. In hospital chapels and nursing homes, over 1,000 Holy Masses are celebrated every Sunday [9]. Patients in hospitals or hospices can be visited by chaplains every day or several times a week. Patients cared for at home are served by parish priests. Over 92% of parishes undertake activities for the sick, including spiritual support (99%), organizing free time for the sick (25%), or nursing (9%) [13]. The problem, however, lies in the lack of specialized education programs for health care chaplaincy in Poland (one of the very few initiatives was organized by John Paul II University in Cracow and the Brothers Hospitallers of St John of God, which trained about 80 members of the clergy and laical volunteers).

Many obstacles to pastoral care emerged during the height of the COVID-19 pandemic. In Poland, as in other countries, chaplains were banned or limited from visiting patients in most hospitals across the country. However, model procedures for safely rendering pastoral care in the time of a pandemic are accessible, and pastoral care should be available [14].

The Role of Medical Staff in Spiritual Care

Studies have reported that health care practitioners who provide spiritual care to their patients significantly contribute to improving their patients' overall well-being. They show the positive effects of spiritual care on cancer patients' quality of life and reveal that a lack of spiritual support by health care teams is associated with poor quality of life, dissatisfaction with care, less hospice utilization, the use of more aggressive treatment, and increased costs [3,4,15,16]. Therefore, physicians, nurses, other medical staff members, and volunteers in hospices and hospitals should be able to provide basic spiritual support. Spirituality is also an important factor in the professional life of medical staff and can shape doctors' attitudes toward patients [17]. However, many doctors and other PC practitioners consider themselves unqualified to provide this type of care, and many express the need for training [18]. The European Association for Palliative Care (EAPC) white paper (2020) defines the core elements of multidisciplinary education for spiritual care in PC [19].

In most Polish hospices, the staff and volunteers are trained to recognize patients' spiritual needs and provide a basic level of spiritual care as well as coordinate further advanced support from relevant specialists. Volunteers who serve in hospices are (mostly) laypeople; however, there are also priests, monks, nuns, and clerics among them. Patients indicate the spectrum of support needed. For patients who declare the need for nonreligious spiritual support or who declare themselves to be atheist, the staff as well as dedicated volunteers provide them with the most suitable individualized support.

One of the most important initiatives for implementation of spiritual care into clinical practice, education, and research was the establishment of the Polish Association for Spiritual Care in Medicine (PASCiM) in December 2015 [20]. Among PASCiM members are doctors as well as other health care professionals, and chaplains (not only from the Roman Catholic Church but from other denominations as well). PASCiM organizes conferences and courses, but first of all makes efforts to initiate and coordinate long-term strategies for changing the health care system in Poland to be more open to incorporating spiritual care as an integral part of caring for patients. One of PASCiM's first achievements was to disseminate the understanding of 'spirituality' among different branches of medicine (e.g., cardiology and lung diseases) as the dimension of human life that relates to transcendence and other important existential values. According to this concept, spirituality entails (1) religiousness of an individual, especially his or her relationship with God, personal beliefs, religious practices, and community interaction; (2) existential quests, especially with regard to the meaning of life, suffering, and death, issues of personal dignity, who one actually is as a person, a sense of individual freedom and responsibility, hope and despair, reconciliation and forgiveness, love and joy; and (3) values by which a person lives, especially with regard to oneself and others, work, nature, art and culture, personal ethical and moral choices, and life at large [19,20]. One of the most valuable PASCiM activities is the educational program compatible with Clinical Pastoral Education requirements, which is planned to be piloted in 2022. PASCiM also supported the introduction in 2018 of the pioneering spiritual care program for medical students in Nicolaus Copernicus University in Toruń, Collegium Medicum in Bydgoszcz (CM UMK). The current program includes 12 hours for second-year students and 12 hours for fifth-year students. Topics related to spiritual needs and spiritual support have been presented in conferences organized by PASCiM and other societies and academic institutions, for example, Winter Summits in PC: "Heart and Spirit in Palliative Care" (2017) and "Breath and Spirit in Palliative Care and Pneumonology" (2018), both under the auspices of EAPC. Important aspects of "spiritual support" were also addressed in conferences organized by bioethicists and psychologists (e.g., the Fifth European Conference on the Research of Spirituality and Health in Gdansk, 2016; the First International Conference on Science, Religiousness and Human Spirituality, 2012). World-recognized leaders in spiritual care were invited to attend these events in Poland (e.g., Prof. Christine Puchalski, Prof. Richard Groves, Prof. Harold Koenig).

Research on the Spirituality/Religiosity of Patients in Poland

Empirical research on spirituality in medical practices, including cancer patient care, has quite a long tradition in Poland. Already in 1968, Prężyna published the scale for measuring religiosity (Scale of Religious Attitudes) [21], which, in the following years, was modified and used in research [22]. In recent years, several tools were also validated in Poland, including the Spiritual Needs Questionnaire (SpNQ) [23], Duke University Religion Index (PolDUREL) [24], Spiritual Attitude and Involvement List [25], and Spiritual and Religious Attitudes in Dealing with Illness (SpREUK) [26].

We found the results of studies concerning cancer patients and those in the advanced stages of the disease to be particularly interesting. A sample of cancer patients and caregivers of Poznan Hospice was included in an international multicenter study based on focus group method [27]. The study revealed a great variety of existential (meaning suffering), psychological (feelings of burden, guilt, helplessness, loss of control), religious (anger at God, questioning God), and social/relational (worry about the future of family members) concerns of participants. Of note, spirituality was primarily perceived as support for coping, but for some individuals it was associated with framing illness as punishment and, for others, spiritual care was reduced to "seeing a priest." Most patients and caregivers confirmed that spiritual care was essential in whole-person care at EOL. Case studies from Polish PC indicate that the physical dimension of pain should not be considered in isolation from the mental, social, and spiritual suffering experienced by patients [28].

Another interesting trend in spiritual care research in Poland is dignity therapy (DT), which is a short-term psychotherapy for patients (and their families) living with life-limiting illness [29]. DT intervention has been well received by Polish patients at the EOL suffering with chronic obstructive pulmonary disease (COPD) and advanced cancer, helping to enhance their sense of dignity, recognize and satisfy their spiritual needs, and reestablish a broken relationship with relatives [30,31]. One study involving home care patients suggested that even one dignity question: "What do I need to know about you as a person to take the best care of you that I can?" can be a brief diagnostic and therapeutic intervention significantly influencing patient care and well-being [32].

Hope is of great importance for patients diagnosed with cancer, especially those nearing EOL. In one study, authors noted varied levels of hope and varied internal structures of hope and observed that the highest levels of patients' hope (measured by the Hope of Cancer Patients Scale developed by Bogusław Block) were situated in the spiritual-religious area and the lowest levels concerned finding a cure [33]. Other authors published studies focusing on religiousness and anxiety in cancer patients [34], coping [35], and quality of life [36]. Differences in cancer perceptions among patients and medical staff also play an important role in medical care [37], and differences in "miraculous healing" beliefs among patients, health care providers, and chaplains can lead to different decisions concerning health care at EOL [38,39].

The results of these studies show that there is still a great need for continued research on topics relating to PC as well as other health care sectors, health education, and public health for the spiritual care of patients with life-limiting diseases.

Conclusions

Spiritual support is a key element of whole-person care that should be addressed to patients with cancer and other life-limiting diseases. Poland exemplifies the idea that the driving force for development of holistic care for patients with advanced cancer and at the EOL may be a religious community and social solidarity. However, with the progressing processes of secularization of society and the medicalization of dying, patients and caregivers increasingly expect spiritual support, not only from chaplains, but also from medical staff. The contemporary challenge, particularly in the field of hospital care for the dying, is to ensure access to whole-person medical care. Therefore, there is a need to educate both chaplains and members of medical staff in the field of spiritual support and whole-person care.

References

1. Puchalski C. Integrating spirituality into patient care: An essential element of person-centered care. *Pol Arch Med Wewn*. 2013;123:491–497.
2. Sepúlveda C, Marlin A, Yoshida T, Ullrich A. Palliative Care: The World Health Organization's global perspective. *J Pain Symptom Manage*. 2002 Aug;24(2):91–6. doi: 10.1016/s0885-3924(02)00440-2. PMID: 12231124.
3. Puchalski CM, Sbrana A, Ferrell B, et al. Interprofessional spiritual care in oncology: a literature review. *ESMO Open*. 2019;4(1):e000465. Published 2019 Feb 16. doi:10.1136/esmoopen-2018-000465
4. Balboni TA, Balboni M, Enzinger AC, et al. Provision of spiritual support to patients with advanced cancer by religious communities and associations with medical care at the end of life. *JAMA Intern Med*. 2013;173(12):1109–1117.
5. Pew Research Center. Surveys conducted 2015–2017 in 34 European countries; 2018. Available online: https://www.pewresearch.org/interactives/how-religious-is-your-country/. Accessed November, 2020.
6. CBOS. Życie religijne w Polsce. Wyniki badania spójności społecznej [Religious Life in Poland]; 2018. Available online: https://stat.gov.pl/obszary-tematyczne/inne-opracowania/wyznania-religijne/zycie-religijne-w-polsce-wyniki-badania-spojnosci-spolecznej-2018,8,1.html. Accessed November, 2020.
7. Krakowiak P, Skrzypińska K, Damps-Konstańska I, Jassem E. Walls and barriers. Polish achievements and the challenges of transformation: Building a hospice movement in Poland. *J Pain Symptom Manage*. 2016;52(4):600–604.
8. Sadłoń W. Differentiation, polarization and religious change in Poland at the turn of XX and XXI century. *Przegląd Religioznawczy—The Religious Studies Review*. 2016;4(262):25–42.
9. Instytut Statystyki Kościoła Katolickiego (ISKK) [Institute for Catholic Church Statistics]; 2020. http://iskk.pl/images/stories/Instytut/dokumenty/Annuarium_Statisticum_2020_07.01.pdf. Accessed November, 2020.
10. Łuczak J, Kotlińska-Lemieszek A, Kluziak M, Bozewicz A. Poland: Cancer pain and palliative care. *J Pain Symptom Manage*. 2002;24(2):215–221.
11. Bogusz H, Pękacka-Falkowska K, Magowska A. Under the British roof: The British contribution to the development of hospice and palliative care in Poland. *J Palliat Care*. April 2018;33(2):115–119.
12. Kubiak R. Patient's right to pastoral care. *Medycyna Paliatywna*. 2019;11(1):33.
13. Sadłoń W. Determinanty funkcjonowania opiekuńczej wspólnoty lokalnej: aktywność parafii w Polsce na rzecz chorych. *Polityka Społeczna*. 2012;5(6):24–29.
14. Hall DE. We can do better: Why pastoral care visitation to hospitals is essential, especially in times of crisis. *J Relig Health*. 2020;59:2283–2287.
15. Balboni T, Balboni M, Paulk ME, et al. Support of cancer patients' spiritual needs and associations with medical care costs at the end of life. *Cancer*. 2011;117:5383–5391.
16. Vallurupalli M, Lauderdale K, Balboni MJ, et al. The role of spirituality and religious coping in the quality of life of patients with advanced cancer receiving palliative radiation therapy. *J. Support Oncol*. 2012;10:81–87.

17. Pawlikowski J, Sak J, Marczewski K. Physicians religiosity and attitudes towards patients. *Ann Agric Environ Med.* 2012;19:503–507.
18. Gijsberts MHE, Liefbroer AI, Otten R, Olsman E. Spiritual care in palliative care: A systematic review of the recent European literature. *Med Sci* (Basel). 2019;7(2):25.
19. Best M, Leget C, Goodhead A, Paal P. An EAPC white paper on multi-disciplinary education for spiritual care in palliative care. *BMC Palliat Care.* 2020;19:9.
20. Polskie Towarzystwo Opieki Duchowej. [Polish Association for Spiritual Care in Medicine.] Available online: https://ptodm.org.pl/ Accessed November 2020.
21. Prezyna W. Skala postaw religijnych [Scale of Religious Attitudes]. *Ann Philos.* 1968;16:75–89. Polish.
22. Jarosz M. (ed). Psychologiczny pomiar religijności [Psychological Measurement of Religiosity]. Lublin: KUL; 2011. Polish.
23. Büssing A, Pilchowska I, Surzykiewicz J. Spiritual needs of Polish patients with chronic diseases. *J Relig Health.* 2015;54(5):1524–1542.
24. Dobrowolska B, Jurek K, Pilewska-Kozak AB, Pawlikowski J, Drozd M, Koenig H. Validation of the Polish version of the Duke University Religion Index (PolDUREL). *Pol Arch Med Wewn.* 2016;126(12):1005–1008.
25. Deluga A, Dobrowolska B, Jurek K, Ślusarska B, Nowicki G, Palese A. Nurses' spiritual attitudes and involvement—Validation of the Polish version of the Spiritual Attitude and Involvement List. *PLoS One.* 2020;15(9):e0239068.
26. Büssing A, Franczak K, Surzykiewicz J. Spiritual and religious attitudes in dealing with illness in Polish patients with chronic diseases: Validation of the Polish version of the SpREUK Questionnaire. *J Relig Health.* 2016;55(1):67–84.
27. Selman LE, Brighton LJ, Sinclair S, et al. InSpirit Collaborative. Patients' and caregivers' needs, experiences, preferences and research priorities in spiritual care: A focus group study across nine countries. *Palliat Med.* 2018;32(1):216–230.
28. Nowakowska-Arendt A, Graczyk M, Gęsińska H, Krajnik M. Total pain in a patient with lung cancer diagnosis. *Palliat Med Pract.* 2020;14(3):211–214.
29. Chochinov HM, Kristjanson LJ, Breitbart W, et al. Effect of dignity therapy on distress and end-of-life experience in terminally ill patients: A randomised controlled trial. *Lancet Oncol.* 201112(8):753–762.
30. Brożek B, Fopka-Kowalczyk M, Łabuś-Centek M, et al. Dignity therapy as an aid to coping for COPD patients at their end-of-life stage. *Adv Respir Med.* 2019;87(3):135–145.
31. Łabuś-Centek M, Adamczyk A, Jagielska A, et al. Application of dignity therapy in an advanced cancer patient—wider therapeutic implications. *Palliat Med Pract.* 2018;12(4):218–223.
32. Łabuś-Centek M, Jagielski D, Krajnik M. The meaning of dignity patient question and changes in the approach to this issue of cancer patients during home hospice care. *Palliat Med Pract.* 2020;14(2):89–94.
33. Baczewska B, Block B, Kropornicka B, et al. Hope in hospitalized patients with terminal cancer. *Int J Environ Res Public Health.* 2019;16(20):3867.
34. Janiszewska J, Buss T, de Walden-Gałuszko K, et al. A. The religiousness as a way of coping with anxiety in women with breast cancer at different disease stages. *Support Care Cancer.* 2008;16(12):1361–1366.
35. Klimasiński M, Theda J, Cofta S, Springer D, Wieczorowska-Tobis K. Spiritual care in medicine: Spiritual perception of illness, spiritual coping with suffering—a quantitative survey study on the Polish population of chronically ill adults. *Sztuka Leczenia.* 2020/1; 35: 9–18. Available online: https://doi.org/10.34938/h1k9-t164 Accessed November 2020
36. Żołnierz J. Quality of life and religiosity in the group of chronically ill people. Medical University of Lublin, PhD thesis, unpublished; 2019.

37. Sagan D, Sak J, Wiechetek M, Pawlikowski J, Olszewska E, Cieślak T. Differences in psycho-logical perception of lung cancer between patients, medical staff and medical students. *Eur J Cardiothorac Surg.* 2012;41(3):607–611.
38. Pawlikowski J. Consequences of the complexity and variety of beliefs about miracles. *Am J Bioeth.* 2018;18(5):71–72.
39. Pawlikowski J, Wiechetek M, Sak J, Jarosz M. Beliefs in miraculous healings, religiosity and meaning in life. *Religions.* 2015;6:1113–1124.

20

The Role of Faith in Coping with Cancer among Palliative Care Patients in Turkey, Turkey

Adem Akcakaya and Gulbeyaz Can

Introduction

Cancer is one of the most significant health problems faced by almost every country in the world in terms of morbidity and mortality [1]. Presently, the incidence of cancer in Turkey is 212.6 in 100.000 [2]; each year approximately 170,000 people are diagnosed as having cancer, and about 600,000 people are currently living with the disease [3].

According to World Health Organization (WHO) statistics, 58 million people die each year and nearly 100 million people need palliative care. In developed countries, palliative care services, which differ from country to country, are mainly provided in three levels of health care services. The first is hospital-based palliative care, where patients with especially complex, high-risk illnesses are cared for. The second is home-based care, where the primary care environment is at the patient's home and the aim is to provide palliative care at the level that can be provided in the hospital. The third is community-based palliative care which takes place at clinics created for outpatients. The common goal in all three levels is to provide the appropriate physical, psycho-social and moral support to the patient and their relatives, based on their cultural values [3].

The first long-term palliative care center for cancer patients in Turkey was founded in 1993. In 2010, there were only nine palliative care centers. Palliative care legislation in Turkey was initiated between 2008 and 2009, with three workshops held in Ankara. The First Palliative Care Action Plan published within the scope of the National Cancer Control Program and the Pallia-Türk Project defined the palliative care approach for the country. The establishment of hospital-based palliative care centers increased rapidly between 2012 and 2013. Legal arrangements were completed with a new regulation published in 2015. As of July 2019, the number of hospital-based palliative care centers reached 410 and the number of beds reached 5,143 [3,4]. This was a very quick breakthrough for Turkey. While these developments were taking place in the field of palliative care, there was not enough progress in the hospice structuring because the families continued to care for their patients during the terminal period at home. In Turkey, 80% of inpatients, 50% of those who are admitted to the outpatient clinic, and almost all relatives of these patients need professional support. Although many patients around the world want to die at home, 80% of patients still die in hospitals. In Turkey, 40% of deaths occur at home, and each patient in the terminal period is hospitalized for an average of 15–20 days [3].

Cancer is a difficult disease. For many, receiving a cancer diagnosis is associated with a peak of emotional distress, negative thoughts, introversion, and restlessness [5]. About 40–50% of cancer patients experience significant clinical distress [6]. Many patients perceive a cancer diagnosis as a death sentence. Elizabeth Kubler-Ross (1969) proposed that a patient with a life-threatening illness progresses through five stages of grief when informed of their illness: denial, anger, bargaining, depression, and acceptance, in that sequence. Each patient has a different way of coping with cancer [7], as their cultural background and beliefs have an important role in the individual's response to the disease [8].

Islam

Protecting life and taking measures against diseases are among the basic principles of Islam. Islam accepts that nothing happens by chance—the heavens, the earth, and everything in between, it teaches, have been created with a purpose (Quran; 44:38) [9]. Worship, in Islam, is not limited to rituals such as prayer, *salat* (obligatory Muslim prayers, performed five times each day), and Hajj (a physically demanding journey required of all Muslims once in a lifetime, that Muslims believe offers a chance to wipe clean past sins and start anew before God). It also involves creating an atmosphere conducive to righteousness in all spheres of life and having consistently good morals while on earth. In other words, for a lifetime, Muslims are expected to strive to do what is best for the planet and its inhabitants. There is also no time limit to fulfill this expectation. It is recommended that Muslims "work for the world as they would never die, for the hereafter as if they would die tomorrow" [10]. Perfect health is a wish that people desire because it is the greatest blessing of the Creator after faith [11]. This belief requires that people take advantage of even their last moments and live every moment of life fully. This is also in full compliance with palliative care principles. Reminding the Muslim patient of these principles helps to increase their coping skills [9]. Islam encourages Muslims to seek treatment when they get sick and forbids hastening death, even if it is claimed to be for pain relief [10].

In Islamic belief, sickness and healing are from Allah. Without Allah's permission, no entity or object has the power to make a person sick or heal them. Islam encourages Muslims to acknowledge that everything good or bad comes from Allah [12,13]. Illness can be the result of our deeds or a divine warning. The sick person is obliged to seek treatment and, for this, they can use spiritual methods such as prayer and material factors such as medicine. However, goodness, healing, or disease-related death decisions are not in our hands but are subject to Allah's permission [14]. In one study, up to 50% of health care workers stated that cancer was an affliction given by Allah [15]. This information makes it easier for palliative care patients in Turkey to use positive coping methods, as sickness and its associated pain and suffering are also perceived as a reason to ask Allah's forgiveness or atone for their wrongdoing.

Spirituality

Spirituality is derived from the Latin word *spiritus*, which means "breathing" or "living." In literature, the dimensions of spirituality are defined as religion, anxiety, hope, and a sense of belonging. Moreover, it includes the individual's efforts to understand and accept their relationship with themselves and others, their place in the universe, and their lives [16]. Spirituality is defined as "a dynamic and intrinsic aspect of humanity in which people seek ultimate meaning, purpose and transcendence, and experience the relationship with themselves, their families, society, nature and the sacred" [17]. Spirituality includes beliefs about health, illness, sin, death, life after death, and responsibility to others [5,18].

Death

Death is one of the most important elements in determining one's orientation toward spirituality. Death is proof of existence. The first comment on whether death is good or bad came from Socrates, who said that "it is perhaps the most beautiful thing that can happen to us, because we do not know what death is," alleviating humans' fear of death. However, Plato's student, Aristotle, defended this thesis: "death is the worst thing that can happen to a man." Epicurus's philosophy was "death does nothing to us, we cannot say that it is bad because there is no death when we are alive and, when death comes, we are absent." Seneca, a late-period philosopher of the Stoics, accepted that a single universe existed but is repeated temporally, and, by synthesizing Plato's and Aristotle's cosmology, he saw death as the separation of the soul and body. His interpretation was, "the soul is immortal and is born with death to a new life." According to Seneca, "death is not the opposite of existing, the opposite of existence is nonexistence. However, death is not a complete absence." Encountering or remembering death, according to Heidegger, brings out the anxiety that questions everything, leads us to question our existence, enables us to find the purpose of life, and reminds us of ourselves and who we are. Jean-Paul Sartre, who claimed that nothingness comes to the world through human consciousness, looked at death similarly to Epicurus. He said, "I was born and I will die, but I will not be aware of either of them". Hegel assessed death differently from Heidegger; he emphasized its unreality and introduced the idea that life encompasses death [19].

Death has taken an important place in the Islamic conception and has been interpreted by different cults in society for millennia. Al-Kindi, one of the early Arab Muslim philosophers, reminds us a bit of Epicurus and narrated death in metaphors, describing death as "a ship that will take us home to our true homeland." On the other hand, Abu Bakr Ar-Razi, a Persian alchemist and philosopher, said that those who do not have eternal belief and desire for eternity find it difficult to get rid of the fear of death, and they are caught in the streams of their passions. He explained that it is not possible for those who know death as nothingness to fear death because there can be no pain and suffering in nothingness, and so he concluded, the fear of death must be replaced by the desire for eternity. Abu Nasr Muhammad al-Farabi, one the earliest Islamic intellectuals, found the fear of death to be based in ignorance and said that the ignorant people are afraid because they think that they will lose their happiness with death but, if they know about the happiness after death, they will not have this fear of losing. Avicenna, the most famous and influential of all the Islamic philosopher-scientists, said that people will realize death by realizing their existence; they will experience ontological problems, and they will meet with pain. He pointed out that humans can only be complete with death; that is, humans will reach their highest horizon with death, and, therefore, it is necessary to desire death, not fear it. When Rumi, a 13th-century poet and philosopher who lived in Anatolia, defined the moment of death as the "wedding night," he explained that it is a moment of reunion rather than a separation. For Yunus Emre, a well-known Turkish folk poet and Sufi mystic, death meant entering the path of eternity and waking up from sleep. In Islam, death is only the death of the body; there is no such thing as the death of the soul.

According to studies, the main features of the "good death" concept in Western cultures are listed as follows [20]: awareness of death and positive acceptance of death, preparedness, physical comfort, especially pain control, peace and dignity, family or family-like environment, feeling like an individual, having a sense that their desires are taken into account, good timing, clarity about when and how death will take place, and, most importantly, the feeling of control by the individual. None of these features are related to medicine except physical comfort, which is one of the features that determines a good death. In other words, the only thing expected from medicine for a good death is to eliminate the symptoms that may disturb the individual, especially pain.

Since the Sumerian period (5th to 3rd millennia BCE), when the first written works appeared, disease has sometimes been defined as a punishment and, at other times, as a test for the elevation of the spiritual position. Divine religions, such as Islam, are not limited to faith, worship, and good morals; they also regulate a person's way of thinking and medical experience.

Faith in Coping

Cancer is a difficult process that individuals cannot control but must go through. Individuals overcome this difficult period by incorporating their personal experiences and spiritual and cultural values to find new meaning for themselves in the world. In Turkey, many patients who receive a fatal diagnosis begin to question their life and its meaning [21]. In times of stress or crisis, religious and spiritual practices that have a positive effect on people can turn into a coping style for patients. They can affect an individual's point of view and provide a source of coping [6].

The two types religious coping are positive and negative. Positive religious coping involves believing in the spiritual meaning of suffering and cooperating with God in solving problems. Positive religious coping helps patients to reduce stress, positively affects the mental and physical health of patients, improves the quality of life, and decreases suicide rates [2,6,22,23]. Praying, evaluating situations, feeling a secure relationship with God, believing in a purposeful life, and hoping for God's help is constructive and beneficial for psychosocial adjustment and is effective in reducing symptoms [22]. However, negative religious coping has worse consequences [2].

They reduce the quality of life, increase symptoms, decrease life satisfaction, increase the psychological distress of patients, and cause the intense desire for death [2,22]. Negative religious coping is associated with feeling sinful, punishment by God, abandonment, psychological problems, and suicide attempts, and it can be viewed as spiritual disconnection, having doubt in the power of and love of God, or excluding God from the solution [6].

In Turkey, palliative care patients, particularly cancer patients, primarily use positive religious coping methods based on Islamic teachings and traditional Turkish culture, although they have regional and sectarian differences [2]. Some non-Islamic superstitious coping strategies may also have negative consequences. For example, if a person adheres to a religious belief or practice, their condition may worsen if they continue to pray without medicine and hope for a miracle [24]. At this point, it is necessary to distinguish between positive and negative religious coping styles [2]. In Turkey, it has been found that negative religious coping, though small in numbers, can include attitudes such as believing that the devil brings on the disease and that being sinister can cause despair [25].

Religious and cultural beliefs have an impact on one's ability to endure illness and remain patient. Praying, attending a religious meeting, and performing certain religious rituals provide significant benefits for the patient to adapt to cancer [26]. There are many religions throughout the world, and each interprets the meaning of suffering and how to manage it differently. For example, in the Middle Eastern Arab countries, patients express their pain aloud. The Chinese, Japanese, and Vietnamese may not outwardly express their pain due to their cultural or religious belief that pain should be endured silently [13]. One study [27] showed that Muslim cancer patients use positive coping approaches such as reciting the Quran, praying, and feeling that Allah is with them as a method of handling pain [27]. These patients understand that illness, suffering, and dying are part of life and are a test from Allah; their knowledge of Allah increases as a result of the disease, and they feel closer to Allah. Seeing their weaknesses, they seek forgiveness from Allah, who is all forgiving [28]. In case of illness, a person seeks shelter in divine power in order to cope with such a difficult situation, and their beliefs are supported by praying and worshipping. Taking refuge in the sacred value to find a solution for problems that are beyond human control and the trend of using religious coping tools are especially common in Turkey [29]. Health professionals should bear in mind that significant individual and religious diversity within spiritual bases can affect how one is able to endure illness and its symptoms [4].

Changes in religious habits and practices may occur after a cancer diagnosis, and people may choose to alter their prayer and religious rituals. In a study from Turkey, it was shown that patients who prayed regularly before the diagnosis of cancer prayed less after the diagnosis; in contrast, it was shown that one-fifth of patients who did not pray before the diagnosis of cancer began to pray after learning of the diagnosis. According to data in the available literature, these changes are usually due to the main factor causing the psychological stress, the character of the patient, the thought that their illness will worsen if they practice (or do not practice) this ritual, the fear of death, or other conditions [30,31]. These changes are common in patients with cancer and are not observed in patients with other chronic medical conditions [32]. Another study of 248 cancer patients showed that when the patients' spiritual needs were met, more than 40% reported that the fear was eliminated, their lives had more meaning, their hope level increased, and they felt more vigorous. The results of a study with colorectal cancer patients showed that a higher level of spiritual well-being resulted in more effective treatment of physical symptoms; they also reported that their experience with cancer increased their spiritual awareness [5,33].

Cancer is a disease for which hope gains importance due to negative perceptions about the future of the disease and life expectancy, and religious beliefs and practices are one of the factors affecting the level of hope [2]. Religious coping in cancer patients is one of the approaches that affects compliance with the disease, psychological health, quality of life, and treatment [34]. In the course of cancer, a quick death of patients in a short time increases despair [2]. Hope is an effective coping strategy that gives the cancer sufferer the power to adapt to changes, increases interest in life and in the future, gives meaning to life, increases motivation, and prevents feelings of pessimism or helplessness during illness. In cancer patients, hope is seen as a means of helping to facilitate coping in times of uncertainty, pain, and difficulty and to show the will to fight against the disease. It has also been found that patients with high levels of hope tend to live longer and have longer disease-free periods [2]. Studies show that patients with diseases such as cancer tend to turn to religion and use positive religious coping, which, in turn, reduces the patient's stress [35]. Some publications show that the effect of religious coping on hope is not clear for diseases such as cancer, which affects the entire lives of both the individual and the family. In clinical practice, health care professionals must become familiar with their cancer patients' physical and mental health, religious coping styles, and hope levels before providing holistic care [2]. Sanatani et al. found that those who received chemotherapy therapeutically had slightly higher levels of hope than those who received only palliative treatment [36]. The high level of hope seen in the patients in this study might be due to the patients' belief that, by receiving chemotherapy in the outpatient clinic, their disease will be treatable [2,36].

Different cultures use spirituality as a coping method in various ways. In some studies, 90% of patients have stated that spirituality is an integral part of coping with cancer [18]. Religious, cultural, and spiritual differences between Turkey and other countries (such as Europe, Japan and the United States) have been studied to examine the impact of these beliefs on patients' coping methods. Results of tests carried out in other countries, which have been modified and adapted to Turkey, showed no significant differences statistically [17].

The coping methods used by cancer patients in Turkey can be divided into four categories: achievements, struggle, support, and religion/belief. On matters of fate and faith, some patients said that they prayed a lot to God and defeated cancer, stating that their belief in God and prayer helped them overcome illness. Some patients stated that their spiritual feelings and beliefs were an effective way of coping, that belief was important, and that one should never lose faith, no matter what. Others saw their illness as a test and said that they would ultimately be free from sin and that their beliefs enabled them to look at every newborn day with hope [37]. In a study performed by Dedeli et al., it was stated that spirituality was an integral part of human life. The study found that spiritual needs and spiritual practices were important parts of cancer patients' lives, relieving their stress and helping them cope [5].

It has been observed that cancer patients who are associated with religious institutions, who participate in religious services and activities, and who are active members in their houses of worship show fewer signs of physical symptom distress [23]. Participating in religious activities also reduces psychological distress in cancer patients. A similar phenomenon was observed in Muslim patients, where an elevated level of faith and spirituality helped to alleviate physical and mental distress [6].

The Quran and *salat* are widely practiced for spiritual support in the Islamic world. Guz et al. found that the most common method used by *hodjas* (teachers or spiritual leaders) in Turkey was to pray on behalf of the patient (27.3%) [7]. A study in Turkey conducted with patients with breast cancer reported that the most prominent alternative treatment methods used by people, after herbal treatment, was prayer and spiritual support. Of these patients, 82% stated that they chose this method of their own free will, without any other guidance [8].

Research findings reveal that cancer patients are more comfortable when they use positive religious coping methods [2]. In this situation, cancer patients have a high tendency to turn to religion when they think death is approaching; they tend to turn to God and pray [35].

Conclusion

Just as immortality is not possible, it is not possible to talk about life without death. The medical community must work to prevent diseases and help those who face death, when the time comes, to die peacefully and in comfort. In Turkish Muslim culture, it is believed that feelings of forgiveness, trusting in Allah, and asking for help from Allah reduce troubles. Spiritual well-being is a fundamental aspect of an individual's inner life and an important determinant of their relationship with the outside world. It is believed that finding meaning in suffering improves the patient's ability to cope [9,38,39]. In combating a life-threatening disease such as cancer, it is necessary to combat all symptoms, especially pain. For the management of pain, the patient, their family, and caregivers should not despair during the care process and should continue care with hope and faith. The patient's life should be made meaningful, and coping skills and problem-solving abilities should be supported [5]. Awareness of one's spirituality is important for both patients and health professionals. While patients need spirituality to cope with diseases such as cancer, health care professionals become more sensitive to understanding the spirituality of patients, speak more comfortably, and provide more benefit to their patients [17]. Spirituality and cultural background affect people's perspectives on death and palliative care differently. It has been found that Middle Eastern people are more interested in receiving training in spiritual care than Americans are [39,40]. Islamic theology fits perfectly with the principles of palliative care, as Islam deals with the details of individuals' lives. Similarly, the integrity of palliative care requires sensitive and sincere consideration of the cultural and spiritual aspects of care for Muslim patients. This demonstrates that it is essential for non-Muslim palliative care professionals caring for Muslim patients to raise their awareness of Islamic principles regarding palliative care [9].

If the medical team does not receive support from spiritual professionals, they should, at the very least, follow the methods of listening to the patient, be aware of their expectations, be respectful, and give referrals when necessary. While collecting data about the patient, a holistic perspective should be adopted, and evaluations should be made regarding physical, social, and psychological problems, along with religious beliefs. Also, patients should be supported in using positive religious coping methods. In this context, Turkey is similar to Western countries in that there are deficiencies in palliative care. When evaluating a Muslim patient, Islamic perspectives regarding the safe journey to death and beyond should be taken into consideration, understanding the religious and spiritual sensitivity of the patient and connecting with the patient. The incidence of questioning patients about their personal religious beliefs, spiritual care, and destiny, as well as conducting studies in this field, have increased in parallel with the whole world. Studies in Turkey have found that spiritual care is conducive to positive religious coping and helps deal with adverse symptoms in both palliative care units and for cancer patients [3]. People seeking a solution and a place of refuge when feeling helpless can turn to spiritual coping, a method that has been used since ancient times. Health professionals have a duty to support the use of this method and understand the individual's cultural past and expectations.

References

1. Kara B, Fesci H. Kanserde öz-bakım ve yaşam kalitesi. (Self-care and quality of life in cancer). *Hematol–Oncol.* 2004;6(3):124–129.
2. Sabanciogullari S, Yilmaz FT. The effect of religious coping on hope level of cancer patients receiving chemotherapy. *J Relig Health.* 2021;60(4): 2756–2769 doi:10.1007/s10943-019-00944-1
3. Akçakaya A, Akçakaya F. Palyatif Bakım Tanımı ve Tarihçesi (History of palliative care). In: Akçakaya A (ed). *Palyatif Bakım ve Tıp (Palliative Care and Medicine).* I. Istanbul: Istanbul Tıp Kitabevleri; 2019:2–6.
4. Göksel F, Şenel G, Oğuz G, et al. Development of palliative care services in Turkey. *Eur J Cancer Care.* 2020;29(6):e13285 doi:10.1111/ecc.13285
5. Dedeli Ö, Karadeniz G. An integrated psychosocial-spiritual model for cancer pain management. *Ağrı (Pain).* 2009;21(2):45–53.
6. Yılmaz Karabulutlu E, Yaralı S, Karaman S. Evaluation of distress and religious coping among cancer patients in Turkey. *J Relig Health.* 2019;58(3):881–890. doi:10.1007/s10943-017-0453-6
7. Guz H, Gursel B, Ozbek N. Religious and spiritual practices among patients with cancer. *J Relig Health.* 2012;51(3):763–773. doi:10.1007/s10943-010-9377-0
8. Kalender M, Buyukhatipoglu H, Balakan O, et al. Depression, anxiety and quality of life through the use of complementary and alternative medicine among breast cancer patients in Turkey. *J Cancer Res Therapeut.* 2014;10(4):962–966. doi:10.4103/0973-1482.138010
9. Al-Shahri MZ. Islamic theology and the principles of palliative care. *Palliat Support Care.* 2016;14(6):635–640. doi:10.1017/S1478951516000080
10. www.islamweb.net 2006; Fatwa no. 91760.
11. Deuraseh N. Health and medicine in the Islamic tradition based on the Book of Medicine (Kitab Al-Tibb) of Sahih Al-Bukhari. *Jishim.* 2006;5:2–14.

12. Mendieta M, Buckingham RW. A review of palliative and hospice care in the context of Islam: Dying with faith and family. *J Palliat Med.* 2017;20(11):1284–1290. doi:10.1089/jpm.2017.0340

13. Can G, Mushani T, Rajhi BH AL, Brant JM. The global burden of cancer pain. *Seminars in Oncol Nurs.* 2019;35(3):315–321. doi:10.1016/j.soncn.2019.04.014

14. Atmaca V. The relationship of illness and sin in old civilizations and the matter of god's revenge. *Atatürk Üniversitesi İlahiyat Fakültesi Dergisi.* 2010;34(1):99–121.

15. Tasci-Duran E, Koc S, Korkmaz M. Turkish social attitudes towards to cancer prevention: A health belief model study. *APJCP.* 2014;15(18):7935–7940. doi:10.7314/APJCP.2014.15.18.7935

16. Aktürk Ü, Erci B, Araz M. Functional evaluation of treatment of chronic disease: Validity and reliability of the Turkish version of the Spiritual Well-Being Scale. *Palliat Support Care.* 2017;15(6):684–692. doi:10.1017/S1478951517000013

17. Bar-Sela G, Schultz MJ, Elshamy K, et al. Training for awareness of one's own spirituality: A key factor in overcoming barriers to the provision of spiritual care to advanced cancer patients by doctors and nurses. *Palliat Support Care.* 2019;17(3):345–352. doi:10.1017/S147895151800055X

18. D'Souza K, Astrow AB. Patient spirituality as a component of supportive care: assessment and intervention. *Curr Treat Options Oncol.* 2020;21(11):1–10. doi:10.1007/s11864-020-0701-y

19. Tan A. Death in Western philosophy and Islamic mysticism. *SD Dergi.* 2020;54(1):16–21.

20. Hayran O. End of life: When, how, where? *SD Dergi.* 2020;54(1):6–11.

21. Hicdurmaz D, Oz F. Spirituality as a dimension of coping. *J Anatolia Nurs Health Sci.* 2013;16(1):50–56.

22. Tarakeshwar N, Vanderwerker LC, Paulk E, Pearce MJ, Kasl SV, Prigerson HG. Religious coping is associated with the quality of life of patients with advanced cancer. *J Palliat Med.* 2006;9(3):646–657. doi:10.1089/jpm.2006.9.646

23. Holt CL, Oster RA, Clay KS, Urmie J, Fouad M. Religiosity and physical and emotional functioning among African American and white colorectal and lung cancer patients. *J Psychosoc Oncol.* 2011;29(4):372–393. doi:10.1080/07347332.2011.582634

24. Haghighi F. Correlation between religious coping and depression in cancer patients. *Psychiatria Danubina.* 2013;25(3):236–240.

25. Uysal V, Goktepe A, Karagoz S, Ilerisoy M. A research about the relationships and interactions between religious coping, hope, life satisfaction and psychological resilience. *J Marmara University Faculty of Divinity.* 2017;52(1):139–160.

26. Woll ML, Hinshaw DB, Pawlik TM. Spirituality and religion in the care of surgical oncology patients with life-threatening or advanced illnesses. *Ann Surg Oncol* 2008;15(11):3048–3057. doi:10.1245/s10434-008-0130-9

27. Shaheen Al Ahwal M, Al Zaben F, Sehlo MG, Khalifa DA, Koenig HG. Religious beliefs, practices, and health in colorectal cancer patients in Saudi Arabia. *Psychooncology.* 2016;25(3):292–299. doi:10.1002/pon.3845

28. Rezaei M, Adib-Hajbaghery M, Seyedfatemi N, Hoseini F. Prayer in Iranian cancer patients undergoing chemotherapy. *Complement Ther Clin Pract.* 2008;14(2):90–97. doi:10.1016/j.ctcp.2008.01.001

29. Ayten A. *A psychosocal research on refuge in God/religious coping (in Turkish).* 2nd ed. Istanbul: Iz Yayıncılık; 2015.

30. Tas F, Karabulut S, Ciftci R, et al. The behavior of Turkish cancer patients in fasting during the holy month of Ramadan. *Jap J Clin Oncol.* 2014;44(8):705–710. doi:10.1093/jjco/hyu070

31. Spilka B, Shaver P, Kirkpatrick LA. A general attribution theory for the psychology of religion. *J Sci Study Relig.* 1985;24(1):1–20. doi:10.2307/1386272

32. Turhal NS, Akinci F, Haciabdullahoglu Y, et al. Changes in lifestyle upon diagnosis of cancer or other chronic illnesses: A Turkish Oncology Group study. *J Health Psychol.* 2018;23(4):561–566. doi:10.1177/1359105316658968

33. Taylor EJ. Spiritual needs of patients with cancer and family caregivers. *Cancer Nurs.* 2003;26(4):260–266. doi:10.1097/00002820-200308000-00002

34. Bonomo A, Gragefe C, Gerbasi A, Carvalho M, Fontes K. Religious/spiritual coping in cancer patients under treatment. *J Nurs UFPE on Line Recife.* 2015;9(Suppl.3):7539–7546. doi:10.5205/reuol.7049-61452-1-ED.0903supl201506

35. Celasin H, Karakoyun R, Yilmaz S, Elhan AH, Erkek B, Kuzu MA. Quality of life measures in Islamic rectal carcinoma patients receiving counselling. *Colorectal Dis.* 2011;13(7):170–175. doi:10.1111/j.1463-1318.2011.02649.x

36. Sanatani M, Schreier G, Stitt L. Level and direction of hope in cancer patients: An exploratory longitudinal study. *Support Care Cancer.* 2008;16(5):493–499. doi:10.1007/s00520-007-0336-6

37. Sercekus P, Baskale H. Living and Coping With Cancer. *Holistic Nurs Pract.* 2015;29(3):144–150. doi:10.1097/HNP.0000000000000082

38. Puchalski CM. Spirituality and end-of-life care: A time for listening and caring. *J Palliat Mede.* 2002;5(2):289–294. doi:10.1089/109662102753641287

39. Baydar Erkoc T, İlkilic I. Ethical evaluation of euthanasia in the Islamic tradition. *Euthanasia and Assisted Suicide.* 2017;1(1):147–166.

40. Bar-Sela G, Schultz MJ, Elshamy K, et al. Human Development Index and its association with staff spiritual care provision: A Middle Eastern oncology study. *Support Care Cancer.* 2019;27(9):3601–3610. doi:10.1007/s00520-019-04733-0

21

The Impact of Culture and Beliefs on Cancer Care

Iranian Perspectives, Iran

*Maryam Rassouli, Azam Shirinabadi Farahan, Leila Khanali Mojen,
and Hadis Ashrafizadeh*

Introduction

Despite significant advances in medical science, cancer is still one of the major diseases of the current century and the third leading cause of death in Iran. Every year, 112,000 people in Iran develop various types of cancer. This disease will be the cause of 80% of deaths in Iran within the next 15 years [1,2].

Given the increasing number of cancer cases in Iran and the importance of improving the level of health and quality of life in cancer patients and their families, the management of this disease, including palliative care provision, is of great importance [3].

Several factors affect cancer care in Iran, the most important of which are specific religious, cultural, and social differences of the Iranian society and the related challenges. These religious and cultural factors influence people's beliefs and attitudes toward health and disease and impact their behaviors in cancer control programs [4]. Therefore, identification and management of these factors can be considered a major factor in the management of cancer in Iran.

This chapter reviews the role of the culture and religious beliefs of Iranian people in cancer care, studies the cultural diversity in the Iranian society, and investigates how culturally related factors affect different stages of cancer. It also reviews Iranian traditional medicine and its undeniable role in cancer treatment, and then refers to the religious beliefs of Iranians and explains the role of religious rituals in cancer management.

The Role of Culture in Cancer Care

Iran is a land of diverse ethnicities with people of different religions and denominations with different languages and dialects, traditions, customs, beliefs, and cultural elements of their own, who despite cultural differences share commonalities that are reflected in the Iranian culture [5].

In different studies, the impact of religious and cultural beliefs on different aspects of cancer care has been investigated, and concepts such as truth-telling, decision making, communication, meanings of suffering, end-of-life care, death and dying, grief, and coping with pain are discussed [6–9].

Given the importance of different periods of cancer, the impact of cultural factors has been studied on the aspects of palliative care during four stages (*prior to the disease*, at *onset of the disease, symptom management,* and *treatment*), as well as the end-of-life care, which are discussed in this chapter.

Cultural Considerations in Prevention, Screening, and Early Diagnosis

Prevention is an important strategy in reducing cancer mortality that is made possible through screening and early diagnosis. Although the three most common cancers—breast cancer, cervical cancer, and colorectal cancer—are screened free of charge, this program is not widely accepted because of cultural, economic, and social differences, which are considered barriers to an effective screening program [10]. Fear of being diagnosed with a serious disease and being rejected by one's spouse, family members, and friends, as well as belief in the destiny and God's will, are considered as cultural barriers and are effective factors in people's attitudes toward screening tests [4].

Cultural Considerations at the Onset of the Disease

Cancer diagnosis has many ups and downs for the family; Problems such as cancer diagnosis in a culture with cancer stigma, the fear of unknown therapies, approaching death, and the fear of losing the patient create a set of challenges for the family at the onset of the disease [4,11]. Accepting a care known as palliative care is a cultural challenge in itself, the reason for which perhaps is associated with the terminology of palliative care, which is rooted in the insufficient knowledge of the public and even the treatment team. This is often perceived by patients and families, as a sign of the doctors' giving up therapeutic efforts, or it may even be seen as a sign of imminent death [7].

One of the most important challenges in this stage is the physician's communication with the patient and the family, as well as telling them the truth. Establishing good communication between the physician, the patient, and the caregivers is the key to success in providing palliative care [12]. Communication is both verbal and non-verbal, and culture is basically an effective factor in providing it [13].

According to cultural and religious beliefs in Iran, touching and looking at the opposite sex is against the social norms [14]. Moreover, gender and culture are considered as barriers to communication [15]. In Iran, 70% of the population of nurses are women [16]; therefore, the number of male nurses is very small. Thus, female nurses need to provide care for male patients while due to the religious background of the country, male patients avoid contact with the opposite sex and challenge the treatment team in examining the patient and providing effective care [15].

Proper communication is associated with better emotional adjustment and higher satisfaction [17]. Therefore, trying to remove cultural barriers in communication seems necessary.

Telling the patient the truth is a cultural challenge in many countries. Although according to ethical principles, knowing the truth is the right of every patient, factors such as different cultural attitudes interfere in expressing the truth and deprive the patient of the right to know the truth and to make decisions [18].

Despite the fact that more than 80% of patients acknowledge that they have the right to know the truth and would like to be told the information about the disease, its complications and its prognosis, still most patients are unaware of the diagnosis of their disease [19]. Most of the time, families avoid revealing the disease in order to reduce the patient's fear and anxiety and to increase the patient's hope [4]. In this way, various studies have shown that the quality of life had been lower in patients who had been aware of their diagnosis. They had also experienced more psychological distress [20].

The impact of this stigma on Iranian culture is so great that even the treatment team may be accused of committing an immoral act by disclosing it [4]. Therefore, physicians prefer to use the word "cancer" less frequently in their communication with the patient and use alternative words such as "tumor" and "mass" more often [6]. In addition, the fear of stigma can be a barrier to the disclosure of cancer diagnosis [21]. In some cases, women hide their disease due to the fear of family members' worries, changes in parental and spousal roles, and the stigma of cancer, as well as the possibility that their children may inherit the disease, all of which will delay the beginning of treatment [4,21].

Patients are interested in being involved in decision making, but what matters most to them is the physician's opinion. Moreover, patients and their families prefer to communicate with physicians and receive all the information only from them [17,22]. Patients allow their physicians to make treatment decisions in their stead because of the communication culture that exists between physician and patient as well as Iran's paternalistic model of communication or "patriarchy" [4,17,19].

Cultural Considerations during the Course of the Disease

After decision making and starting the treatment process, palliative care starts as a comprehensive care approach that will last until the end of life. During this period, one of the most important challenges is pain management, which is largely influenced by culture.

Pain management, as the most common symptom in cancer, is influenced by culture and has challenged it extensively [23]. Religious and spiritual beliefs in Iran, as a strategy for coping with pain, represent a cultural challenge. In some cases, despite the emphasis of health care providers on pain relief, not only do people not seek medicine and treatment, but they also voluntarily accept pain. They believe that pain is a kind of treatment, and they regard suffering from pain as a value. They view suffering from disease as atonement for their sins and a means of purifying themselves and the society as well [23]. Some even believe that pain and disease arise from divine wisdom, fate, and predestination [4]. In the Iranian culture, sometimes not expressing pain is due to the family structure. Since parents are the pillar of the family, they tolerate their pain and refuse to express it in order to maintain family unity and not place pressure on the family [24].

Misconceptions such as fear of addiction and drug dependence are other cultural challenges involved in pain management [25]. Iran's low ranking in drug use according to the statistics provided by the International Narcotics Control Board (INCB) is also evidence of this claim [24]. In 2014, the INCB reported that Jordan, Lebanon, Turkey, Egypt, and Iran had the highest morphine consumption among middle eastern countries, respectively, which is considered low in comparison with the global amount of consumption [6,24,26].

Providing care for caregivers is one of the principles of palliative care, ignoring another important cultural challenge in Iran [27]. In the Iranian culture, which has traditionally espoused strong family feelings and relationships, it is a human duty to shoulder the burden of caring for family members. Therefore, patients keep silent, and their inner pain is never to be expressed [28]. Frequent hospitalization of the patient and long-term care with their accompanying problems on one hand, and the inability to solve these problems owing to the lack of financial and social support provided by the health care system and other family members on the other hand, put immense pressure on caregivers, to the point that they no longer have a normal life [29].

Cultural Considerations in End-of-Life Care and Death

In the end-of-life stage, cultural and religious variables are important factors in providing palliative care services. The main goal of end-of-life care is to provide a good and calm death for the patient with cancer, as well as bring peace and comfort to the patient's family [30].

In the Iranian culture, families often expose the patient to treatments whose harmful effects may outweigh their benefits to satisfy their own feeling of guilt and denial and because of the stigma of cancer [31,32]. Decisions regarding the received interventions, omission of useless treatments, and the place of care provision (hospital or home) are mostly made by the family. However, the patient may have other preferences, including receiving care at home [4].

In Islamic culture, special emphasis is placed on preparation before death. The last days of life can be a good opportunity to make amends, returning the borrowed, seeking forgiveness, and reconciliation. Moreover, the right to make out a will is emphasized in the Quran (Verse 180 of Surah al-Baqarah). However, because of Iran's cultural beliefs, including the fear of worsening the patient's spiritual and psychological condition, the patient is deprived of such a right [18].

End-of-life care may be provided in the home, hospice, or hospital, based on the patient's preferences. Nevertheless, according to reports from the World Health Organization (WHO), end-of-life care in the Middle East is very limited and requires special attention. One reason for this limitation is the lack of awareness and the absence of a positive attitude toward hospices, which is rooted in the culture [33]. In the Iranian culture, putting a patient in these centers would be like leaving an elderly person in a nursing home. It is considered an action that forgets the patient and may lead to the family being labeled as irresponsible.

A Do Not Resuscitate (DNR) order issued in the end-of-life stages is also frowned on for both cultural and religious reasons. Most Iranians are Muslims and believe that life and death are in the hands of God. Thus, Islam's attitude toward the issue of life has a direct impact on the DNR order [34].

A good death, that is, a death that takes place in peace, has different definitions in different cultures [35]. Iran follows various customs for death and dying such as placing the Quran above or beside the patient's bed; turning the dying patient toward the city of Mecca; reciting Shahadah; not leaving the dying patient alone; and not overly conversing with the patient [4,36,37]. The more respectfully the rituals are performed for the dying person, the better will the emotional and mental reactions of the family be [38,39].

Another aspect of end-of-life care is mourning care. Mourning is one of the most common human reactions in all cultures [40]. In the Iranian culture, various mourning ceremonies and rituals support the family of the deceased, alleviating the family's loneliness and helping the survivors adapt to the loss of their loved one [40]. Iran's ceremonies are rooted in their religious beliefs and include funerals, special prayers for the dead member, prayer of the burial night, three-day mourning rituals, recitation of the Quran and prayers, charitable donations, visits to the grave, and saying the Al-Fatiha (a surah of Quran which is read for happiness of the soul of the decedent) [4,36]. Despite all these opportunities, the evidence suggests that spiritual or religious people are present without spending any special training to support the patient and the family in hospitals, and the need for mourning care and guidelines to support the family is deeply felt [41].

The Role of Traditional Iranian Medicine in Cancer Management

Medicine in Iran has an ancient history. Traditional Iranian medicine, dating back to 10,000 years ago, considers not only the human being's material aspects, but also takes in other aspects of a person's existence as a divine creation. From this perspective, maintaining health precedes treatment. The focus of traditional Iranian medicine is on a person's way of life and specifically on providing healthy air, proper diet, adequate physical activities, sufficient rest, and a balanced mental status [42].

Since traditional Iranian medicine has a holistic approach and emphasizes curing the patient, not the disease, by understanding the general principles of cancer treatment and the possible mechanisms of medications, the same treatments can be generalized to new known malignancies [43].

Traditional Iranian medicine refers to the four types of nature (Khelt) in human being that if they become more than normal, they will overcome the body and cause illness. Studies in this field discuss cancer under the topic of a type of cold swelling attributed largely to the accumulation of abnormal black bile (soda) in the body. In some cases, phlegmatic swelling can be considered an equivalent of malignancy [44–46].

In traditional Iranian medicine, disease treatment follows a number of general principles, which are also followed for the treatment of cancer. Initially in the treatment, the diet is modified, then the pharmacological treatment is instituted, and finally, practical measures, such as phlebotomy and surgery, are taken. If the cancer is dormant, that is, neither growing nor metastasizing, it is not subjected to any manipulation or to the use of toxic and stimulant drugs; instead, the goal is to gradually diminish the tumor and prevent its growth [43,47].

Oral traditional medicine in Iran includes the experiences and the data that have been passed down from generation to generation, chest to chest, and includes various medical and treatment approaches. Thanks to its ancient history as well as its many different ethnicities, races, languages and climates, Iran is a country with innumerable medical experiences, as well as oral medical opinions and ideas [48].

In general, Iranians have a positive attitude toward complementary medicines, and the demand for such treatments is increasing [49]. Numerous studies have been conducted in the country, which have examined the frequency of practice or knowledge in the field of complementary medicine and herbal medicine as well [50,51]. A study conducted in Khorramabad in the western part of Iran, whose inhabitants belong to a certain cultural group (Lors), showed that 79.8% of the subjects had used complementary and traditional medicine methods at least once. Medicinal plants and prayer therapy had the highest consumption, 69.2% and 37.2%, respectively [52].

Most patients in Iran use complementary therapies for cancer or have used them in the past [53]. In order to avoid the frequent problems caused by chemotherapy, radiotherapy, and bone marrow transplantation, cancer patients look for interventions such as complementary (alternative) medicine and traditional medicine, which can be performed outside medical clinics [53]. The two most common methods of implementing complementary medicine are using medicinal herbs and seeking nutritional advice in order to select the correct type of food and its proper cooking method. Other complementary therapies include massage therapy [54], reflexology [55,56], acupuncture [57, 58], acupressure [59], touch therapy [60,61], aromatherapy [62–64], yoga and meditation therapy [65,66], music therapy [67,68], and prayer therapy [69,70]. Most cancer patients believe that using complementary medicine increases their general ability to resist the disease, improve daily functioning, and reduce the side effects of chemotherapy. They often seek to reduce symptoms of anxiety, fatigue, depression, spiritual distress, pain, difficulties in performing daily tasks, shortness of breath, weight change, and sleep problems, and to improve the quality of life through complementary therapies [53].

The most common reasons for using complementary medicine, in order of importance, are previous familiarity with these methods, the need to gain hope in life, an increased feeling of physical recovery, and the safety of these methods. Patients with breast and gastrointestinal cancers [71] were the most receptive cancer patients to complementary medicine.

People who suffer from serious diseases such as cancer are attracted to traditional medicine because of their opposition to the chemical side effects of drugs [53]. They believe that chemical drugs have a great impact on general health. Nevertheless, traditional methods have not yet produced the result that may give patients hope either. In addition to their benefits, chemical drugs prescribed by doctors to treat diseases sometimes have both short-term and long-term side effects that can directly affect a person's life [72,73].

One of the misconceptions of advocates of traditional medicine is "that medicinal herbs cause no complication"; this belief leads many people to use any medicinal herbs relentlessly. The minimum risk this belief poses is that those who consume medicinal herbs with abandon will not be protected against their complications and the harmful impacts of their abusing [74]. As a result, this trend can put patients at risk [75]. In some cases, these patients will not feel the need for medical treatment protocols and will stop following them prematurely [76].

The Role of Spiritual and Religious Beliefs in Cancer Management

Spirituality is related to seeking meaning and purpose and communication with a superior power. It helps one act in line with their purpose in life [77]. Spirituality is believed to be one of the major factors helping cancer patients cope with their disease during treatment, survival, disease recurrence, and dying. It can also control the worse effects of the disease and life's pressures [78,79]. Since spirituality is one of the important components of individual-centered and holistic care, spiritual intervention should be considered and included in the care plans of every patient with cancer [78]. One goal of palliative care is spiritual counseling designed to boost the patient and their family members; these strategies are effective in well-being and lead to psychological adjustment and adaptation [80–83].

In the Muslim holy book, religiosity is defined as the color and the smell of God (Al-Hadid, verse 4; Al-Baqara, verse 115). The contemporary Iranian philosopher, Motahari (1989), frequently refers to moral values and virtues in his discussion of spirituality [84].

In some societies, especially Islamic societies such as Iran, spirituality is overshadowed by religion; this superiority of religion is seen in all affairs of life, especially in treatment of diseases. Therefore, it seems necessary to address this issue, especially in regard to incurable diseases. Most Iranian patients possess a strong faith and consider themselves religious, for religious rituals have been part of their lives since childhood. These religious beliefs also influence medical decisions. In other words, religious beliefs, more than spiritual and cultural attitudes, overshadow patients' decision making in critical situations [85–87].

Spiritual interventions in Iran include religious practices, traditions, and customs such as performing prayers and reciting the Quran and other sacred texts, repentance, and forgiveness, focusing on the innermost needs of individuals. It seems that the threatening nature of cancer increases both the spiritual and religious needs of patients [88]. In this regard, religious and spiritual interventions give hope to Iranian patients in most situations and best meet these spiritual needs. These interventions are either performed individually by the patient alone and with the family or by formal care providers, given the multidisciplinary nature of cancer care and treatment.

Pilgrimages to Mecca and religious places, sacrificing animals in order for the sick person to be healed, saying prayers and participating in religious ceremonies, and helping the poor to please God and be healed are classified under those spiritual interventions, which are used to cure diseases by the patient and the family [23,89].

After being diagnosed with the disease, the cancer patient and the family may consider going on a pilgrimage. Pilgrimage and religious trips have their roots in the culture and ideology of many human societies. Islam emphasizes religious trips, especially pilgrimage to holy places. According to the Quran's commandments, Muslims always have an obligation to undertake religious travel. Patients therefore will visit holy shrines and pilgrimage sites in the hope of miracles and healing [90].

Sacrificing animals is a religious ritual that has a special place and importance in worship traditions. In all parts of Iran, sacrificing animals is a common practice intended to find healing for incurable patients; it is a practice that all Iranians have long accepted [91].

During illness, the followers of all the religions of the world turn to prayers and worship to seek healing for the sick and their recovery. In some religions, a word spoken for the worship of God may be expressed in the form of a carol or sermon. Praying and performing religious activities are among the main activities Iranian Muslims perform at the time of diagnosis or during end-of-life care [89,92,93].

The main theme of the most famous prayers used for treatment is seeking forgiveness and offering gratitude. The content of this prayer is a kind of cognitive therapy based on religious facts that subdues the destructive mental processes caused by facing the disease. In this way, the level of the individual's mental health improves, and then through psychosomatic mechanisms, the physical symptoms also improve [94].

Helping people is one of the valued human traits that Islamic teachings emphasizes. Paying obligatory alms, such as khums and zakah, is considered a way to help fellow human beings, the product of which is the pleasure of God, which plays an important role in healing the sick. Therefore, following the diagnosis, Iranian patients and families try to facilitate God's pleasure and the healing of their patients by paying alms and other financial aids [95].

With regard to actions taken by official care providers, spiritual therapy and the use of clinical guidelines for spiritual care are examples of the efforts providers make in performing religious and spiritual interventions at the patient's bedside. As a result, Iran is ranked among the top four developing countries after India, Brazil, and Israel with the most interventions and research in this field [96].

Conclusion

The management of cancer requires focus on all factors affecting the knowledge, attitudes, and behaviors of the society in order to prevent and treat the disease, as well as providing palliative care. Therefore, it is very important to consider cultural and religious variables. In some cases, these variables are considered barriers. It is necessary to turn threats into opportunities by being aware of them. Thus, sometimes they are considered facilitators that can be upgraded for the use of their synergistic power. It is important to adopt strategies with the aim of educating and increasing the health care professional's awareness of the importance of providing culture-based care; improving public awareness of the need to participate in screening programs; changing attitudes toward the disease and its causes; expanding integrative oncology in the country's cancer management programs; and including care in care programs to ensure their effectiveness.

Acknowledgments

The authors hereby express their gratitude to Professor Michael Silbermann, who eliminated all geographical boundaries through his amazing efforts and patience. He helped the countries in the region mobilize and take action toward attaining a single goal: notably, the provision of palliative care to cancer patients, regardless of their culture, language, and religion. The authors also thank Professor Mohammad Esmaeil Akbari for his guidance and knowledgeable support of the establishment of palliative care in Iran.

References

1. Rouhollahi MR, Mohagheghi MA, Mohammadrezai N. Situation analysis of the National Comprehensive Cancer Control Program in the I. R. of Iran; assessment and recommendations based on the IAEA imPACT mission. *Arch Iran Med.* 2014;17(4):222–231.
2. Ministry of Health and Medical Education. Cancer in iranian people. 2020; http://www.behdasht.gov.ir/news
3. Rahmani A, Ferguson C, Jabarzadeh F, Mohammadpoorasl A, Moradi N, Pakpour V. Supportive care needs of Iranian cancer patients. *Indian J Palliat Care.* 2014;20(3):224–228.
4. Fallahi S, Rassouli M, Mojen LK. Cultural aspects of palliative cancer care in Iran. *Palliat Med Hosp Care Open J.* 2017;1(2):44–50.
5. Culture Ca. Iranian Culture.2020; https://www.everyculture.com/Ge-It/Iran.html
6. Kirby E, Lwin Z, Kenny K, Broom A, Birman H, Good P. "It doesn't exist … ": Negotiating palliative care from a culturally and linguistically diverse patient and caregiver perspective. *BMC Palliat Care.* 2018;17(1):90–98.
7. Six S, Bilsen J, Deschepper R. Dealing with cultural diversity in palliative care. *BMJ Support Palliat Care.* 2020;2(1):1–5.
8. Schim SM, Doorenbos AZ. A three-dimensional model of cultural congruence: Framework for intervention. *J Soc Work in End-of-Life Palliat Care.* 2010;6(3–4):256–270.
9. Cain CL, Surbone A, Elk R, Kagawa-Singer M. Culture and palliative care: Preferences, communication, meaning, and mutual decision making. *J Pain Symptom Manage.* 2018;55(5):1408–1419.
10. Education MoHaM. Screening for three common cancers for early detection and diagnosis. 2018; https://dme.behdasht.gov.ir/
11. Mehrabi E, Hajian S, Simbar M, Hoshyari M, Zayeri F. The lived experience of Iranian women confronting breast cancer diagnosis. *J Caring Sci.* 2016;5(1):43–55.
12. Campos VF, Silva JMd, Silva JJd. Comunicación en cuidados paliativos: equipo, paciente y familia. *Revista Bioética.* 2019;27(4):711–718.
13. Hartog J, Hartog EA. Cultural aspects of health and illness behavior in hospitals. *West J Med.* 1983;139(6):910–916.

14. Rassouli M, Zamanzadeh V, Abbaszadeh A, et al. Patient-centered communication barriers: experiences of patients with cancer, their family members and nurses. *J Urmia Nurs Midwifery Faculty.* 2014;11(10):1–10.

15. Norouzinia R, Aghabarari M, Shiri M, Karimi M, Samami E. Communication barriers perceived by nurses and patients. *Glob J Health Sci.* 2016;8(6):65–70.

16. Sajjadi M, Mojen L. Nursing education in palliative care in Iran. *J Palliat Care Med.* 01/01 2015;s4(1):S4-001. doi:10.4172/2165-7386.1000S4001

17. Motlagh A, Yaraei N, Mafi AR, et al. Attitude of cancer patients toward diagnosis disclosure and their preference for clinical decision-making: A national survey. *Arch Iran Med.* 2014;17(4):232–240.

18. Zahedi F. The challenge of truth telling across cultures: a case study. *J Med Ethics Hist Med.* 2011;4(1):4–11.

19. Rozveh AK, Amjad RN, Rozveh JK, Rasouli D. Attitudes toward telling the truth to cancer patients in Iran: a review article. *Int J Hematol Oncol Stem Cell Re.* 2017;11(3):178–183.

20. Montazeri A, Tavoli A, Mohagheghi MA, Roshan R, Tavoli Z. Disclosure of cancer diagnosis and quality of life in cancer patients: Should it be the same everywhere? *BMC Cancer.* 2009;9(1):39–47.

21. Shiri FH, Mohtashami J, Manoochehri H, Rohani C. Explaining the meaning of cancer stigma from the point of view of Iranian stakeholders: A qualitative study. *Int J Cancer Manage.* 2018;11(7):5–15.

22. Lashkarizadeh M, Jahanbakhsh F, Samareh Fekri M, PoorSeyyedi B, Aghaeei Afshar M, Shokoohi M. Views of cancer patients on revealing diagnosis and information to them. *Iran J Med Ethics Hist Mede.* 2012;5(4):65–74.

23. Rassouli M, Sajjadi M. Palliative care in the Islamic Republic of Iran. In: Silberman M (ed). *Palliative Care to the Cancer Patient: The Middle East as a Model for Emerging Countries.* Nova; 2014:317–336. vol. 1.

24. Heydarpour SZE, Mehrabi E, Heidarpour F, Kolivand M. Comparison of primipara's women perception of pain, fear and anxiety of vaginal delivery among Persian, Kurdish and Turkish women. *J Clin Res Paramed Sci.* 2015;4(3):e82039.

25. Givler A, Maani-Fogelman PA. The importance of cultural competence in pain and palliative care. *StatPearls [Internet].* Treasure Island (FL):StatPearls Publishing; [Updated 2021 July 26]. https://www.ncbi.nlm.nih.gov/books/NBK493154/

26. Mojen LK, Rassouli M, Eshghi P, Sari AA, Karimooi MH. Palliative care for children with cancer in the Middle East: A comparative study. *Indian J Palliat Care.* 2017;23(4):379–381.

27. Abbasnezhad M, Rahmani A, Ghahramanian A, et al. Cancer care burden among primary family caregivers of Iranian hematologic cancer patients. *APJCP.* 2015;16(13):5499–5505.

28. Mobasher M, Nakhaee N, Tahmasebi M, Zahedi F, Larijani B. Ethical issues in the end of life care for cancer patients in Iran. *Iran J Public Health.* 2013;42(2):188–195.

29. Nemati S, Rassouli M, Ilkhani M, Baghestani AR. Perceptions of family caregivers of cancer patients about the challenges of caregiving: a qualitative study. *Scand J Caring Sci.* 2018;32(1):309–316.

30. Ghaljeh M, Rezaee N. Experiences of nurses about end-of-life care for cancer patients in Iran: A qualitative study. *Iran J Nurs.* 2018;31(114):65–75.

31. Mobasher M, Aramesh K, Zahedi F, Nakhaee N, Tahmasebi M, Larijani B. End-of-life care ethical decision-making: Shiite scholars' views. *J Med Ethics Hist Med.* 2014;7(1):4–11.

32. Shayestefar S, Mardani-Hamooleh M, Kouhnavard M, Kadivar M. Ethical challenges in pediatrics from the viewpoints of Iranian pediatric residents. *J Comprehens Pediatr.* 2018;9(1):e62747.

33. Zarea K, Rassouli M, Hazrati M, Molavynejad S, Beiranvand S. Comparison of the hospice palliative care delivery systems in Iran and selected countries. *Int J Cancer Manage.* 2020;13(6):e101635.

34. Rassouli M, Sajjadi M. Palliative care in the Islamic Republic of Iran. *Palliative Care to the Cancer Patient: The Middle East as a Model for Emerging Countries.* In: Silberman M, editor. New York: Nova Scientific Publisher. 2014:39:317–336.

35. Murray S. The 2015 Quality of Death Index. Ranking palliative care across the world. A report by The Economist Intelligence Unit. Line D (ed). Accessed on December 8, 2015 Pp. 56–72. http://www.lienfoundation.org/sites/default/files/2015%20Quality%20 of%20Death%20Report.pdf.

36. Ghasemzadeh N, Asghari F, Shirazi M, Razini FF, Larijani B. Jurisprudential and ethical considerations of practicing medical Islamic procedures on nearly dead patients: Part II (Shiite jurisprudents' viewpoints). *J Med Ethics Hist Med.* 2018;15(11):5–10.

37. Sotoudeh S, Mahdavi H, Tahmasebi M. Crises in caring for dying patients regarding cancer within Iranian cultural backgrounds: A systematic review of qualitative studies. *Int J Cancer Manage.* 2019;12(2):e87245.

38. Hojjati H, Hekmati Pour N, Nasrabadi T, Hoseini S. Attitudes of nurses towards death. *J Health Care.* 2015;17(2):146–153.

39. Ghaljeh M, Iranmanesh S, Nayeri ND, Tirgari B. Organizational challenges: A major obstacle at end of life care in Iran. *J Adv Med Med Res.* 2016;16(7):1–12.

40. marzie sharifi saa, maryamosadat fatehizade. Psychometric properties of the Hogan Grief Reaction Checklist in Iranian bereaved families. *Knowledge Res Applied Psychol.* 2013;14(53):69–79.

41. Pakseresht M, Baraz S, Rasouli M, Reje N, Rostami S. A comparative study of the situation of bereavement care for children with cancer in Iran with selected countries. *Int J Pediatr.* 2018;6(2):7253–7263.

42. Naseri M RH, Chupani Zanjani R, Anoshirvani M. *An overview of general Iranian traditional medicine.* Vol. 12. Iranian Traditional Medicine Publications; 2005:100.

43. Motavalizadeh Ardekani A, Hashemi M, Safakish M, Alem Bagheri A, Baradaran Shokoohi S, Mosaddegh M. Medical treatment of cancer in traditional Iranian medicine. original tesearch. *J Islam Iran Tradit Med.* 2012;3(1):3–18.

44. Akhawinei ReA. *Hedayate ol Moteallemin* vol 1. Ferdosi University of Mashhad 1992;1(1):15–25.

45. alTabari AiSR. *Firdaus al-Hikma.* Dar Al-Kitab Publications;1001;81(1):811–825.

46. Chaghmini Me-MeO. Ghanooncheh (cancer). In: Publications IUoMS, ed. *Ghanooncheh.* Iran University of Medical Sciences Publications; 1000 AH(Anno Hegirae);4(15): 2820–2840.

47. Moeini R, Gorji N, Rezaeizadeh H, Pasalar P, Nazem E, Kamalinejad M. Etiology and treatment of cancer; view point of Persian medicine. *Med Hist Jl.* 2017;9(30):55–82.

48. Sezik E, Tabata M, Yesilada E, Honda G, Goto K, Ikeshiro Y. Traditional medicine in Turkey I. Folk medicine in northeast Anatolia. *J Ethnopharm.* 1991;35(2):191–196.

49. Tehrani Banihashemi m, Asgharifard H, Haghdoost A, Barghmadi M, Mohammadhosseini N. The use of complementary/alternative medicine among the general population in Tehran, Iran. *Payesh (Health Monitor).* 2008;7(4):355–362.

50. Sedighi J MF, Zeaii A. Herbal medicine: Knowledge, attitude and practice among people of Tehran. *J Herb Mede.* 2005;13(4):61–67.

51. Golshadi IM AR, Asgari S, Sarafzadegan T, Beshtam M. Knowledge, attitude and practice about herbal medicine among Isfahan's people. *J Herb Med.* 2003;1(2):21–28.

52. Anbari K, Ghanadi K. Use of complementary and alternative mediecine methods and its related factors in person referred to health centers in khorramabad. *Complementary Medicine Journal.* 2015;4(4):987-999.

53. Farahani AS, Salmani N, Khoubbin Khoshnazar TAS, et al. The perspective of cancer patients on the use of complementary medicine. *Int J Cancer Manage*. 2019;12(2):e89916.

54. Bossak S DB, Hosseini SM, Latifi M. The influence of massage therapy on vomiting in under chemothrapy patient with breast cancer. *Iran Q J Breast Dis*. 2010;3(1):14–18. http://ijbd.ir/article-١-٧-١-fa.html

55. Haghighat S. The effect of reflexology on quality of life of breast cancer patients during chemotherapy. *Iran Q J Breast Dis*. 2013;6(1):23–34.

56. Pedramrazi S. The effect of reflexology on quality of life in Iranian patients with breast cancer. *J Clin Oncol*. 2016;34(26 suppl):90. doi:10.1200/jco.2016.34.26_suppl.90

57. Beikmoradi A, Najafi F, Roshanaei G, Pour Esmaeil Z, Khatibian M, Ahmadi A. Acupressure and anxiety in cancer patients. Research Article. *Iran Red Crescent Med J*. 2015;17(3):e25919. doi:10.5812/ircmj.25919

58. Sharif Nia H, Pahlevan Sharif S, Yaghoobzadeh A, et al. Effect of acupressure on pain in Iranian leukemia patients: A randomized controlled trial study. *Int J Nurs Pract*. April 2017;23(2):1–7 doi:10.1111/ijn.12513

59. Eghbali M, Varaei S, Jalalinia SF, Aalam Samimi M, Sa'atchi K, Yekaninejad MS. Effect of auricular acupressure on acute nausea and vomiting induced by chemotherapy among breast cancer patients. *Hayat*. 2015;21(2):29–39.

60. Matourypour P, Vanaki Z, Zare Z, Mehrzad V, Dehghan M, Ranjbaran M. Investigating the effect of therapeutic touch on the intensity of acute chemotherapy-induced vomiting in breast cancer women under chemotherapy. *Iran J Nurs Midwifery Res*. May-Jun 2016;21(3):255–260. doi:10.4103/1735-9066.180373

61. Tabatabaee A, Tafreshi MZ, Rassouli M, Aledavood SA, AlaviMajd H, Farahmand SK. Effect of therapeutic touch in patients with cancer: A literature review. *Med Arch*. / 2016;70(2):142–147. doi:10.5455/medarh.2016.70.142-147

62. Khalili Z, Khatiban M, Faradmal J, Abbasi M, Zeraati F, Khazaei A. Effect of cardamom aromas on the chemotherapy-induced nausea and vomiting in cancer patients. *Avicenna J Nurs Midwifery Care*. 2014;22(3):64–73.

63. Eghbali M, Varaei S, Hosseini M, Yekaninejad MS, Shahi F. The effect of aromatherapy with peppermint essential oil on nausea and vomiting in the acute phase of chemotherapy inpatients with breast cancer. *J Babol University Med Sci*. 2018;20(9):66–71. doi:10.18869/acadpub.jbums.20.9.66

64. BabashahiKohanestani F, Ahmadi F, Memarian R. The effect of lavender aromatherapy program on the pain intensity of patients with AML undergoing chemotherapy. *Nurs Midwifery J*. 2013;11(3):1–10.

65. Yazdani F. The effects of yoga on symptom scales quality of life in breast cancer patients undergoing radiotherapy. *Iran Q J Breast Dis*. 2015;7(4):33–42.

66. Yazdani F. The effect of yoga program on the quality of life in breast cancer patients *Nurs Midwifery J*. 2014;12(6):444–453.

67. Naseri P, Shirazi M, Gholamreza Sanagouye Moharer G. Comparison of the effect of music therapy and writing therapy on the anxiety and depression of students with cancer. *Iran J Rehabil Res Nurs*. 2020;7(1):55–65. doi:10.29252/ijrn.7.1.55

68. Jasemi M, Aazami S, Zabihi RE. The effects of music therapy on anxiety and depression of cancer patients. *Indian J Palliat Care*. 2016 Oct-Dec 2016;22(4):455–458. doi:10.4103/0973-1075.191823

69. Seyedfatemi N., Rezaie M., Givari A., Hosseini F. Prayer and spiritual well-being in cancer patients. *Health Monitor J Iran Inst Health Sci Res*. 2006;5(4):295–303.

70. Rezaei M, Adib-Hajbaghery M, Seyedfatemi N, Hoseini F. Prayer in Iranian cancer patients undergoing chemotherapy. *Complement Ther Clin Pract*. 2008;14(2):90–97. doi:10.1016/j.ctcp.2008.01.001

71. Sajadian A.S, Kaviani A, Montazeri A, et al. Complementary medicine use among Iranian cancer patients. *Health Monitor J Iran Inst Health Sci Res.* 2005;4(3):197–205.

72. Paryab M, Raeeszadeh M. The study of the rate and reasons of medical herb use by the patients visiting the specialized treatment centers in Fars Province in 2014. *Commun Health J.* 2017;10(2):62–71.

73. Hatami Varzaneh M. Secret health with herbs. *Fahmideh Shahid Publishing.* 2002;254(1):22–25.

74. Naja F, Abi Fadel R, Alameddine M, et al. Complementary and alternative medicine use and its association with quality of life among Lebanese breast cancer patients: a cross-sectional study. *BMC Complement Altern Med.* 2015;15(1):444.

75. Yarney J, Donkor A, Opoku SY, et al. Characteristics of users and implications for the use of complementary and alternative medicine in Ghanaian cancer patients undergoing radiotherapy and chemotherapy: a cross-sectional study. *BMC Complement Alt Med.* 2013;13(1):16–23.

76. Styczynski J, Wysocki M. Alternative medicine remedies might stimulate viability of leukemic cells. *Pediatric Blood Cancer.* 2006;46(1):94–98.

77. Lee Y-H, Salman A. The mediating effect of spiritual well-being on depressive symptoms and health-related quality of life among elders. *Arch Psychiatr Nurs* 2018;32(3):418–424.

78. Puchalski CM, King SD, Ferrell BR. Spiritual considerations. *Hematol/Oncol Clin.* 2018;32(3):505–517.

79. Puchalski CM. Spirituality in the cancer trajectory. *Ann Oncol.* 2012;1(23):iii49–iii55.

80. Koopman C, Angell K, Turner-Cobb JM, et al. Distress, coping, and social support among rural women recently diagnosed with primary breast cancer. *The Breast J.* 2001;7(1):25–33. doi:https://doi.org/10.1046/j.1524-4741.2001.007001025.x

81. Al-Azri MH, Al-Awisi H, Al-Rasbi S, Al-Moundhri M. Coping with a diagnosis of breast cancer among Omani women. *J Health Psychol.* 2014;19(7):836–846. doi:10.1177/1359105313479813

82. Danhauer SC, Crawford SL, Farmer DF, Avis NE. A longitudinal investigation of coping strategies and quality of life among younger women with breast cancer. *J Behav Med.* 2009;32(4):371–379. doi:10.1007/s10865-009-9211-x

83. Sajjadian AS, Haghighat S, Montazeri A, Kazem Nejad A, Alawi FA. Post diagnosis coping strategies patients with breast cancer. *Iran Q J Breast Dis.* 2011;4(3):52–58.

84. Motahari M. *Collection of Works.* Vol. 22. Sadra Publications; Tehran.1989, pp. 41–52.

85. Faranak Farzadi, Meroe Vameghi, Jila Sadighi, Farahnaz Mohammadi, Batool Mohtashami, Batool Ahmadi. Religion and spirituality in a health model for Iranian women: Farmehr model. *Health Monitor J Iran Inst Health Sci Res.* 2017;16(5):587–594.

86. Memaryan N, Ghaempanah Z, Seddigh R. Spiritual interventions in Iran: A review article. *SOJ Psychol.* 02/25 2017;3(1):1–5.

87. Boalhari J, Dos Ali Vand H, Mirzaei M. Spiritual approach in medical education and humanities. *Med Ethics.* 2014;6(20):101–125

88. Hatamipour K, Rassouli M, Yaghmaie F, Zendedel K, Alavi Majd H. Development and psychometrics of a "spiritual needs assessment scale of patients with cancer": A mixed exploratory study. *Int J Cancer Manag.* 2018;11(1):e10083. doi:10.5812/ijcm.10083

89. Abedi M. Palliative care within the Iranian context: Re-defining palliative care, deploying spirituality as a support measure and need for cultural sensitivity. Year of access 2012.

90. Saghaei M AEM. Tourism from the perspective of the Quran and hadiths. *Q J Quran Human.* 2014;3(2):93–105.

91. Sacrificing for health and repelling evil in Islam, 2012. available in: https://zaya.io/b44zy.

92. Ghali H. Cultural challenges in implementing palliative care services in Iraq. *Palliat Med Hospice Care Open J.* 2017;SE(1):S19–S23.Special edition. doi:10.17140/PMHCOJ-SE-1-105

93. Ahmadifaraz M, Mosavizadeh SR, Reisi-Dehkordi N, Ghaderi S. The effect of group spiritual intervention based on the Quran and prayer on spiritual health of patients with cancer. *J Isfahan Med School*. 2015;32(320 (Special Issue Complementary Medicine)):2454–2463.

94. Hamid N, Rigi AS, Marashi SA. The efficacy of spiritual/religious psychotherapy-emphasizing the importance of 15th and 23th prayers of Sahifeh Sajjadiyeh-on quality of life and attitude toward disease in cancer patients in Ahvaz City. *Iran J Psychiatr Nurs*. 2018;6(5):34–41.

95. Gaining God's approval is a lasting factor in helping others. 2017. Available in: https://btid.org/fa/news/106553.

96. Lucchetti G, Lucchetti A. Spirituality, religion, and health: over the last 15 years of field research (1999–2013). *Int J Psychiatry Med*. 12/10 2014;48:199–215. doi:10.2190/PM.48.3.e

22

Spiritual Healing in Cancer Care

A Hindu Perspective, India

Seema Rajesh Rao, Vidya Viswanath, and Srinagesh Simha

Introduction

The burden of cancer is rising globally, as one in five people are likely to develop cancer during their lifetime [1]. For patients and their families, the diagnosis and treatment of cancer or chronic illness threaten the intactness of the person and open the doorway to unbridled suffering that encompasses the physical and psychosocio-spiritual domains [2–4]. Mainstream medicine has long adopted a reductionist model and confined itself to the care of the human body [5]. With the advent of patient-centered whole-person care (PCC), the focus has shifted beyond Engel's biopsychosocial model to the biopsychosocio-spiritual model. A growing body of evidence supports the beneficial role of spirituality in the health and well-being of patients with chronic illnesses [6]. Studies have shown that spiritual well-being improves patient outcomes, helps patients cope with stress, aids difficult medical decision making, improves patient quality of life (QOL), reduces healthcare disparities, and enhances clinical care [7–9]. Spiritual issues are important determinants of QOL and warrant inclusion into QOL measures [10–11]. However, addressing spirituality can be challenging given the lack of a common language, the variations in cultural and religious practices, and the limitations of service provision.

Spirituality and religion, though independent constructs, are intricately intertwined. Personal religiosity is an aspect of a person's spirituality and interacts in varying degrees with organized religion. The cognitive-existential, experiential, and behavioral dimensions of spirituality are influenced by religious beliefs and have to be understood within that context [12]. Spiritual suffering can occur in any of these three dimensions, either alone or in conjunction with each other. Religious and cultural perspectives influence how the patient copes with the disease, views death and dying, and derives meaning and purpose. This chapter will familiarize health care providers with the basic tenets of Hinduism and the various nuances of suffering in Hinduism. It will also help them understand how these concepts can be utilized to provide whole-person care and promote spiritual healing among Hindu patients and their families.

Basic Tenets of Hinduism

With over 1.25 billion followers, Hinduism is the third largest religion in the world [13]. Hinduism originated in and is practiced predominantly in the Indian subcontinent. It is not an organized religion, but a conglomeration of various religious, cultural, and philosophical principles and practices [14]. Hindus worship multiple gods/goddesses and practice polytheism. Hindus believe these gods and goddesses to be different manifestations of one supreme God, the Brahman [15], as well as in the interconnectedness of the universe, with the Brahman representing the universal spirituality to which every Hindu remains connected [16]. There are multiple holy books in Hinduism, the most popular of which is the *Bhagavad Gita* [17]. The core principles, values, and beliefs of Hinduism are embedded in this book. The framework for spirituality in this chapter has been derived from the teachings of the *Bhagavad Gita*.

The basic tenets of Hinduism revolve around *samsara, karma, dharma,* and *moksha*.

The cycle of *samsara* [18] (see Figure 22.1): All living beings go through a cycle of birth, life, death, and rebirth or reincarnation. While the physical body perishes, the *atman*, the soul, is considered imperishable and is reborn in a new life form. This cycle is termed *samsara*. Hindus believe that the universe undergoes an endless cycle of creation, preservation, and dissolution.

The principle of *karma* [19]: *Karma* is the law of cause and effect, which states that every action has a consequence. Acts that are morally good will produce positive consequences; bad acts will produce negative consequences. Thus, individuals are architects of their fate and create their destiny by their thoughts, words, and deeds. The effects of these acts may be experienced in the present life or carried over to future lives. The form an individual assumes in the next life is determined by one's *karma*.

The path of *dharma* [20]: In Hinduism, *dharma* signifies the right way of living, that is, behaviors that are culturally appropriate, legally correct, and morally upright. It encompasses moral values, duties, rights/laws, and rituals/customs and prescribes a code of conduct that Hindus need to follow. Hindus believe that by following the path of righteousness, good *karma* ensues, and *moksha* can be attained.

The goal of *moksha* [21]: In Hinduism, the final and ultimate goal of human existence is *moksha*, or liberation from the cycle of *samsara*. The soul is reincarnated through many births until *moksha* is attained. *Moksha* is transcendence and unity with the Ultimate Consciousness, in line with the Unity model and the nonduality in the Hindu religion [12] (see Figure 22.1).

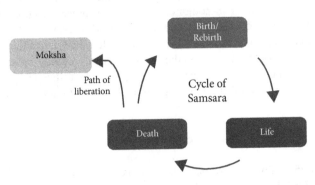

Figure 22.1 The cycle of *samsara*

The Concept of Pain, Suffering, and Death in Hinduism

Pain and suffering in Hindu tradition are viewed from multiple perspectives. The concepts of *karma, dharma, ṛta, ṛna,* and *moksha* are interwoven and explain how Hinduism views and understands the concept of suffering.

Hindus believe that mental and physical suffering does not occur at random but is the consequence of past inappropriate actions (thoughts, words, deeds) in either the current or past life. Suffering is not punishment, but rather a consequence of one's actions. Hindu philosophy views suffering as atonement for one's actions and urges individuals to accept full responsibility for their suffering without blaming others.

While the psychophysical being (the physical body and the mind) experiences pain and suffering, the inner Self or *atman* remains unharmed. Birth, existence, growth, decay, disease, and death are the six changes that are experienced by the mortal body. The Self is impervious to these changes and immutable. "*Weapons cleave it not, Fire burns it not, Water moistens it not, Wind dries it not*" [21] *(Bhagavad Gita 2:23).* Hindus believe in enduring suffering with fortitude, accepting it as a temporary and inevitable malady of the perishable body by developing an attitude of nonattachment and by viewing it as an opportunity for spiritual growth [22].

Hindus are born with obligatory duties to themselves and to the universe. For all Hindus, this sense of duty (personal and collective) takes precedence over their rights *(adhikara)* [23]. Ṛta is the natural order of the universe and encompasses cosmic and ethical components. As the cosmic order, it sustains all natural phenomena like planetary orbits, the day–night cycle, tides, seasons, sleep, digestion, and so on. As an ethical principle, it sustains all beings, both living and nonliving, to coexist in harmony. A Hindu is born with a duty to preserve this natural order through various activities. Righteous living *(dharma)* for a Hindu involves repayment of the debts *(ṛna)* of the universe by practicing an attitude of gratefulness and through various rites and rituals as prescribed in the religious texts. The five debts enumerated in Hindu texts are debts to God/universe/environment, ancestors, culture/knowledge, living beings, and other humans. Inability to fulfill one's duties and repay the *karmic* debts can be a source of spiritual suffering for Hindus.

Hinduism describes four goals of human life that provide a framework within which one can live peacefully and develop spiritually: enjoyment of sensual pleasure *(kama),* economic security or worldly success *(artha),* righteous living *(dharma),* and liberation *(moksha). Dharma* provides the moral framework within which pleasure and success can be pursued [17]. Hindus believe that their journey on earth is in stages, going through the period of education *(brahmacharya),* the responsibilities of family life *(grihastha),* the gradual retreat from worldly ties *(vanaprastha),* and the wait for liberation through death *(sanyasa)* [14] (see Table 22.1). Individuals may be in different phases of spiritual development in their present lifetime. For a Hindu, the ultimate purpose of human life is to unite with the divine and attain ultimate liberation.

Hindus believe in a graceful unification with death at the right auspicious time, at the right place (preferably at home or by the banks of the Ganges), at the right age, and surrounded by family and friends [24]. A good death is conceptualized as one that

Table 22.1 Traditional Social System in Hinduism

Life Stage	Tasks Achieved	Life Goals or *Purusharthas*
Brahmacharya Student Life	Knowledge	*Dharma* (Moral and Ethical Values, Piety, and Duty)
Grihastha Householder	Wealth and Progeny	*Kama* (Pleasure of senses) *Artha* (Wealth and Success)
Vanaprastha (Retirement)	Wisdom	*Moksha* (Liberation)
Sanyasa (Renunciation)	Disinterest and Detachment	*Moksha* (Liberation)

occurs in a conscious state, with the person's mind on God, after fulfilling all worldly duties and repaying worldly debts (*rna*) [24]. Premature, uncontrolled, violent deaths occurring in unsuitable places symbolize bad death [25].

Spiritual Concerns and Healing in Hinduism

Various studies have explored the spiritual concerns and coping of Hindu patients with chronic illness. Spiritual distress occurs when individuals experience a loss of meaning in life and feel alienated from themselves, their families, the society or community, and God [26]. For a Hindu, the concept of *dharmic* living and *moksha* provides meaning and purpose in life; *karma* attributes a positive meaning to the suffering; pursuit of *purusharthas* helps in maintaining connectedness to the family, the society, and the community; rituals reestablish connectedness with the transcendent or God, while nonattachment and yoga help in reconnecting with oneself, and the understanding of *samsara* promotes acceptance of death. This section will discuss how these principles of Hinduism facilitate spiritual healing.

The Role of Rituals

In Hinduism, religious rituals, rites of passages for different life stages, and practice of austerities are commonplace and considered important for righteous living. These rituals are passed down from one generation to the next through oral inheritance and by demonstration within families and in the community and are part of collective spiritual practises [16]. Praying to the ancestors and seeking their blessings are part of any major festivity in families. Religious observances such as fasting, vegetarianism, specific food offerings to the deities, marking auspicious timings for important activities including treatment planning, wearing a talisman or the holy ash, keeping a sacred icon or a picture of a favorite deity on the cell phone or adjacent to the hospital bed, prayer and chanting of holy hymns (*mantras*), and ritualized worship (*pooja*) are some of the practices observed by Hindu patients [27]. Placing holy Ganges water on the lips of the dying person along with *tulasi* (basil) leaf is an important end-of-life ritual in Hinduism [24]. Rituals also form an integral part of the mourning period, extending over a fortnight, with monthly and annual remembrances.

These religious practices are important spiritual coping mechanisms that help Hindu patients transcend their physical and mental pain and reduce the stress associated with chronic or terminal illness [28]. Ritualistic behaviors foster a sense of mastery and discipline. Prayers and religious chanting foster connectedness with God. Ritualistic worship along with the family or the spiritual community eases anxiety, allays the sense of loneliness, and helps patients feel valued. Austerity practices like vegetarianism represent retributive penance, reduce feelings of guilt, and foster mental well-being. Routine activities like eating when connected to the divine become blessed and offer therapeutic benefits. Religious imagery and paraphernalia are considered to be symbols of God's protection and good luck and foster a sense of security, hope, and connectedness [29]. These activities help patients rise beyond their physical pain and mental anxieties to connect with one's true self. Health care providers need to be sensitive to these sociocultural and religious concerns as they contribute to mental as well as physical well-being in patients with terminal illnesses. Enabling and upholding these traditions in the sterile hospital environment will foster temporary transcendence and facilitate spiritual healing among Hindu patients [16].

The Concept of *Karma*

Spiritual distress is almost universally defined by the question, "Why me?" [22]. This is a sign of despondency when the long years gone by become meaningless and faith is questioned. Hindus with chronic illnesses utilize the concept of *karma* to reconcile with this distress. Teachings in Hinduism reiterate that *karma* is not binding and that individuals can influence the future by their present actions [17,30]. *Karma* is not to be misunderstood as a fatalistic attitude, it has restorative and retributive aspects, making one the master of one's destiny.

Suffering in Hinduism is considered to be the repercussion of past negative deeds and is to be endured [16]. Hindu patients and their families may use various austerity practices and rituals to atone for their bad *karma*—repentance is an important aspect of spiritual healing. Health care providers, by allowing time and space for these activities, can enhance spiritual healing and well-being in patients with life-limiting illnesses and their families.

The concept of *karma* facilitates better coping and acceptance of pain and suffering [16]. Acceptance alleviates existential anxieties and enhances psychospiritual well-being [31]. Hinduism espouses the notion that passive acceptance is akin to resignation and leads to psychopathology and should be avoided. "Neither let there be in thee any attachment to inaction" [21] (*Bhagavad Gita 2:47*). Hinduism propagates active acceptance. It encourages Hindus to acknowledge the existing reality, focus on achievable meaningful goals, and abandon futile actions aimed at changing the unchangeable reality [16]. Acceptance, forgiveness, and compassion (to self and others) are spiritual activities that foster healing in Hinduism.

Partial and misplaced understanding of *karma* can precipitate spiritual distress. Some patients perceive suffering as punishment for their sins [27]. This can trigger feelings of guilt, regret, anger, hopelessness, and abandonment by God and give rise to irrational ritualistic behaviour [16,20]. Some patients may blame their family members' *karma* for their suffering, causing disruption within family systems. Also, some Hindu patients may refuse treatment for pain or other symptoms in an attempt to repay their *karmic* debts, which can cause conflicts with the treating team [32]. Understanding the concept of *karma* will help health care providers address these concerns.

The Path of Nonattachment

According to Hindu philosophy, attachment to worldly things is the root cause of pain and suffering [22]. The ultimate goal of a Hindu is to develop a dispassionate attitude, which is the key to liberation. It is the ability to observe the nature of worldly events neutrally without being affected by them [15]. Existential fulfillment and spiritual well-being are achieved when patients can relegate the pain and suffering to the mortal body while maintaining connectedness to their true Self and God or higher power [16]. Realizing the Self is to dwell on it and nurture the ability to discern and choose well. The Self is considered to be the powerhouse that propels the physical, mental, and intellectual faculties. Strengthening the Self is training to be balanced in the vicissitudes of life, be it in physical changes, health and disease, youth and aging, handling emotions, or dealing with relationships.

Hindu scriptures aid in healing from within as they focus on realizing the inner Self and the importance of living in equanimity and finding one's equipoise. In medical practice, these concepts cannot be relegated to being just an intellectual understanding or an escape from reality. It means that patients in pain should continue their attempt to relieve suffering [22]. The goal lies in achieving neutrality, where a lack of immediate success and inability to control symptoms completely should not dishearten the patients or allow them to give up trying; rather, it is in continuing the healing process without being frustrated by failure. It is the ability to disengage from struggling with pain to a realistic approach in managing the pain and engaging in daily activities to the best possible extent [22]. From the practitioner's point of view, working with equanimity involves pursuing one's calling *(dharma)*, continuing to care and heal the patient with empathy, keeping in mind the limitations of the treatment, and accepting all the outcomes [22]. It is acknowledging reality and working toward meaningful goals.

Finding equipoise, the ability to concentrate and live with intelligent moderation, requires a steady mind, withdrawn from preoccupations. The patient strives to raise the mind from the preoccupation with physical and mental suffering to a spiritual plane where they can reconnect with the Self and God [16]. Rituals, yoga, meditation, prayer, art, and creativity are some practices that aid in developing this attitude, albeit temporarily [16]. Enduring nonattachment and equipoise is the conscious incorporation of these techniques into one's life on a day-to-day basis, while realistically accepting the limitations of the body and the mind, and maintaining neutrality to the happenings in life.

Mind–Body Techniques

To enable spiritual coping and mental strengthening in the face of adversity and chronic illness, Hinduism uses mind–body techniques such as yoga and meditation [22]. Yoga is an ancient Indian science with therapeutic benefits widely recognized today. The techniques include postures done with awareness *(asanas)*, voluntary, regulated nostril breathing techniques *(pranayama)*, guided relaxation with imagery *(yoga nidra)*, and meditation techniques *(dhyana)* [33]. Growing evidence-based research indicates that yoga promotes healing of the body, mind, and spirit (see Figure 22.2). Techniques of *asanas* and *pranayama* aid focus and concentration, and promote calmness and relaxation, contributing to physical and mental well-being [33]. Patients with cancer reported reduction in fatigue and sleep disturbances and improvement in anxiety, depression, and health-related quality of life [34,35]. The techniques of self-restraint *(yama)*, self-discipline *(niyama)*, and introspection *(pratyahara)* enable spiritual healing [33]. Suffering results when an individual overidentifies with the body and mind, to the exclusion of the Self. The techniques in yoga help the patient to refocus on their selfhood, while disidentifying from the sufferings of the physical body and mind [36]. Yoga utilizes a comprehensive holistic approach to well-being, tailored

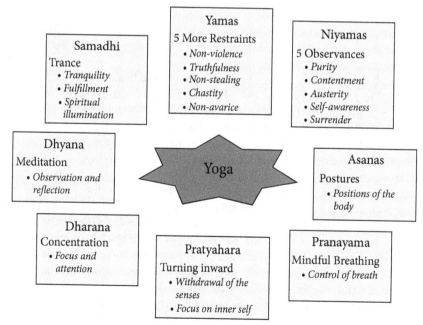

Figure 22.2 The Eight Limbs of Yoga

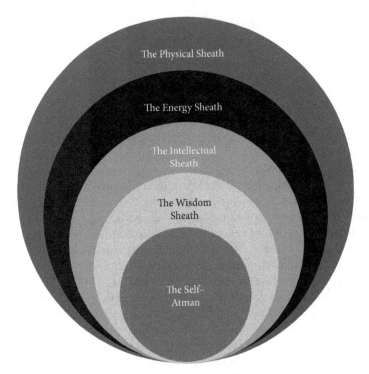

Figure 22.3 The Five Sheaths (Koshas) in the Human Body

to individual patient needs. Yoga is self-empowering and requires individuals to participate in their own healing. The individual's state of mind is crucial to healing, and a positive attitude fosters quicker healing [37].

Ayurveda is an ancient Indian indigenous system of medicine that is based on Vedic literature. Health in Ayurveda is viewed as a state of physical, psychological, social, and spiritual well-being. The nervous system (*Vata*), the venous system (*Pitta*), and the arterial system (*Kapha*) are the three life forces that are considered important for normal body function [38]. The human body is made up of five sheaths: the physical sheath, the energy sheath, the emotional sheath, the intellectual sheath, and the causal body that includes the *atman* (see Figure 22.3). Treatment in Ayurveda brings about a balance between these life forces and aims to heal the body, mind, and soul. The therapeutic approach in Ayurveda is divided into four categories: maintenance of health (*prakritisthapani chikitsa*), cure of the disease (*roganashani chikitsa*), restoration of normal function *(rasayana chikitsa)*, and restoration of the spirit (*naishthiki chikitsa*) [39]. It provides personalized recommendations for the type of food, lifestyle changes, symptom control, and psychological and spiritual practices for healing. There are reports of successful integration of Ayurveda with modern medicine in cancer management. However, the challenge of these forms of therapy is the paucity of high-quality intensive research. The safety, efficacy, and cost-effectiveness of these therapies need to be explored further [38].

Death and Bereavement

"As a man casts off his worn-out garments and takes on new ones, so does the embodied Self cast away worn–out bodies and enters another new" [21]
—Bhagavad Gita 2:22

Hindus consider death as an evolution of the soul, and this thought can bring solace to the patient and the family. Elaborate rituals are performed before and after death to enable good death. Hindus believe in natural death; any attempt to shorten life (euthanasia or suicide) or artificially prolong life will *accrue* karmic debts and are to be avoided [24]. Some dying patients may refuse food and medications to enable spiritual purification and a good death. Although the Hindu way of life is death-accepting and advocates preparation for dying, collusion is commonplace in Indian culture [23]. Collusion can impact patient autonomy, decision making, and preparedness for death. In Indian culture individual autonomy is considered isolating, and health care decisions are taken on by the family who considers it their duty to protect their loved ones [23]. These beliefs are contradictory to Western views and are sources of conflict among health care providers, patients, and loved ones.

Coping with anticipatory grief, loss, and bereavement is a transition for the family and follows a long trajectory. The healing gradually comes from within the Self and is supported by the community through rituals. Culturally sensitive care by health care providers can aid this process of healing.

Conclusions

Religion and spirituality are important domains in the care of patients with cancer but are seldom discussed in health care settings. They are important predictors of quality of life and play a major role in how patients and their families cope with and heal from suffering and pain. Sociocultural and religious beliefs that are at odds with the Western system of medicine may create conflicts among health care providers, patients, and their loved ones. This conflict not only impedes adjustment to illness but also causes significant distress. Understanding the nuances of patients' spirituality and religious beliefs can enable health care providers to deliver more comprehensive, culturally competent care. Hinduism is rightly described as a way of life, with wide variation in practice and tradition. However, some commonalities bind every Hindu and influence their way of dealing with pain and suffering. This chapter attempts to acquaint health care providers with Hindu traditions and beliefs so that spiritual care harmonized to patient's preferences can be provided.

References

1. Ferlay J, Ervik M, Lam F, Colombet M, Mery L, Pineros M, et al. Global Cancer Observatory: Cancer Today [Internet]. Lyon, France: International Agency for Research on Cancer. Available from:https://gco.iarc.fr/today [cited December 16, 2020].

2. Cassell EJ. *The Nature of Suffering and the Goals of Medicine*. 2nd ed. New York: Oxford University Press; 2004: 1–334.

3. Cassel EJ. The nature of suffering and the goals of medicine. *N Engl J Med*. 1982;306(11):639–645.

4. Sulmasy DP. A biopsychosocial-spiritual model for the care of patients at the end of life. *The Gerontologist*. 2002;42(Suppl_3):24–33.

5. Ramsey P, Jonsen AR, May WF. *The Patient as Person: Explorations in Medical Ethics. New Haven*. New Haven, CT: Yale University Press; 2002:1–283.

6. King DE. *Faith, Spirituality and Medicine: Toward the Making of a Healing Practitioner*. Binghamton, NY: Haworth Pastoral Press; 2000.

7. Yates JW, Chalmer BJ, James PS, Follansbee M, McKegney FP. Religion in patients with advanced cancer. *Med Pediatr Oncol*. 1981;9(2):121–128.

8. Vincensi B. Interconnections: Spirituality, spiritual care, and patient-centered care. *Asia-Pac J Oncol Nurs*. 2019;6(2):104–110.

9. Puchalski CM. Integrating spirituality into patient care: An essential element of person-centered care. *Pol Arch Med Wewn*. 2013;123(9):491–497.

10. Gotay CC. The experience of cancer during early and advanced stages: The views of patients and their mates. *Soc Sci Med*. 1984;18(7):605–613.

11. Donovan K, Sanson-Fisher RW, Redman S. Measuring quality of life in cancer patients. *J Clin Oncol*. 1989;7(7):959–968.

12. Anandarajah G. The 3 H and BMSEST models for spirituality in multicultural whole-person medicine. *Ann Fam Med*. 2008;6(5):448–458.

13. Hackett, Conrad & Grim, Brian & Stonawski, Marcin & Skirbekk, Vegard & Potančoková, Michaela & Abel, Guy. The Global Religious Landscape: A Report on the Size and Distribution of the World's Major Religious Groups as of 2010; 2012. 10.13140/2.1.4573.8884, Available from: https://www.pewforum.org/2012/12/18/global-religious-landscape-exec [cited December 18, 2020].

14. Das, Subhamoy. "Hinduism for Beginners." Learn Religions, Sep. 3, 2021, learnreligions.com/hinduism-for-beginners-1770069. [Cited December 18, 2020]

15. Thrane S. Hindu end of life: Death, dying, suffering, and karma. *J Hosp Palliat Nurs*. 2010;12(6):337–342.

16. Singaram VS, Saradaprabhananda S. Cultural thanatology: An exploration of the religious, spiritual, and existential concerns of elderly terminally-ill diasporic Hindus. *J Relig Spiritual Aging*. 2020;54:1–21.

17. Anandarajah G. Hinduism. In: Peteet JR, D'Ambra MN (eds). *The Soul of Medicine: Spiritual Perspectives and Clinical Practice*. Baltimore, MD: Johns Hopkins University Press; 2011: 59–79.

18. Firth S. Death, dying and bereavement among British Hindus, Religion Today. 1988;5(1/2):4–7.

19. Clooney FX. Evil, divine omnipotence, and human freedom: Vedānta's theology of karma. *J Relig*. 1989;69(4):530–548.

20. Wezler A. Dharma in the veda and the dharmaśāstras. *J Indian Philos*. 2004;32(5–6):629–654.

21. Radhakrishnan S. *The Bhagavad Gita*. New York: HarperCollins; 2014: 136 p.

22. Whitman SM. Pain and suffering as viewed by the Hindu religion. *J Pain*. 2007;8(8):607–613.

23. Viswanath V, Rao SR. Chapter Palliative care: The Hindu perspective. In: Benton KD, Pegoraro R, (eds). *Finding Dignity at the End of Life A Spiritual Reflection on Palliative Care*. 1st edition. New York: Routledge; 2021: 45–52.

24. Firth S. End-of-life: A Hindu view. *The Lancet*. 2005;366(9486):682–686.

25. Choudry M, Latif A, Warburton KG. An overview of the spiritual importances of end-of-life care among the five major faiths of the United Kingdom. *Clin Med J R Coll Physicians London*. 2018;18(1):23–31.

26. Selman, LE, Harding-Swale, R, Agupio, G, Fox, PT, Galimaka, D, Mmolendi, K, Higginson, IJ & Spiritual Care in sub-Saharan Africa Advisory Group, T 2010, *Spiritual care recommendations for people receiving palliative care in sub-Saharan Africa: With special reference to South Africa and Uganda*. Cicely Saunders International, London. http://www.nccd-crc.issuelab.org/resources/17251/17251.pdf

27. Simha S, Noble S, Chaturvedi S. Spiritual concerns in Hindu cancer patients undergoing palliative care: A qualitative study. *Indian J Palliat Care*. 2013;19(2):99–105.

28. Lang M, Krátký J, Xygalatas D. The role of ritual behaviour in anxiety reduction: An investigation of Marathi religious practices in Mauritius: The role of ritual in anxiety reduction. *Philos Trans R Soc B Biol Sci*. 2020;375(1805):20190431.

29. Hodge DR. Working with Hindu clients in a spiritually sensitive manner. *Soc Work*. 2004;49(1):27–38.

30. Gupta VB. How Hindus cope with disability. *J Relig Disabil Heal*. 2011;15(1):72–78.

31. Bhatia SC, Madabushi J, Kolli V, Bhatia SK, Madaan V. The *Bhagavad Gita* and contemporary psychotherapies. *Indian J Psychiatry*. 2013;55(6):S315–S321.

32. Thrane S. Hindu end of life: Death, dying, suffering, and karma. *J Hosp Palliat Nurs*. 2010;12:337–342.

33. Rao RM, Amritanshu R, Vinutha HT, et al. Role of yoga in cancer patients: Expectations, benefits, and risks: A review. *Indian J Palliat Care*. 2017;23(3):225–230.

34. Cramer H, Lauche R, Klose P, Lange S, Langhorst J, Dobos GJ. Yoga for improving health-related quality of life, mental health and cancer-related symptoms in women diagnosed with breast cancer. *Cochrane Database Syst Rev*. 2017;1(1):CD010802.

35. Naveen S. Integrating AYUSH into palliative care. *Indian J Palliat Care*. 2017;23(3):219–220.

36. Holte A, Mills PJ. Yoga and Chronic Illness. In: Stoltzfus MJ, Green R, Schumm D (eds). *Chronic Illness, Spirituality, and Healing: Diverse Disciplinary, Religious, and Cultural Perspectives*. 1st edition. New York: Palgrave Macmillan; 2013: 141–163.

37. Desikachar K, Bragdon L, Bossart C. The yoga of healing: Exploring yoga's holistic model for health and well-being. *Int J Yoga Ther*. 2005;15:17–39.

38. Balachandran P, Govindarajan R. Cancer—An Ayurvedic perspective. *Pharmacol Res*. 2005;51(1):19–30.

39. Thatte U, Dhahanukar S. Ayurveda, the natural alternative. *Sci Today*. 2001 (1991):12–18.

23

The Impact of Chinese Culture and Faith in Cancer Care, China

Lili Tang, Ying Pang, and He Yi

Introduction

Family members' withholding of bad news from cancer patients is a very common phenomenon in China, as cancer is a life-threatening disease and is even considered to be equal to death by most Chinese people. Many family members of cancer patients believe that by withholding the bad news from their sick relative they can protect them from overwhelming emotional harm. For this reason, family members usually ask their physicians not to disclose the diagnosis and prognosis information directly to the patient. Additionally, according to the Law of the People's Republic of China on Medical Practitioners, medical personnel should tell the truth to patients and their families, but they are obligated to be cautious in order to avoid adverse consequences of telling the truth. To avoid medical disputes, many physicians also adopt the "family consent disclosure" approach instead of the "patient consent disclosure" approach and make the family members play a principal role in the process of receiving bad news and decision making.

A recent study [1] showed that over 60% of patients in China did not know about their cancer diagnosis before chemotherapy. Although most patients (91%) wanted to be informed about their diagnosis of a terminal disease, only half of family members wanted their ill relative to be informed in this situation. This study also found that patients of a younger age and higher educational and economic level were more likely to want to be informed about the bad news; elders with lower educational or economic standing were usually thought to be too vulnerable to receive the bad news and needed to be protected.

Cultural Factors that Affect Breaking Bad News

In traditional Chinese culture, a dead person will transform into a ghost. The description of the ghost world in Chinese ancient literary works nearly always gives people a mysterious and horrible feeling, which causes many Chinese people to fear death and ghosts in particular [2].

In today's Chinese society, most people have no religion, so these people feel uncertain about the process of dying and what will happen to them after death. The uncertainty about dying and death causes a feeling of death anxiety. For all these reasons, death is a taboo topic that most Chinese people feel uncomfortable talking about openly. A survey conducted in China showed that only 28% of medical students were able to talk about death openly and that 72% of them felt uncomfortable talking about death and either avoided talking about it or never talked about it at all [3]. So, breaking the bad news of a poor prognosis and talking about death and dying are very tough tasks in the Chinese clinical oncology setting.

Self-concept and Filial Piety Culture

The self-concept construction in Chinese culture differs fundamentally from that of Western cultures; notably, in China, the family unit has been integrated into the self-concept. Therefore, the family relationship in China is much closer than what is found in Western countries [4].

Filial piety culture is an essential component of Chinese culture [5]. "When a young bird grows up, it feeds its mother." Chinese culture uses this saying figuratively to mean that the grown child should reciprocate to their parents. Another saying in Chinese culture is "Treating the elders as if they were little kids": In Chinese society, aged parents are considered to be fragile and vulnerable, and when they contract a life-threatening disease such as cancer, their adult children usually undertake the responsibilities of caring for their sick elders and try to protect them from receiving any bad news or facing any tough choices. This picture changes if the elder parent has more than one child. The siblings may well have different opinions about breaking bad news or decision making, which may lead to family conflict. If the conflict continues to the bereavement period, the siblings may blame each other for a bad decision regarding medical treatment and care. Most Chinese couples with only one child are in their 60s or 70s, since the one-child policy was adopted in the late 1970s. Once the disease occurs, the only child will bear the double burden of providing financial and care assistance; facing the bad news and tough choices alone may put a lot of pressure on the only child [6]. If the treatment fails or the patient dies, the only child will be likely to ruminate the whole course of treatment and caring, and feel regret or guilty about the decisions made.

Family's Role in the Patient's Spiritual Care

Spirituality can be defined as the existence of God, spiritual practices and rituals, connectedness with others, nature and God(s), self-transcendence, feelings of communion and mutuality, peace, strength, energy, meaning, purpose, beliefs, values, faith, hope, conscious and reflective aspects of spirituality, motivation, forgiveness, love, guiding life and death, supernormal and mystical belief, peak experiences, and so on [7]. As previously mentioned, most Chinese do not follow any religion. When they face death, most of their spiritual distress comes from their connectedness with others. In our recent study of advanced breast cancer patients, we found that "becoming burden to others" and "the impact of my death on my loved ones" are the top two items that patients rated with the highest score in the Death and Dying Distress Scale (DADDS) (the research article on this study is currently being prepared). In addition, these two items are the only two that refer to family/intimate relationships. The results indicated that open communication and mutual support are most important for alleviating patients' spiritual distress.

Breaking Bad News to the Whole Family

Most Chinese cancer patients would like to know the truth, even if it is bad news, and studies show that there are no significant differences between patients in the disclosure group and those in the nondisclosure group [1]. It is essential to explore an appropriate way for breaking bad news to Chinese cancer patients. According to Chinese culture, the family is an indispensable part of the entire medical process. So, breaking bad news to the whole family would be a better way of proceeding. First, it offers the patient the right to know their true condition and gives them the autonomy to participate in medical decision making. Second, it reduces the burden attached to having too much responsibility. Third, it provides a safe environment to talk about the bad news, dying, and death openly among the whole family, and it also gives them an opportunity to talk about their feelings and to support one another.

How to break bad news to the whole family? The following four steps can be followed:

Step 1: Define Who Is in the Family

This step should be taken by the patients themselves. Sometimes the family is defined as a nuclear family composed of only the spouse and their children. But the family may be more extended, including spouse, children, parents, siblings, and even other relatives who are very important to the patient.

Step 2: Set the List of Participants

First, ask the patient if they would like to attend the meeting. It is very important to ask this question prior to every family meeting, as patients sometimes change their mind. If the patient says, "Just tell my family, don't tell me," you need to ask who, instead of the patient, they would like to appoint to make the medical decision. Generally, family members younger than 18 years old are not asked to participate in the meeting.

Step 3: Organize a Family Meeting

The medical team participating in the family meeting should include the doctor in charge, the principal nurse, and a psychologist, who can provide more professional emotional support and facilitate communication and support among family members. The purpose of the family meeting is to break bad news to the whole family clearly and frankly, to facilitate communication and support among all the family members, and to reach an agreement on a plan for treatment and care.

Step 4: Identify the Family's Unmet Psychological Needs and Provide a Referral

Sometimes the family needs to be referred to a psychologist for additional family therapy when the family's functioning is not strong enough or when the family finds it too difficult to cope with the bad news effectively.

Shortcomings in Current Clinical Practice

Although there has been some meaningful exploration in some of the larger cancer centers [8], China is vast (one of the most populous countries on Earth) and the medical resources in the different areas are uneven. Many physicians and nurses in oncology settings still lack the training to convey bad news, and in many places, psychological services are unavailable. A hopeful development is that some academic platforms on psycho-oncology have launched an ongoing effort to provide skilled training for communication of breaking bad news and for how to provide psychological support to cancer patients and their families. The continuous development of internet technology and some professional publications (such as the Chinese Psychosocial Oncology Clinical Practice Guidelines) has also boosted this process.

Decision Making: The Role of Doctor and Family

Since the 1980s, there has been a shift in patient-centered care (PCC) and shared decision-making (SDM) in Western medical literature and clinical practice. This change occurred in response to criticisms of the traditional doctor–patient relationship being too paternalistic and one-directional. The definition of SDM advocates increasing patient participation and transparency in treatment and care. One definition of SDM is "a process in which clinicians collaborate to help patients obtain evidence and value consistent medical decisions." In the SDM model, patients are encouraged to form a consensus on the preferred treatment. There is also overlap in PCC, which is usually based on the implementation of certain care principles that "respect and respond to patients' personal preferences, needs and values, and ensure that patients' values guide all clinical decisions."

Decision Making: The Role of Doctor and Family

The doctor-patient relationship has undergone a transition throughout the ages in Western medical literature and clinical practice. This change occurred in response to criticisms of the traditional doctor–patient relationship based on paternalistic model

[9]. The shared decision-making (SDM) advocates increasing patient participation and transparency in treatment and care. One definition of SDM is "a process whereby clinicians collaboratively help patients to reach evidence-informed and value-congruent medical decisions" [10]. In the SDM model, patients are encouraged to form a consensus on the preferred treatment. There is overlap in patient centered care (PCC), which is usually based on the implementation of certain care principles that "respect and respond to patients' personal preferences, needs and values, and ensure that patients' values guide all clinical decisions" [11].

Decision Making in China

Different countries have different decision-making process in cancer care, which are formed according to the culture, laws, traditions, religious beliefs, and ethical views of different backgrounds. Although, in Western clinical practice it is ultimately the patient's choice, patients are usually encouraged to include family members in the decision-making process. In China, Confucianism is the main philosophical basis , which focuses on the close relationship between family members and emphasizes that family members should not only share happiness, but also share responsibility. When family members are ill or disabled, this is a priority for the whole family, especially in the medical decision-making process.

Research on Decision Making in China

One study found that family members of 50% of Chinese cancer patients make important decisions for them [12]. Also, research shows that family members of Asian patients with lung cancer and colorectal cancer are more involved in treatment decisions [13].

In one cross-sectional study conducted in China, a total of 542 doctors and 619 patients were investigated [14]. Self-report questionnaire on patient-doctor SDM, satisfaction with treatment decisions were completed. The results showed that SDM was the most important predictor of patients' satisfaction with decision making. Therefore, it is suggested to strengthen the communication between doctors and patients to improve their SDM and improve patient satisfaction.

Another cross-cultural study conducted in China and Australia showed that, in both countries, the desire for medical information is influenced by the culture and personal values at the individual level [15]. This finding points to the potential benefits of customized health communication based on personal thinking to promote informed decision making. In both countries, the ideal level of self-participation in decision making is relatively independent of other cultures and personal values, which indicates that cultural stereotypes should be treated with caution. The results also show that the participation preference in the decision-making process in clinical contact should be considered separately from information needs.

A survey-based study on decision making among Chinese patients and their family members used the Decision-Making Preferences Questionnaire (DMPQ) and the

Disclosure of Information Preferences Questionnaire (DIPQ) [16]. The results of these measures found that about 27.3% of patients and families preferred SDM, and that there was a discrepancy between information disclosure beliefs and family members' decisions.

A study investigated the characteristics and related factors of decision-making details in Chinese patients with advanced cancer [17]. This study reflects some characteristics of Chinese terminal cancer patients' decision-making regarding hospice care. The main decision makers were primarily arranged in the following order: spouse, children, parents.

In medical practice, it is very important to treat each family individually and explore the family's beliefs and values for every issue. Medical staff should formulate their own methods of truth-telling according to the needs of the individual in each situation. Narrative ethics should be used to coordinate teamwork among medical staffs and family caregivers to support cancer patients and ensure their autonomy and hope [18].

Spiritual Care in China

Spiritual Care

Spirituality is a basic element of the human experience. It involves our relationship with the meaning of life, our understanding of goals, our connection with others, and our inner peace [19]. Spiritual care refers to the cognition and response to human spiritual needs when an individual is faced with trauma, disease, or sadness. Providing spiritual support is one of the core contents of holistic care because it is closely related to the quality of life of patients. Spiritual care should be offered to all patients and their families regardless of their religious belief [20].

Spiritual Care in Chinese Culture

The Chinese mainland population, belonging to any of 56 ethnic groups, has rich and varied cultural tradition and values. China's pluralistic society is influenced not only by the early confucian philosophy, but also by the later modern Communist China, and recently by the spread of materialism stemming from the rapid economic development [21]. Taoism and Buddhism are still dominant religious traditions. Nonreligious theists are very common in China and the religious population is small. In the health care system, there is a wide range of spiritual care requirements for nonreligious people. A study of nonreligious theistic families shows that they prefer a particular religion when faced with life-threatening diseases [22]. Parents seek religious care as an important way to gain psychological and spiritual comfort after their children's death. Parents' spiritual needs require further support, such as bereavement care for families, and death education.

In China, the concept of spirituality lies in the word "Jingshen." This Chinese word originated from Jing, Qi and Shen, which can be traced back to taoist philosophy and traditional Chinese medicine. Jing is "essence" and Shen is "spirit", which refers to a meta-mental entity seated in the mind. Qi is an important energy behind Jing and Shen. With the development of culture and language, Jingshen has added new meanings of "a state of mind" and "purpose" in modern society. It can also have various meanings in the social and cultural context of individuals, such as the "unity of being" as an individual entity of the unity of yin-yang, and the compassion of the group influenced by Confucius social ethics and Buddhist morality [23,24]

Therefore, medical staff need to consider cultural background to support the spiritual needs of patients. Especially in the implementation of spiritual care, they need to realize that when the Chinese understand these terms, they integrate Confucianism, Buddhism, and Taoism, which may provide information inconsistent with their religious beliefs.

Spiritual Care Training in China

Spiritual care is the basic content of holistic care, but the spiritual care knowledge and ability of clinical staff often cannot meet the needs of patients. Accordingly, the medical community is reluctant to broach the topic of spirituality, as it is either unknown to them or they believe that the provision of spiritual care is beyond their capabilities. Therefore, medical staff is in urgent need of relevant training to enhance their abilities to provide patients with spiritual care.

A descriptive cross-sectional survey was conducted among 2,970 Chinese nurses [25]. The Spiritual Care Competence Scale and General Self-Efficacy Scale were used in this survey. The results showed that spiritual care competence was related to their self-efficacy. Appropriate ways and trainings to enhance this competence are needed to address the spiritual care needs of patients.

China has begun to develop this training and research. One study [26] included spiritual care training mainly based on expert lectures, group interventions, clinical practice, case sharing, and a framework to clarify the components of spiritual care competence through the synthesis of existing empirical and theoretical work. This proposed framework can be used as a model to promote spiritual care competence of oncology health care professionals in China. More research evidence and training are needed to better develop spiritual care in China.

References

1. Liu Y, Yang J, Huo D, Fan H, Gao Y. Disclosure of cancer diagnosis in China: The incidence, patients' situation, and different preferences between patients and their family members and related influence factors. *Cancer Manage Res.* 2018;10:2173–2181.
2. Yang L. Analysis of Chinese and Western Culture's attitude towards death. *Chizi.* 2016;(11X):2. (Chinese)
3. Xia Y, Zou Y, YE L. Analysis of medical students' attitude towards death and their educational needs for life and death. *J Chinese Higher Med.* 2011(1):38–39. (Chinese)

4. Jia Z, Li X, Chang Z. Why do Chinese people attach importance to interpersonal relationship? *Soc Psychol Sci*. 2012;27(140):1328–1331. (Chinese)

5. Chen F. The practice of Chinese filial piety culture. *People's Forum*. 2019:140–141. (Chinese)

6. Yang X, Hao Y, George SM, Wang L. Factors associated with health-related quality of life among Chinese caregivers of the older adults living in the community: A cross-sectional study. *Health and Qual Life Outcomes*. 2012;10:143–143.

7. Hsiao S, Gau M, Ingleton C, et al. An exploration of spiritual needs of Taiwanese patients with advanced cancer during the therapeutic processes. *J Clin Nurs*. 20:950–959.

8. Pang Y, Tang L, Zhang Y, et al. Breaking bad news in China: Implementation and comparison of two communication skills training courses in oncology. *Psychooncology*. 2015;24:608–611.

9. Kaba R, Sooriakumaran P. The evolution of the doctor-patient relationship. *Int J Surg*. 2007;5(1):57–65.

10. Grad R, Légaré F, Bell NR, Dickinson JA, Singh H, Moore AE, KasperaviciusD, Kretschmer KL.Shared decision making in preventive health care: what it is; what it is not. *Can Fam Physician*. 2017; 63(9):682–684.

11. Kane HL, Halpern MT, Squiers LB, Treiman KA, McCormack LA. Implementing and evaluating shared decision making in oncology practice. *CA Cancer J Clin*. 2014;64(6):377–88.

12. Zhai H, Lavender C, Li C, Wu H, Gong N, Cheng Y. Who decides? Shared decision-making among colorectal cancer surgery patients in China. *Support Care Cancer*. 2020;28(11):5353–5361.

13. Hobbs GS, Landrum MB, Arora NK, Ganz PA, van Ryn M, Weeks JC, Mack JW, Keating NL. The role of families in decisions about cancer treatments. *Cancer*. 2015; 121(7):1079–1087.

14. Wei Y, Ming J, Shi L, Ke X, Sun H, Chen Y. Physician–patient shared decision making, patient satisfaction, and adoption of new health technology in China. *Int J Technol Assess Health Care*. 2020;36(5):518–524.

15. Dolan H, Alden DL, Friend JM, et al. Culture, self, and medical decision making in Australia and China: A structural model analysis. *MDM Policy Pract*. 2019;4(2):2381468319871018.

16. Wei S, Chen F, Chen H, et al. Patients' and family members' decision-making and information disclosure preferences in a single-center survey in China: A pilot study. *Am J Hosp Palliat Care*. 2016;33(8):733–741.

17. Gu X, Chen M, Liu M, Zhang Z, Cheng W. End-of-life decision-making of terminally ill cancer patients in a tertiary cancer center in Shanghai, China. *Support Care Cancer*. 2016;24(5):2209–2215.

18. Ling DL, Yu HJ, Guo HL. Truth-telling, decision-making, and ethics among cancer patients in nursing practice in China. *Nurs Ethics*. 2019;26(4):1000–1008.

19. Puchalski C, Ferrell B, Virani R, et al. Improving the quality of spiritual care as a dimension of palliative care: the report of the consensus conference. *J Palliat Med*. 2009;12(10): 885–904.

20. Best M, Butow P and Olver I. The doctor's role in helping dying patients with cancer achieve peace: a qualitative study. *Palliat Med*. 2014; 28(9): 1139–1145.

21. Yuan H, Porr C. Integrating spiritual care into a baccalaureate nursing program in mainland China. *J Holist Nurs*. 2014;32(3):240–243.

22. Cai S, Guo Q, Luo Y, et al. Spiritual needs and communicating about death in non-religious theistic families in pediatric palliative care: A qualitative study. *Palliat Med*. 2020;34(4):533–540.

23. Niu Y, McSherry W, Partridge M. The perceptions of spirituality and spiritual care among people from Chinese backgrounds living in England: A grounded theory method. *J Transcult Nurs*. 2021;32(4):350–359.

24. Da'an Pan. The Tao of a peaceful mind: the representation of emotional health and healing in traditional Chinese literature, Mental Health, Religion & Culture, 2003;6(3): 241–259.

25. Cheng Q, Liu X, Li X, et al. Spiritual care competence and its relationship with self-efficacy: An online survey among nurses in mainland China. *J Nurs Manage.* 2021;29(2):326–332.
26. Hu Y, Jiao M, Li F. Effectiveness of spiritual care training to enhance spiritual health and spiritual care competency among oncology nurses. *BMC Palliat Care.* 2019;18(1):104.

24

Sociocultural Influences on Cancer Care in Sub-Saharan Africa

Use of Traditional and Complementary Medicines

Amos Deogratius Mwaka

Introduction

Culture has been defined as the norms, values, beliefs, and behaviors that are common in a society and that one needs to know in order to function appropriately in each particular society at any given time. It is necessary to understand the local culture in order for an individual to adapt to a new environment, to survive and flourish. Cultures are cognitive, adaptive, structural, and symbolic systems that determine a society's way of life [1]. Culture can explain an individual's beliefs regarding health, healing, and wellness; how illness, disease, and its causes are perceived; the ways in which health care is sought; and the views and values of those delivering the health care [2]. Cultural beliefs regarding health and illness affect one's ability to understand and respond to health care providers' instructions, thus affecting the degree of compliance and treatment outcomes [3]. How we perceive, experience, and cope with disease is based on our understanding of sickness [4], which, in turn, influences our perception of symptoms [5] and the way we label particular diseases and respond to illnesses [6]. The culture of any given society helps determine what it means to be healthy; acceptable methods for attaining, maintaining and regaining health; and what sources of care are available for various diseases [7]. Thus, culture plays a significant part, both positively and negatively, when it comes to seeking access to health care.

Culture's Impact on Help-Seeking

When people perceive and/or recognize symptoms of illness, the help they seek depends on a multitude of factors, including affordability, accessibility, acceptability, and convenience, as well as what they believe will heal the particular illness. Recognizing illness and the potential benefits of and need for treatment are prerequisites for help-seeking. When appraising abnormal physical feelings that could be symptoms of an illness, there is a process of assigning remedies based on the perceived cause(s) of the illness [8,9]. These remedies can be provided by friends, relatives, traditional and complementary medicine healers, faith-based healers, and/ or biomedical healthcare providers. Help-seeking is, therefore, broader and entails health-seeking, which is a complex intellectual and emotional process beginning with the detection of a symptom, then inferring illness, and, finally, deciding to seek medical care from a preferred source, such as a health care provider [10,11]. Scholars have sought and proposed models to facilitate understanding the processes of help-seeking and the factors leading up to them. These include (1) Fabrega's model, which assesses the logic of how and why patients decide on a source of care and move from one form of care system to another [12]; (2) Freidson's model, which explains the role of lay referrals in health-seeking, draws a link between the society and the health professionals in the care system, and considers the progression and continuum of care from kin referral to professional care, which can be used to understand and strengthen care [13]; (3) Frankenberg's model, which considers the sociocultural aspects of illness and health-seeking and demonstrates that health-seeking is not merely an individual affair, but is also a social action that concerns and involves, to varying degrees, other members of the sick individual's society [14]; and (4) De Nooijer's model, which assesses health-seeking through a stage-by-stage process referred to as delay, as patients traverse the health system upon recognizing symptoms of a disease [10,11].

There are, however, some gaps in these models, primarily in those that relate to modern Western medicine. For example, Igun notes that Fabrega's model disregards the influence of sociocultural factors in health-seeking; Freidson's model does not adequately explain the factors that lay referrals take into considerations when recommending or advising the use of a particular system of care; and Frankenberg's model does not adequately account for the fact that patients, their relatives, and close friends monitor, in an ongoing pattern, effects of the treatments and, depending on their interpretations of these patterns, may decide to move from one source of care to another [15]. Low demand for modern health care interventions that often arise from negative cultural and social views regarding a disease condition and/or its treatments may delay health-seeking [16]. In many sub-Saharan African countries, cultural beliefs and socioeconomic and other factors influence help-seeking [17]. In the United States, studies have shown that sociocultural and religious beliefs explain, in part, the persistent health disparities and poorer health outcomes among certain ethnic/racial groups, especially for African Americans. Consequently, interventions based on culture and religious affiliations have resulted in improved cancer survival rates among African Americans [18].

Spirituality and Religiosity Influence Help-seeking for Cancer

The concepts of spirituality and religiosity are similar and intricately related to the sacred [19]. However, in a stricter sense, spirituality is understood as the way people find meaning and purpose in life and involves their interconnectedness with other people and the sacred being [20]. Spirituality has been associated with social, emotional, and functional well-being among cancer patients and provides a sense of meaning in the lives of those suffering with severe illness [21]. On the other hand, religiosity/religion is a set of organized beliefs about the sacred and involves participation in religious and social structures [22]. Religion, therefore, refers to that which binds together humankind to the supernatural and humankind to humankind [23]. Religion is a form of motivation, a source of value in life, of health and well-being and of coping; but religion could also become a source of distress and death when its tenets are not adhered to [19]. Religion is intricately intertwined with the culture of a people; by its nature, religion is cultural and provides the foundation for human judgment [24–26]. Indeed, religion and culture interchangeably influence each other and provide sources of values, purpose, and moral strength for any given society [27–29]. The concepts of religiosity and spirituality support patients and their families in coping with illnesses and their consequences [30]. Addressing a patient's spiritual needs may promote recovery, while unmet spiritual needs and/or spiritual distress can become a barrier to health-seeking and adherence to prescribed treatments [31]. Unmet spiritual needs and concerns can also delay recovery and lead to reduced quality of life among patients [32,33]. For example, prostate cancer patients with low spirituality experienced poorer physical and mental health outcomes [34]. Cancer patients with greater spiritual needs or concerns are more likely to be dissatisfied with the quality of their care [35]. On the other hand, patients with high spirituality and fulfilled spiritual needs are more likely to experience improved health outcomes, higher quality of life, and a better subjective state of wellness, and they are less likely to experience depression and more likely to enjoy life [33,34,36–38]. A meta-analysis also showed that higher spirituality in cancer patients significantly correlated with better physical and functional well-being [39]. Religion and spirituality, therefore, have important positive impacts on cancer care [40].

Sociocultural Influences on Cancer Stage at Diagnosis in sub-Saharan Africa

A majority of cancer patients in sub-Saharan Africa, when diagnosed, are already in advanced stages of cancer and, therefore, have poor chances for survival [41–43]. Several factors can contribute to delayed health-seeking and advanced-stage diagnoses, including the interaction of cultural background and beliefs and how this influences symptom awareness, appraisal, interpretations and attributions, and sources of care [7]. A systematic review showed that sociocultural factors, such as believing in the superiority of T&CM and fearing a diagnosis of breast cancer and the assigned stigma that accompanies it, reduce the incidence of prompt health-seeking for breast cancer in SSA [44,45]. In Asia, the following reasons contribute to the long intervals between help-seeking for women with cervical cancer and account, in part, for the advanced stages at which cervical cancer is diagnosed: lack of awareness, low level of education, being divorced or widowed, and, for reasons of modesty, not sharing information regarding symptoms affecting the women's genitals [46–48]. In general, a number of sociocultural factors have been shown to operate in concert to hinder recognition of symptoms, prolong appraisal and help-seeking intervals, and lead to advanced-stage cancers at diagnoses. For example, people who trust the effectiveness of traditional medicine, believe in their own potential for self-management, and/or perceive that there are multiple barriers to accessing biomedical care take longer to seek biomedical care for cervical cancer symptoms [49–51]. Even in high-income countries like the United States, sociocultural beliefs among African Americans and Hispanics, such as cancer fatalism, have been linked to advanced stage at diagnosis, inadequate utilization of treatments, lower tendency to seek help early, and fear about symptoms suggestive of cancer, thereby benefiting less from the advances that have been made in cancer biomedicine [52,53]. In Australia, the factors found to negatively influence prompt help-seeking for cancer symptoms included misunderstanding the symptoms, fear of death, fatalism, and preference for traditional healing [54]. Socio cultural factors may interact with structural challenges in health care systems and increase the time until diagnosis, obviating the goal of early detection of cancers [55].

Use of Traditional and Complementary Medicines by Cancer Patients

The World Health Organization defines traditional and complementary medicine (T&CM) as "the sum total of the knowledge, skills and practices based on the theories, beliefs and experiences traditional to different cultures, whether explicable or not, used in the maintenance of health as well as in the prevention, diagnosis, improvement or treatment of physical and mental illness." Complementary medicine has also been defined as "a broad set of healthcare practices that are not part of that country's own tradition or conventional medicine and are not fully integrated into the dominant healthcare system" [56]. Worldwide, there is increasing preference for traditional medicines or alternative therapies, especially among cancer patients [57–59]. The proportion of cancer patients who use traditional/alternative and complementary medicine practices in both high-income countries (HICs) and low- and middle-income countries (LMICs) range from 50 to 80% [51,60–64]. Some cancer patients use traditional and/or alternative and complementary medicines concurrently with modern medicines, while other patients undertake traditional medicines as the main mode of therapy for their cancers [57,58,65]. A systematic review and meta-analysis from Australia, Canada, Europe, New Zealand, and the United States showed an increase in use of T&CM from 25% in the 1970s and 1980s to about 49% in the 2000s [59]. In a systematic review of 21 studies regarding the prevalence of T&CM use, 11–95% of cancer patients reported using some form of T&CM [66].

In the LMICs, use of T&CM by cancer patients is equally common. A systematic review on the use of traditional, complementary, and alternative medicine in sub-Saharan Africa showed that T&CM use by cancer patients ranged from 34.5 to 79% [45]; in sub-Saharan Africa, use of T&CM was highest in Ethiopia [67,68]; in Nigeria, 34.5–65% of cancer patients reported use of T&CM; while in Ghana, up to 73.5% used T&CM [64,68–70]. In Uganda, 55–77% of cancer patients at the Uganda Cancer Institute used T&CM concurrently with conventional cancer therapies [71,72]. A scoping review of 12 studies on the use of T&CM by cancer patients in sub-Saharan Africa showed that 14.1–79.0% of cancer patients reported use of T&CM for treating their cancers [73].

Reasons for Cancer Patients' Use of Traditional and Complementary Medicines

Cancer patients have used T&CM for a multitude of reasons and with various expectations, including finding a cure, managing symptoms, boosting the immune system, and improving physical and psychological well-being. Other reasons include fear of surgery, recommendation by friends and family, and trust in T&CM providers. In the United States, cancer patients use T&CM to boost the immune system, improve their quality of life, prevent recurrence, and feel more in-control of their own lives [74]. In Malaysia, breast cancer patients reported that they use traditional medicines for the following reasons: the therapies were recommended by family members or friends; therapies could be obtained on credit from the traditional healers; traditional medicines had perceived benefits over modern medicines; and they wanted to avoid the side effects of modern medicines [75]. Cancer patients at the Uganda Cancer Institute use T&CM to cure cancer, strengthen the immune system, relieve pain, reduce cancer symptoms and treat the side effects of conventional cancer therapies [71]. Another reason patients are drawn to T&CM has to do with the convenient methods of payment for services; ooften, T&CM practitioners offer either partial payment, payment in kind, or payment after a favorable outcome; for example, cure has been achieved [76,77]. In a scoping review of studies on cancer patients' use of T&CM in sub-Saharan Africa, Mwaka et al. [73] showed that patients also use T&CM because of their dissatisfaction with conventional medical care, their fear of surgery, and the multiple side effects of conventional cancer medicines. Moreover, T&CMs are readily available and cheaper than conventional medicines [68,70,78,79]. Therefore, in sub-Saharan Africa, T&CM continues to be used because they have always been part of the people's culture, patients trust T&CM providers, and payment methods for T&CM are convenient [80,81].

Disclosure of Use of Traditional and Complementary Medicines by Cancer Patients

Most cancer patients undergoing conventional cancer therapy do not disclose use of T&CM to their health care providers. In a systematic review of 21 studies on the use of T&CM, it was found that 20–77% of cancer patients who use T&CM do not disclose this fact to their doctors, either because the doctors do not inquire, the patient anticipates the doctor's disapproval, or the patients perceive that disclosure of T&CM use is irrelevant to their conventional care [66]. Similarly, a systematic review of studies in sub-Saharan Africa on general T&CM use showed that 55.8–100% did not disclose use of T&CM primarily due to fear of negative attitudes from health care providers, fear of rebuke and mistreatment by health care providers, or not being asked about use of T&CM [67]. A scoping review of studies on T&CM use among cancer patients in sub-Saharan Africa showed that a majority of cancer patients never disclosed use of T&CM to their health care providers, with the exception of two studies where more than half of patients disclosed use of T&CM (85.7% in Monicah et al., 2019; and 55.0%

in Ong'udia et al., 2019) [82,83]. Patients did not disclose their use of T&CM for the same reasons mentioned above, in addition to their perception that health care professionals have little knowledge regarding T&CM and, therefore, there was no need to discuss this with them [73].

Traditional and Complementary Medicine and Cancer Outcomes

There is evidence that cancer patients who seek care from traditional health practitioners (THPs) and engage in the use of T&CMs or other means of unproven therapies tend to delay presentation to established biomedical facilities for diagnoses of histological types of cancer. For example, in low-income countries, seeking care from traditional health practitioners and the use of T&CMs have been associated with delayed presentation for symptomatic female breast cancers [84–88]. Cancer patients who use T&CM are often in advanced stages at diagnoses [71], as they are more likely to desperately seek any sort of care, including T&CM, or because the cancer has progressed into advanced stages during the patients' prolonged usage of T&CM that were, perhaps, ineffective.

In Uganda, a majority of patients who self-reported T&CM use had started using them immediately upon symptom onset and prior to visiting a health care professional, while some continued to use T&CM concurrently with conventional therapy [71]. In Cameroon, 76.1% of 213 symptomatic patients with Burkitt lymphoma who reported T&CM use had initially consulted traditional health practitioners (THPs) before seeking care in biomedical facilities [89]. A similar finding was reported in Nigeria, where cancer patients at a radiotherapy unit revealed that they would seek Western medical care only when their symptoms did not improve with T&CM [70]. In Malaysia, 35.5% (87/245) of patients with hematologic malignancy had already been using T&CM before cancer diagnoses, while 70.2% (172/245) continued to use T&CM together with conventional therapies [90]. The use of T&CM prior to seeking care at biomedical facilities potentially delays health-seeking. Other studies have shown that cancer patients who employ T&CM often delay diagnosis by several months and are often in advanced stage disease at presentation [91–94]. In the United States, patients who reported use of T&CM were statistically more likely to not adhere to conventional cancer therapies and experienced poorer survival rates compared to nonusers [95,96]. There is limited data on the survival statistics of cancer patients using T&CM in SSA. These findings have important implications for interventions targeting THPs who are visited earlier on in the disease trajectory for promoting early detection of cancer.

Future Research Directions

There is need for appropriately designed research studies in sub-Saharan African countries to better understand the sociocultural underpinnings regarding use of T&CMs in order to inform health interventions that are embedded in people's beliefs and cultures. Gaps in knowledge remain regarding the extent of use, types, and reasons for using T&CM, safety and risk profiles of the various T&CMs, predictors of use among adult cancer patients, and benefits of T&CM treatment, including recovery. There is also limited data on the T&CM's mechanism of actions for cancer patients in SSA. Cancer patients who use T&CMs do not disclose use to health care professionals for various reasons, including fear of reprimand and their perception that health care professionals are ignorant regarding T&CMs. To date, there is limited data from healthcare professionals on why cancer patients use T&CMs but prefer not to disclose this to their healthcare team.

Conclusions

Cultural beliefs guide most of our thoughts and behaviors and may determine what preventive measures we take and what we perceive causes of illnesses to be. Cultural beliefs also influence who gets ill, directs our treatment decisions, and recovery, and it has the potential to protect the population from getting ill [97,98]. Culture, therefore, influences our state of health and illness in many ways; specifically, help-seeking behaviors through culturally specific illness explanatory models direct people's thinking, conduct, and responses to poor health [9,99,100,4]. Beliefs and culture are, thus, important determinants of health and illness, as well as contributing factors to the outcomes of cancer treatments by influencing decisions and practices regarding prevention, help-seeking, choice of cancer treatment, and adherence to conventional cancer therapies.

References

1. Romney AK, Weller SC, Batchelder WH. Culture as consensus: A theory of culture and informant accuracy. Am Anthropol. 1986;88:313–338.
2. Szczepura A. Access to health care for ethnic minority populations. Postgrad Med J. 2005;81:141–147.
3. Shaw S, Huebner C, Armin J, Orzech, K, Vivian J. The role of culture in health literacy and chronic disease screening and management. J Immig Minor Health. 2009;11:460–467.
4. Kleinman, A., Eisenberg, L. & Good, B. Culture, illness, and care: clinical lessons from anthropologic and cross-cultural research. Ann Intern Med, 1978; 88, 251–8.
5. Mechanic D. Social psychologic factors affecting the presentation of bodily complaints. N Engl J Med, 1972; 286:1132–1139.
6. Waxler NE. Culture and mental illness. A social labeling perspective. J Nerv Ment Dis. 1974; 159:379–395.
7. Kagawa-Singer M, Kassim-Lakha S. A strategy to reduce cross-cultural miscommunication and increase the likelihood of improving health outcomes. Acad Med, 2003; 78:577–587.
8. Kleinman A. Concepts and a model for the comparison of medical systems as cultural systems. Soc Sci Med. 1978; 12:85–95.
9. Kleinman A. Patients and Healers in the Context of Culture: An Exploration of the Borderland between Anthropology, Medicine, and Psychiatry. Berkeley, University of California Press; 1980.

10. De Nooijer J, Lechner I, de Vries H. Help-seeking behaviour for cancer symptoms: perceptions of patients and general practitioners. Psychooncology. 2001a; 10:469–478.

11. De Nooijer J, Lechner I, de Vries H. A qualitative study on detecting cancer symptoms and seeking medical help: An application of Andersen's model of total patient delay. Patient Educ Couns. 2001b;42:145–157.

12. Fabrega H, Jr. Toward a model of illness behavior. Med Care. 1973;11:470–484.

13. Friedson E. Client control and medical practice. Am J Sociol. 1960;65:374–382.

14. Frankenberg R. Medical anthropology and development: A theoretical perspective. Soc Sci Med Med Anthropol. 1980;14B:197–207.

15. Igun UA. Stages in health-seeking: A descriptive model. Soc Sci Med. 1979;13A:445–456.

16. O'Donnell O. Access to health care in developing countries: Breaking down demand side barriers. Cad. Saúde Pública (Rio de Janeiro). 2007;23(12):2820–2834.

17. Dzator J, Asafu-Adjaye J. A study of malaria care provider choice in Ghana. Health Policy. 2004;69:389–401.

18. Hamilton JB. 2017. Cultural beliefs and cancer care: Are we doing everything we can? Cancer Nurs. 2017, 40(1):84–85.

19. Pargament, K. I., Magyar-Russell, G. M. & Murray-Swank, N. A. The Sacred and the Search for Significance: Religion as a Unique Process. J Soc Issues, 2005; 61, 665–687.

20. Puchalski, C., Ferrell, B., Virani, R., et al. Improving the Quality of Spiritual Care as a Dimension of Palliative Care: The Report of the Consensus Conference. J Palliat Med, 2009; 12, 885–904.

21. Bai, J., Brubaker, A., Meghani, S. H., et al. Spirituality and Quality of Life in Black Patients With Cancer Pain. J Pain Symptom Manag, 2018; 56, 390–398.

22. Thomas, T., Blumling, A. & Delaney, A. The Influence of Religiosity and Spirituality on Rural Parents' Health Decision Making and Human Papillomavirus Vaccine Choices. Adv Nurs Sci, 2015; 38, E1–E12.

23. Steinhauser, K. E., Fitchett, G., Handzo, G. F., et al. State of the Science of Spirituality and Palliative Care Research Part I: Definitions, Measurement, and Outcomes. J Pain Symptom Manag, 2017; 54, 428–440.

24. Cohen AB. Religion's profound influences on psychology: Morality, intergroup relations, self-construal, and enculturation. Curr Dir Psychol Sci. 2015;24:77–82.

25. Aranoff D. Religion as culture. Dialog. 2020;59:193–194.

26. Lukoff D, Lu FG, Turner, R. Cultural considerations in the assessment and treatment of religious and spiritual problems. Psychiatr Clin North Am. 1995;18:467–485.

27. Hordern, J. Religion, culture and conscience. Medicine. 2020;48:640–643.

28. Abdulla MR. Culture, religion, and freedom of religion or belief. Rev Faith Int Affairs. 2018;16:102–115.

29. Ahmadi F, Hussin NAM, Mohammad MT. Religion, culture and meaning-making coping: A study among cancer patients in malaysia. J Relig Health. 2019;58:1909–1924.

30. Peteet JR, Balboni J. Spirituality and religion in oncology. CA: A Cancer Journal for Clinicians. 2013;63:280–289.

31. Choumanova I, Wanat S, Barrett R, Koopman C. Religion and spirituality in coping with breast cancer: perspectives of Chilean women. Breast J. 2006;2:349–352.

32. Winkelman WD, Lauderdale K., Balboni MJ, et al. The relationship of spiritual concerns to the quality of life of advanced cancer patients: preliminary findings. J Palliat Med. 2001;14:1022–1028.

33. Zavala MW, Maliski, SL, Kwan L, Fink A, Litwin MS. Spirituality and quality of life in low-income men with metastatic prostate cancer. Psychooncology.2009;18, 753–761.

34. Krupski TL, Kwan L, Fink A, Sonn GA, Maliski S, Litwin MS. Spirituality influences health related quality of life in men with prostate cancer. Psychooncology, 2006;5:121–131.

35. Astrow AB, Wexler A, Texeira K., HE, MK, Sulmasy, DP. Is failure to meet spiritual needs associated with cancer patients' perceptions of quality of care and their satisfaction with care? J Clin Oncol, 2007;25, 5753–5757.

36. Kang J, Shin DW, Choi, JY, et al. Addressing the religious and spiritual needs of dying patients by healthcare staff in Korea: Patient perspectives in a multi-religious Asian country. Psychooncology, 2012;21:374–381.

37. Brady MJ, Peterman AH, Fitchett G, Mo M, Cella D. A case for including spirituality in quality of life measurement in oncology. Psychooncology. 1999;417–428.

38. Kristeller JL, Sheets V, Johnson T, Frank, B. Understanding religious and spiritual influences on adjustment to cancer: individual patterns and differences. J Behav Med. 2011;34:550–561.

39. Jim, HSL, Pustejovsky JE, Park, et al. Religion, spirituality, and physical health in cancer patients: A meta-analysis. Cancer, 2015;121:3760–3768.

40. Palmer Kelly E, Paredes AZ, Tsilimigras DI, Hyer JM, Pawlik TM. The role of religion and spirituality in cancer care: An umbrella review of the literature. Surg Oncol. 2020; 101389.

41. Mwaka AD, Garimoi CO, Were E.M, et al. Social, demographic and healthcare factors associated with stage at diagnosis of cervical cancer: Cross-sectional study in a tertiary hospital in Northern Uganda. BMJ Open, 2016; 6, e007690.

42. Sengayi-Muchengeti M, Joko-Fru, WY, Miranda-Filho A., et al. 2020. Cervical cancer survival in sub-Saharan Africa by age, stage at diagnosis and Human Development Index: A population-based registry study. Int J Cancer. 2020; 147:3037–3048.

43. Joko-Fru, W. Y., Miranda-Filho, A., Soerjomataram, et al. Breast cancer survival in sub-Saharan Africa by age, stage at diagnosis and human development index: A population-based registry study. Int J Cancer. 2020;146:1208–1218.

44. Akuoko, C. P., Armah, E., Sarpong, T., et Al. Barriers to early presentation and diagnosis of breast cancer among African women living in sub-Saharan Africa. Plos One, 2017; 12, e0171024.

45. Gebremariam, A., Addissie, A., Worku, A., et al. Perspectives of patients, family members, and health care providers on late diagnosis of breast cancer in Ethiopia: A qualitative study. PloS one,2019; 14, e0220769.

46. Yu, C. K., Chiu, C., Mccormack, M. & Olaitan, A. Delayed diagnosis of cervical cancer in young women. J Obstetr Gynaecol., 2005; 25, 367–370.

47. Gyenwali, D., Pariyar, J. & Onta, S. R. Factors Associated with Late Diagnosis of Cervical Cancer in Nepal. APJCP, 2013; 14, 4373–4377.

48. Kaku M, Mathew A., Rajan B. Impact of socio-economic factors in delayed reporting and late-stage presentation among patients with cervix cancer in a major cancer hospital in South India. APJCP. 2008; 9:589–594.

49. Were, E. O. & Buziba, N. G. Presentation and health care seeking behaviour of patients with cervical cancer seen at Moi Teaching and Referral Hospital, Eldoret, Kenya. East Afr Med J, 2001; 78, 55–59.

50. Kazaura, M. R., Kombe, D., Yuma, S., et. al. Health seeking behavior among cancer patients attending Ocean Road Cancer Institute, Tanzania. East Afr J Public Health, 2007; 4, 19–22.

51. Birhanu, Z., Abdissa, A., Belachew, T., et al. Health seeking behavior for cervical cancer in Ethiopia: a qualitative study. Int J Equity Health, 2012; 11, 83.

52. Powe, B. D. Fatalism among elderly African Americans: Effects on colorectal cancer screening. Cancer Nurs, 1995; 18, 385–392.

53. Beeken, R. J., Simon, A. E., Von Wagner, C., et al. Cancer fatalism: deterring early presentation and increasing social inequalities? Cancer Epidemiol Biomarkers Prev, 2011; 20, 2127–2131.

54. Shahid, S., Finn, L., Bessarab, D. & Thompson, S. C. Understanding, beliefs and perspectives of Aboriginal people in Western Australia about cancer and its impact on access to cancer services. BMC Health Serv Res, 2009; 9, 132.

55. Weller, D., Vedsted, P., Rubin, G., et al. The Aarhus statement: improving design and reporting of studies on early cancer diagnosis. Br J Cancer, 2012; 106, 1262–7.

56. WHO. WHO Traditional Medicine Strategy: 2013–2023. World Health Organization, Geneva. 2013;15.

57. Ernst, E. The role of complementary and alternative medicine in cancer. Lancet Oncol, 2000; 1, 176–80.

58. Shen, J., Andersen, R., Albert, P. S., et al. Use of complementary/alternative therapies by women with advanced-stage breast cancer. BMC Complement Alt Med, 2002; 2, 8.

59. Horneber, M., Bueschel, G., Dennert, G., et al. How many cancer patients use complementary and alternative medicine: a systematic review and metaanalysis. Integr Cancer Ther, 2012; 11, 187–203.

60. Klafke, N., Eliott, J. A., Wittert, G. A. & Olver, I. N. Prevalence and predictors of complementary and alternative medicine (CAM) use by men in Australian cancer outpatient services. Ann Oncol, 2012; 23, 1571–8.

61. Yildiz, I., Ozguroglu, M., Toptas, T., et al. Patterns of complementary and alternative medicine use among Turkish cancer patients. J Palliat Med, 2013; 16, 383–90.

62. Nazik, E., Nazik, H., Api, M., et al. Complementary and alternative medicine use by gynecologic oncology patients in Turkey. APJCP, 2012; 13, 21–5.

63. Ku, C. F. & Koo, M. Association of distress symptoms and use of complementary medicine among patients with cancer. J Clin Nurs, 2012; 21, 736–44.

64. Ezeome, E. R. & Anarado, A. N. Use of complementary and alternative medicine by cancer patients at the University of Nigeria Teaching Hospital, Enugu, Nigeria. BMC Complement Alt Med, 2007; 7, 28.

65. Sparber, A., Wootton, J. C., Bauer, L., et al. Use of complementary medicine by adult patients participating in HIV/AIDS clinical trials. J Alt Complement Med, 2000; 6, 415–22.

66. Davis, E. L., Oh, B., Butow, P. N., et al. Cancer patient disclosure and patient-doctor communication of complementary and alternative medicine use: a systematic review. Oncologist, 2012; 17, 1475–81.

67. James, P. B., Wardle, J., Steel, A. & Adams, J. Traditional, complementary and alternative medicine use in Sub-Saharan Africa: a systematic review. BMJ Global Health, 2018; 3, e000895.

68. Erku, D. A. Complementary and Alternative Medicine Use and Its Association with Quality of Life among Cancer Patients Receiving Chemotherapy in Ethiopia: A Cross-Sectional Study. Evidence-Based Complement Alt Med, 2016, 8.

69. Yarney, J., Donkor, A., Opoku, S. Y., et al. Characteristics of users and implications for the use of complementary and alternative medicine in Ghanaian cancer patients undergoing radiotherapy and chemotherapy: a cross- sectional study. BMC Complement Alt Med, 2013; 13, 16.

70. Asuzu, C. C., Elumelu-Kupoluyi, T., Asuzu, M. C., et al. A pilot study of cancer patients' use of traditional healers in the Radiotherapy Department, University College Hospital, Ibadan, Nigeria. Psychooncology, 2017; 26, 369–376.

71. Mwaka, A. D., Mangi, S. P. & Okuku, F. M. Use of traditional and complementary medicines by cancer patients at a national cancer referral facility in a low-income country. Eur J Cancer Care, 2019; 28, e13158.

72. Kiwanuka, F. Complementary and Alternative Medicine use: Influence of Patients' Satisfaction with Medical Treatment among Breast Cancer Patients at Uganda Cancer Institute. Advances Biosci Clin Med, 2018; 6, 24–29.

73. Mwaka, A. D., Abbo, C. & Kinengyere, A. A. Traditional and Complementary Medicine Use Among Adult Cancer Patients Undergoing Conventional Treatment in Sub -Saharan Africa: A Scoping Review on the Use, Safety and Risks. Cancer Manag Res, 2020; 12, 3699–3712.

74. Nahleh, Z. & Tabbara, I. A. Complementary and alternative medicine in breast cancer patients. Palliat Support Care, 2003; 1, 267–73.

75. Muhamad, M., Merriam, S. & Suhami, N. Why breast cancer patients seek traditional healers. Int J Breast Cancer, 2012; 689168.

76. Muela, S. H., Mushi, A. K. & Ribera, J. M. The paradox of the cost and affordability of traditional and government health services in Tanzania. Health Policy Plan, 2000; 15, 296–302.

77. Leonard, K. L. & Zivin, J. G. Outcome versus service based payments in health care: lessons from African traditional healers. Health Econ, 2005; 14, 575–593.

78. Aliyu, U. M., Awosan, K. J., OChe, M. O., et al. Prevalence and correlates of complementary and alternative medicine use among cancer patients in usmanu danfodiyo university teaching hospital, Sokoto, Nigeria. Niger J Clin Pract, 2017; 20, 1576–1583.

79. Aziato, L. & Clegg-Lamptey, J. N. A. Breast Cancer Diagnosis and Factors Influencing Treatment Decisions in Ghana. Health Care Women Int, 2015; 36, 543–557.

80. Falisse, J.-B., Masino, S. & Ngenzebuhoro, R. Indigenous medicine and biomedical health care in fragile settings: insights from Burundi. Health Policy Plan, 2018; 33, 483–493.

81. Rutebemberwa, E., Lubega, M., Katureebe, S. K., et al. Use of traditional medicine for the treatment of diabetes in Eastern Uganda: a qualitative exploration of reasons for choice. BMC Int Health Hum Rights, 2013; 13, 1.

82. Monicah K, Mbugua G, Mburugu R. Use of complementary and alternative medicine among cancer patients in Meru County, Kenya. Int J Profess Pract. 2019; 7:24–33.

83. Ong'udi M, Mutai P, Weru U, I. Study of the use of complementary and alternative medicine by cancer patients at Kenyatta National Hospital, Nairobi, Kenya. J Oncol Pharm Pract. 2019; 25:918–928.

84. Pace, L. E., Mpunga, T., Hategekimana, V., et al. Delays in Breast Cancer Presentation and Diagnosis at Two Rural Cancer Referral Centers in Rwanda. Oncologist, 2015; 20, 780–788.

85. Ezeome, E. R. Delays in presentation and treatment of breast cancer in Enugu, Nigeria. Niger J Clin Pract, 2010; 13, 311–6.

86. Ermiah, E., Abdalla, F., Buhmeida, A., et al. Diagnosis delay in Libyan female breast cancer. BMC Res Notes, 2012; 5, 452.

87. Malik, I. & Gopalan, S. Use of CAM results in delay in seeking medical advice for breast cancer. Eur J Epidemiol, 2003; 18, 817–822.

88. Hill, J., Mills, C., Li, Q. & Smith, J. S. Prevalence of traditional, complementary, and alternative medicine use by cancer patients in low income and lower-middle income countries. Glob Public Health, 2019; 14, 418–430.

89. Afungchwi, G. M., Hesseling, P. B. & Ladas, E. J. The role of traditional healers in the diagnosis and management of Burkitt lymphoma in Cameroon: understanding the challenges and moving forward. BMC Complement Alt Med, 2017; 17, 209.

90. Gan, G. G., Leong, Y. C., Bee, P. C., et al. Complementary and alternative medicine use in patients with hematological cancers in Malaysia. Support Care Cancer, 2015; 23, 2399–2406.

91. Kerdpon, D. & Sriplung, H. Factors related to delay in diagnosis of oral squamous cell carcinoma in southern Thailand. Oral Oncol, 2001; 37, 127–31.

92. De Boer, C., Niyonzima, N., Orem, J., et al. Prognosis and delay of diagnosis among Kaposi's sarcoma patients in Uganda: a cross-sectional study. Infect Agent Cancer, 2014; 9, 1750–9378.

93. Maghous, A., Rais, F., Ahid, S., et al. Factors influencing diagnosis delay of advanced breast cancer in Moroccan women. BMC Cancer, 2016; 16, 356.

94. Broom, A., Nayar, K., Tovey, P., et al. Indian Cancer Patients' use of Traditional, Complementary and Alternative Medicine (TCAM) and delays in presentation to Hospital. Oman Med J, 2009; 24, 99–102.

95. Johnson, S. B., Park, H. S., Gross, C. P. & Yu, J. B. Complementary Medicine, Refusal of Conventional Cancer Therapy, and Survival Among Patients With Curable Cancers. JAMA Oncol, 2018a; 4, 1375–1381.

96. Johnson, S. B., Park, H. S., Gross, C. P. & Yu, J. B. Use of Alternative Medicine for Cancer and Its Impact on Survival. JNCI, 2018b; 110, 121–124.

97. Helman, G., Cecil. Culture, Health and Illness. Hodder Arnold, an imprint of Hodder Education, part of Hachette Livre UK, Easton Road, London, 2007; 5th Edition, 128–143.

98. Hruschka, D. & Hadley, C. A glossary of culture in epidemiology. J Epidemiol Commun Health, 2008; 62, 947–951.

99. Asbridge, M., Tanner, J. & Wortley, S. Ethno-specific patterns of adolescent tobacco use and the mediating role of acculturation, peer smoking, and sibling smoking. Addiction, 2005; 100, 1340–1351.

100. Luby, S. P., Agboatwalla, M., Feikin, D. R., et al. Effect of handwashing on child health: a randomised controlled trial. The Lancet, 2005; 366, 225–233.

25

Barriers to Addressing Emotional and Psycho-Social Needs in Cancer Care, Turkey

Gülçin Şenel

Introduction

The diagnosis of cancer is an event that makes people question the meaning of life and changes the course of their lives. The patient and the family would likely face many new emotional and psychosocial difficulties that begin with the diagnosis of cancer. Many factors, such as the biological effects of malignancy and the burden of physical symptoms including pain, fatigue, weakness, anorexia, nausea, and vomiting (all of which may be due to the illness or difficult cancer treatments), sleep disturbances, fear of death, grief regarding the current situation, and grief for anticipated losses contribute to psychiatric morbidity [1,2].Impairment of physical, psychological, and social functionality, along with problems related to daily life [3], working life [4], and finances [5] may arise. These emotional, psychological, social, or spiritually unpleasant experiences prevent the ability to cope with cancer and create emotional distress. The rate of patients experiencing emotional stress is suggested to be 40–60% [6]. The continuous feelings of vulnerability, combined with experiencing sadness and fear, can lead to adjustment disorders, depression, and anxiety. Specific measured techniques can reveal the presence of possible adjustment disorders, anxiety, or depression in 40–50% of cancer patients [7–9]. The incidence of clinically significant anxiety is reported to be 12–30% [10]. Depression is a common condition in patients who have undergone cancer surgery [11] chemotherapy, adjuvant therapy, or radiotherapy [12,13], and it is reported to be at a rate of 40% in those patients under palliative care [14]. With the recognition and appropriate treatment of the emotional distress and psychiatric disorders in patients and their families, their quality of life [15–17], treatment compliance [18,19], and life span [20,21] can be increased.

Today, two-thirds of patients diagnosed with invasive cancer can live more than five years due to the advancements in cancer diagnosis and treatment [22]. With many cancer patients, fear of cancer's recurrence, symptoms of posttraumatic stress, anxiety, or depression can be encountered following completion of treatment [23]. Untreated psychological problems can lead to increased physical and emotional pain [24], decreased physical functionality [24], higher medical costs, and prolonged hospital stays [25].

Many consensuses and guidelines recommend providing appropriate psychosocial care for cancer patients and their families in order to obtain better quality of life. Psychosocial care should be handled broadly, including identifying the needs of the patient and the family, facilitating communication with cancer caregivers, providing a safe care environment, educating the family/caregivers, assisting with access to the health care system and community resources, and physical, social, and vocational rehabilitation services [26,27]. A care system that accords with the patient's personal, spiritual, and cultural values in terms of illness, life, and death should be planned [28]. For best results, this care system should be integrated as soon as possible and should be implemented at all stages of the disease, including the hospitalization period, outpatient environments, and routine cancer care [17]. For a dying patient, whose possible life span is limited to weeks/days, the patient's comfort requests should be evaluated and supported. Emotional support should be provided to patients and family members to prevent family conflicts related to palliative care interventions. Psychosocial support for family members should be continued during the grieving process following death. In a recent systematic review of advanced cancer patients, psychosocial resources are identified as among the factors that promote personal development during the cancer experience [29].

The uncertainties and multiple decisions may raise spirituality-related issues more often in persons diagnosed with cancer than with other long-term illnesses. The current clinical practice includes psychosocial screening; spiritual inquiry also is needed in recognition that each cancer patient's history and illness are unique and will affect all dimensions of that person in unique ways. Spirituality is defined as the way people find meaning and purpose in life, and how they experience their connectedness to self, others, the significant, or sacred [30]. In cancer care, spirituality interacts with the physical and psychosocial domain. Untreated spiritual suffering may worsen the pain experience [31]. Spiritual and/or psychosocial support may be required in the treatment of depression diagnosed with unhappiness, hopelessness, and meaninglessness [32]. Spirituality can be a powerful positive force in helping patients reframe their illness, find greater meaning in life, and recognize what is ultimately important and of value to them. Unresolved spiritual distress can lead to poorer quality of life and poorer health outcomes [33].

Adequate identification and management of psychosocial problems of cancer patients remain the major unmet requirements in the delivery of oncology services [34–36]. Almost 40% of these patients worldwide are deprived of the necessary psychosocial interventions, independent of the average income level of their respective countries [37]. Barriers to meeting the spiritual, emotional, and psychosocial needs of cancer patients can be multiple and diverse. Although it may vary by region, even a single barrier may be the reason for not being able to provide proper psychosocial care.

Barriers Originating from the Patient and Family

Unawareness, Refusing the Need

Patients report that the main barrier to receiving psychosocial care is the perception that it is not needed [38,39]. Lack of information, negative thoughts, insecurity, and disbelief about psychosocial services prevent patients from benefiting from these services. Promoting services and providing accessible, effective, and sustainable support would bring increased awareness and would benefit patients and their families [39].

Cultural Structure and Fear of Stigmatization

Cultural beliefs and values related to cancer are considered important determinants for psychological and behavioral outcomes of the cancer diagnosis and treatment process [40,41]. In Western cultures, individuals are expected to participate in an active struggle to "fight cancer" and regain health, while in Eastern cultures the disease is often perceived as one's destiny. By avoiding naming cancer (not calling cancer "cancer") and not talking about it, it will be more difficult to express the needs of the patient and to comply with the recommended treatments, especially in societies where the authority for decision making and consent is held by the family rather than the patient.

Cancer is considered not just an individual, but also a family, experience. However, the degree and style of family involvement differ across cultures [42]. In traditional societies, the family reduces the patient's personal responsibility by avoiding the presence and contribution of this individual in the decision-making processes. Family members aim to protect the patient by keeping cancer information confidential or by giving the patient selective information, thus preventing the patient from getting psychosocial support by causing isolation. On the other hand, positive aspects of strong family ties such as emotional support, participation in medical care, and sharing the financial burden can be beneficial to the patient.

Although each country is different, cancer continues to carry significant amounts of stigma, myth, and taboo all around the world [43,44]. Other negative preconceptions about cancer are that it is often synonymous with death, suffering, disaster, bad destiny, worthlessness, and punishment [45,46]. Cancer is considered a taboo subject in some parts of Asia [47]. Studies have shown that stigma related to cancer is present in many countries [48–50]. Stigmatizing is a powerful social process that starts with labeling, causing unfair action against the individual or group, and leads to discrimination and loss of status [51]. Cancer stigma can be more difficult and even more unbearable than cancer treatments and the disease itself [52]. Fear of stigmatization can prevent the disclosure of a cancer diagnosis, causing isolation and depression [53] and is known to be especially high in gynecological and breast cancers [54,55]. The perception that a person diagnosed with cancer is too sick to be employed is also common. The disease is often kept secret due to the difficulties of returning to work or finding a new job. In addition to cancer stigma, cancer patients often fear the stigma surrounding mental health care, and thus, they hide their feelings or refuse to seek help [56].

Cultural values and spiritual and religious beliefs can affect the end-of-life care, which is very difficult for the patient, their family, and health care professionals. If limitations are placed on sharing information about the disease and its prognosis, then there cannot be self-determination, autonomy, priority planning, advance care planning, and informed consent in end-of-life care. In belief systems where maintaining life is prioritized over quality of life, difficulties may be encountered in terms of discontinuing treatments that are not beneficial to the patient or when making end-of-life decisions [57]. When the patients' desire to die at home in order to be with their loved ones and prepare for a peaceful death is respected, passing this period at home can also mean being left to die. Knowing the rituals in different cultures is also important to help increase access to emotional and psychosocial care during the grieving process. Health professionals should try to give the best possible psychosocial care during the planning and preparation process, in accordance with cultural norms and belief systems, through open communication and evaluation of each patient's and family's connotation of death.

Communicational Difficulties, Distrust in the System

The sociodemographic characteristics of both patients and health professionals can significantly impact communication in cancer care. Patients with advanced age, a low level of education, socioeconomic weaknesses, and/or origin from racial or ethnic minorities request less information about their disease from their doctors and share less of their own disease experience [58]. Elderly patients may have multiple communication problems, as their attitudes and beliefs regarding cancer may be different from those of young adults, and they may have less health literacy and more cognitive or sensory weaknesses [59]. It has been reported that women generally seek and receive more information and emotional support than men [60].

Being a minority or immigrant in the community can also limit psychosocial support due to communication difficulties and distrust in the health system, causing conflicts between health care professionals and care recipients [61,62]. Other important barriers for immigrants to obtain effective emotional and psychosocial support in cancer care are lack of support from family, language barriers, cost of care, and fear of deportation. [63]. Trying to communicate in different languages impedes asking questions and speaking freely, putting an additional burden on both patient and provider.

Cancer Care Barriers for Health Care Professionals

Attitudes and Beliefs of Health Professionals

Feeling valued can affect the delivery of psychosocial care. Clinicians and health care professionals need to be aware that psychosocial problems are a significant burden on patients and their families and that psychosocial care is presently inadequate. Attitudes and beliefs of health care providers toward psychosocial issues affect the way they communicate with patients. Though rare, some physicians believe that their patients expect them to provide only medical care, not psychological care [64]. Although many physicians accept the importance of meeting psychosocial needs, they expect the request to come from the patients [65]. Patients, on the other hand, think that the doctor should inquire about their needs [66]. Physicians who express positive attitudes about psychosocial care show more empathy toward their patients, and, in so doing, their patients are more willing to report emotional problems [67].

Lack of Education

Communication Skills

In cancer care, it is necessary to have a sufficient level of communication skills to pass on information clearly, as well as a positive attitude to facilitate and support interpersonal communication. Because cancer is often associated with suffering, difficult treatments, bodily changes, and stigmatization, the form of communication can be even more complicated. A safe and compassionate communication that provides appropriate information at the patients' developmental and educational level forms the basis for management of psychosocial needs [68].

Starting from the medical and nursing curricula, education models that help physicians and nurses to develop their communication skills and recognize emotional and psychological distress should be applied. Education modules that provide problem-based learning depending on clinical cases have been shown to be effective in providing psychosocial knowledge, communication skills, and positive attitudes toward patients [69–71].

Evaluation Skills

Identifying emotional distress among patients with cancer is the first step to providing holistic psychosocial care. Recognizing emotional distress as early and accurately as possible is the basis of the treatment. It is very important to make timely and systematic evaluations in order to identify psychiatric disorders in patients and to distinguish normative emotional responses from psychopathology.

Although health professionals have many scales and diagnostic methods whose validity and reliability are defined, they are reluctant to investigate psychiatric disorders in cancer patients or often cannot correctly diagnose them [72,73]. In oncology centers, only one-third of patients with serious psychological problems are recognized by their oncologists [35]. Sadness is perceived as a normal response to cancer, and it is difficult to distinguish between psychological distress and disease symptoms.

Oncology nurses spend more time with patients and family members while providing care and play an important role in recognizing and guiding psychological distress [74,75]. Despite this important role in potentially identifying the problem, research to date has shown that oncology nurses, similarly to other health care professionals, often do not correctly detect the psychological problems of patients and tend to underestimate serious symptoms [76,77]. It has been reported that nurses who use screening tools to recognize psychological distress can more often direct the patient to appropriate psychosocial services than psychologists [78].

Intervention Skills

It is not enough for cancer caregivers to recognize the psychosocial needs of their patients; they also need to know how to manage these requirements. Physicians and nurses working in cancer care should receive basic education in psychosocial care.

They should convey the appropriate information to support and encourage patients to accept treatment. Patients at high risk of psychological distress should be directed to special care that can provide evidence-based treatments. High-risk patients should be directed to specialized mental health services that can apply individualized evidence-based psychosocial (cognitive-behavioral therapy, awareness-based therapy, psychoeducation, etc.) and psychopharmacological treatments. Even when psychological distress is identified, it has been reported that as low as 15–50% of cancer patients receive treatment [35,79]. Clinicians' lack of knowledge about how to provide appropriate psychosocial care creates a potential barrier to quality care. More than 70% of health professionals working in the field of oncology reported that they do not have the ability to provide psychosocial care and would like to receive training on this subject [80]. The lack of skills for providing psychosocial care may prevent patients from discussing psychosocial issues for fear they will not be able to cope if Pandora's box is opened.

Cancer patients with high spiritual well-being reported better quality of life, lower levels of depression and anxiety, and less death anxiety [33]. It has been shown that the spiritual care provided to cancer patients by the medical team provides emotional support and improves treatment compliance, quality of life, and patient satisfaction. As spirituality is a critical component of holistic and person-centered care, spiritual care should be considered along with psychosocial care and be included in the care plan of each cancer patient [81]. Although physicians and nurses accept the necessity of providing spiritual care for patients, it is, in fact, less common in clinical practice [82]. The biggest barrier to spiritual care is, again, the lack of education [83–85].

Workload and Lack of Time

Cancer treatment units have a high workload. This burden is due to the number of patients, the complexity of the diseases and their treatments, and the lack of staff. The focus of both the clinician and the patient on the cancer treatment during the limited time allotted for consultation often leads to overlooking psychosocial needs. Oncology nurses frequently mention workload and lack of time among the obstacles for identifying psychological problems and providing psychosocial care [86,87]. Training for integrating communication skills and the recognition of psychosocial distress in daily practice can reduce the perception of lack of time.

Lack of Role and Job Description

Although all health care professionals are obliged to provide basic psychosocial support, whose role it is to participate in psychosocial care and the timing and extent of this care should be clarified. Role definition at the organizational and institutional level provides accountability, along with meeting both the physical and psychosocial needs of patients. It promotes a more holistic approach in which it is the individual who is treated, not the disease.

Inadequacy of Support Systems for Health Care Professionals

Health professionals regard psychosocial care services as an emotional burden that can lead to stress and burnout [88]. Being appointed as a decision maker by the patient and/or family for the treatment process and at the end-of-life stage further increases the burden on clinicians. In addition, understanding cancer caregivers' fears regarding the concepts of disease and death should be addressed. Psychology, psychiatry, and social working specialties may better cope with stress than other health care workers. Skilled professional development programs, communication strategies, counseling, and rewarding all health care professionals providing psychosocial care can be supported by specialist and health organizations, thus reducing the perceived burden.

Lacking Cultural Competence

Attitudes toward disease, suffering, treatment decisions, and all oncology care framed by cultural factors are important when both screening and evaluating psychosocial problems. Cultural practices and beliefs should be considered when providing diagnostic and prognostic information, as it can affect the patient and family concerning decision making, doctor–patient communications, psychological responses to cancer, and coping mechanisms. There may be a need to adapt the validation and reliability analyses for screening and assessment tools to different languages and cultures. A therapeutic relationship can be established through communication that respects cultural values and beliefs so that true patient/family-centered care is provided equally to all members of the community [89,90]. Therefore, multidisciplinary oncology and palliative care teams should strive to reach cultural competence [91].

Barriers of the Health System

Not Valuing and Prioritizing/Limited Resources

The level of adequacy of staff and systems to support new implementations and allow for more time and access to health facilities can affect the behavior of both individuals and organizations. Clinical settings may not always be suitable for good psychosocial care. Limited budgets and resources lead to ignored multidisciplinary and psychosocial care. This emphasizes the value and priority of psychosocial care at the organizational and governmental levels. Limited resources require psychosocial care systems to be both sustainable and cost effective.

Standards Not Being Set

The absence of national and institutional standards and clinical practice guidelines that define psychosocial care processes and goals may be the cause of poor awareness in clinical practices. The detection of psychosocial distress will not turn into action when there is a lack of resources designated to providing care. In addition to determining psychosocial screening and treatment procedures, these standards should include the organization and structure of psychosocial services and appropriate training of psychosocial care providers.

Integrated Systems Not Being Constituted

Perhaps the main challenge to the health care system arises from the lack of coordinated evidence-based psychosocial services for the active cancer treatment process, palliative care and survivor follow-up. Existing systems are often fragmented and poorly coordinated. Units such as psychiatry, social services, palliative care, pain treatment, and rehabilitation work independently from one another and do not allow for a collaborative approach in accordance with patient needs [92]. In psychosocial care, there is a need for better collaboration among fields of expertise and systems to ensure continuity and to respond to needs that change over time [93].

Collaborative care programs go beyond positioning health care professionals in oncology centers. Better and lasting results can be achieved with active cooperation for solving complex problems that are difficult to manage. Collaborative care also includes measurement-based care. It uses care management records and clinical rating scales to identify patients in need of treatment or at risk and then it provides measurement-based cascading care to those who need treatment. Five basic elements are emphasized within the framework of the integrated model for psychosocial care [94]:

1. Identification of patients with psychosocial health needs
2. Planning to address these needs
3. Mechanisms to link patients with psychosocial health services
4. Supporting self-management of the illness
5. Follow-up on care delivery

In many cancer centers, there is no psychosocial care system that can be integrated into patients' cancer care. There is inadequate communication and sharing of information among the oncology, psychosocial care, and primary care providers regarding the psychosocial needs of the patient [95–97]. Cancer care should be integrated (from screening to palliative care) in all care settings (inpatient/outpatient cancer services and primary/home care). It is recommended to establish common care protocols between oncology and primary care during the transition from hospital to home care or during survivor follow-up [98]. Patients with psychological problems do not usually admit themselves into psychiatric clinics; most of the time the cancer treatment team directs them. A system that coordinates the maintenance of both physical and psychosocial problems for a large population in need of oncology care facilitates access to timely and appropriate psychosocial care. At the same time, more effective interventions can be made with more efficient use of limited resources. In addition, long-term problems can be averted by timely and appropriate psychosocial care [99]. Mental and behavioral stigma can also be overcome by integrating psychosocial care into oncology and primary care.

Social Inequality and Difficulty in Accessing Services

Insufficient health insurance systems are a barrier both for access to cancer treatment and for elimination of physical and psychosocial problems. The difficulty of accessing monetary settlements and the fact that the resources are found only in certain centers make access to the services difficult.

How to Deal with Barriers

Barriers to emotional and psychosocial support in cancer care may differ between communities and institutions and should, first of all, be determined, It is not enough to eliminate a single barrier in order to obtain positive results, as strategies must be developed that combat all barriers simultaneously.

Conclusion

In order to offer better psychosocial care, health systems must help patients and health professionals to change their behavior. Information on available community resources should be provided, and access to them should be facilitated. Organizational structures that encourage an innovative and collaborative approach are needed to change the established cancer care culture. Early and effective integration of psychosocial care in cancer care should be among the primary goals of health systems, and all individual, organizational, and cultural factors should be considered. Education of patients and health professionals on the value and effectiveness of psychosocial interventions should be supported by national health policies. As cancer and palliative care environments are becoming increasingly multiracial and multicultural, specific requirements of the cultural structure should be taken into consideration for legal directives and individualization of care to be facilitated.

References

1. Carlson LE, Bultz BD. Efficacy and medical cost offset of psychosocial interventions in cancer care: Making the case for economic analyses. *Psychooncology.* 2004;13:837–849.
2. Geinitz H, Zimmermann FB, Thamm R, et al. Fatigue in patients with adjuvant radiation therapy for breast cancer: Long-term follow-up. *J Cancer Res Clin Oncol.* 2004;130:327–333.
3. Malone M, Harris AL, Luscombe DK. Assessment of the impact of cancer on work recreation, home management and sleep using a general health status measure. *J R Soc Med.* 1994;87:386–389.

4. Schulz R, Williamson GM, Knapp JE, Bookwala J, Lave J, Fello M. The psychological, social, and economic impact of illness among patients with recurrent cancer. *J Psychosoc Oncol.* 1995;13:21–45.

5. Van Tulder MW, Aaronson NK, Bruning PF. The quality of life of long-term survivors of Hodgkin's disease. *Ann Oncol.* 1994;5:153–158.

6. Zabora J, Brintzenhofeszoc H, Curbow B, Hooker C, Piantadosi S. The prevalence of psychological distress by cancer site. *Psychooncology.* 2001;10:19–28.

7. Grassi L, Gritti P, Rigatelli M, Gala C. Psychosocial problems secondary to cancer: An Italian multicentre survey of consultation-liaison psychiatry in oncology. Italian Consultation-Liaison Group. *Eur J Cancer.* 2000;36:579–585.

8. Kissane DW, Grabsch B, Love A, et al. Psychiatric disorder in women with early stage and advanced breast cancer: a comparative analysis. *Austr NZ J Psychiatry.* 2004;38:320–326.

9. Singer S, Szalai C, Briest S, et al. Co-morbid mental health conditions in cancer patients at working age-prevalence, risk profiles, and care uptake. *Psychooncology.* 2013;22:2291–2297.

10. Bodurka-Bevers D, Basen-Engquist K, Carmack CL, et al. Depression, anxiety, and quality of life in patients with epithelial ovarian cancer. *Gynaecol Oncolol.* 2000;78:302–308.

11. Fallowfield LJ, Hall A, Maguire GP, et al. Psychological outcomes of different treatment policies in women with early breast cancer outside a clinical trial. *BMJ.* 1990;301:575–580.

12. Jenkins C, Carmody TJ, Rush AJ. Depression in radiation oncology patients: a preliminary evaluation. *J Affect Disord.* 1998;50:17–21.

13. Jacobsen PB, Bovberg DH, Redd WH. Anticipatory anxiety in women receiving chemotherapy for breast cancer. *Health Psychol.* 1998;12:469–475.

14. Bukberg J, Penman D, Holland JC. Depression in hospitalized cancer patients. *Psychosom Med.* 1984;46:199–212.

15. Breitbart W, Rosenfeld B, Pessin H, et al. Meaning-centered group psychotherapy: An effective intervention for improving psychological well-being in patients with advanced cancer. *J Clin Oncol.* 2015;33:749–754.

16. Carlson LE, Waller A, Mitchell AJ. Screening for distress and unmet needs in patients with cancer: Review and recommendations. *J Clin Oncol.* 2012;11:1160–1177.

17. Stagl JM, Bouchard LC, Lechner SC, et al. Long-term psychological benefits of cognitive-behavioral stress management for women with breast cancer: 11-year follow-up of a randomized controlled trial. *Cancer.* 2015;121:1873–1881.

18. Kennard BD, Stewart SM, Olvera R, et al. Nonadherence in adolescent oncology patients: Preliminary data on psychological risk factors and relationships to outcome. *J Clin Psychol Med Set.* 2004;11:31–39.

19. Roter DL, Hall JA, Merisca R, et al. Effectiveness of interventions to improve patient compliance: A meta-analysis. *Med Care.* 1998; 36:1138–1161.

20. Hjerl K, Andersen EW, Keiding N, et al. Depression as a prognostic factor for breast cancer mortality. *Psychosomatics.* 2003;44:24–30.

21. Loberiza FR. Jr Rizzo JD, Bredeson CN, et al. Association of depressive syndrome and early deaths among patients after stem-cell transplantation for malignant diseases. *J Clin Oncol.* 2002;20: 2118–2126.

22. Miller KD, Siegel RL, Lin CC, et al. Cancer treatment and survivorship statistics, 2016. *CA Cancer J Clin.* 2016;66(4):271–289.

23. Lu D, Andersson TM, Fall K, et al. Clinical diagnosis of mental disorders immediately before and after cancer diagnosis: A nationwide matched cohort study in Sweden. *JAMA Oncol.* 2016;2(9):1188–1196.

24. Wells KB, Stewart A, Hays RD, et al. The functioning and well-being of depressed patients. Results from the Medical Outcomes Study. *JAMA.* 1989;262(7):914–919.

25. Simon GE, VonKorff M, Barlow W. Health care costs of primary care patients with recognized depression. *Arch Gen Psychiatry*. 1995;52:850–856.

26. Northouse L, Williams AL, Given B, et al. Psychosocial care for family caregivers of patients with cancer. *J Clin Oncol*. 2012;30:1227–1234.

27. Applebaum AJ, Kulikowski JR, Breitbart W. Meaning-centered psychotherapy for cancer caregivers (MCP-C): Rationale and overview. *Palliat Support Care*. 2015:13(6):1–11.

28. Keall RM, Clayton JM, Butow PN. Therapeutic life review in palliative care: A systematic review of quantitative evaluations. *J Pain Symptom Manage*. 2015;49:747–761.

29. Moreno PI, Stanton AL. Personal growth during the experience of advanced cancer: A systematic review. *Cancer J*. 2013;19:421–340.

30. Puchalski CM, Ferrell B, Virani R, et al. Improving the quality of spiritual care as a dimension of palliative care: The report of the consensus conference. *J Palliat Med*. 2009; 12(10): 885–904.

31. Delgado-Guay MO, Bruera E. Management of pain in the older person with cancer part 1. *Oncology*. 2008; 22(1): 56–61.

32. Norris L, Pratt-Chapman M, Noblick JA, et al. Distress, demoralization, and depression in cancer survivorship. *Psychiatr Ann*. 2011; 41(9):433–438.

33. Puchalski CM. Spirituality in the cancer trajectory. *Ann Oncol*. 2012;23(Suppl 3):49–55.

34. Holland JC, Alici Y. Management of distress in cancer patients. *J Support Oncol*. 2010;8:4–12.

35. Sollner W, Devries A, Steixner E, et al. How successful are oncologists in identifying patient distress, perceived social support, and need for psychosocial counselling? *Br J Cancer*. 2001;84:179–185.

36. Nakash O, Levav I, Aguilar-Gaxiola S, et al. Comorbidity of common mental disorders with cancer and their treatment gap: Findings from the World Mental Health Surveys. *Psychooncology*. 2014;23:40–51.

37. Endo C, Akechi T, Okuyama T, et al. Patient- perceived barriers to the psychological care of Japanese patients with lung cancer. *Jpn J Clin Oncol*. 2008;38(10):653–660.

38. Steele R, Fitch MI. Why patients with lung cancer do not want help with some needs. *Support Care Cancer*. 2008;16(3):251–259.

39. Barney L, Griffiths K, Christensen H, et al. Exploring the nature of stigmatising beliefs about depression and help-seeking: implications for reducing stigma. *BMC Public Health*. 2009;9(1):61.

40. Kreuter MW, Haughton LT. Integrating culture into health information for African American women. *Am Behav Sci*. 2006; 49:794–811.

41. Yilmaz M, Dişsiz G, Demir F, et al. Reliability and validity study of a tool to measure cancer stigma: Patient version. *Asia Pac J Oncol Nurs*. 2017;4:155–161.

42. Surbone A. Cultural aspects of communication in cancer care. *Support Care Cancer*. 2008;16:235–240.

43. Keusch GT, Wilentz J, Kleinman A. Stigma and global health: developing a research agenda. *The Lancet*. 2006;367:525–527.

44. Ling BG, Phelan JC. Stigma and its public health implications. *The Lancet*. 2006;367:528–529.

45. Sette CP, Capitão CG, Carvalho DFL. Depressive symptoms in patients with cancer. *Open J Med Psychol*. 2016;5:7–16.

46. Wilson K, Luker KA. At home in hospital? Interaction and stigma in people affected by cancer. *Soc Sci Med*. 2006;62:1616–1627.

47. Karbani G, Lim J NW, Hewison J, et al. Culture, attitude and knowledge about breast cancer and preventive measures: A qualitative study of south Asian breast cancer patients in the UK. *APJCP*. 2011;12:1619–1626.

48. Fujisawa D, Hagiwara N. Cancer stigma and its health consequences. *Curr Breast Cancer Rep*. 2015;7:143–150.

49. Suwankhong D, Liamputtong P. Breast cancer treatment experiences of changes and social stigma among Thai women in southern Thailand. *Cancer Nurs*. 2015;15:1–8.

50. Badihian S, Choi EK, Kim I-R, et al. Attitudes toward cancer and cancer patients in an Urban Iranian population. *Oncologist*. 2017;22(8):944–950.

51. Marlow LAV, Wallar J, Wardle J. *Does lung cancer attract greater stigma than other cancer types? Lung Cancer*. 2015;88:104–107.

52. Tang PL MDK, Chou FH, Hsiao KY. The experience of cancer stigma in Taiwan: A qualitative study of female cancer patients. *Arch Psychiatr Nurs*. 2015;30:204–209.

53. Cho J, Choi EK, Kim SY, et al. Association between cancer stigma and depression among cancer survivors: a nationwide survey in Korea. *Psychooncology*. 2013;22:2372–2378.

54. Suwankhong D, Liamputtong P. Breast cancer treatment: Experiences of changes and social stigma among Thai women in southern Thailand. *Cancer Nurs*. 2016;39(3):213–220.

55. Botti M, Endacott R, Watts R, et al. Barriers in providing psychosocial support for patients with cancer. *Cancer Nurs*. 2006;29(4).309–316.

56. Shrank WH, Kutner JS, Richardson R, et al. Focus group findings about the influence of culture on communication preferences in end-of-life care. *J Gen Int Med*. 2005;20:703–709.

57. Bullock K. The influence of culture on end-of-life decision making. *J Soc Work End-of-Life Palliat Care*. 2011;7(1):83–98.

58. Siminoff LA, Graham GC, Gordon NH. Cancer communication patterns and the influence of patient characteristics: disparities in information-giving and affective behaviors. *Patient Educ Couns*. 2006;62:355–360.

59. Greene MG, Adelman RD. Physician-older patient communication about cancer. *Patient Educ Couns*. 2003;50:55–60.

60. Fujimori M, Uchitomi Y. Preferences of cancer patients regarding communication of bad news: A systematic literature review. *Jpn J Clin Oncol*. 2009;39:201–216.

61. Schmid B, Allen RS, Haley PP, et al. Family matters: Dyadic agreement in end-of-life medical decision making. *The Gerontologist*. 2010;50(2):226–237.

62. Smith AK, Sudore RL, Perez-Stable EJ. Palliative care for Latino patients and their families: Whenever we prayed, she wept. *JAMA*. 2009;301(10):1047–1057.

63. Girgis A, Sanson-Fisher R, McCarthy W. Communicating with patients: Surgeons' perceptions of their skills and need for training. *Aust NZ J Surg*. 1997;67:775–780.

64. Detmar SB, Aaronson NK, Wever LD, et al. How are you feeling? Who wants to know? Patients' and oncologists' preferences for discussing health-related quality-of-life issues. *J Clin Oncol*. 2000;18(18):3295–3301.

65. Levinson W, Roter D. Physicians' psychosocial beliefs correlate with their patient communication skills. *J Gen Intern Med*. 1995;10(7):375–379.

66. Nandi PL, Chan JN, Chan CPK, et al. Under- graduate medical education: Comparison of problem-based learning and conventional teaching. *Hong Kong Med J*. 2000;6(3):301–306.

67. McParland M, Noble LM, Livingston G. The effectiveness of problem-based learning compared to traditional teaching in undergraduate psychiatry. *Med Educ*. 2004;38(8):859–867.

68. Song L, Weaver MA, Chen RC, et al. Associations between patient-provider communication and socio-cultural factors in prostate cancer patients: a cross-sectional evaluation of racial differences. *Patient Educ Couns*. 2014;97:339–346.

69. Dilworth S, Higgins I, Parker V, et al. Patient and health professional's perceived barriers to the delivery of psychosocial care to adults with cancer: A systematic review. *Psychooncology*. 2014;23:601–612.

70. Werner A, Stenner C, Schüz J. Patient versus clinician symptom reporting: How accurate is the detection of distress in the oncologic after-care? *Psychooncology*. 2012;21:818–826.

71. Miyajima K, Fujisawa D, Hashiguchi S, et al. Symptoms overlooked in hospitalized cancer patients: Impact of concurrent symptoms on overlooked by nurses. *Palliat Support Care.* 2014;12:95–100.

72. Estes JM, Karten C. Nursing expertise and the evaluation of psychosocial distress in patients with cancer and survivors. *Clin J Oncol Nurs* 2014;18:598–600.

73. Vitek L, Rosenzweig MQ, Stollings S. Distress in patients with cancer: Definition, assessment, and suggested interventions. *Clin J Oncol Nurs.* 2007;11:413–418.

74. Kaneko M, Ryu S, Nishida H, et al. Nurses' recognition of the mental state of cancer patients and their own stress management: A study of Japanese cancer-care nurses.. 2013;22:1624–1629.

75. Nakaguchi T, Okuyama T, Uchida M, et al. Oncology nurses' recognition of supportive care needs and symptoms of their patients undergoing chemotherapy. *Jpn J Clin Oncol.* 2013;43:369–376.

76. Musiello T, Dixon G, O'Connor M, et al. A pilot study of routine screening for distress by a nurse and psychologist in an outpatient haematological oncology clinic. *Appl Nurs Res.* 2017;33:15–18.

77. Mehta RD, Roth AJ. Psychiatric considerations in the oncology setting. *CA: A Cancer J Clin.* 2015;65:299–314.

78. Strömgren AS, Groenvold M, Pedersen L, et al. Does the medical record cover the symptoms experienced by cancer patients receiving palliative care? A comparison of the record and patient self-rating. *J Pain Symptom Manage.* 2001;21:189–196.

79. Jones JM, James J, Rodin G, et al. A province-wide needs assessment of oncology health care professionals in psychosocial oncology. *J Cancer Educ.* 2001;16(4):209–214.

80. McCaughan E, Parahoo K. Medical and surgical nurses' perceptions of their level of competence and educational needs in caring for patients with cancer. *J Clin Nurs.* 2000; 9(3):420–428.

81. Balboni MJ, Sullivan A, Enzinger AC, et al. Nurse and physician barriers to spiritual care provision at the end of life. *J Pain Symptom Manage.* 2014;48:400–410.

82. Balboni MJ, Sullivan A, Amobi A, et al. Why is spiritual care infrequent at the end of life? Spiritual care perceptions among patients, nurses, and physicians and the role of training. *J Clin Oncol.* 2013;31:461–467.

83. Epstein-Peterson ZD, Sullivan AJ, Enzinger AC, et al. Examining forms of spiritual care provided in the advanced cancer setting. *Am J Hosp Palliat Care.* 2015;32:750–757.

84. Phelps A, Lauderdale KE, Alcorn S, et al. Addressing spirituality within the care of patients at the end of life: Perspectives of patients with advanced cancer, oncologists, and oncology nurses. *J Clin Oncol.* 2012;30:2538–2544.

85. Bar-Sela G, Schultz MJ, Elshamy K, et al. Training for awareness of one's own spirituality: A key factor in overcoming barriers to the provision of spiritual care to advanced cancer patients by doctors and nurses. *Palliat Support Care.* 2019;17(3):345–352.

86. Güner P, Hiçdurmaz D, Kocaman Yıldırım N, et al. Psychosocial care from the perspective of nurses working in oncology: A qualitative study. *Eur J Oncol Nurs.* 2018;34:68–75.

87. Turner J, Mackenzie L, Kelly B, et al. Building psychosocial capacity through training of front-line health professionals to provide brief therapy: Lessons learned from the PROMPT study. *Support Care Cancer* 2018;26:1105–1112.

88. Ramirez AJ, Graham J, Richards M, et al. Mental health of hospital consultants: The effects of stress and satisfaction at work. *The Lancet.* 1996;347(9003):724–728.

89. Kumagai AK, Lypson ML. Beyond cultural competence: critical consciousness, social justice, and multicultural education. *Acad Med.* 2009;84:782–787.

90. Teal CR, Street RL. Critical elements of culturally competent communication in the medical encounter: a review and model. *Soc Sci Med.* 2009;68:533–543.

91. Surbone A. Cultural competence in oncology: where do we stand? *Ann Oncol.* 2010;21:3–5.

92. Pincus HA, Patel SR. Barriers to the delivery of psychosocial care for cancer patients: Bridging mind and body. *J Clin Oncol.* 2009;27:661–662.

93. Gagliardi AR, Dobrow MJ, Wright FC. How can we improve cancer care? A review of interprofessional collaboration models and their use in clinical management. *Surg Oncol.* 2011;20:146–154.

94. Adler NE, Page AEK (eds). *Cancer Care for the Whole Patient: Meeting Psychosocial Health Needs.* Washington, DC: National Academies Press;2008.

95. Pirl WF, Muriel A, Hwang V, et al. Screening for psychosocial distress: A national survey of oncologists. *J Support Oncol.* 2007;5:499–504.

96. Hodges L, Butcher I, Kleiboer A, et al. Patient and general practitioner preferences for the treatment of depression in patients with cancer: How, who, and where? *J Psychosom Res.* 2009;67:399–402.

97. Lis CG, Rodeghier M, Gupta D. Distribution and determinants of patient satisfaction in oncology: A review of the literature. *Patient Prefer Adherence.* 2009;3:287–304.

98. Earle CC. Failing to plan is planning to fail: Improving the quality of care with survivorship care plans. *J Clin Oncol.* 2006;24:5112–5116.

99. Whitley E, Valverde P, Wells K, et al. Establishing common cost measures to evaluate the economic value of patient navigation programs. *Cancer.* 2011;117:3616–3623.

26

A Jewish Israeli Case Study in End-of-Life Spiritual Care for a Cancer Patient, Israel

"So that there will be one good and true thing to say about me in my eulogy"

Michael Schultz

An earlier version of this chapter was published in Hebrew; Bentur N, Schultz M, eds. *Meeting in the Midst: Spiritual Care in Israel.* Jerusalem: JDC Eshel; 2017.

Introduction

The case study that follows presents an example of spiritual care in the palliative care setting. Despite widespread recognition of the importance of the spiritual dimension in palliative care [1,2], as well as in other settings, professional spiritual care and the efficacy of spiritual interventions have not been well studied [3]. This includes, and in part results from, a dearth of published case studies. Case studies are a necessary preliminary step to identifying and detailing the interventions to be studied [4], and spiritual caregivers have begun to address this literature gap [4–7]. Among other benefits, these case studies aid colleagues in other health care professions, health care decision makers, and the public at large understand the work done by spiritual care providers [8].

Integrative medicine understands the key impact that culture has on how we experience a given situation as well as the importance of understanding a patient's cultural identity for providing the best care possible. This is especially true in spiritual care [9–11]. The present case study is one of the first ever written from within the Israeli setting.

The Context

This case study is about Reuven, 55 years old, divorced, with a teenage son, and about Reuven's sister, Ayala, divorced with an adolescent son. At the time I met him, Reuven had advanced pancreatic cancer. In his words, his life has been a waste because of his drug addiction, though he has stopped using since taking ill and is trying to be a positive influence in his sister's and nephew's lives. Reuven and Ayala describe themselves as traditional, not religious, Jews. Their parents both died of cancer in recent years, their father in the past year, and Ayala is scared that, after Reuven, she will be next.

Rambam Health Care Campus is a public, academic 1,000-bed hospital in Haifa, Israel. It is the tertiary care hospital serving the whole of northern Israel's diverse 2 million residents and 12 district hospitals. The six-member spiritual care service, part of the palliative care unit, serves over 2,200 patients, family members, and staff, annually.

I have been working as a spiritual accompanier at Rambam since 2009 and am the director of the spiritual care service. I grew up in the Boston area, was ordained as an Orthodox rabbi, and, in 2009, made *aliyah* to Israel, joining the young, growing Israeli profession of spiritual care. One of the interesting aspects of moving to Israel was transitioning from the American setting, where the vast majority of spiritual care-givers are men and women of faith and religion figures more prominently in spiritual care provision, to the Israeli setting, where, from its foundation, the profession thinks broadly about spirituality and spiritual caregivers come from all different professional backgrounds [9,11].

In a country like Israel, where interreligious tensions and the tension between secular and religious are so strong, it has been crucial to base the profession on open-minded spiritual caregivers not charged with representing their religious group. Israelis of all ethnic and religious backgrounds are increasingly searching for a deeper sense of spirituality, often traveling the world over in their quest [10]. But it is a kaleidoscopic spirituality they are often searching for, drawing from multiple sources and allowing for constant growth.

Israeli spiritual care has offered new innovations to the larger field of spiritual care. The broad-based approach to spirituality, considering all aspects of what can move our spirits, including art, literature, and personalized ritual, ensures that everyone's spiritual needs can be addressed, from the most religious to the most secular [12–14].

Spiritual Care Visits

The following four visits took place over the course of three weeks.

Reuven, the Patient

The First Visit
The nurses told me that Reuven was stressing them out, expressing a lot of worries about his treatment. I met Reuven for the first time on a Monday. He told me that over the weekend he experienced acute shortness of breath. This put him in a panic, and he thought he was going to die. He told me that he turned to God and said, "Take me, I can't stay like this. I want to be healthy, but I'm also ready to die, I just can't stay like this." Sadness fell over him, and he said:

Reuven: What a waste. What a waste of a life. I latched onto a bad group of friends, and from there to an even worse group and then an even worse group. I was a star soccer player, I was on Maccabi Tel Aviv's junior team. But I didn't have that inner quiet I needed to avoid making those bad decisions. I don't really understand why I did it. I could've been a star (*imagining it*). A champ ...

Spiritual Accompanier: Your picture in the paper.

Reuven: The President calling to congratulate me!

And Reuven started laughing, laughing, a great, dark black laugh, black, when he caught himself imagining these things. He said that laugh did him good. Now, he continued, he's trying to write his life's story anew, so that at least there will be one good and true thing to say about him in the eulogy they deliver for him. He wants to share the wisdom that he gained from his experiences. He wants to help out his sisters, both of them divorced, and he's worried that men will take advantage of them when he's not around. And he wants to help out his son.

We got to talking about forgiveness. Reuven said that he now understands that he also needs to forgive himself. I tried encouraging him, by saying that from what I can see he's already begun writing a new chapter in the story of his life. He listened, and accepted what I was saying, but very wisely added, "It's too early to know. If I were to get better," he said, "would I really manage to stop smoking, like I want to? Succeeding to change while you're hospitalized is not the same thing. The moment of truth is when you're healthy—I'm not in the clear yet."

Reuven wondered out loud what verse would be inscribed on his tombstone. Once he brought the subject up, I pulled out my book of Psalms and suggested that we read Psalm 30 together, since his story reminded me of that psalm, I told him. As I read, I added some commentary and made connections between the text and his story, and he also responded out loud to our joint reading:

1. A psalm of David. A song for the dedication of the House.
2. I will extol you, O Lord, for You lifted me up and did not let my enemies rejoice over me
3. O Lord, my God, I cried out to You, and You healed me. [Reuven: like on the Sabbath, I thought I was dying, and I cried out to God and He saved me]
4. O Lord, You lifted my soul up from *Sheol*, kept me alive from going down into the pit [MS (*explaining the difficult Hebrew*): I was almost dead] [Reuven: exactly, almost dead!]
5. O you faithful of the Lord, sing to Him, and acknowledge His holy name. [Reuven: yes, you need to give thanks]
6. For He is angry but a moment, and when He is pleased there is life. One may lie down weeping at nightfall; but at dawn there are shouts of joy. [Reuven: On the Sabbath the tears, yesterday the joy]
7. When I was untroubled, I thought, "I shall never be shaken" [MS: When everything was going fine, I said to myself that nothing could ever happen to me] [Reuven: Oy, what a waste, I fell so far]
8. For You, O Lord, when You were pleased, made [me] firm as a mighty mountain. When You hid Your face, I was aghast [Reuven: I was aghast, all these years, oy look where I've gotten]
9. I called to You, O Lord, to my Lord I appealed [Reuven: I'm calling out to Him!]
10. What is to be gained from my death, from my descent into the pit [MS: what good is there in it if I die]. Can dust praise You? Can it declare your faithfulness? [Reuven: I don't want to die, God, please!]
11. Hear, O Lord, and have mercy on me; O Lord, be my help!

12. You turned my lament into dancing, You undid my sackcloth and girded me with joy [Reuven starts to smile once more, almost laughing].
13. That [my] whole being might sing hymns to You endlessly; O Lord my God, I will praise you forever.

At the end of our joint reading, Reuven was very moved and felt a sense of wonder: "It's like I wrote those words myself!" From his weekend experience of thinking this was the end to having been a youth who thinks nothing bad could ever happen to him, to his fall, to God's hidden face, to his prayer for healing, even to his great dark laugh a few minutes prior ("you have girded me with joy"), all the way to his desire to give thanks—he felt like this was exactly his own story, and yet King David wrote it thousands of years prior.

He was very happy we had met. We said goodbye while he was still feeling a sense of wonder, joy, and release.

The Second Visit

I saw Reuven again two days later. He told me that our visit had done a great deal for him. Seeing his exact words in the verses of Psalms made him feel like there was a connection between him and God. He felt like that channel, previously closed, had been opened up.

Reuven told me about his sister. He really appreciates her, and wants to show her how much he appreciates her. I encouraged him to do so. He's very worried about her health. When their parents were sick and ultimately died, he was at home and became the primary caretaker. He saw how much their every cough affected him. He thinks that might have been a major contributing factor in him becoming sick with cancer, and now he's worried that this might happen to his sister, too.

He told me that he wants to return to synagogue. For the year of saying the *kaddish* prayer for his mother, he went to synagogue regularly. But when his father passed away, he didn't make it to the synagogue. "I was lazy," he told me. He had already started cancer treatments at that point. He told me that he wanted to return to the synagogue, but I heard it as "When I get better—I hope there will be a miracle and I'll get better—then I plan on going back to the synagogue."

Toward the end of the visit, Reuven told me that the previous night, in the middle of the night, he was lying awake in bed and composed a song. I asked if he would sing it to me. He sang a slow song, in a very deep voice, of yearning for a different past.

The Third Visit

Reuven was discharged home. A week later, he returned to the ED because of shortness of breath and was hospitalized in one of the internal medicine wards. I saw him in the hallway in Oncology, while his sister was talking with the head of the department in his office, expressing her anger at his being placed in Internal Medicine and not in Oncology. They had explained to him that in Internal Medicine he could get better treatment for his shortness of breath. But Reuven didn't feel the same inner confidence in Internal Medicine that he felt in Oncology, and that's what we spoke about. It was a short conversation, in which I tried to lend a listening ear in a scary time.

After he calmed down, Reuven told me that while he had been at home he managed to sit down with his son and with his ex-wife. He asked them to forgive him for all he had done, and they forgave him. He still feels like he has more things to speak about with them, and he's hoping they'll come visit him while he's hospitalized. He told me that he also sat down with his sister and told her how much he appreciates her.

The Fourth Visit

The following week, I checked to see if Reuven was still hospitalized and came to visit him. He was very happy to see me, and I realized I had found him at a fortunate moment.

Reuven was experiencing a kind of inner struggle and debate regarding what kinds of thoughts he should allow himself to entertain. He called it a game he was playing. In the past, he would hold himself back from saying good things, lest it bring on the evil eye. Now he was wondering if he had to say only positive things, like people were suggesting to him, in order to cause positive things to happen. He was worried that he had to act in a precise manner in order to bring about the right result from heaven. And he added that actually, he'd like to just say things like they are, in one direction or the other, without being afraid of failing to find the right formulation .

What Reuven was describing, the pressure from the thought that if we just think a certain way or behave in the right way, we can bring about a specific result, resonated with me. In my personal life that year, I found myself playing that same game, trying to find the "key" to the heavenly gates in order to bring about my desired result. I decided to make use of my personal experience.

I spoke from the heart, that that past year I had also caught myself trying all kinds of things so that God would do the thing I wished for. That if I just spoke like this, or thought like that, or did this or that, then undoubtedly I would get my wish. He began laughing, a laugh of release and of identifying with me. I told him about a Torah talk I had heard that week, on the topic of prayer. The rabbi giving the talk examined various approaches to prayer, from seeing prayer as something supernatural, to being a means of adding to one's merits. At the end, he concluded that the essence of prayer is truly saying to God whatever is weighing on our hearts, setting those things before God. Just to open up a dialogue and tell God what's in our hearts.

Reuven said that hearing what I had shared really relieved him, to hear that someone else had found himself in that same corner and that he wasn't the only one.

Then Reuven told me about another spiritual matter that was distressing him. He has the sense that no matter what he does, he'll receive a further punishment. He connected this to what he had told me in our first visit, how it's hard for him to forgive himself. He doesn't feel okay with his life. I told him a *midrash* (Jewish didactic story) which speaks to this subject. At the time I summarized it to the best of my memory, but here I'll cite it:

[The great men of Rome] found Rabbi Hanina ben Teradion sitting and occupying himself with the Torah, publicly gathering assemblies, and keeping a scroll of the Law in his bosom. Straightaway they brought him [to judgment], wrapped him in the Scroll of the Law, placed bundles of branches round him and set them on fire.

They then brought tufts of wool, which they had soaked in water, and placed them over his heart, so that his soul should not depart quickly.... The executioner then said to him, "Rabbi, if I strengthen the flame and take away the tufts of wool from over your heart, will you bring me into life in the world to come?" "Yes," he replied. "Then swear unto me." He swore unto him. He then strengthened the flame and removed the tufts of wool from over his heart, and his soul departed speedily. The executioner then jumped and threw himself into the fire. And a heavenly voice called out: Rabbi Hanina ben Teradion and the executioner have been assigned to the world to come. When Rabbi heard it he wept and said: "One may acquire eternal life in a single hour, another after many years."

(Babylonian Talmud, Avodah Zarah 18a, based on the Soncino translation)

Just like in the first visit, Reuven said that he wished he could believe he would make the change, but the true test will only be if he does the right thing when he's healthy. It's too easy to make the change now, while he's sick. I suggested we try guided imagery. After a short exercise, paying attention to his breathing, I guided him to imagine that he was healthy. To imagine that he was considering returning to drugs, or someone offers him a drug. To imagine his response, and to pay attention to what is giving him the ability to respond in that way. We'll never know how he would have responded if he had really gotten better, but at least in this guided imagery exercise he found that he was up to the test.

Ayala, Reuven's sister

The First Visit
As I left Reuven's room after that fourth visit, I found his sister, Ayala, waiting in the hallway, and accompanied her out to the smoking area. Ayala told me that she was falling apart. She really hadn't had a moment to recover from her father's death before Reuven got sick, and traumatic memories of his illness keep cropping up.

"What am I supposed to do?" she cried out. "Be here with Reuven all the time? Or go to work? And no matter what I do, it doesn't help, and his condition just gets worse and worse! And will I be next in line? If I get sick, what'll happen with my son? And how will he even manage without Reuven, Reuven's like a father to him?!" She was feeling tremendous stress from these doubts and fears. "Does it really not matter what I do?" she asked herself, and me. "How much suffering can I take!?"

After about half an hour, we moved to a quieter location, the porch at the end of the departmental hallway, and I suggested that we do a relaxation exercise. As part of the exercise, we practiced releasing the need to do, and the thought that things depend on us. At the end, she said that she felt some peace and calm, something that she almost never feels lately, even though she really wants to feel it more. We returned to Reuven's room, she told me I was an angel, and we said goodbye.

The Second Visit
Very sadly, I never saw Reuven again. The week after these visits, I was sick. During that time, his condition continued to deteriorate, and he was discharged to a hospice facility, where he died within 24 hours.

Some while later, as the holidays approached, I called Ayala. She told me that it was very hard for her. She caught herself calling Reuven on the phone, forgetting that he was no longer alive to answer her. In a very vivid dream she saw him, as if he was really there next to her, and she felt that that meant that he's guarding over her. But still, even the knowledge that he was guarding over her didn't take away her feeling of loss.

She told me more about him and about their relationship. They were very close. He would always give her strength if she started falling apart and she, in turn, had been like a mother to him. She said, "It's not the same thing, losing a brother [as compared to other losses]. He was caring, he was smart." She said she forgives him for everything he did. Her sense is that his main flaw was that he was too curious and didn't stop himself from trying things out. But he always made sure that the damage didn't reach them, that it was only inflicted on himself.

Ayala told me that she didn't go to the funeral; she just fell apart and couldn't. I asked her, "What would you have said about him if you had been there?" She began imagining it, and the first thing that came out was a pure wail, a strong wordless wail. Then she continued: "Reuven, you were caring, you were smart, I forgive you." She went on and said that he knew something about every subject, he had a very high IQ, he would sit and explain all sorts of things to her. With her son, hours upon hours, he would drive home the importance of physical activity. Her son is a bit overweight, and she might have thought he wasn't listening to Reuven at all. But after Reuven died, he joined a gym, and Ayala thinks he did it for Reuven.

When I asked her about her spiritual life in these months, Ayala told me that she's a spiritual person, that she believes in that. Suddenly she called out, "God, enough!" Then she said that it seems like she's a strong woman, after all she didn't get into drugs despite all that's happened to her in her life. I joined her in that place of hope, that she won't fall down, and that there will be good things in her future. I began to give her my blessings for the New Year, and, in effect, we created a prayer space which she entered into entirely. She wished for herself: "Maybe now things can be good, and maybe my son's lot in life can be a good one, and maybe he could even have a good life. It doesn't have to be just more bad things and more bad things."

Discussion: Assessment, Interventions, Outcomes

Reuven

Once Reuven's physical suffering abated slightly, he was able to focus more on the question of how he had lived his life and how he could still hope to live it. He was deeply saddened to look at his life and conclude that he wasted it. If only he had managed to find an "inner quiet" that would enable him to not make the wrong decisions, maybe he could have realized his potential. When he sang his song, he expressed this same sadness, but in a softened way, singing a song of wishing, if only things could have been different.

In our first visit, when Reuven began recalling his youthful potential to be a sports star, I joined him in imagining. He was telling his story, but it was more than that; he was entering into a different kind of space. The laugh, the extended, full-bodied, bitter—but not entirely—laugh—it was a transformative laugh. It wasn't a laugh of beating himself up for his mistakes. It was a moment of being deeply true. In reimagining those youthful dreams, it was also a moment of experiencing the feeling of hope, even just remembered hope. And that left him filled with a feeling of potential, the potential for life, rather than just the sense of what a waste. That laugh, that wonderful dark laugh, led right into his expressing a desire to still do something with his life. That it wasn't too late to rewrite his story, from a life that was entirely wasted to a life that was largely wasted, but that at the end was used well.

He did, in fact, try to use his remaining time well. He showed care and appreciation for his sister. He spoke openly and honestly with his ex-wife and son, asked for and received their forgiveness. Yet, he continued struggling with the question of whether he could truly change his story. The final time I saw Reuven, he expressed the sense that he was bad. Or to be more precise, that he was unforgiveable. That any good he might try to do now won't be good enough, given all the mistakes and bad that he has already done.

When I brought the *midrash* of how the executioner earned his place in heaven with one good deed, I was trying to create a space, drawing on the Jewish tradition that I knew generally speaks to him, for believing that atonement, that heavenly forgiveness, is possible even when the bad outweighs the good.

Reuven wanted to be able to be forgiven, and he wanted to be able to forgive himself, but he wouldn't do so casually, without feeling he had really earned it. And he couldn't earn it unless he did the right thing when he was healthy, not just when he was sick. Maimonides, a leading medieval rabbi, teaches that repentance is not complete until one faces the same circumstance and resists the temptation. I believe that is what Reuven was saying. "If I were to get better, and not have death hovering in the near future, would I actually be able to make a change? Do the good deeds that I am doing now really count, since I haven't proven that I could change if I was really put to the test? Has my story really been rewritten?"

In spiritual care, all we have is the moment. For this reason, I suggested the guided imagery. This was a way to try to give him an opportunity to face the test and pass it. I thought he would pass the test, as indeed he felt he did, but I couldn't know for certain and, if he hadn't, then we would have been present just the same with the experience of not being able to change.

The second key spiritual issue for Reuven was the question of expressing himself truly. He asked me about people telling him he needed to think positively, while he really wanted to just be able to express himself honestly. He was not only speaking about how he expressed himself to others, but even about how he allowed himself to express his thoughts internally, or in prayer. Earlier in his life, he hadn't allowed himself to express positive thoughts, for fear of bringing on the evil eye, a common traditional belief. Now he was being told that he couldn't express negative thoughts, for fear of worsening his condition. As with forgiving himself, so too here—he just wanted to be able to be honest with himself.

My key intervention here was the use of self, and it really took a load off him to hear that he wasn't the only one struggling with the pressure of not allowing certain thoughts to be expressed, as well as to hear my affirmation of his desire to speak his personal truth without worrying about the metaphysical effects of his words.

Similarly, our reading of Psalm 30 was a powerful experience, making him feel as if he was not alone in his specific struggles. Reuven felt like it precisely described everything he had gone through, in the past week and throughout his entire life. But the fact that his life, his words, were being expressed in a holy text, turned this into a religious experience for him. He began straightaway dialoguing with the text, in effect restating it in his own words, making it his own. One of the themes of the chapter is God hiding God's face, God closing the connection, leading the Psalmist to cry out to God. At the moment that we read of the Psalmist praying, crying out in a time of divine concealment, Reuven himself began crying out, "I'm crying out to Him, I don't want to die! Please, God!" Reading this Psalm together, making it his own, turned it into a process of praying the Psalm, of experiencing God's hidden face becoming visible, and of God opening up the closed channel.

Ayala

Ayala's primary spiritual concerns were a sense of guilt that she was unable to stop the endless run of family suffering, the fear that one member of her family after another would fall, and an inability to find even a moment of inner calm. In effect, I wanted to help separate these concerns, to separate the importance of giving space to her sadness over multiple losses, from the internal feeling of being lost and powerless in trying to find the way to change things. I tried to use my authority, as a member of the staff, to help her accept our own limitations in changing our circumstances. In place of powerlessness, to become empowered to accept that if things don't work out, it's not because we didn't try our hardest or because we didn't find the key. If nothing else, the relaxation exercise helped her experience some calm for the first time in a long time.

In our phone call, Ayala's primary need was to mourn her loss. She offered her sense of how Reuven's life had gone wrong ("he was too curious") and, in that sense, could better make sense of her loss. Because she hadn't been up to eulogizing him at his funeral, I wanted to offer an opportunity for her to do so, even just on the phone with me, to enable another kind of closure. Her wail, long and pure, seemed to come from such a deep and true place and, in that sense, reminded me of Reuven's dark, deep laugh.

When I asked Ayala directly about the spiritual component of her experience since Reuven's passing, she fairly quickly entered into a dialogue with God where she asserted her place: "God, enough!" Now she was ready to address the other concern she had shared with me – that the family's run of suffering could not be stopped. In speaking about spirituality, she found within herself the means of meeting that fear head on and not letting it dominate her any longer. She could speak directly to God, and she could stand up to God. Enough! In place of the certain continuing chain of tragedy, she found the hope that she and her son would continue to survive and even to thrive.

Conclusion

Spiritual care is at its best when it is experiential, and I would suggest that for it to be transformative, it must contain that experiential element. Reuven's laugh, Ayala's wail, Reuven's praying the psalm and making it his own and Ayala's asserting, but in the form of a prayer, her right to hope, were all moments of spiritual experience that seemed to be transformative, opening the way for true expression of self and for redis-covering hope, despite it all.

There is also great power in enabling a person to tell their story. We can see here two narratives, that of Reuven and of Ayala, being told and then, in the context of the spiritual care relationship, retold. Reuven's narrative begins as a simple tale of a wasted life, while Ayala's feared narrative is of a family beset by tragedy that will never cease. Whereas ultimately Reuven chooses to add a coda, reframing his narrative as "My life was a waste, until I turned things around," Ayala finds the inner reserve to reframe her life's story as "I'm strong, and despite all the bad things that happened to me and my family and that may or may not continue to happen, I've always found the way to con-tinue on and do the right thing."

I am grateful, in presenting this case study, to play my part in fulfilling Reuven's wish that touched my heart so deeply, that there will be one good and true thing to say about him in his eulogy. In Ayala's words:

"Reuven, you were caring, you were smart."

References

1. National Consensus Project for Quality Palliative Care. *Clinical Practice Guidelines for Quality Palliative Care.* 4th edition. Richmond, VA: National Coalition for Hospice and Palliative Care; 2018. https://www. nationalcoalitionhpc.org/ncp

2. Puchalski C, Vitillo R, Hull S, Reller N. Improving the spiritual dimension of whole person care: Reaching national and international consensus. *J Palliat Med.* 2014; 17(6):642–656.

3. Kelley AS, Morrison RS. Palliative care for the seriously ill. *N Engl J Med.* 2015;373:8.

4. Fitchett G, Nolan S(eds). *Spiritual Care in Practice: Case Studies in Healthcare Chaplaincy.* London: Jessica Kingsley Publishers; 2015.

5. Cooper R. Case study of a chaplain's spiritual care for a patient with advanced metastatic breast cancer. *J Health Care Chaplaincy.* 2011;17:19–37.

6. King S. Facing fears and counting blessings: A case study of a chaplain's faithful compan-ioning a cancer patient. *J Health Care Chaplaincy.* 2012;18:1–22.

7. Redl N. "What can you do for me?" In: Fitchett G, Nolan S (eds). *Spiritual Care in Practice: Case Studies in Healthcare Chaplaincy.* London: Jessica Kingsley Publishers; 2015:223–241.

8. King S. Touched by an angel: A chaplain's response to the case study's key interventions, styles, and themes/outcomes. *J Health Care Chaplaincy.* 2011;17:38–45.

9. Bar-Sela G, Bentur N, Schultz M, Corn B. [Spiritual care in hospitals and other health serv-ices in Israel—a profession in formation]. Hebrew. *Harefuah.* 2014 May;153(5):285–288.

10. Margolin R. The Israeli yearning for a spiritual life. In: Bentur N, Schultz M (eds). *Meeting in the Midst: Spiritual Care in Israel.* Jerusalem: JDC Eshel; 2017:21–33.

11. Pagis M, Tal O, Cadge W. What do non-clergy spiritual care providers contribute to end of life care in Israel? A qualitative study. *J Relig Health.* 2017;56:614–622.

12. Ettun R, Schultz M, Bar-Sela G. Transforming pain into beauty: On art, healing, and care for the spirit. *Evid Based Complement Alternat Med.* 2014;2014:789852.

13. Schultz M, Bentur N, Rei-Koren Z, Bar-Sela G. [From pastoral care to spiritual care—trans-forming the conception of the role of the spiritual care provider]. Hebrew. *Harefuah.* 2017 Nov;156(11):735–739.

14. Thiel MM, Robinson MR. Spiritual care of the nonreligious. *PlainViews.* 2015;12(7):1–12.

27

Existentialism and Spirituality in the Healing Process of Cancer Patients, United Kingdom and United States

Eve Namisango, Lawrence Matovu, Richard Harding, and Ann Berger

Introduction

A cancer diagnosis may elicit fear, anguish, suffering, existential loss, and worry about death, a trauma that may lead to adverse outcomes [1]. To cope with the trauma, it is common for patients and their families to look for sources of existential/spiritual support for meaning, comfort, and hope. For this reason, the relationship between existential/spiritual well-being and health is gaining increasing attention and has culminated in the recognition of spirituality as a core domain of health and an important outcome of interest in terminal illness, palliative care and health at large [2]. At the 2013 African Palliative Care International Conference, which was held in Kampala Uganda [3], 85 palliative care professionals were asked about their definition of spirituality, and the following main themes emerged: relationship with supernatural being, the meaning of sickness, health, life and death, the source of one's internal power, beliefs, norms and values, inner integrity and beliefs, meaning, and purpose of life. These themes are in line with the definition of spiritual distress, "an intimate, deep and suffering experience in life, which requires coping strategies and involves spiritual values and beliefs" [4], which is now a recognized symptom in terminal illness.

Usually, the most pressing priority when faced with the diagnosis of cancer is to regain good health; if this is successful, the implications of mortality might once again slip into the background. Sometimes the illness is regarded as only a temporary bump in the road of life, as opposed to a stark reminder of life's fragility. But more often than not, cancer has a way of capturing our attention, deepening our reflection on what is important, and causing us to live with more awareness of our ultimate priorities.

Spiritual distress and spiritual crisis occur when a person is "unable to find sources of meaning, hope, love, peace, comfort, strength and connection in life or when conflict occurs between their beliefs and what is happening in their life" [5]. The estimated point prevalence for spiritual distress ranges between 16 and 63% and the majority of cancer patients (about 96%) experience some form of spiritual pain in their lives [6]. In a study of 113 cancer patients in an acute palliative care unit , 44% reported spiritual distress during the initial chaplain visit. Moreover, patients with spiritual distress were more likely to report pain and depression [7]. In another study conducted among cancer patients in an outpatient setting in Israel, 23% of the 202 cancer patients reported spiritual distress [8]. The study also highlighted key parameters of spiritual distress, including "not feeling peaceful," "feeling unable to accept that this is happening," and "the perceived severity of one's illness. Spiritual distress has also been noted in a population of cancer patients in India. Among the 300 adult patients interviewed, over 73% reported some form of spiritual distress; 76.3% of the participants felt their illness was unfair; and 83.3% kept wondering why the illness had happened to them [9]. Even for children with cancer, existential/spiritual well-being is a priority as children with cancer have expressed existential/spiritual needs that predispose them to spiritual distress [10]. Notable is the fact that children may not be able to speak about their spiritual/existential needs due to their age, advanced disease, or cognitive impairments; engaging carer-proxy reporting (having a carer report about the patient's well-being) may therefore be necessary [11].

In my (EN) 20 years' experience of working with palliative care patients and their families, spiritual distress commonly affects the patient's attitude toward life, the care, and their family members, and this attitude is usually negative. They may question the value of care if it cannot heal and if they commonly feel they are a burden to their carers. In my (EN) personal communication with a theology/culture specialist who provides end-of-life religious rites to dying patients (Father Augustine Mpagi), he observed that dying patients tended to face the away from people at the dying moment which he thinks shows some form of rejection of other people and may cause caregivers psychological distress and poor bereavement outcomes. Although this may be explained by spiritual distress, Father Mpagi also noted that this moment is spiritual and brings the dying closer to the supernatural being. This may bring peace to bereaved caregivers who are saddened by such acts at their beloved ones' moment of death. In the existing literature, existential/spiritual distress has been associated with negative health outcomes. These outcomes include: worsening physical pain [12], psychological distress [5], diminishing quality of life [12], and low satisfaction with quality of life for several reasons [13]. While existential/spiritual well-being is defined as being sound in body, mind, and spirit, it also concerns being in harmony with one's beliefs, values, philosophical and religious beliefs, as well as cultural norms and practices. This stems from the realism of culture being the window through which values, norms, practices, preferences, and behavior are expressed and its role in shaping the meanings of life events (these may include illness, health-related suffering, death, and dying) [14]. For example, in a systematic review that examined the relationship between culture and the experience of breast cancer among women in South Asia, a cancer diagnosis being associated with "a weak body system" reportedly led to rejection of testing services and nondisclosure [15]. Notably, this theme was consistent among diverse religious groups, including Sikhs, Muslims, Hindus, and Christians.

Failure to provide culturally sensitive care may, therefore, introduce stressors and negatively impact the expected outcomes. This reality upholds the World Health Organization's premise that culturally sensitive care is an important aspect of quality palliative care [16]. Culturally sensitive existential/spiritual care is the pathway to a spiritual healing process that relieves the associated distress and further improves patient care outcomes. Healing is an "inner agency that gives a degree of relief from suffering, an inner agency that the patient must find within the depths of his or her own psyche" [17].

Benefits of Existential/Spiritual Well-being

Although existential/spiritual well-being is recognized as an important domain of health, it is not given the attention it deserves in cancer care in most settings. Positive spiritual/existential perspectives empower cancer patients to make sense of the illness and health-related suffering, relieve anxiety, and strengthen their relationship with the larger self, hence improving their general well-being [18]. Literature further advances that religion, and spiritual practices are associated with better physical and mental health outcomes [18].

The barriers to advance care planning in palliative care include fear of being judged and inability to handle potential psychological distress or crises that may arise following the conversations. In my (EN) ongoing research on difficult conversations in cancer care, issues of advance care planning and how to deliver person-centered care to cancer patients in Uganda (ethics approval ref HS1000ES), one of my respondents expressed concerns about breaking bad news to patients.

> I cannot deliver devastating news to my patients, even if I know that I am giving this chemotherapy and that I am not going to be with this patient for long, I do not tell them. I fear being judged, I also do not know how they may take it and how it may affect them. We do not have support groups here, so the onus will be on me, I cannot talk about the pending bad news. I will say, "let me treat you, then your God will heal you." It would be an opportunity for them to look into their end-of-life wishes, but how do I know about their spiritual/existential state? This helps me in judging their ability to cope with the news.—Health Worker #7

It is clear that knowing the patient's existential/spiritual status may also provide an opportunity or pathway for easing difficult conversations concerning the terminal nature of the diagnosis, advance care planning, and end-of-life care. This is because such conversations require existential/spiritual tranquility and are deeply rooted in the patient's and family's cultural, religious beliefs, values, norms, philosophies, and practices. For example, as commonly argued, in line with most religious values, only the supernatural power knows one's hour of death, a belief that should be respected. For this reason, most health workers commonly avoid discussions pertaining to death and dying and advance care planning [19]. Regrettably, denial of the reality and psychological defense mechanisms are commonly used to affirm life for the dying patient, even when death may be imminent. This may explain the low level of prognosis awareness among patients with advanced cancer [20].

In some instances, patients may recognize on their own that death is imminent, and, in preparation, some may resort to giving the traditional verbal instructions regarding their end-of-life wishes [21]. Unfortunately, these verbal instructions may not be respected under the legal frameworks, which poses a crisis from a legal and human rights perspective. As such, while we have a duty to respect these boundaries, some patients appreciate the initiation of difficult conversations about advance care planning as it helps them to prepare for reality by tending to priorities of unfinished business. Given that the lived experience of human beings is largely connectedness, people have relationships that matter to them and these deserve good closures. Part of what we can do to help our loved ones in case we die is to "put our house in order," and supporting patients through this process is a key indicator for good quality of care [22]. The African Palliative Care Association[1] is promoting the integration of legal services into palliative care services in Africa in response to such needs. Having highlighted why existential/spiritual well-being matters in cancer care, we now discuss the construct of existential/spiritual healing, which has potential to alleviate existential/spiritual distress.

Existential/Spiritual Healing in Terminal Illness

In our ongoing work on existential/spiritual healing in Uganda (ethics approval ref HS1000ES), we interviewed 35 patients with advanced cancer about the meaning of existential/spiritual healing. The emerging themes included acceptance of the situation and of the idea that the cancer is an accident and hence the patient should not be angry with anyone or even God; total cure of body and mind; divine hope; and overcoming the cancer and its effects. It is evident that, although a clinical cure of a terminal illness may not happen, spiritual healing is possible when patients experience positive life-transforming changes [23], thus improving quality of life for patient and family both. Spiritual healing manifests as positive psychological, social, and spiritual changes and strengthening of inner resources, regardless of the disease's outcome [24]. The healing may also come with changes in personal values, standards, and the whole experience of conceptualizing the construct of quality of life [25]. For example, in an anthropological study among patients with advanced cancer who had a very small chance of surviving beyond five years, patients who received spiritual support from indigenous spiritual healers survived beyond the five years. They also showed notable improvements in the person-centered dimensions of forgiveness, release of blame, bitterness and chronic anger, sense of humor, and refusal to accept death as an immediate prognosis. With supportive communities, faith, and a sense of meaning and purpose, patients experienced changes that transformed the quality of their relationships and self-esteem and led to a spiritual transformation [26]. This is now a recognized complementary/alternative treatment for psychological distress [27,28].

This may be a good entry point for initiating difficult conversations regarding palliative care. Culturally sensitive existential/spiritual care provides a strong foundation for initiating difficult conversations, even in collective cultures such as those in Africa, India, and Japan, where breaking bad news may be misinterpreted as disrespect for the supernatural being, elder, or families [20]. Furthermore, even in settings where families continue to play a major role in receiving the bad news on behalf of the patient, for example, in Saudi Arabia [29] and the Republic of Singapore [30], the difficult conversations may be more strategic and may require good planning and favorable pathways for initiation. Spiritual healing offers a favorable ground, for it enhances coping and adjustment and improves quality of life. It is, therefore, pivotal [31].

Another important consideration is the aspect of preference regarding how patients may wish to receive resources and support for meeting their existential/

spiritual needs. The key issues to be addressed are similar; these issues include forgiveness, reconciliation, managing anger, finding meaning or purpose, quality of relationships, hope, and letting go. The approaches to existential/spiritual healing vary according to culture and may use paranormal forces involving the soul and one's energies [32]. Patients and their families commonly request a room to make consultations elsewhere; in most cases, this may be an expression of preference for consulting ancestral spirits or witch doctors. It may also include the use of mental or spiritual activities, such as the laying on of hands or other special religious rituals. Religious rituals may include administering last rites, mediating forgiveness as a sacrament, relying on scriptures for support, giving hope and encouragement, offering continued prayer and meditation, as well as revering iconic saints who have endured suffering. The approaches may further include healing through guided imagery and dreams [33], the therapeutic touch [34], dedicated intercessions or healing prayers, intercessory or petition prayers, and energy-healing practices [33]. Spiritual healing uses paranormal forces such as the soul and energies [32]. The spiritual healing may be implemented remotely by mediums or other spiritual care providers, relieving patients of the need to travel long distances to receive care and healing [35].

The religious approach may also involve administration of a holistic and inclusive approach to providing existential/spiritual care, recognizing the importance and complementarity of self-appropriation and self-transformation. Practically, it means recognizing what is going on inside ourselves: knowing who we are, why we choose what we choose, do what we do, and what are our feelings and desires. Self-transformation, on the other hand, refers to the gradual transformation of our ego-centered vision and choices. The dynamic of palliation is to move beyond self-concern and to reach out to the higher power and others through compassion and care. Cancer patients are vulnerable, and the ethos of religion calls upon us to deliver compassionate holistic care that goes beyond the physical aspects. Believers are always encouraged to pray to God or a higher power, especially when they face difficult circumstances, including adversity, which offers an opportunity for spiritual healing and growth. For example, in Iran, faith therapists visit patients and recommend relevant prayers to them [36], and these can alleviate anxiety and improve physical functioning [37]. Similar structures exist in many other religious faiths. Indeed, evidence highlights the association between faith and religion as key ingredients for spiritual healing [36,37]. Therefore, religion under palliative care can be a pathway for meeting some existential/spiritual needs.

In many cultures, health, illness, and healing are believed to be divine, or bestowed upon us by a supernatural being, and it is also common for patients to seek healing through cultural spiritual actors [38]. Some patients may wish to seek reconciliation with their deceased relatives with whom they would soon be meeting and trust to welcome them and support them in settling into the new world. Culturally, reconciliation and forgiveness may be brought about through healing symbols such as healing rocks or water [39], through communal rituals such as shared meals, or through communal, extended-family prayers. It is thus plausible to engage traditional healers in cancer care if we are to implement culturally sensitive, person-centered existential/spiritual care.

Accelerating Access to Existential/Spiritual Care in Oncology Services

To integrate existential/spiritual care into palliative care, we must first address the major priorities for health systems. A global survey of 807 palliative care providers from 87 countries ranked spiritual screening tools as the number one priority for spiritual care research [40]. Spiritual care is an essential domain of palliative care, which focuses on the needs of the whole person and family. Existential/spiritual care is (and can be) a very sensitive area, and there are (and can be) common pitfalls for both the palliative care team and the spiritual advisors. These pitfalls include, but are not limited to:

- Lack of mutual respect resulting in 'forced' conversations.
- Lack of balance where spiritual care undermines other aspects of care: patient may be advised to stop medical consultations, medications, and treatment.
- Lack of sensitivity resulting in feelings of guilt and fear.
- Inappropriate philosophizing, theologizing, moralizing, and sermonizing.
- Inappropriate use of rituals such as shouting and loud prayers in hospital wards or with a very ill patient.
- Health care workers are very suspicious of spiritual advisors.

The lack of appropriate outcome measures can be a significant barrier to measuring constructs such as spirituality. On a positive note, progress has been made in shaping the strategic direction for assessing spiritual well-being and integrating spiritual care into overall patient care. For example, in sub-Saharan Africa, the Spirit 8 [41] and two of the items on the African Palliative Care Outcome Scale (APCAPOS)—peace and life being worthwhile [42]—are some of the measures available for assessing and screening for spiritual distress in palliative care patients. In addition, guidelines for the integration of spiritual care into routine care have also been developed for different settings [43]. These form a good foundation for developing spiritual care as an integral discipline to the palliative care discipline. Although religion is a recognized platform for the expression of spirituality and, as so, provides a proximate opportunity for initiating discussion about spiritual/existential well-being, it may not always be the best approach for initiating conversations, inasmuch as it could put off those who do not subscribe to the theory. The care provider must therefore take a person-centered approach to initiating such conversations; the needs and concerns are cross-cutting, but personal preferences, norms, beliefs, and culture largely shape how patients and their families may wish the care to be delivered. Spirituality relates to our souls; it involves the deep inner essence of who we are. It is an openness to the possibility that the soul within each of us is somehow related to the soul of all that is. Spirituality is what happens to us that is so memorable that we cannot forget, yet we find it hard to talk about as words fail to describe it. Spirituality is the act of looking for meaning in the very deepest sense and looking for it in a way that is most authentically ours.

The National Institutes of Health Healing Experience of All Life Stressors (NIH-HEALS) is a 35-item measure developed to assess spiritual healing in cancer patients [31]. It consists of main factors: connection, reflection/introspection, trust and acceptance. The measure was developed and validated in the United States [44]. The work to adapt the measure for use in lower- and middle-level settings is underway, and cognitive interviewing to provide further evidence for face and content validity is ongoing in Uganda. Once the psychometric evaluation is completed, this will provide another useful tool for assessing patient spiritual well-being in cancer patients as part of routine clinical care.

In addition capacity-building for spiritual care providers to address barriers to delivering this care, some of which include lack of skills, inability to maintain boundaries, lack of awareness, negative staff attitudes, and lack of robust evidence for effectiveness and appropriate models of care is also critical [40]. Training to address these barriers is, therefore, critical in order to prepare and recognize the need for these services and to support the integration of spiritual/existential care into routine palliative care services. In terms of service development, some existential/spiritual health-inclined models have been proposed. For example, we should be promoting community-based participatory survivorship interventions that are culturally, spiritually, and peer-based [45]. These interventions would allow survivors to draw on spiritual/existential resources and to take part in meeting their own needs and those of other patients through a participatory action learning approach. Such models of care have been found to be acceptable among Spanish and Latina women. A pilot of this model of service delivery was developed in the United States, where First Nations people incorporated spirituality into cancer survivorship by giving thanks, attending places of spiritual connectedness, singing, praying, speaking to the Creator, and engaging the sun and moon [46]. The pilot demonstrated a strong link between culture and how the women viewed themselves, as well as how they viewed the cancer, with "praying to win the battle" being a dominant metaphor [46]. This is a promising model for providing culturally sensitive spiritual care to patients and their families and within their communities.

Increased access to spiritual care should be prioritized in cancer care, and the core facets include screening, history-taking, assessment, and documenting and evaluating interventions. The training of spiritual caregivers has been increasingly recognized by academic institutions, professional associations, and faith communities, and care providers should prepare to integrate spiritual services into the core palliative care services and into the human resource structures. Spiritual care providers should ideally be personnel with core competencies to diagnose spiritual needs or spiritual distress, who are skilled in spiritual communication and know how to use any available resources from both a cultural and religious perspective. However, these resources must be appropriately aligned. To optimize outcomes of care, cancer services should prioritize the integration of existential/spiritual care services, hinging the service development on the highlighted health system and, thus, strengthening priorities. Therefore, the assessment and attention to the existential/spiritual needs of patients center around relationships that make them feel safe and loved, especially when things turn out to be complicated and scary. Listening to patients, trying to understand their world and what they think is happening, is key to understanding what their spiritual needs are. Unaddressed existential/spiritual issues may frustrate one's attempts to treat other symptoms and have an adverse effect on quality of life. As each dimension is addressed in turn, distressing symptoms may be alleviated.

Note

1 (https://africanpalliativecare.org/resources-centre/legal-resources/)

References

1. Moeini M, Taleghani F, Mehrabi T, Musarezaie A. Effect of a spiritual care program on levels of anxiety in patients with leukemia. *Iran J Nurs Midwifery Res.* 2014;19(1):88–93.

2. Selman L, Harding R, Gysels M, Speck P, Higginson IJ. The measurement of spirituality in palliative care and the content of tools validated cross-culturally: A systematic review. *J Pain Symptom Manage.* 2011;41(4):728–753.

3. Downing J, Namisango E, Kiyange F, et al. The net effect: Spanning diseases, crossing borders—highlights from the fourth triennial APCA conference and annual HPCA conference for palliative care. *Ecancermedicalscience.* 2013;7:371.

4. Martins H, Caldeira S. Spiritual distress in cancer patients: A synthesis of qualitative studies. *Religions.* 2018;9(10):285.

5. Puchalski CM. Spirituality in the cancer trajectory. *Ann Oncol.* 2012;23(Suppl 3):49–55.

6. Roze des Ordons AL, Sinuff T, Stelfox HT, Kondejewski J, Sinclair S. Spiritual distress within inpatient settings—A scoping review of patients' and families' experiences. *J Pain Symptom Manage.* 2018;56(1):122–145.

7. Delgado-Guay MO, Hui D, Parsons HA, et al. Spirituality, religiosity, and spiritual pain in advanced cancer patients. *J Pain Symptom Manage.* 2011;41(6):986–994.

8. Schultz M, Meged-Book T, Mashiach T, Bar-Sela G. Distinguishing between spiritual distress, general distress, spiritual well-being, and spiritual pain among cancer patients during oncology treatment. *J Pain Symptom Manage.* 2017;54(1):66–73.

9. Bhatnagar S, Gielen J, Satija A, Singh SP, Noble S, Chaturvedi SK. Signs of spiritual distress and its implications for practice in Indian palliative care. *Indian J Palliat Care.* 2017;23(3):306–311.

10. Hart D, Schneider D. Spiritual care for children with cancer. *Seminars Oncol Nurs.* 1997;13(4):263–270.

11. Stein A, Dalton L, Rapa E, et al. Communication with children and adolescents about the diagnosis of their own life-threatening condition. *Lancet.* 2019;393(10176):P1150–1163.

12. Delgado-Guay MO, Parsons HA, Hui D, De la Cruz MG, Thorney S, Bruera E. Spirituality, religiosity, and spiritual pain among caregivers of patients with advanced cancer. *Am J Hosp Palliat Care.* 2013;30(5):455–461.

13. Namisango E, Katabira E, Karamagi C, Baguma P. Validation of the Missoula-Vitas Quality-of-Life Index among patients with advanced AIDS in urban Kampala, Uganda. *J Pain Symptom Manage.* 2007;33(2):189–202.

14. Dancy J, Davis W. Family and psychosocial dimensions of death and dying in African Americans. *Key Topics on End-of-Life Care.* 2006:187–211.

15. Bedi M, Devins GM. Cultural considerations for South Asian women with breast cancer. *J Cancer Survivorship.* 2016;10(1):31–50.

16. World Health Assembly. WHO Strengthening of palliative care as a component of comprehensive care throughout the life course; 2014. http://apps.who.int/gb/ebwha/pdf_files/WHA67/A67_R19-en.pdf year of publication 2014; Accessed October 2020)

17. Puchalski C, Ferrell B. *Making Health Care Whole: Integrating Spirituality into Patient Care.* Philadelphia: Templeton Foundation Press; 2011.

18. Panzini R, Bandeira D. Spiritual/religious coping. *Revista Psiquiatria Clínica.* 2007;34:126–135.
19. Lanre-Abass B. Cultural issues in advance directives relating to end-of-life decision making. *Prajna Vihara J Philos.* 2008;9:23–49.
20. Applebaum AJ, Kolva EA, Kulikowski JR, et al. Conceptualizing prognostic awareness in advanced cancer: A systematic review. *J Health Psychol.* 2014;19(9):1103–1119.
21. Ekore R, Lanre-Abass B. African cultural concept of death and the idea of advance care directives. *Indian J Palliat Care.* 2016;22:369–372.
22. Donabedian A. The quality of care: How can it be assessed? *JAMA.* 1988;260:1743–1748.
23. Li L, Sloan DH, Mehta AK, Willis G, Weaver MS, Berger AC. Life perceptions of patients receiving palliative care and experiencing psycho-social-spiritual healing. *Ann Palliat Med.* 2017;6(3):211–219.
24. Mount BM, Boston PH, Cohen SR. Healing connections: On moving from suffering to a sense of well-being. *J Pain Symptom Manage.* 2007;33(4):372–388.
25. Hefferon K, Grealy M, Mutrie N. Post-traumatic growth and life threatening physical illness: a systematic review of the qualitative literature. *Br J Health Psychol.* 2009;14(Pt 2):343–378.
26. Mehl-Madrona L. Narratives of exceptional survivors who work with aboriginal healers. *J Alt Complement Med* (New York). 2008;14(5):497–504.
27. Levin J, Taylor RJ, Chatters LM. Prevalence and sociodemographic correlates of spiritual healer use: findings from the National Survey of American Life. *Complement Ther Med.* 2011;19(2):63–70.
28. CJ. B. Public health implications of spiritual healing practice, in conditions such as depression. *Public Ment Health.* 2013;12:6–9.
29. Mobeireek AF, Al-Kassimi F, Al-Zahrani K, et al. Information disclosure and decision-making: The Middle East versus the Far East and the West. *J Med Ethics.* 2008;34(4):225–229.
30. Tan MS, Narasimhalu K, Ong SY. Letting the cat out of the bag: Shifting practices of cancer disclosure in Singapore. *Singapore Med J.* 2012;53(5):344–348.
31. Ameli R, Sinaii N, Luna MJ, Cheringal J, Gril B, Berger A. The National Institutes of Health measure of Healing Experience of All Life Stressors (NIH-HEALS): Factor analysis and validation. *PLoS One.* 2018;13(12):e0207820.
32. Levin J, Taylor RJ, Chatters LM. Prevalence and sociodemographic correlates of spiritual healer use: Findings from the National Survey of American Life. *Complement Ther Med.* 2011;19(2):63–70.
33. Jonas WB, Crawford CC. Science and spiritual healing: A critical review of spiritual healing, "energy" medicine, and intentionality. *Alt Ther Health Med.* 2003;9(2):56–61.
34. Wirth DP. The significance of belief and expectancy within the spiritual healing encounter. *Soc Sci Med.* 1995;41(2):249–260.
35. Javaheri F. Prayer healing: An experiential description of Iranian prayer healing. *J Relig. Health.* 2006;45(2):171–182.
36. Rafii F, Javaheri F, Saeedi M. Spiritual healing from Iranian cancer patients' viewpoints: A hybrid concept analysis. *J Edu Health Promot.* 2020;9(32):1–9.
37. Simão T, Caldeira S, Campos De Carvalho E. The effect of prayer on patients' health: Systematic literature review. *Religions.* 2016;7(1):11.
38. Kahissay MH, Fenta TG, Boon H. Religion, spirits, human agents and healing: A conceptual understanding from a sociocultural Study of Tehuledere Community, Northeastern Ethiopia. *J Relig Health.* 2020;59(2):946–960.
39. van Leeuwen R, Tiesinga LJ, Jochemsen H, Post D. Aspects of spirituality concerning illness. *Scand J Caring Sci.* 2007;21(4):482–489.

40. Selman L, Young T, Vermandere M, Stirling I, Leget C. Research priorities in spiritual care: An international survey of palliative care researchers and clinicians. *J Pain Symptom Manage.* 2014;48(4):518–531.

41. Selman L, Siegert RJ, Higginson IJ, et al. The "Spirit 8" successfully captured spiritual well-being in African palliative care: Factor and Rasch analysis. *J Clin Epidemiol.* 2012;5(4):434–443.

42. Selman L, Speck P, Gysels M, et al. "Peace" and "life worthwhile" as measures of spiritual well-being in African palliative care: A mixed-methods study. *Health Qual Life Outcomes.* 2013;11:94.

43. Selman L, Harding R, Agupio G, et al. *Spiritual Care Recommendations for People Receiving Palliative Care in Subsaharan Africa: With Special Reference to South Africa and Uganda.* London: King's College; 2011.

44. Luna MJ, Ameli R, Sinaii N, Cheringal J, Panahi S, Berger A. Gender differences in psychosocial-spiritual healing. *J Women's Health.* 2019;28(11):1513–1521.

45. Yan AF, Stevens P, Holt C, et al. Culture, identity, strength and spirituality: A qualitative study to understand experiences of African American women breast cancer survivors and recommendations for intervention development. *Eur J Cancer Care* (England). 2019;28(3):e13013.

46. Magaña D. Praying to win this battle: Cancer metaphors in Latina and Spanish women's narratives. *Health Commun.* 2020;35(5):649–657.

28

Psychosocial-Spiritual Healing

An Impression of the Impact of Culture and Faith in Cancer Care in Africa, Kenya, Sub-saharan Africa, Culture, Beliefs, Traditional Healers, Herbal Treatment, Religion, Spirituality, Ethnic Groups, Ancestors

John K. Weru and Esther W. Nafula

Introduction

Culture has been defined in several ways in the literature. It is commonly defined as a way of life of a given community or group of people. It is characterized by a set of patterns of knowledge, beliefs, and behaviors. Cultural groups share thoughts, communication styles, views, and values, and their lifestyle is defined by common practices and customs [1]. Many different communities and ethnic groups exist in sub-Saharan Africa with major cross-cultural differences. The cultural variations exist among patients and health care providers and greatly influence health-seeking behavior and treatment choices [2]. Culture determines the way in which individuals respond to a cancer diagnosis and associated symptoms. Some responses may be judged as abnormal when they are in fact culturally appropriate—hence the increased need for knowledge on culture in health care providers [3]. The concept of culture and its relation to cancer is poorly understood. There is unequal distribution of resources, with more screening and treatment programs for cancer being available in urban compared to rural areas in Africa [4].

Common reactions to a cancer diagnosis are denial, anger, depression, or anxiety, but these emotions are expressed differently depending on who the patient is. Cultural competence is defined as the ability to have basic knowledge of different cultural practices and attitudes across the world and the influence of these practices and attitudes on patient decision making [2].

Religion and *spirituality* are terms that have been used interchangeably in the literature [2]. However, they are different, with spirituality aiming at giving meaning to life which is experienced through meditation, nature, or art [5,6]. Spirituality is best described as that which gives us strength to go on with life and to go on creatively [7]. On the other hand, religion has been defined as a connection to a higher being with set beliefs and associated with set rituals [8]. Religion is a big part of many cultures and varies from one to another [2].

There are many racial groups living in Africa, and not surprisingly then, a variety of religious groups from all over the world coexist on the continent. In many instances, religion and culture overlap. The main religious groups in Africa include the traditional African religion, Christianity, Islam, Hinduism, Buddhism, and Sikhism. In this chapter we will look at the dominant religions: Christianity, Islam, Hinduism, and the traditional African religion [9].

Noncommunicable diseases are responsible for over 60% of deaths worldwide, with over 80% of these deaths occurring in low- and middle-income countries. In Africa, most patients with cancer are diagnosed at a late stage of the disease when cure is impossible due to poor screening programs, poorly structured referral systems, and negative cultural influences. A study conducted in Ghana [10] showed that 64.1% of patients with breast cancer presented at late stages because of a lack of knowledge and because of a widespread culture of consulting traditional healers first. Cancer of the cervix is rampant in sub-Saharan Africa, with many cases of human papilloma virus (HPV) infections documented as being attributed to the culture of polygamy [11].

Cultural Influences on Care

Through specific beliefs, sickness and death are made comprehensible and manageable [12]. A cancer diagnosis carries a negative implication and is often thought to be a death sentence [2]. There is a lot of uncertainty associated with cancer, and understanding of the illness is very poor among many societies. There is limited data on the way culture influences perceptions of patients regarding risks of developing cancer, as it is not a widely studied topic [2]. Adjustment problems are very common among patients receiving a cancer diagnosis, with anxiety levels being high at the time of initial investigations, when a bad prognosis is revealed or when the patient is noted to be at the end of life [8]. It is important to be aware of cultural and religious differences when examining patients' patterns of adjustment to a cancer diagnosis.

Asobayire and Barley [4] carried out a qualitative study using focus groups of women from the local communities to understand the practices in breast cancer screening and treatment. The study revealed that there was no word for cancer in the local language and in many African languages. Overall, there was little knowledge about cancer, with many people believing that it was caused by witchcraft or supernatural powers inherited from ancestors. Traditional healers are often the first point of contact for cancer patients, as has been corroborated in other studies across Africa [13]. Traditional healers use an array of herbs, some of which are applied to cancer wounds, and incarnation of ancestral spirits to treat cancer. Many patients in Africa believe that traditional healers are able to cure their cancer, and they only seek hospital treatment as a last resort. Some patients conclude that they have been cursed, that they are being punished by God for past errors [14], or that they are bewitched when the traditional healer is unable to sort out their problem [4,15]. Traditional healing has existed since time immemorial in Africa. This tradition cuts across all facets of life, whether physical, psychological, social, or spiritual.

Spirituality and Faith Healing

In many studies, the spiritual needs of patients have been defined as both distressing spiritual struggles and seeking of the meaning of cancer. Some patients harbor anger toward God as they seek to understand why they have to suffer while others turn to God as their source of hope during difficult times. Steinhauser et al. [16] found that patients viewed being at peace with God as a means of coping with their pain, especially in terminal phases of illness. Religious coping has generally been associated with better psychological well-being among cancer patients [6].

Various denominations of Christianity have different beliefs, but their common belief is that Jesus is the son of God who was sent to earth as a savior. Christians believe that repentance of sins through belief in Jesus is important in order to obtain a reward after death. Many patients who embrace Christianity fix on repentance, especially when they realize cure is not possible; repentance, they feel, is the way they can get a new life in heaven. Those who die without repenting of their sins, they believe, are condemned to a life in hell [17]. African Christians are found to be more likely to opt for life-sustaining treatments even when there is little hope of survival. Many would rather pray for a miracle to happen as they try to prolong life than choose end-of-life care.

Islam is made up of sects and subsects that are heavily influenced by culture. In Africa, Muslims are from different races—Arabs, Asians, and Africans. Muslims believe the afterlife is one of the stages in God's overall plan for humanity. Islam, they feel, is a way of life, and many who profess this faith live in a culture largely defined by the religion. Muslims pray five times a day at set times, and their dress easily distinguishes them from others. Ramadan is a holy month of fasting that is important to them [17]. Serious illness and death are considered to be God's will, and it is one's duty to accept whatever God sends them. Muslim patients are more receptive to news of advanced cancer compared to their Christian counterparts and are often unwilling to receive life-sustaining therapies because these therapies are against God's plans [17].

Hinduism is characterized by beliefs in reincarnation, which is a constant never-ending circle of life, death, and rebirth. The philosophy of Karma largely influences the life of a Hindu with the belief that what one does in this life will determine what happens to them in the next life. Prayer and meditation are important parts of their spirituality. Many Hindu patients with cancer are often concerned about their time for prayer and meditation and spend much time reflecting on their actions prior to illness [17].

The traditional African religion focuses on moral and spiritual values and is taught from a young age. The emphasis is on living life in a way that is just and pleasing to God. Prayers are offered by designated elders in the society, and sometimes sacrifices are carried out to appease God, who is represented by objects in nature such as trees and mountains. God is considered powerful and is able to answer prayers [18]. In many African societies, people still cling to their traditional religions and seek treatment from traditional healers who are believed to have divine connection with the gods [4]. Most people do not connect African traditional healing to spirituality or even traditional African religious practices. There is a broad belief that most people worship ancestors and not the Almighty God. This conviction is far from the truth, as most traditional healers believe their power emanates from a superior being. Furthermore, African traditional healers are believed be to custodians of the traditional African religion and customs, educators about culture, counselors, social workers, and psychologists among many more roles [19]. There are as many names for God as there are tribes in Africa. To cite just a few, the

Kikuyus of Kenya call Him *Ngai*, the Maasais of East Africa call Him *Enkai*, and the Yoruba of West Africa call Him *Oludumare*, while in South Africa names such as *Inkosi* and *Unkulunkulu* are used [20,21].

In addition to the Almighty God, Africans also traditionally believe in the intercession and influence of ancestors for their well-being. These are also referred to as the living dead and are direct blood relatives of the living. It is believed that they continue to influence the daily lives, experiences, and well-being of those who are still alive [22]. Just as the name of the Higher Being varies from tribe to tribe, so do the names of the ancestors, with the Bapedi, Batswana, and Basotho of South Africa calling them *badimo* and the Amazulu referring to them as *amadlozi* [19]. The most common language in East Africa, Swahili, refers to ancestors as *wahenga* [23].

Thus, the traditional African religion can be described as tribal-based, and its practice varies from tribe to tribe. However, the substance remains the same all over the continent. It is therefore important to understand that the concept of God was not introduced to Africans by the West but has been in existence over the ages. In fact, there are no atheists in traditional Africa. This common tradition sees the divinities, the traditional healers, and their practice as those who receive authority from the Supreme Being to serve their people.

It is thus important to understand that African religious beliefs still largely influence cancer care in the continent, even as Western religions take great root within. As stated earlier, it is still believed that a cancer diagnosis is due to wrongs done to ancestors or other relations. It is believed to be a test by God or even a punishment by God as a consequence of human misdeeds. But God's punishment is not taken as a misdeed by one member of the tribe but by the entire community. Thus, the community searches to cleanse the wrongdoer or its own deeds by sacrificing animals or rituals to cleanse the concerned person first. This may take quite some time, and by the time the patient and family seek treatment, the cancer is already advanced to an incurable stage. Further, it is common to find people visiting traditional healers first before visiting the conventional treatment centers. They do so only when the traditional healers' interventions have failed. It is important to note that the traditional healers' understanding of cancer is not scientific but rather is in keeping with traditional beliefs. In their study, Asuzu et al. [24] found out that the traditional healers reported cancer as being caused by "eating foods like cassava, poor personal hygiene and infection with bacteria" and another healer said that "cancer is caused by viruses and body impurities." Still others said that "cancer is a life, it is a spirit of infirmity caused by satanic and demonic attacks."

With these beliefs, treatment modalities will thus have to be in response to the same beliefs and be tailored to understanding their foundational ethos. These include herbs for drinking, preparations for skin applications, divination, incantation, and sacrifice. The faith-based healers use the spoken word, prayers, holy water, anointing oil, and fasting on behalf of the patient. Unlike conventional treatment modalities, which are considered costly and out of reach of the majority in the continent, many traditional and faith-based healers believe that the power to heal was freely given by God. So healing is free, but if patients recover and decide to give anything in appreciation, it is accepted. This is a significant factor influencing many people to opt for these alternative ways of treatment rather than visit cancer treatment centers from the beginning of illness. 24] also found that most patients in their study had used either herbal or spiritual remedies for their cancer before going to the hospital. Some of them only went to the hospital because the traditional treatment was not as effective as they had hoped or because the healer advised it.

Conclusion

Collaboration between African traditional and faith healers with the Western physicians is important to both the effectiveness and efficiency of cancer treatment within the continent. It will assist patients in accessing conventional treatment in the early, curable stages of the disease. It will also ensure that patients and families commence and complete treatment as advised by their doctors. However, this will only be possible if this partnership between Western medicine and traditional African healing is accepted. For this endeavor to succeed, traditional and faith healers must be seen as equal partners and must be recognized as important players in cancer treatment. Their buy-in is key to eventually managing the cancer malady in its entire trajectory. Otherwise, there will always be a discrepancy in how early patients access treatment and are compliant to their treatment. Unless traditional healers are engaged in the care of patients, they will continue mistrusting conventional treatment modalities which they will continue considering as a way of lack of faith in their healing powers and also the importance of God in the healing process.

The engagement of these important stakeholders in health care delivery can also enrich cultural interpretations of medical actions by exploring the potential of plants. There is a need to take another look at cancer public health campaigns in the face of competing demands for the meagre resources in the continent. Using these healers as public health advocates and remunerating them for their efforts would greatly assist the continent's public health system. These efforts should will help break the vicious cycle of late presentation, nonadherence to treatment, poor trust of conventional treatment modalities, adverse treatment outcome, and reluctance of patients to present to health facilities because of poor outcome.

Success depends on use of constructive alternativism, which challenges the notion of a single objective reality across the globe. Reality can be constructed, interpreted, and understood in different ways. For example, the traditional African healer has a different construction and etiology of cancer compared to the Western trained doctor. The Western physician primarily looks at the biological and physiological basis of cancer and adheres to the pharmacodynamics and pharmacokinetics of Western medicine. However, the traditional African healer might look at witchcraft and ancestors as possible causes of the disease and thus view its cure as a correction of the wrongs that could have caused it. The question that arises is which of the constructions is superior, especially if the two constructions of reality seem to be very different, as is the case with cancer? We believe neither one nor the other is superior. Rather, the context demands that the two approaches merge and supplement each other, for there is no single given universally accepted assessment and management of any malady that bedevils humanity.

References

1. Betancourt JR. Cross-cultural medical education: Conceptual approaches and frameworks for evaluation. *Acad Med,* 2003;78(6):560–569.
2. Surbone A. Cultural aspects of communication in cancer care. *Support Care Cancer,* 2008;16(3):235–240. Accessible: https://doi.org/10.1007/s00520-007-0366-0
3. Mystadikou K, Parpa E, Tsilika E, et al. Cancer information disclosure in different cultural contexts. *Support Care Cancer,* 2004;12:147–154.
4. Asobayire A, Barley R. Women's cultural perceptions and attitudes towards breast cancer: Northern Ghana. *Health Promot Int.* 2015;30(3):647–657. Accessible: https://doi.org/10.1093/heapro/dat087
5. Kellehear A. Spirituality and palliative care: A model of needs. *Palliat Med,* 2000;14(2):149–155. Accessible: https://doi.org/10.1191/026921600674786394
6. Peteet JR, Balboni MJ. Spirituality and religion in oncology. *CA: Cancer J Clin.,* 2013;63(4), pp. 280–289.
7. Merton T. What Is Spirituality? 2020. Accessible: https://www.takingcharge.csh.umn.edu/what-spirituality
8. Dien S. Screening and cancer prevention across cultures: Moving beyond culture. *Culture and Cancer Care Anthropological Insights in Oncology,* 2006; 15(2): 147–149.
9. Platvoet JG. The religions of Africa in their historical order. *Platvoet, Cox & Olupona,* 1996; 6(2): 46–102.
10. Kantelhardt J, Muluken G, Sefonias G, et al. A Review on Breast Cancer Care in Africa. Breast Care (Basel), 2015;10(6):364–370. Accessible: https://doi.org/10.1159/000443156
11. Anorlu RI. Cervical cancer: The sub-Saharan African perspective. *Reproduct Health Matters.* 2008;16(32):41–49. Accessible: https://doi.org/10.1016/S0968-8080(08)32415-X
12. Kagawa-Singer M, Valdez Dadia A, Yu MC, Surbone A. Cancer, culture, and health disparities: Time to chart a new course? *CA: Cancer J Clin,* 2010;60(1):12–39. Accessible: https://doi.org/10.3322/caac.20051
13. Walter T. Spirituality in palliative care: Opportunity or burden? *Palliat Med.* 2002;16(2):133–139. Accessible: https://doi.org/10.1191/0269216302pm516oa
14. Mousavi SR, Akdari ME. Spirituality and religion in cancer. *Ann Oncol,* 2010;21(4):907–908. Accessible: https://doi.org/10.1093/annonc/mdp604
15. Johnson Taylor E. Spirituality, culture, and cancer care. *Seminars in Oncol Nurs,* 2001;17(3):197–205.
16. Steinhauser KE, Christakis NA, Clipp EC, McNeilly M McIntyre, L, Tulsky JA. Factors considered important at the end of life by patients, family, physicians, and other care providers. *JAMA.* 2000;284(19):2476–2482.
17. Schultz CA. Cultural aspects of death and dying. *J Emerge Nurs.* 1979;5(1):24–27.
18. Kasongo A. Impact of globalization on traditional African religion and cultural conflict. *J Alt Perspect Soc Sci,* 2010;2(1):309–322.
19. Mokgobi M. Understanding traditional African healing. *Afr J Phys Health Educ Recreat Dance.* 2015;2, 24–34. Accessible: https://www.ncbi.nlm.nih.gov/pmc/articles/PMC4651463/
20. Chris. Shadows of Africa. KENYAN TRIBES & RELIGIONS. 2016. Accessible: https://www.shadowsofafrica.com/blog/kenyan-tribes-religions
21. Kalumbu I. Exploring Africa: Africa Names of God. 2021. Accessible: http://exploringafrica.matrix.msu.edu/african-names-for-god/
22. Walt J. *Understanding and Rebuilding Africa: From Desperation Today to Expectation for Tomorrow.* Potchefstroom: The Institute for Contemporary Christianity in Africa; 2003.

23. Mohamed, A, Gebe B, Dill C, Massaba J, Babalola S, Karim S. *Wahenga: The Queen's University Black History Journal.* Wahenga Journal. 1994. Accessible: https://www.africa.upenn.edu/Publications/Wahenga.html

24. Asuzu C, Akin- Ondanye E, Asuzu M, Holland J. A socio-cultural study of traditional healers' role in African health care. 2019. Accessible: https://infectagentscancer.biomedcentral.com/articles/10.1186/s13027-019-0232-y

29

Psychosocial Aspects of Breast Cancer
The Turkish Experience, Turkey

Sedat Ozkan

Introduction

Cancer is a chronic, life-threatening disease that greatly impacts all spheres of life. Cancer patients develop various and differing emotional, mental, and behavioral reactions toward their illness throughout the diagnosis, treatment, and palliative periods [1].

The experience of cancer cannot be understood independent of the specific culture [2]. The beliefs and values of a society influence perceptions about the meaning of an illness, the types of treatment or remedies that are useful, and the likely outcome. Cross-cultural differences may lead to ethical dilemmas regarding communication, decision making, treatment choices, and end-of-life decisions.

What Is Culture?

Culture is the sum total of a society's way of life, constituting values, beliefs, standards, language, thinking patterns, behavioral norms, and communications styles, and influences many different aspects of daily life, including perceptions, emotions, belief systems, and behaviors. A society's culture also significantly influences religion, family structure, gender relationships, and social organization, as well as diet, dress, body image, and one's perception of illness and medical treatment.

The most important issues that dominate cultural variations in symptom presentation, health care-seeking behavior, and illness perception are:

- Variations in family systems and structures (e.g., patriarchal families)
- Variations in age and gender role
- Educational factors
- Socioeconomic factors
- Environmental factors (rural or urban)
- The meaning and perceived cause of illness [3]

A culture-specific understanding and approach is necessary for delivering optimum psychiatric and physical care [4].

Turkish Culture

Turkish culture began in Central Asia 20,000 years prior to the advent of Islam. Beginning in Turkey, the Turks spread over an extensive geographical area to the Caucasus, Anatolia, the Middle East, the Balkans, and Central Europe and established various states and empires. With their acceptance of Islam, a new age began. Modern Turkey is the focal point of this culture. The modernization and Westernization movement that took place during the last 150 years of the Ottoman Empire was institutionalized by Kemal Atatürk (1881–1938), the founder of the republic, who formed the basis for a new synthesis and prospects for this culture. Turkish culture is a composite of historical depth and geographical expanse. Perhaps, too, it is a new model for the Central Asian Turkic republics, the Caucasus and the Middle East, as well as some Balkanic countries that share a common culture and civilizational past with the Turks. Atatürk declared that the basis of the Turkish republic was culture.

"Turkish culture" should be understood as the interaction and synthesis of pre-Central Asian Turkish culture with Islam, the cultures of Anatolia, the Balkans, the Middle East, and the Caucasus, into which they spread, as well as other areas that were part of the Seljuk and Ottoman Empires, and the modern reformism of Atatürk. It is a fusion of conservative, traditional, and religious values with modern Western culture.

The Sufi movement takes a traditional medieval Turkish approach, teaching spirituality through near-mysticism and using song and dance to induce an altered state and a closer connection to God. This new attitude toward the mind, freeing mental illness from implications of wrongdoing, paved the way for a more scientific examination of the causes and symptoms of mental illness.

Turkish cultural traditions developed a humanistic orientation that is concerned with treating the "whole person," thus emphasizing the integrity of the individual—both the mind and the body. Through the centuries, all the "Houses of Healing" established in the Turkish world integrated mental and physical health (Gevher Nesibe, built in the 1200s, is the first hospital that served both physically and mentally ill patients) [5].

Illness Perception

The Turkish version of the Revised Illness Perception Questionnaire (IPQ-R) was adapted by Kocaman, Özkan, Armay, Özkan, et al. in 2007 and is a reliable and valid tool used to study cultural aspects of cancer patients [6].

After translating and adapting the language to suit the Turkish population, the scale was applied to 203 cancer patients at Istanbul University, Oncology Institute. The study revealed that patients lacking knowledge and information regarding cancer had underlying fatalistic and passive attitudes. The IPQ-R cause scale showed that most of the cancer patients strongly attributed causes such as "stress" or "chance/bad luck" to their illness, with "accident/injury" being the least ascribed attribution. In the section of the questionnaire inquiring about the perceived cause, the majority of the participants proposed that "destiny" is the cause of illness. The less educated patients in Turkey attributed their illness more to issues of faith [7].

Erbil et al.'s 1996 [8] findings suggest that psychosocial distress is expressed differently in Belgium and Turkey. Turkish patients more frequently express their anxiety through somatic complaints. According to the authors' experience, illness perception, a culturally dependent factor, appears to influence psychological adjustment; a clearer perception of illness led to more anxiety in the Belgian patients compared to the Turkish patients [8]. Similarly, a 1983 study analyzed the perceptions, causal attributions, and attitudes toward illness among a group of 33 Jewish Israeli cancer patients and found two distinct response patterns: (1) the 'Western' patients (science-oriented, active) and (2) the "Oriental" ones (fatalistic, passive) [9].

Special Issues in Communication: Telling the Truth

Revealing the diagnosis of terminal cancer to a patient is still not fully accepted in some countries without an Anglo-Saxon cultural background. In a country such as Turkey, where family hierarchy dominates, often the patient's family makes all decisions concerning treatment. Physicians discuss the cancer diagnosis with the family before discussing it with the patient and frequently comply with the family members' requests. A similar paternalistic approach exists in Arab and Islamic cultures. While the tendency now is to disclose the truth more often than was the case in the past, full openness is still not a common practice.

There is a polarity in perceptions, causal attributions, and attitudes toward cancer: Western style (science oriented, participating) and Eastern style (fatalistic, passive). In Western countries, where medicine is taught and practiced using a full disclosure model, regulations are in place to protect the patients' right to participate in decision making and to be fully informed about their treatment prior to giving consent. At the opposite end of the spectrum is the nonmaleficence model, whereby the patient is not told of a poor prognosis in the belief that this will protect the patient against unnecessary physical and emotional harm. In some Eastern cultures, discussing serious illness and death is even viewed as impolite and provokes unnecessary anxiety, depression, and a sense of helplessness, thereby eliminating all hope.

Somewhere in the middle of the spectrum is the model of beneficence, where family members actively participate in the communication, share the burden of a poor prognosis with the patient, and encourage hope. This is the general attitude in Turkey. In the last two decades, Turkey's population growth, urbanization, and changes in education have been rapid, complex, and irregular, together bringing about a participatory model. A silent attitude was once the general norm in Turkey, but this attitude appears to have changed in accordance with changes in the society and culture.

The stigmatization of cancer is more prevalent in rural areas where there is lack of knowledge concerning disease. Studies have generally revealed that lack of information and knowledge regarding cancer results in fatalistic and passive causal attributions [4]. A study performed by Şener, Günel, and Akçalı in 1999 showed that the higher the degree of information and knowledge about one's illness, the better the chances for positive problem-solving strategies [10].

The author's clinical experience and research findings, obtained through our liaison psychiatry practice and carried out with the breast surgery unit, show that the primary basis for distress in breast cancer patients who had undergone mastectomy was the cancer itself, whereas aesthetical concerns and cancer's effects on their quality of life was secondary [11,12]. Feeling under threat, these patients were found to have a greater fear about death and its associated anxiety than about losing one or both breasts [4]. Fertility and motherhood are still of utmost importance for women in rural and more traditional parts of the society. A study by Kulakaç et al. implied that the women's "mother" role was considered more fundamental than the female role [13].

Most adult and elderly patients state that their main concern is not facing death, but rather becoming a burden on the family and dying in unbearable pain. Adjustment to cancer is better in a family environment characterized by open expression of feelings and an absence of family conflict. Clearly, the most challenging and difficult management issues for the family arise with the loss of a child.

Regarding the effect of cancer on the perception of life, Öner and İmamoğlu reported optimistic findings [14]. In this 1994 study, 80% of the participants reported that cancer had a great impact on their lives, and 48% of them evaluated the impact as a positive, life-enhancing experience. Patients reported that experiencing cancer had been a catalyst, forcing them to see their lives more positively, offering them a chance to restructure their lives and to change their perspective toward people and the world. The authors reviewed 24 studies on breast cancer, published from 1990 to 2010, which revealed that a relatively small percentage of women experienced posttraumatic stress disorder, whereas the majority reported posttraumatic growth. Age, education, economic status, subjective appraisal of the threat of the disease, treatment, support from significant others, and positive coping strategies were among the most frequently reported factors associated with these phenomena.

Bayraktar's 2008 thesis [15], written in our department, was entitled "Post Traumatic Growth in Cancer Patients and Related Factors." The results displayed a relationship between posttraumatic growth and confrontive coping, self-control, accepting responsibility, escape-avoidance, intentional problem solving, positive reappraisal, and seeking social support. Coping strategies and perceptions of illness were important variables affecting posttraumatic growth. Parry and Chesler [16] found that coping processes, creating meaning and spiritual/moral development were particularly associated with long-term psychosocial well-being.

The manner in which pain is perceived, manifested, and treated by patients and families is another area affected by culture. Cancer patients who are more confident about coping and controlling cancer define less pain. An association has been found between the severity of pain, depression, and quality of life [17].

Taking into consideration and integrating our experience at the Department of Psychooncology, Institute of Oncology, University of Istanbul (the main pioneering department in the country), the results of nearly 50 master theses conducted at our department, and the general psychooncology studies and experiences shared in major scientific meetings throughout the country, I would like to summarize my thoughts, based on the above, as follows:

- In the past 40–50 years, prosperity, democratization, and participatory culture have expanded in Turkey.

- Urban migration and Westernization have contributed to a higher social consciousness.
- Until the 1970s and 1980s, cancer was perceived as equivalent to death and was referred to as a "cruel illness," with a silent attitude being most prevalent.
- Cancer has become less of a taboo subject in Turkish society; increased social awareness regarding cancer has become more prevalent.
- The discussion of cancer in academia and the media has become increasingly multifaceted.
- The perception of cancer as a catastrophe has declined in society. More emphasis is now placed on the importance of psychological and social support.
- Psycho-oncology practice has helped decrease prejudice, such as the belief that only insane people receive treatment from psychiatrists or psychologists. The culture now more readily accepts the necessity of psychological support of cancer patients.
- The fear of recurrence is still the most prevalent source of anxiety among cancer patients.
- The old-fashioned way of thinking was strongly influenced by religion and arose from within a traditional, feudal social structure. The ongoing Westernization and an increasingly institutionalized process of modernization have given rise to a brand-new structure and sensibility.
- Religious or spiritual approaches to illnesses and cancer, with respect to both cause and treatment, have gradually diminished.
- However, the impact of religion on reactions to cancer can still be seen. A fatalistic approach can be anxiety-relieving for some; for others, it can impede treatment. Nevertheless, a fairly widespread and functional way of perceiving and style of coping are characterized by the attitude "first do what you can, then leave it to God."
- The approach "if it's cancer, take the entire organ" is common.
- Society and the family still prioritize longevity over quality of life.
- There is a widespread impact of belief systems pertaining to death and the basic acceptance of death.
- In Turkey, with regard to cancer, religion, strongly tied to a belief in Islam, is associated with a reduction in loss of hope, suicidal thinking, and dying in the hospital.
- In the terminal phase of cancer, there is an increased turning toward religion and resort to prayer.
- Religious thought and rituals are prevalent in the processes of saying goodbye.
- There are conflicting reports on the effects of religion on (better) health [18].
- Observation of Turkish patients with cancer reveals that a diagnosis of cancer makes people more faithful, even those who do not regularly practice religion.
- There is an increase in perceptions of meaningfulness in life and hope: "There is always hope with God."
- The association of religion and spirituality with cancer has not been systematically studied in Turkey. We do not know the impact of religion and spirituality on the outcome of cancer.

- With regard to grief, concerns about death, and the afterlife, patients and families turn more to religion for guidance, without sacrificing scientific treatments.
- In Turkish culture, cancer care is more family-oriented than individualistic. Similar to catastrophic events such as earthquakes, when there is a diagnosis of cancer, all the family members congregate and face the situation together. This family solidarity is generally supportive for the patient and may act as a protective factor.
- Grief and bereavement are experienced more collectively and religiously. The grief process is not experienced as individualistically and silently as it is in some Western countries; wailing and crying out is more common in Turkey No formal or routine religious assessments are made of cancer patients in clinics in Turkey.
- Patients' religious concerns and needs are not routinely addressed.
- On the other hand, the practice of psychotherapy does not always integrate spirituality unless the patient actively requests it. Spirituality is more the realm of families.

The integration of traditional Turkish culture with modern Western values concerning the impact and continued functionality of the family, a sense of social solidarity, religious beliefs, and a humanistic understanding rooted in culture has given rise to a synthesis of two views: "health is more important than anything else" and "with God, there is hope." Our culture has had a positive impact on outcomes by taking a holistic approach to treating the cancer and the patient simultaneously, incorporating the mind, body. and spirit.

References

1. Ozkan M. Psychosocial adaptation during and after breast cancer. In: Aydıner A. İğci A, Soran A (eds). *Breast Disease: Management and Therapies*. Istanbul: Springer International Publishing Switzerland; 2016:821–852.
2. Brown R, Bylund C, Kissane D. Principles of communication skills training in cancer care. In: Holland WHJ (ed). *Psycho-Oncology*. New York: Oxford University Press; 2010: 597–604.
3. Anuk D, Özkan M, Kizir A, Özkan S. The characteristics and risk factors for common psychiatric disorders in patients with cancer seeking help for mental health. *BMC Psychiatry.* 2019:1–11.
4. Özkan S, Özkan M, Armay, Z. Cultural meaning of cancer suffering. *Pediatr Hematol Oncol.* 2011:102–104.
5. Özkan S. The historical development of mental health in Turkish culture. *Gevher Nesibe Hospital and Medical Academy.* 2007:77–83.
6. Kocaman N, Özkan M, Armay Z, Özkan S. The reliability and the validity study of Turkish adaptation of the Revised Illness Perception Questionnaire. *Anadolu Psikiyatri Dergisi.* 2007:271–280.
7. Armay Z, Özkan M, Kocaman N, Özkan S. Hastalık Algısı Ölçeği'nin Kanser Hastalarında Türkçe Geçerlilik ve Güvenilirlik Çalışması. *Klinik Psikiyatri.* 2007:192–200.

8. Erbil P, Razavi D, Farvacques C. Cancer patients psychological adjustment and perception of illness: Cultural differences between Belgium and Turkey. *Support Care Cancer.* 1996:455–461.

9. Baider L, Sarell M. Perceptions and causal attributions of Israeli women with breast cancer concerning their illness: The effect of ethnicity and religiosity. *Psychother Psychosom.* 1987:136–143.

10. Şener Ş, Günel N, Akçalı Z. Meme Kanserinin Ruhsal ve Sosyal Etkileri Üzerine Bir Çalışma. *Klinik Psikiyatri Dergisi.* 1999:254–260.

11. Özkan S, Turgay M. Masektomi Olgularında Psikiyatrik Morbidite Psikososyal Uyum ve Kanser—Organ Kaybı—Psikopatoloji İlişkisi. *Nöropsikiyatri Arşivi.* 1992:207–215.

12. Isıkhan V, Güner P, Kömürcü S. The relationship between disease features and quality of life in patients with cancer. *Cancer Nurs.* 2001:490–495.

13. Kulakaç O, Buldukoglu K, Yılmaz M. An analysis of the motherhood concept in employed women in South Turkey. *Soc Behav Personal.* 2006:837–852.

14. Öner H, İmamoğlu O. Meme kanseri olan Türk kadınlarının hastalıklarına ve uyumlarına ilişkin yargılar. *Kriz Derg.* 1994:261–268.

15. Bayraktar S. Kanser hastalarinda travma sonrasi gelisim olgusunun ve etkileyen faktörlerin incelenmesi. İstanbul Üniversitesi Saglık Bilimleri Enstitüsü, Yüksek lisans tezi; 2008.

16. Parry C, Chesler M. Thematic evidence of psycho-social thriving in childhood cancer survivors. *Qual Health Res.* 2005:1055–1073.

17. Uzun Ö, Aslan F, Selimen D. Quality of life in women with breast cancer in Turkey. *J. Nurs Scholarship.* 2004:207–214.

18. Fitchett G, Canada A. The role of religion/spirituality in coping with cancer: evidence, assessment, and intervention. In: Holland J, Breitbart W, Jacobsen P, Lederberg M, Loscalzo M, McCorkle R (eds). *Psychooncology.* New York: Oxford University Press; 2010:440–446.

30

Cancer Pain Care in French-speaking African Countries and Access to Analgesics

Barriers and Cultural and Emotional Aspects, France

Yacine Hadjiat, Serge Perrot, Jallal Toufiq, and Christian Ntizimira

Introduction

"Cancer pain is one of the most common, feared, debilitating and often undertreated symptoms among cancer patients. It needs attention since it has a significant impact on the quality of life of the patients" [1]

The incidence of cancer in Africa is estimated to increase by 89% between 2020 and 2040 [2] due to an increasing population and aging [3]. In the later stages, it is estimated that two out of every three cancer patients experience moderate to severe pain [4]. However, the barriers to treating and managing pain—not just as a result of cancer—are significant, especially in emerging economies [5]. In a 2013 review of the availability of palliative care in 25 African countries, it was found that opioids were made available in only 15 countries. However, this did not guarantee access when needed [4]. In 2014, the World Health Organization (WHO) passed the resolution Strengthening of Palliative Care as a Component of Comprehensive Care Throughout the Life Course [6] to specifically address the need for palliative care (including pain management) in countries' universal health coverage. The WHO 2002 definition of palliative care states that "palliative care is an approach that improves the quality of life of patients (adults and children) and their families who are facing the problems associated with life-threatening illness through the *prevention and relief of suffering by means of early identification and correct assessment and treatment of pain* and other problems, whether physical, psychosocial or spiritual" (emphasis added) [6].

This chapter covers the barriers to care and treatment of cancer pain in French-speaking African countries. (While cancer pain is the focus, the information is relevant and applicable to all causes and types of pain.) Most French-speaking countries are in West Africa and include 26 of the 54 African countries [7]. Overall, there is a dearth of research in this area, making recommendations for policy, regulation, aid, and support difficult. Further, the lack of comprehensive evidence provides a challenge for tracking and evaluating public health programs across the continent in a standardized manner and in accordance with international guidelines such as those provided by the WHO [1].

The use of opioid analgesics for clinical pain management in Africa remains among the lowest globally, with 50 daily doses per million per day, compared with the Americas, which have the highest consumption, 14,320 daily doses per million per day [8,9,10]. Within Africa, the use of opioids varies significantly. The International Narcotics Control Board (INCB) has determined that less than 200 S-DDD (defined daily doses for statistical purposes) is inadequate for a population's pain management. South Africa has an estimated S-DDD of >500, while French-speaking countries, such as Cote d'Ivoire (S-DDD = 1) and the Democratic Republic of Congo (S-DDD = 2), face massive shortages [9].

Figure 30.1 shows the rank order of opioid consumption in various African countries for 2010. Research published by the African Palliative Care Association Atlas of Palliative Care in Africa suggests that these consumption levels experienced little change in the following years (2010–2017) [11].

Indications of levels of pain associated with cancer can be gleaned from research on palliative care. Palliative care, though broader in scope, includes access to pain medication for treating conditions such as cancer and HIV/AIDS. The WHO Global Atlas of Palliative Care notes that Africa is ranked highest for the number of adults in need of palliative care [12]. Although funding for antiretroviral treatment for HIV/AIDS has been made available by donors such as PEPFAR (the United States President's Emergency Fund for AIDS Relief) and the Global Fund, the funding does not extend to pain control and thus leaves a gap.

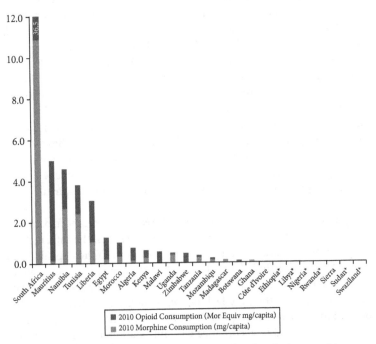

Figure 30.1 Rank order of 2010 opioid consumption (mg/capita in morphine equivalence without methadone) for surveyed African countries.

Access to and the comprehensiveness of palliative care varies throughout Africa and within African countries. It is not possible to generalize about access to pain care and management for the entire continent as a whole; one must consider examples for each specific country separately. Comprehensive reviews of each African country's public health policies and their implementation are necessary to get a continental view. Notably, Africa is socioeconomically underdeveloped, and access to resources remains a challenge [4].

The main barriers to accessing pain care and management include:

- Strict regulations which are often overprescriptive and prohibitive
- Limitations on access to pain medications, especially opioids
- Limitations on which health care workers can prescribe medications
- Fear of criminalization regarding opioids [4]

In addition to these barriers, culture, attitude, and beliefs negatively impact the use of opioids.

Barriers to Cancer Pain Care in Africa

"The current situation regarding Cancer in Africa is quite deplorable. Many patients do not seek medical advice. Those who do, do so when the cancer is at an advanced stage when cure is no longer possible. There is a lack of oncologists of all kinds, nurses and the necessary health professionals and technicians to support their work. There is a lack of treatment centres. There is a lack of treatment. Most countries do not have access to opioid drugs for palliative care and pain control. The situation is bound to get worse as the population grows and ages and cancer risk factors imported from high-[13] resource countries begin to have their effect." [13]

The range of barriers to the access and use of opioids and other pain medications varies across African countries and within the countries. Table 30.1 lists the barriers most commonly experienced.

WHO policy guidelines [14,15] and palliative care strategies advocate for an increase in the availability of medication and education and for government policies to adapt in order to enable more effective palliative care. With pain being a very frequent symptom in cancer, there is a need for clinical and nonclinial management. The WHO's analgesic ladder, though published in 1986, remains a relevant classification and treatment plan for cancer pain. However, lack of access to medication or an enabling environment that allows opioids to be included in treatment regimens render the above guidelines moot.

There are multiple barriers to the use of opioids in Africa. The most underresearched area is the population's various attitudes, beliefs, and culture. Data does exist on policies and regulatory environments, which, on the whole, are unsupportive, but this does not describe or analyze the roots and antecedents of legal and policy issues or what drives a particular policy or law to be implemented. While it is true that, in many

Table 30.1 Barriers to the Optimal Treatment of Physical Pain in Developing Countries [32,34]

Structural and knowledge barriers	Sociocultural and attitude barriers	Economic barriers
1. Pain is not recognized as a public health priority 2. General practitioners do not have the required knowledge and expertise to treat pain 3. There is a scarcity of qualified pain specialists 4. Many schools of medicine and of pharmacy have very limited time included in their curricula for the treatment of pain 5. Resources and medical personnel are unevenly distributed 6. Administrative requirements to access pain medications are significant and deter usage 7. Regulation of pain medication may be restrictive at a country level due to fears of misuse, abuse, and diversion 8. No national policy, strategy or implementation plans 9. Bureaucratic process for legislation 10. Punitive regulations 11. Inadequate ability to report consumption to the narcotics board 12. Lack of political will 13. Postcolonial legacies in many African countries regarding opioids	14. Cultural beliefs impact the understanding and treatment of pain 15. Many accept pain as a natural and unavoidable part of aging and disease 16. Traditional medicines (including herbal medicines and spiritual rituals and practices) may be the preferred treatment, to the exclusion of Western medicines, in some countries 17. Religious beliefs in some countries see pain as part of atonement, and this mindset leads to reduced help-seeking behavior and treatment 18. Patients, health care workers, and governments may have a fear of using opioids for treatment 19. The concept of "total pain" (physical, psychological, social, and spiritual aspects) is not familiar in many African societies	20. Competing demands for resources at a country level have impact negatively on health care spending in general, and on the treatment of pain specifically 21. The cost of medicines and other treatments could be high or not be seen as priority 22. Vulnerable subgroups and people with lower socioeconomic status have less access to resources to seek and pay for treatment 23. Limited or no medical insurance in many African countries to cover pain treatment 24. Lack of cost and benefit analyses related to physical pain and outcomes

instances, access to medications and health care professionals is scarce due to socioeconomic conditions, these resource constraints do not lead to a regulatory framework that is punitive toward opioid treatments. Policymakers are driven by culture, beliefs, and lived experiences. It is for this reason that an investigation into the social, cultural, and emotional barriers to opioids is so important. Any change in policy rests on changes in attitudes, belief systems, and culture conducive to their use. Without this, access to opioids as a pain treatment will remain limited and the socioeconomic impact on moderate to severe pain will continue.

The Influence of Beliefs and Culture on Pain Management

Cultural factors and beliefs remain a barrier to treating pain, especially when pain management, a large part of palliative care, and where death and dying remain stigmatized [16]. In a review of palliative care, Cleary et al. (2020) discuss the cultural and belief-related barriers to gaining access to treatment and care, which include the belief that certain pain medications are associated with end of life and, thus, are related to the fear of death [17]. People may refuse to come to health centers, may refuse care, or may not adhere to medication regimens. If such beliefs are pervasive in a community or society, health care workers will also demonstrate a reluctance to suggest or prescribe pain medications.

While one cannot generalize about cultural barriers to pain management across the continent, as rich cultural differences do exist and may influence attitude and behavior toward pain and pain management, some studies have proposed that African cultures have a general view of pain, emphasizing stoicism and not complaining [18,19]. Patients are discouraged from reporting pain to health care workers, whether they be traditional or nontraditional health workers [18]. In some instances, families may request that diagnoses are not disclosed to patients in order to prevent further pain and suffering [20].

The causes of pain are often informed by culture and belief systems [11]. For instance, ill will, revenge, or witchcraft may be viewed as responsible for pain. In such instances, traditional medicines and healers are the first points of contact for pain relief. One study found that 80% of people first consult a traditional healer, and only much later do they seek help from modern medicine providers [21]. While this may place less stress on health centers, it does provide a challenge to ensuring adequate care and access to optimal treatment, including opioids [22].

In a discussion regarding barriers to treatment, Benin and Okanla (2018) note that cancer is perceived as a "death threat" and this perception stops people from accessing treatment. This problem is compounded by the finding that cancer patients are often stigmatized in their communities; cancer is taboo, and any illness is seen as disrespect for the divinities [23].

When considering treatment of cancer pain and use of opioid analgesics, it is important to adopt a holistic approach and to include a review of cultural beliefs. For instance, understanding and being sensitive to cultural norms, such as women not being allowed to bathe men; a patient's sense of purpose and peace (versus religion, a set of organized beliefs in a group); personal beliefs concerning how pain is perceived and responded to; and, for patients who are spiritual in nature, the benefit of including elements of spirituality in their treatment plans [24]. A study by Givler, Bhatt, and Maani-Fogelman (2020) argues that culture determines how someone responds to and reports pain. Some cultures may avoid discussing severe pain and death, focusing instead on maintaining hope and lessening the family's suffering. Pain may be described in spiritual or emotional terms rather than in its physical aspects, making it challenging to determine the intensity of the pain [25].

Fear of Opioid Use

Opiophobia is the fear of addiction from opioids and is the main reason for cancer patients refusing and being refused opioids [26], in part arising from the belief that opioids are only used at the end of life or that dependencies may easily occur. Fear of misuse or abuse and negative attitudes toward opioids impact their use for managing cancer pain in Africa [27], likely exacerbated by the opioid crisis in the United States where misuse and addiction to opioids—including prescription pain relievers, heroin, and synthetic opioids such as fentanyl—have become a national crisis, affecting public health as well as social and economic welfare. The global media coverage of this opioid crisis creates an additional barrier for policymakers to consider opioid strategies, when appropriate, in their own countries. Research conducted in Ghana found a fear of dependency on opioids and the association of opioids with the end of life as major barriers to treatment [28]. Healthcare workers are also apprehensive about the use of opioids for fear that their patients may become dependent on them or have negative side effects, as well as the diversion, abuse, or misuse by the general public. These fears persist despite findings to the contrary, such as the fact that there are very low levels of dependency when used appropriately and carefully by people with no history of substance abuse [18]. This fear does not take into consideration the use of opioids in acute versus chronic treatment for cancer sufferers.

A Help the Hospices report, though published some time ago (in 2007), indicates levels of opiophobia among health workers:

- Over 50% of health care workers feared patients would become addicted.
- 25% believed that the public would misuse opioids, thus making their prescription too high risk.
- 35% of policymakers believed that people may abuse opioids.
- 45% of patients fear the side effects of opioids, while 20% fear addiction.
- Similarly, 20% of relatives fear the patient will become addicted [29].

Education and Skills Training on Palliative Care

Economic constraints present a challenge to accessing cancer pain care and management. Cleary et al.'s 2003 review of 25 African countries found that only five countries included palliative care in their health curricula; insufficient formal training is likely to lead to a deficit in standardized, comprehensive, and evidence-based skills training [4]. The distrust of opioids and the unwillingness to use them may be both a cause and a result of lack of education and training in the use of opioids as a treatment. Furthermore, the lack of efficacy and proper protocols for opioid usage promotes negative beliefs and attitudes towards the use of opioids. If no credible challenge to these beliefs is presented, they will persist and, similarly, will perpetuate the reluctance to include opioid treatment in medical education curricula. A study on Nigerian hospitals found that 90% of health care workers had not received any training in pain treatment and only 20% used opioids in cancer treatment [4]. Education is required at all levels, from community workers to specialists, and access to educational material in local languages is essential [17].

Education and training must address the fear of opioid addiction and dependency. Restrictions on the use of opioids have resulted in a lack of training in pain management and treatment for physicians and health care workers [30], reflected in policy frameworks (or lack thereof) dealing with opioid treatment.

Policies and Regulations for Opioid Use

Any form of intervention, whether palliative or not, requires a supportive policy environment. The basis of any public health program for cancer is a set of policies and regulations that specifically outline the requirements for cancer care while facilitating access to medications and treatment for pain. Without these, educational programs and access to medication and treatment protocols cannot be set or assessed for effectiveness. Even in instances where nongovernmental treatment centers are set up (usually through donor agencies, religious groups, and nongovernmental organizations), there is a need for clear government policy to permit operation and access of certain medications [17]. In a review of countries' policies on palliative care, Clelland et al. (2020) found that only 55 countries had a policy already in place, including Côte d'Ivoire, and some countries had policies in progress, such as Ghana and Mauritius. Burundi, Camaroon, Eritrea, Liberia, Senegal, and Tunisia had no policy at all. Many countries had no available data to analyze [31].

Conclusion

Access to analgesics in the treatment of cancer pain and palliative care is an area that needs to be addressed. The social, emotional, and physical outcomes for the patient and their families are significantly worse when treatment is ineffective or nonexistent [30]. Considering that pain management is recognized as a human right [32], there is a need to review and update the structures that restrict access to pain management. Policies and regulations that are evidence-based and suit the context must be put in place. There are existing guidelines that can be followed and adapted to each country. The WHO's recommendations for palliative care are also relevant for cancer pain treatment and include policies and regulations to ensure access to analgesics and other treatments, as well as educational and training programs for health care workers, community workers, and the public [33].

The use of opioids in the treatment of pain must be evaluated and applied in the context of each French-speaking African country in order to build up a base of evidence for policymakers to consider. Palliative care and pain treatment can be integrated into primary health care settings to increase access, safety, monitoring, and efficacy. It is important to acknowledge that culture, beliefs, and misconceptions affect not only patients, but health care workers and policymakers as well. Supplementary education should address cultural barriers and concerns regarding pain management and treatments [33]. Successful examples of this exist in Kenya and Uganda, where programs have integrated policy changes, professional education, and access to analgesic opioids into the public health system [16].

The destigmatization of death and dying, palliative care, and pain treatment in communities is essential. Health care workers trained in palliative care and pain treatment, who can generate trust from community workers, will help address this problem [16].

Finally, the matter of the affordability of opioids must be addressed—from ensuring that the registration of medications is not too costly to trade agreements and manufacturing capability on the continent. These changes are especially urgent given that the burden of noncommunicable diseases continues to rise in Africa.

The paucity of research on the treatment of cancer pain and the use of analgesics throughout Africa, and more specifically in French-speaking African countries, is clear. As long as treatment, research, and education remain poor, cancer patients will continue to suffer.

References

1. African Health Observatory. WHO, 2014. Accessed February 10, 2021: http://www.aho.afro.who.int/profiles_information/index.php/AFRO:Analytical_summary_-_Health_Status_and_Trends
2. Ervik M, Lam F, Ferlay J, Mery L, Soerjomataram I, Bray F. *Cancer Today*. Lyon, France: International Agency for Research on Cancer. Cancer Today; 2016. Accessed February 13, 2021 http://globocan.iarc.fr/old/burden.asp?selection_pop=218991&Text-p=WHO+Africa+region+%28AFRO%29&selection_cancer=290&Text-c=All+cancers+excl.+non-melanoma+skin+cancer&pYear=18&type=0&window=1&submit=%C2%A0Execute%C2%A0
3. Jemal F, Bray F, Forman D. Cancer burden in Africa and opportunities for prevention. *Cancer*. 2012;118(18): 4372–4384.
4. Cleary J, Powell RA, Munene G, et al. Availability and regulatory barriers to accessibility of opioids for cancer pain in Africa: A report from the Global Opioid Policy Initiative (GOPI). *Ann Oncol*. 2013;24(Suppl 11):xi14–xi23, 2013.
5. GBD 2017 Disease and Injury Incidence and Prevalence Collaborators. Global, regional, and national incidence, prevalence, and years lived with disability for 354 diseases and injuries for 195 countries and territories, 1990–2017:Aa systematic analysis for the Global Burden of Disease Study 2017. *The Lancet*. 2018;392(10159):1789–1858.
6. World Health Assembly, WHA67.19, May 24 2014. Accessed February 10, 2021. http://apps.who.int/medicinedocs/en/m/abstract/Js21454ar
7. French Consulate General. French language facts. Accessed January 10, 2021: https://za.ambafrance.org/French-language-facts
8. International Narcotics Control Board. Report of the International Narcotics Control Board on the Availability of Internationally Controlled Drugs: Ensuring Adequate Access for Medical and Scientific Purposes. 2010. Accessed January 10, 2021: http://www.incb.

org/documents/Publications/AnnualReports/AR2010/Supplement-AR10_availability_English.pdf

9. International Narcotics Control Board. Availability of internationally controlled drugs: Ensuring adequate access for medical and scientific purposes. 2015 (Chapter II):15–16. Accessed January 22, 2021: http://www.incb.org/documents/Publications/AnnualReports/AR2015/English/Supplement-AR15_availability_English.pdf

10. Maurer MA. New online tool for exploring global opioid consumption data. J *Pain Palliat Care Pharmacother*. 2017;31(1):45–51.

11. Olaleye O, Ekrikpo U. Epidemiology of cancers in sub-Saharan Africa. In: Adedeji O (eds). *Cancer in Sub-Saharan Africa*. Springer, Cham; 2017. https://doi.org/10.1007/978-3-319-52554-9_1

12. Knaul F, Radbruch L, Conner S, et al. How many adults and children are in need of palliative care worldwide? WHO, Atlas, 2020. Accessed February 9, 2021: http://www.thewhpca.org/resources/global-atlas-on-end-of-life-care

13. Boyle P, Ngoma T, Sullivan R, Brawley O. Cancer in Africa: the way forward. *eCancer*. 2019; 13:953. doi: https://doi.org/10.3332/ecancer.2019.953

14. World Health Organization Briefing Note—April 2012. Access to Controlled Medications Programme. Improving access to medications controlled under international drug conventions. Accessed January 12, 2021: http://www.who.int/medicines/areas/quality_safety/ACMP_BrNote_PainGLs_EN_Apr2012.pdf

15. World Health Organization. Ensuring balance in national policies on controlled substances: Guidance for availability and accessibility of controlled medicines. 2011. Accessed January 29, 2021: https://apps.who.int/iris/handle/10665/44519

16. Fraser BA, Powel RA, Mwangi-Powell FN, et al. Palliative care development in Africa: Lessons from Uganda and Kenya. *J Glob Oncology*. 2017. doi:10.1200/JGO.2017.010090

17. Cleary J, Hastie B, Harding R, Jaramillo E, Conner S, Krakauer E. What are the main barriers to palliative care development? WHO, Atlas, 2020. Accessed February 9, 2021: http://www.thewhpca.org/resources/global-atlas-on-end-of-life-care

18. Namekwaya E, Leng M, Downing J, Katabira E. Cancer pain management in resource-limited settings: A practice review. *Pain Res Treat*. 2011. doi:10.1155/2011/393404/

19. Walters MA. Pain assessment in sub-Saharan Africa. *IASP Pediatric Pain Letter*. 2009; (3):22–26.

20. Lunn JS. Spiritual care in a multi-religious context. *J Pain Palliat Care Pharmacother*. 2003;17(3-4):153–66.

21. Harding R, Kraus D, Easterbrook P et al. Does palliative care improve outcomes for patients with HIV/AIDS? A review of the evidence. *Sex Transm Infect*. 2005;81(1):5–14.

22. Rhee JY, Garralda E, Namisango, E, et al. Factors affecting palliative care development in Africa: In-country experts' perceptions in seven countries. *J Pain Symptom Manage*. 2018;55(5):1313–1320.

23. Okanla K. Unaffordable treatment. Development and Cooperation. Accessed February 16, 2021: https://www.dandc.eu/en/article/because-poverty-fear-ignorance-and-taboos-cancer-normally-diagnosed-late-benin.

24. Weinstein F, Bernstein A, Kapenstein T, Penn E, Richeimer S. Spirituality assessments and interventions in pain medicine. *Pract Pain Manage*. Accessed February 13, 2021: https://www.practicalpainmanagement.com/treatments/psychological/spirituality-assessments-interventions-pain-medicine.

25. Givler A, Bhatt H, Maani-Fogelman PA. The importance of cultural competence in pain and palliative care. In: StatPearls [Internet]. Treasure Island (FL): StatPearls Publishing; 2020. Available from: https://www.ncbi.nlm.nih.gov/books/NBK493154

26. Cella IF, Trindade LCT, Sanvido et al. Prevalence of opiophobia in cancer pain treatment. *Rev Dor.* 2016;17(4):245–247.

27. Sepulveda C. Quality care at the end of life in Africa. *BMJ.* 2003;327(7408):209–213.

28. Fisch MJ. Palliative care education in Ghana: reflections on teaching in West Africa. *J Support Oncol.* 2011;9(4):134–135.

29. Adams V. Worldwide Palliative Care Alliance. Access to pain relief: an essential human right. A report for World Hospice and Palliative Care Day 2007. Help the hospices for the Worldwide Palliative Care Alliance. *J Pain Palliat Care Pharmacother.* 2008;22(2):101–129.

30. Nchakoa E, Bussella S, Nesbetha C, Odohb C. Barriers to the availability and accessibility of controlled medicines for chronic pain in Africa. *Int Health.* 2018;10:71–77. doi:10.1093/inthealth/ihy002

31. Clelland D, Van Steijn D, Whitelaw S, Conner S, Centeno C, Clark D. Palliative care in public policy: Results from a global survey. *Palliat Med Repts.* 2020; 1(1). doi: 10.1089/pmr.2020.0062.

32. Lohman D, Schleifer R, Amon JJ. Access to pain treatment as a human right. *BMC Medicine.* 2010;8(8) https://doi.org/10.1186/1741-7015-8-8.

33. World Health Organization. Palliative care. 2020. Accessed February 12, 2021: https://www.who.int/news-room/fact-sheets/detail/palliative-care

34. Harding R, Powell R, Kiyange F, Downing J, Powell F. Pain relieving drugs in 12 African PEPFAR countries: mapping current providers, identifying current challenges, and enabling expansion of pain control provision in the management of HIV/AIDS. *Afr Palliat Care Assoc.* 2007. Kampala, Uganda.

31

Support and Palliative Care for Cancer Patients in Mexico, Mexico

Maricela Salas Becerril and Noemi Hernández Cruz

Introduction

The World Health Organization (WHO) reports that, annually, 10 million people die from cancer-related causes and 20 million are confirmed with an oncological diagnosis, many of whom are in advanced and/or terminal stages. These statistics depict the necessity for strategies to improve palliative care education for health care workers, especially for nursing professionals. In Mexico, the picture is very similar: cancer is the third-leading cause of death in Mexico, accounting for 12% of all deaths [1–4].

Cancer is a disease that limitates on people's lives and well-being and, at some point, requires palliative care due to the great amount of suffering it causes to both the patients and their families, as well as the presence of constantly changing and multifaceted symptoms generated by the treatments and/or the disease itself. Thus, total, active, and continuous care is needed to help patients live the most comfortable life possible and to provide them with quality of life and a dignified death. The participation of a multidisciplinary team in addressing and meeting their physical, psychological, social, and spiritual needs is essential in order to achieve the objective: of accompanying and assist them in coping with the disease in an effective and dignified manner and to extend this support to the family even during the period of mourning [5,6].

The Pillars of Palliative Care

Palliative care enables patients with incurable diseases such as cancer to be accompanied, comforted, and relieved as much as possible. It is important that the care be based on its essential pillars in order to improve the quality of life of this vulnerable group [7]. These pillars allow the palliative care team, especially nurses, to address the needs of patients and caregivers. For palliative care to be effective, the following pillars must apply: (1) symptom control, (2) communication, (3) relief from suffering, and (4) emotional support. It is imperative that nursing professionals understand the role they play in each pillar so that they can track their own actions, offer the care guaranteeing the maximum well-being of the patient, and educate and train the patient and their caregiver regarding the type of care they require [7,8].

Symptom Control

Symptom control is a priority and one of the basic principles of palliative care. During the evolution of the disease, patients present with multiple symptoms of varying intensities and of multifactorial origins. The symptoms act as an alarm, indicating that the body is not well and requires care; the more intense and persistent the symptoms, the more patients feel their lives are threatened.

It is therefore vital for caregivers to be trained to perform homecare and to fully understand the pharmacological plan, especially during the end-of-life phase. Caring for a suffering patient is not easy and is often physically and mentally overwhelming for the primary caregiver; providing this training aims to reduce the burden. This education and training is the responsibility of the nursing team, who should always be kept informed in order to resolve any questions that may arise. Nurses should take part in the decision-making process along with the patient and family.

General Principles of Symptom Control

Symptom control should follow these basic principles:

- *Assessment before treatment.* A thorough patient assessment must be performed in order to determine the cause of the symptom, its physical and emotional impact, its intensity, and what is exacerbating it.
- *Explanation of the causes.* The patient and family should always be informed about what triggers symptoms and should be given management guidelines with clear, simple, truthful terminology.
- *Individualized treatment.* Each patient is unique, as are the symptoms they present; therefore, formulating a therapeutic and pharmacological plan will be similar to creating a custom-made suit.
- *Monitoring of symptoms.* It is necessary to teach the patient and their family how to measure the intensity of each symptom by using standardized scales, such as the visual analog scale (EVA), the numerical scale (EN), and the scale of Edmonton symptoms. When choosing which scale to use, the patient's and/or caregiver's cognitive level should be taken into consideration. It is advisable to teach them how to log symptoms and pain levels in a daily chart; this will allow the physician to adjust the therapeutic plan in the next review visit.
- *Participation of the entire multidisciplinary team.* This is essential in order to address all the patient and family needs and to provide the most comprehensive treatment and care possible [9].

A reassessment of symptoms should be done periodically to adjust the therapeutic plan, if needed, and maintain symptom control. The role of the nursing professional is to provide information and clarify any doubts concerning the pharmacological therapy in order to achieve better compliance with the treatment.

Further guidelines should be followed for prescription medications: assess if the drugs have little or an undesirable effect; if the drugs are to be administered orally and large or bad-tasting pills are to be avoided; and if it is feasible to continue with the oral route. If the patient shows signs of dysphagia, an alternative route such as subcutaneous injection should be considered to provide continuity of pharmacological treatment. Another guideline to consider is the ease with which a drug may be administered, in both drug presentation and schedules and whether to withdraw all drugs that are no longer needed, such as antihypertensives and hypoglycemic agents [10].

Some of the most common symptoms experienced by an oncology patient with advanced and/or terminal disease are as follows:

Pain is one of the most frequent and severe symptoms experienced by patients. Pain is a subjective experience, and, therefore, patients should always be believed when expressing what hurts them; in no case should a placebo be used. It is important for patients to learn to describe the severity of their pain in order to ensure that the pharmacological treatment is appropriate. The drug, most commonly opioids, will be chosen from the World Health Organization (WHO) analgesic ladder; the use of adjuvant therapies is usually necessary. Nonpharmacological measures such as massage, relaxation techniques, cold or heat applications, acupuncture, and active or passive mobilization will be of great importance [11].

Dyspnea is the symptom that most frightens patients and caregivers, for it produces the sensation of drowning, causing high levels of distress. The drugs commonly used for dyspnea are potent opioids (morphine) and bronchodilators. The care required may entail supplemental oxygen with nasal tips while placing the patient in a Semi-Fowler position and respiratory relaxation techniques to return breathing to a slow pace, using a fan or opening windows to allow natural ventilation of the room. It is advisable to keep the patient at rest and to avoid any effort that demands excessive expenditure of energy and, therefore, higher oxygen consumption. It is also advisable not to leave them alone in order to avoid distress.

Coughing for cancer patients can be chronic and bring with it other symptoms, such as fatigue, social problems, pain, dyspnea, and insomnia that further diminish their quality of life. Potent opioids like morphine and steroids may be prescribed; suggested treatments to minimize coughing are vibratory pulmonary physiotherapy; an electric humidifier or nebulizer used with saline solution or medication, and promotion of passive mobility in bed and changes in position.

Anorexia is a frequent occurrence in terminal illness, increasing anxiety in both patients and their caregivers. It is common for the appetite to be altered by the presence of pain, nausea, mucositis, xerostomia, and the like; therefore, it is important to control any unmitigated symptoms in order to improve appetite. Unfortunately, as the disease continues to advance, anorexia reappears. Medications such as corticosteroids are available to help improve appetite, but their prescription should be assessed. It is recommended that small, appealing meals be offered and that the patient not be forced to eat [10,12].

Constipation is common for the oncologic patient with advanced disease who is prescribed morphine for the control of pain. Additional risk factors precipitating constipation include inactivity, weakness, and decreased water intake. For this reason, prescribing laxatives will almost be the rule. Even when the patient does not present with bowel movement difficulties, laxatives should be considered as a preventative treatment. Nursing care for patients with, or at risk for, constipation include raising awareness about the importance of administering laxatives on schedule; offering abundant liquids throughout the day; facilitating changes in position and encouraging mobility/walking; teaching the caregiver how to perform colonic massage; administering an enema; or carrying out manual extraction of feces (with this last-named remedy being an exception) [10].

Nausea and vomiting are symptoms that have a significant impact on nutrition and quality of life for patients with advanced cancer and may derive from the disease itself, the treatments they receive, perceived odors, and/or the pressure to eat food. Therefore, an appropriate assessment should be made to identify the causes and provide the best pharmacological plan and care. The drugs usually indicated for control of nausea and vomiting are antiemetics, preferably by subcutaneous injection, in line with established hours and with rescue doses. To enhance the effect of these drugs, the following care can be provided: encouraging the intake of cold food and drinks, chunks of pineapple, and frozen orange slices; offering savory cookies; avoiding cooking near the patient to avert an adverse reaction to smells; avoiding highly seasoned foods; and reminding patients to eat slowly. If the patient vomits, remove it from the room, change the soiled clothing and bedsheets, air out the room, and offer mouth freshener [10].

Fatigue, an overwhelming sensation in the final phase of an illness, is described by patients as a lack of energy that does not disappear and cannot be alleviated with rest. It is usually accompanied by decreased strength, difficulty concentrating, increased dyspnea, tachycardia with exertion, and the need to reduce or halt the pace. A number of causes can trigger fatigue, including ill-controlled symptoms, excess or lack of activity, mood disorders, nutritional imbalance, and anemia. Psychostimulants may be prescribed upon appropriate assessment to diminish fatigue and improve the feeling of well-being. Some aspects of nursing care will focus on enabling sleep and/or rest, encouraging controlled exercise, using aids such as walkers or wheelchairs, explaining the causes of fatigue, and setting priorities in the activities that the patient should perform.

Other than the physiological symptoms, patients commonly experience psychological and neurological indications such as depression, anxiety, delirium, agitation, and confusion, which should be treated by psychologists and psychiatrists who will decide the best pharmacological treatment. The nurse's part is to provide nonpharmacological remedies that promote psychological well-being and try to preserve the patient's quality of life. Some measures that will promote stress management are performing a thorough assessment of symptoms and a timely referral to a specialist; clarifying any doubts that patients may have about the information provided by the doctor; and motivate the patient to participate in decision making regarding their own treatment and family situation. Some patients prefer not to be alone and want the company of their loved ones, so harmonious visitations from family and friends, who can provide support as they accompany their loved one, should be encouraged.

Communication

In palliative care, it is essential to establish good communication, initially among the team itself and then with the patient and the family, in order to help them to cope with advanced disease which frequently causes internal strife. The patient and family often experience a sense of threat, feeling defenseless in the face of something they cannot control; as the symptoms become more persistent, the situation may exceed their coping resources. It is common for patients to face difficulties in communication due to their disease, their medication, their health, their mood, and so on, causing them to become anxious or depressed. In addition, if the patient has a tendency to be introverted, this can hinder receiving aid [13].

When faced with this situation, it is necessary to assess the needs of the patient and to provide only the information that the patient requires, that is, details that they have the right to know and the right not to know. The basis of good communication is to convey information in a clear and empathetic way, enabling the patient to assimilate the information in the best way possible and acknowledging what the patient is experiencing without losing sight of the objectives of communication: to inform, guide, and support the patient and the family [13].

It is key for the nursing professional to develop an empathic relationship with patients from the outset, utilizing effective and active listening skills in order to assist and accompany them throughout their journey.

Alleviation of Suffering

During advanced disease, the patient experiences high levels of uncertainty due to the precariousness of the disease and the presence of various symptoms; this uncertainty may cause fear when the perception of their future is compromised. Many symptoms may trigger and/or exacerbate signs of depression and anxiety, leading to even more suffering. This feeling is experienced uniquely by each patient; their personal life story has been interrupted by the presence of an incurable disease, which will inevitably forge concerns such as: easing pain, managing the situation, not becoming a burden, and avoiding a prolonged death. In order to help these patients, it is important to provide timely palliative care by forming a multidisciplinary team that addresses their needs, manages their symptoms, and alleviates their suffering.

One objective of palliative care is to prevent and alleviate suffering through early identification and providing appropriate treatment from a holistic perspective, that is, to cover all areas—physical, psychological, social, and spiritual—with support and respect during care. It should be noted that pain, dyspnea, and delusion are the symptoms that cause the highest levels of distress and fear. When this distress becomes too difficult to bear, the intense suffering will lead to deterioration in quality of life [14,15].

Chronic pain and its accompanied suffering is the symptom that most frightens the patient as, in many cases, its origin is unknown or it is not alleviated. This implies that pain must be treated in all its dimensions. As Cicely Saunders states in her theory of total pain, there is a conjugation of physical pain with spiritual, psychological, and social suffering. Pain is what affects the body, whereas suffering affects the spiritual and psychic spheres. In other words, transcendence, the ultimate sense of life, their values, moral consciousness, relationship with God, and mental health, are all affected [16].

In order to better understand the meaning of suffering, Cassell defined it as the state of severe distress, associated with events that threaten the integrity of the person and that demand awareness of themselves, in which emotions are involved and will impact their body [17]. This emphasizes the need for a thorough assessment by a multidisciplinary team who can provide the patient and their caregivers with adequate management and treatment plans.

When carrying out patient assessment, it is necessary to identify the stage of the disease and accept the poor probability of finding a cure. This will provide the guidelines for the treatment approach. The five phases of disease are incubation, prodromal, illness, decline, and convalescence periods [16].

These circumstances imply that suffering is a complex concept that requires an adequate assessment. Although there are no instruments to expressly assess suffering, several scales are available that assist in assessing symptoms and other aspects in order to gauge the patient's level of suffering. Some instruments include:

- The Distress Thermometer (DT)
- The Edmonton Assessment Scale (ESAS)
- The Brief Symptom Inventory (BSI) [18]

In order to achieve the best approach to alleviate suffering, each care team will choose the scale that is most suitable for their patient. However, these scales should be supported by a clinical interview, which will allow direct, personalized, and effective interaction with the patient, leading to an empathetic and compassionate relationship.

The role of the nursing professional is to accompany and maintain a close relationship with the patient and to provide supportive care in controlling the symptoms for optimum well-being. Unfortunately, the disease has a greater impact in some situations, and, as a result, the patient experiences refractory symptoms and/or situations that produce uncontrollable suffering, especially when all of the usual possibilities for treatment have been exhausted. At present, this suffering can be avoidable, without speeding up death, by resorting to palliative sedation as a viable and exceptional alternative for maximum physical, psychological, and spiritual comfort [19,20].

Palliative sedation is the administration of medications at the minimum doses and combinations necessary to lower the level of consciousness of a patient with advanced or terminal disease presenting with refractory symptoms to help alleviate suffering. In order to offer this treatment option, the physician will have already provided all information on palliative sedation to the patient while in their full cognitive capacity as well as to the family. Clarifying all doubts and inviting the patient to make a decision at the time when it is required will help them die peacefully. This decision must be reflected in an advance directive and become part of the medical file, thus exercising the patient's rights [8].

When the decision to initiate palliative sedation has been made, the role played by the nursing professional is key, as it is the nurse who provides the supportive care required to promote the patient's comfort, as well as being the one who will prepare and administer the appropriate medicines while simultaneously assessing the patient's responses and, above all, offering accompaniment at the end of life.

Emotional Support

Accompanying patients and family members during advanced illness aims to improve their quality of psychosocial and spiritual life as much as possible by easing their suffering and helping them strengthen their personal and psychosocial resources. As they are bound to experience devastating feelings that are difficult to address and treat, it is essential to support them in coping with the disease [21].

Nursing professionals must offer emotional support to the patient, family, and/or caregiver with appropriate conversations addressing their psychological and spiritual needs. It should be noted that, although a multiprofessional team provides care, this area is the responsibility of the psychologist. However, nurses must also be able to address these needs as they are the first contact when making the initial assessment; nurses must first be able to discern these needs, initiate containment wisely, and then channel it through to the experts.

Upon evaluation, nurses should address the psychological state of the patient and assess aspects of personality, behavior, and motivation, as well as be alert to whether the patient shows signs of depression and anxiety, or emotions such as anger, distress, hopelessness, loneliness, fears of abandonment, and death. Situations that cause conflict such as guilt, stress, responses to coping, and, of course, self-esteem and self-image [22] should not be ignored.

Another dimension to be evaluated is the patient's social situation, which includes cultural values, beliefs, relationships, roles within the family, friends, community, as well as rituals, economic resources, expenses, legal aspects, leaving a will, and the relationship with the caregiver. These are some of the points that need to be investigated upon initial contact with the patient and the family in order to establish a closer and more empathetic connection. It is also important to explore the spiritual dimension to get to know the patient's values and beliefs, as well their spiritual advisors [22].

These are not easy tasks. Nurses are part of the health care team to whom the patient imparts important moments of their life, thus facilitating the care and resulting in a shared experience of empathy and compassion [23].

Assessing the cultural, social, and spiritual values and needs of patients and families allows nursing professionals to offer careful, culturally safe palliative care, which is important for overcoming communication barriers. As linguistic barriers are often encountered (Mexico has a wide range of indigenous languages), it is sometimes difficult to understand patients and their families, further inhibiting them from expressing their beliefs, needs, wishes, and cultural values [22].

Although psychosocial interventions are key for effectively helping patients, in some cases pharmacological measures may be necessary to control anxiety. The most commonly used drugs are benzodiazepines, which are unique in their anxiolytic effect. The nurse also has a role as an educator: nurses must understand the goals of treatment and medicine for their patients' improved quality of life.

Influence of Culture on Cancer Cure

Cancer affects a large number of people, effecting significant changes in their emotional, physical, spiritual, and social spheres that lead them to remodel their identity by the incentive to win the battle. However, when seeking an explanation for the origin of the disease, patients sometimes resort to "magical thinking," finding unrealistic cures (which they refer to as "alternative and complementary therapies"). These cures falsely claim to achieve complete healing; this belief is confusing for them, turning something so serious into something so simple [24]. Faced with this yearning to find a cure, patients are attracted to these therapies, using their body, mind, or elements of nature to improve their quality of life. However, these methods provide false hope for the prevention or cure of cancer, and there is no scientific evidence of their efficacy [25].

This magical thinking is very popular among the Mexican population, and it is common for people to turn to alternative and/or complementary therapies as well as "miracle drugs" that promise to cure cancer. One option frequently used by patients is temazcal, which is an old-fashioned steam bath with plants that detoxify the body—"entering the place which symbolizes the belly of the mother earth, slowly regenerating the body, taking out all the bad things that come with it and, thus, it is reborn" [26]. Another option is the therapeutic bed, which functions as a massage-thermos that helps ease muscle pain by unlocking energy channels, relaxing muscles and improving circulation. "Miracle drugs" can be found in a sundry of presentations such as pills, capsules, creams, or oil infusions. Some examples of potions promising a cure are "cat's claw," curcuma, shark oil, and noni juice. These "medicines" are often recommended by someone who has gone through a similar situation where these apparently worked for them while, in the meantime, the patient and family are frustrated seeing no improvement in health and resort to another one of these therapies. In addition, by then the family has exhausted their resources and are unable to afford conventional treatments to regain health.

Frequently, behind these "miracle drugs" are actors who are looking to make a profit by taking advantage of people's desperation to prolong life. Unfortunately, the patient and family often decide to abandon medical treatments, and so the oncologic disease continues to worsen. As time passes and they do not see any real improvement, they may decide to return to the hospital in search of specialized care. By this time, the patient presents with advanced stages without the possibility of receiving curative care. These bad decisions lead to complicated health issues that cause great suffering and, with them, a major deterioration in the quality of life for both patient and family.

Basic Comfort

Palliative care for patients with advanced and/or terminal disease focuses on providing care that helps improve the patient's well-being, that is, comfort care aimed at meeting basic needs such as breathing, eating, hydration, elimination, hygiene, rest, and activity.

Patients in their last days of life and facing their own death have more than one need that must be supported and fulfilled; what they most want is to be at peace, without pain or its accompanied suffering. This can be achieved by offering them comfort care, the goal of palliative care. Palliative care can be performed in the hospital or at home, by nurses, health care professionals, and instructed caregivers who support the nursing staff. The integration of family members in the care tasks promotes a harmonious relationship between patient and caregiver.

References

1. WHO: World Health Organization. 2020 [citado 23 ago 2020]. Disponible en: https://www.who.int/es/news-room/fact-sheets/detail/cancer

2. WHO: Organización Mundial de la Salud. 58ª Asamblea Mundial de la Salud. Punto 13.12 del orden del día provisional. 7 de abril de 2005. Disponible en: https://apps.who.int/gb/archive/pdf_files/WHA58/A58_16-sp.pdf?ua=1

3. Globocan, International Agency for Research on Cancer 2017. Disponible en: https://juntoscontraelcancer.mx/panorama-del-cancer-en-mexico/

4. Infocancer – México, junio 2019. Disponible en: https://www.infocancer.org.mx/?c=conocer-el-cancer&a=estadisticas-mundiales-y-locales

5. WHO: Organización Mundial de la Salud, control del cáncer: Cuidados Paliativos. 2007. Disponible en: https://apps.who.int/iris/bitstream/handle/10665/44025/9789243547343_spa.pdf?sequence=1

6. Worldwide Palliative Care Alliance. Global Atlas of Palliative Care. 2a Edition. London, UK. 2020. [actualizado 6 nov 2020; citado 30 nov 2020] Disponible en: http://www.thewhpca.org/resources/global-atlas-on-end-of-life-care

7. Velasco VM. Cáncer: Cuidado continuo y manejo paliativo. *Rev. Med. Clin. Condes*, 2013; 24(4):668–676. Disponible en: www.elsevier.es › es-revista-revista-medica-clinica-las-con.

8. Astudillo AW, Mendinueta AC. Principios generales de los cuidados paliativos. 1ª sección. Disponible en: file:///c:/users/hp/downloads/principios%20generales%20de%20los%20cuidados%20paliativos.pdf

9. SECPAL: Sociedad Española de Cuidados Paliativos. Guía de Cuidados Paliativos [Internet]. Madrid, España. SECPAL 2014. [Actualizado mayo 2018]. Disponible en:https://www.secpal.com/biblioteca_guia-cuidados-paliativos_4-principios-generales-de-control-de-sintomas

10. Gómez SM, Ojeda MM. Cuidados paliativos, Control de síntomas [Internet]. Las Palmas de Gran Canaria. Laboratorios MEDA; 2009; [citado 3 nov 2020]. Disponible en: https://paliativos.uy/wp-content/uploads/2018/08/Libro-CONTROL-DE-SINTOMAS-EN-CUIDADOS-PALIATIVOS-MINISTERIO-DE-SALUD-1.pdf

11. Consejo de Salubridad General. Guía de manejo integral de cuidados paliativos. [Internet]. Ciudad de México. Early Institute e Instituto Nacional de Cancerología; julio de 2018. [citado 7 nov 2020]. Disponible en: http://www.geriatria.salud.gob.mx/descargas/publicaciones/Guia_cuidados_paliativos_completo.pdf

12. Nervi OF. Síndrome caquexia—anorexia. En: Palma BA, Taboada RP, Nervi OF. Medicina paliativa y cuidados continuos. Santiago, Chile: edicionesuc;2010:139–145.

13. SECPAL: Sociedad Española de Cuidados Paliativos. Guía de Cuidados Paliativos [Internet]. Madrid, España. SECPAL 2014. [Actualizado mayo 2018]. Disponible en: https://www.secpal.com/biblioteca_guia-cuidados-paliativos_12-informacion-y-comunicacion

14. SECPAL: Sociedad Española de Cuidados Paliativos. Madrid: 2014 [actualizado mayo 2018]. Disponible en: https://secpal.com/grupo-espiritualidad_itinerario-de-la-persona_2-a-que-llamamos-sufrimiento

15. Wilson A. Casado da RC. Mendinueta AC. Alivio de las situaciones difíciles y del sufrimiento en la terminalidad. Sociedad Vasca de Cuidados Paliativos. Ed. SOVPAL. España 2005. Disponible en http://www.sovpal.org

16. Celedón LC. Suffering and death in a terminal patient. *Rev. Otorrinolaringol. Cir. Cabeza Cuello.* 2012;72(3):261–266. Disponible en: https://scielo.conicyt.cl/pdf/orl/v72n3/art08.pdf

17. Cassel EJ. The nature of suffering and the goals of medicine. *N Engl J Med.* 1982 Mar 18;306(11):639–645. doi: 10.1056/NEJM198203183061104. PMID: 7057823

18. Krikorian A. Valoración del sufrimiento en pacientes con cáncer avanzado. *Psicooncología.* 2008;5(2-3):257–264. Disponible en: file:///C:/Users/HP/Downloads/Valoracion_del_sufrimiento_en_pacientes_con_cancer.pdf

19. Antueno P. Silberberg A. Eficacia de los cuidados paliativos en el alivio del sufrimiento. *Pers. Bioét.* 2018;22(3): 367–380. doi: 10.5294/pebi.2018.22.2.12 Disponible en: http://www.scielo.org.co/pdf/pebi/v22n2/0123-3122-pebi-22-02-00367.pdf

20. AECC: Asociación Española Contra el Cáncer. Madrid: 2018. Disponible en: https://www.aecc.es/es/todo-sobre-cancer/viviendo-con-cancer/final-vida/sedacion-paliativa.

21. Agámez IC. Álvarez TH. Mera GMV. Paliación y cáncer. Ladiprint Editorial. S.A.S. Bogotá, Colombia. 2012. Disponible en: file:///C:/Users/HP/Downloads/LIBROPALIACIONCANCERFINAL.pdf

22. Grinspun D., Moreno T. Registered Nurses' Association of Ontario. Guía de buenas prácticas clínicas. Enfoque paliativo de los cuidados en los últimos 12 meses de vida. Marzo 2020. Disponible en: https://www.bpso.es/wp-content/uploads/2020/10/D0046_Enfoque-Paliativo_12-Meses-de-Vida.pdf

23. SECPAL: Sociedad Española de Cuidados Paliativos. Monografías. Espiritualidad en Clínica. Una propuesta de evaluación y acompañamiento espiritual en Cuidados Paliativos. No. 6, noviembre 2014. Disponible en: http://www.secpal.com//Documentos/Blog/Monografia%20secpal.pdf

24. Nácar-Hernández VM, Palomares-González A, López-Vega M, Ochoa-Carrillo FJ, Alvarado-Aguilar S. Cáncer: mitos relacionados con la enfermedad. *Gaceta Mexicana de Oncología*;2012, 11(6):835–391. Disponible en: https://www.elsevier.es/es-revista-gaceta-mexicana-oncologia-305-pdf-X1665920112839877

25. American Cancer Society, 2019. Disponible en: https://www.cancer.org/es/noticias-recientes/la-verdad-sobre-los-tratamientos-de-la-medicina-alternativa.html

26. Secretaria de pueblos y barrios originarios y comunidades indígenas residentes, febrero 2018. Disponible en: https://www.sepi.cdmx.gob.mx/comunicacion/nota/medicina-tradicional-mexicana-una-alternativa-complementaria-para-tratar-el-cancer

32

Islamic Cultural-Spiritual Guidance in Caring for Cancer Patients, Iraq

Samaher A. Fadhil and Hasanein H. Ghali

Iraqi Culture: Beliefs and Attitude toward Well-being, Illness and Death

Modern Iraq, the ancient Mesopotamian civilization, lies in the Middle East, which is the place of origin of the world's three major religions: Islam, Christianity, and Judaism. Iraq is an Islamic country, with Islamic cultural beliefs and norms that shape its people's values and their perceptions of life events. Although the largest ethnic groups in Iraq are Arab, followed by Kurds, there are other ethnic groups including Assyrians, Turkmen, Shabaki, Armenians, Mandeans, and other minorities. The Arab population is divided between Shiite Muslims and Sunni Muslims. These mixtures of ethnicity and religious groups among the people are linked with large diversities in norms, beliefs, and lifestyles.

Iraqi families are large and the relationships are close; appreciation and loyalty are expected toward the extended family and the tribe and are of great importance. This intimate nature of relations with relatives and neighbors affects the individual's health and decisions regarding diagnosis of disease and treatment outcome. Family kindship is the basis for offering philanthropy to poor extended family members. The extended family is the core of Muslim society; hence, the extended family is deeply involved in decision making regarding treatment, health, and end-of-life care.

In Islam, health and well-being are considered the best gifts and blessings from God. Illness and suffering are part of life and are perceived as a test of faith by God, whereas physical pain is viewed as a penance for past sins. Most Iraqi people think of wellness in terms of physical health and, to a lesser extent, about mental and spiritual well-being, although in recent years and due to the increased use of the Internet, Iraqi youths and adolescents show an interest in exercise, diet, and even spirituality, along with mental health.

The Quran, the holy book of Muslims, together with the hadiths (the sayings and teachings of the Prophet Muhammad), provide directives toward health and guidance for mental, emotional, social, and spiritual well-being. To a majority of Iraqis, spirituality is connected to religion, and there is no separation between religion and spirituality. Spirituality is an important element of health, and people and patients depend primarily on Islamic rituals, prayers, fasting, charity and supplication to God to improve their health and face illness and suffering.

Islamic teachings also provide guidance on nutrition, lifestyle, and social relationships. Muslims do not eat pork or its by-products, and they do not drink alcohol or products containing alcohol. The majority of Muslims fast during Ramadan, although sick and ill patients are advised not to fast over Ramadan. There is an emphasis on eating certain type of foods such as honey, olive oil, and dates, because these foods are mentioned in the holy Quran and are considered to be of great benefit. Islamic teachings emphasize modesty in every daily activity, including eating, self-care, and dealing with other people.

There are some minor differences in rituals and beliefs between the two major Islamic groups, Shiite and Sunni, and in the perception of and coping with chronic illness and suffering. Shiites, aside from reading the Quran and reciting prayers, believe that visiting the holy places where the bodies of their imams are buried can help their ill relatives; they take their patients to these holy places, mainly in Najaf and Karbala, that hold the graves of the Imam Ali (Prophet Muhammad's cousin) and his son, Al-Hussein, to pray and ask for healing and cure. Some people in smaller cities and rural areas refuse Western medicine and believe that their imams can heal their patients, especially those with chronic illnesses and cancer. There is also particular reliance on herbal and nutritional medicine for cancer, and it is these beliefs that are responsible for later-stage diagnoses of cancers and poorer survival outcomes.

Death is embraced as the end of the Divine Plan, and the exact time of a person's death is known only by God. Expressions of grief vary in different provinces and among different families, but, in general, large numbers of relatives and friends are present at the time of death or at the funeral to lend moral, spiritual, and financial support to the family.

Islam and Medicine

"There is no disease that Allah has created, except that He also has created its remedy"

—Prophet Muhammad

Before Islam, medicine was based on local practices derived from the old traditions of ancient nations. Historically, religion has had a notable impact on medical practices. Islam prioritizes prevention over treatment, and so its teachings are rich with preventive measures, including an emphasis on cleanliness, personal hygiene, sexual hygiene, and environmental cleanliness. Circumcision is mandatory in Islam and is meant to prevent urinary tract infections. Islam also recommends avoiding overeating, psychological stress, and overthinking to maintain sound mental health. Dietary restrictions of specific ingredients (pork, alcohol, and their by-products) are also advised and recommended.

The Islamic heritage is also rich with various treatment measures such as traditional natural remedies, honey, olive oil, and the use of cup suction (Hijama, widely used in Iraq). These measures are still used in many Islamic countries for treating symptoms such as headaches.

With the spread of Islam, medicine along with other sciences was influenced by well-established cultures and older Greek, Roman, Indian, and Persian civilizations. Muslim scientists, primarily during the Abbasid Caliphate age in Baghdad, translated much scientific work, especially medicine, into Arabic. In the decades following, Muslim scholars contributed to many different aspects of the sciences during the Islamic Golden Age from the 8th through the 13th centuries. Remarkable progress was made in numerous scientific fields, including algebra, calculus, geometry, chemistry, biology, medicine, and astronomy.

In medicine, two Muslim physicians became very famous in Europe during this period: Al-Razi (c. 865–925) and Ibn Sina (Avicenna; c. 980–1037). Al-Razi identified smallpox and measles and also recognized fever as part of the body's defense mechanism. He wrote a 23-volume compendium of Chinese, Indian, Persian, Syrian, and Greek medicine [1]. Avicenna was known in the West as "the prince of physicians." His masterpiece work about Islamic medicine, *al-Qanun fi'l tibb* (The Law of Medicine), had full sovereignty in medical fields in Europe until 17th century. For 1,000 years, Avicenna remains known as one of the greatest thinkers and medical scholars in history. His most important medical works are the *Qanun (Canon) of Medicine* and a treatise on cardiac drugs [2].

Another eminent physician during this period was Ibn Al-Nafis, a 13th-century physician, who discovered pulmonary circulation [3].

Abu Al-Qasim Al-Zahrawi was considered the father of modern surgery. The old reports tell that there was great advancement in the fields of anesthesia and surgery. They used cannabis and opium for anesthesia and alcohol as an antiseptic [4].

During the Islamic Golden Age, a significant evolution took place in medicine and education. Hospitals became affiliated with universities. Despite the later decline of Islamic civilization, its effect on Western and modern medicine remained and is still evident today.

In general, there are no visual differences between Islam and modern medicine. Currently, there are advanced medical centers in some Islamic countries, and many Muslim scholars and physicians are working and practicing medicine in well-established medical centers around the world. Yet, a considerable number of Muslims continue to seek or practice traditional or complementary medicine. Prophetic medicine (Al-Tib Al-Nabawi) refers to a collection of sayings and actions of the Prophet Muhammad that are related to illness, diet, hygiene, and general health. Still, a majority of Muslims believe in the healing power of reading the Quran and reciting prayers that, in turn, impact spiritual and emotional health.

Truth Disclosure of Cancer in Islamic Culture

Cancer is considered to be a leading global health challenge, based on the rapid increase in incidence rates, high prevalence, and belated diagnoses. The poor outcome of cancer in developing countries has emanated from these above-mentioned facts. Offering treatment for cancer is witnessing a significant rise internationally, with an estimated $458 billion as the total spending budget by the year 2030 [5].

The truth disclosure for cancer or other life-threatening and grave medical conditions is now considered to be an essential issue in contemporary medical ethics in developed countries. Applying these ethical facts as equal fundamental principles to both Western and non-Western countries is truly challenging and may even be preposterous, given the context of the paramount and significant cultural diversity in truth-telling attitudes and practices.

Historically, many families of Islamic cultures tend to avoid telling newly diagnosed patients with cancer about the nature of their disease. Those with known cases of cancer may face the same attitude when malignancy becomes advanced and progresses rapidly, as their families tend to avoid telling them about the disease's progression. Families prefer to talk to their ill relatives about cure, even when it is unattainable, rather than about the real facts of the illness. Some health care professionals, in accord with the families, hide information from patients and, instead of talking with the patient, talk to other family members, given the nature of extended families in the community. For Iraqis, breaking bad news is the best example for this issue, as many people know about the new diagnosis of their family member before the patient knows. Parents, siblings, cousins, uncles, and so on believe that the truth might put further pressure on patients and make them feel hopeless and helpless, their dreams shattered and lost. Thus, decisions regarding treatment are made by the family and not the patient.

Screening reveals similar results. A considerable percentage of cancer patients in Turkey (44%) do not have any idea about their diagnosis. Approximately half of the physicians in Lebanon tell the patient facts about their cancer. Likewise, in Kuwait ,79% of physicians respect the family's request and hide the diagnosis from the patient. Seventy-five percent of Saudi Arabian physicians favor discussing information about the disease with close relatives rather than with the patients themselves, even if the mental capacity of those patients is stable [6].

Recently, the inclination to tell the truth underwent marked changes with further exposure of health care professionals to the external world and with increasing evidence confirming the benefits of sharing information about diagnosis, treatment and prognosis of diseases and future plans. It is now clear that, in the less developed regions, these acts may strengthen the relationship between patients and medical professionals and hiding information can further impact the anxiety of those patients.

One setback in this step is competing with the family's preference and will to hide information. The physician is caught in the middle between evidence-based medicine and cultural or family preferences.

In 2017, a cross-sectional study of cancer disclosure conducted in Saudi Arabia among a population aged 20 years and above showed the following results: the majority (86.5%) received information about cancer, 58% of them from media sources. Furthermore, 93% of the participants believed that it conceivable to recover from cancer. A significant number (82.5%) preferred that the patient be told about the disease, 37.8% of them believing that informing the patient would help in the course of treatment, whereas fewer participants (16.9%) had a negative response to disclosure [7].

In Iraq no data can be found pertaining to diagnosis disclosure among cancer patients. Current limited observations show that most adult patients are often informed about their diagnosis. Good communication between patient and caregiver has been viewed to be associated with better emotional coping and higher levels of satisfaction with symptom management. However, a large controversy remains concerning revealing news of terminal illness and progressive disease. Informed consent is required before starting treatment, and families tend to hide information from their elderly and children in an effort to avoid anxiety, dissatisfaction, and treatment rejection.

A Usual Case Scenario

UZ, a 38-year-old woman with terminal breast cancer and a mother of four teenage kids, requested to see her friend and neighbor, Dr. SA, a physician and pediatric oncologist. She brought along her medical records and asked her friend to clarify her medical condition. Dr. SA asked her if she had had any opportunity to meet with her physician and to know more details about the disease. She stated that her physician had told her she was responding and doing well. The next question was about how she was feeling. UZ answered, "I am doing well, but I have some pain." Her medical reports and investigations showed that her breast cancer had spread and was in the terminal stage. UZ looked insecure and was not sure about the information she had received from her physician. She observed her friend's reaction closely and silently tried to get some information. She was feeling that she had something worse than what she had been told by her physician. A few weeks later she passed away. She did not get the chance to discuss her feelings; she did not get the opportunity to be told the truth or to explain her hidden, but debilitating, anxiety. Her husband later told Dr. SA that he knew her condition was terminal and had asked her physician not to tell her the truth about the disease's progression, as he thought that secrecy would help to alleviate her anxiety. Furthermore, UZ did not have the chance to discuss her feelings with her husband or kids. Everyone surrounding her was hiding the truth. This scenario is most familiar and common in Iraqi culture.

Spiritual Care in an Islamic Context

Spirituality is defined as "an individual's sense of peace, purpose and connection to others, and beliefs about the meaning of life" that may be expressed through religion or other means, while religion is defined as a "set of beliefs and practices associated with a particular religious tradition or denomination" [8]. Spirituality is related to the aspect of humanity that refers to how individuals look for and express the meaning of life, and to the way they experience their connectedness to the moment, self, others, nature, and the significant or sacred [9].

In Iraq and many other similar cultures, religion and spirituality are intimately linked together by roots, aims, and applications. Spirituality can be expressed through an organized religion or can be related in another way to the individual's beliefs. For many people, religion and spirituality are synonymous; those who work through spirituality are generally known to be religious and vice versa. A smaller number of people practicing spirituality are nonreligious. The concept of spirituality centers around the relationship between the individual and God (Allah) and, therefore, elucidates the individual's sense of meaning, self-dignity, satisfaction, and relationship to others.

The roots of spirituality in Islam are clearly cataloged in the Quran and in Islam's two main sects, Sunni and Shiite. In the Quran, the term *pure heart* appears many times to emphasize that it is the source of worship and moral values. "But only one who comes to Allah with a sound heart, will be saved" (*Surah Ash-Shu'ara* [The Poets], Chapter 26: verse 89). The Quran says that people with a clean, unblemished heart can stand confidently in front of God at doomsday. Those who have a deep faith and a strong capacity to cope with disease and hard times are tested for the true beliefs they carry.

According to Islamic teaching, one way a person's own spirituality is realized is by observing religious rituals. Muslim patients believe that prayers, remembrance of God, repentance, and giving alms will increase their tolerance and patience [10].

Many Muslims believe that they can find all the answers to their existential questions in the Quran. They believe that the Quran is the solution for all kinds of physical, psychological, and even spiritual issues. Additionally, many doctrines postulate that the Quran protects them from black magic, the "evil eye," and envy, all of which can cause physical and emotional illnesses.

Spiritual care in Islam applies the skills and practices necessary to help patients achieve a good mental, physical, social, and emotional life, and it helps people cope with suffering. Through better understanding of the concepts of illness, terminal care, and death, they can seek and find hope.

Another aspect of spiritual care involves encouraging visitations to patients; these visits are considered to be indispensable and fundamental through offering help, comfort, and conversational companionship (Sohba). The Prophet Muhammad encouraged Muslims to say positive words to patients to help reduce their anxiety and bring mental relief. The concept of God being near to those who suffer from their illnesses and the concept of pain purifying them from sin and impurities are the most common coping mechanisms for Muslims. In Islamic ideology, being near to God (Allah) during illness has many meanings. This is considered to be a decisive step in the process of tolerating pain, as well as healing and curing, and it provides a magnificent coping mechanism.

The word "Ehsan," which denotes offering the sick or people with special needs assistance through financial, social, or, at least, pleasant utterances, is frequently mentioned in the Quran and in Islamic sayings. It also implies showing generosity and mercy to the grieving family of a deceased loved one through comfort and support during the funeral and burial processes.

The best way to express remembrance of God and read the Quran is to attend funerals, as they relieve distress and represent the ultimate opportunity to offer help, through solace and condolences, to those who have lost a loved one. Constructive spiritual care is applied in most developed countries and medical institutions of excellence. Culturally competent care, including Islamic-based care for Muslims with cancer or terminal illnesses, is offered in United States, Canada, and some European countries in addition to the Islamic countries. This care relies on religious practices and beliefs.

Generally, many low- and middle-income countries have no formal, dedicated, and structured spiritual care or even palliative care. Iraq lacks any well-planned spiritual care in most of its health institutions. The burden of care and social support lies with the family, and no governmental or official institutions practice or implement it as part of their services.

Along with the enormous pressures and work responsibilities of health care professionals in cancer units, spiritual and palliative care must be offered to patients with progressive malignancies and terminal illnesses. A major impediment facing physicians working in cancer units is their inability to incorporate spiritual care practices in the hospital setting when they have no background for what to offer and how to apply it. Therefore, it is imperative that they educate themselves about rituals and rites in the sector in which they work in order to help patients cope. This imperative is greatly hampered by the lack of spiritual and palliative care training available to physicians and health care professionals during their studies and clinical practice.

Some hospitals have established mosques in their setting, and sometimes, albeit infrequently, imams, the Muslims' spiritual leaders, come to hospitals to provide support and spiritual care to patients. However, in Iraq, this is a matter for the individual and is not officially sanctioned.

In areas of ethnic diversity, culturally based spiritual needs may vary depending on the social, cultural, and religious backgrounds of the population. Thus, promoting hope for some and emotional relief for others at a time of pain or at end of life may represent the structure of spiritual care in these settings.

Cancer Care in Iraq

As of 2020, Iraq's population was estimated at around 40 million. Data from Iraq's national cancer registry indicate that there were 33,873 newly diagnosed cancer cases in Iraq in 2020. Cancer is one of the leading causes of mortality in the country, contributing to an estimated 11% of total deaths. This figure does not reflect the true incidence of cancer in Iraq, for a significant number of cancer patients receive treatment abroad, mainly in neighboring countries such as Jordan, Lebanon, and Turkey, with a rising number being treated in India.

Iraq is an upper-middle-income country with profound political and economic instability, owing to its dependence on oil as their major financial source and the labile international price of oil barrels. It shares with most low- and middle-income countries (LMICs) the burden of a rise in cancer cases with all its consequences, including the readiness of diagnostic tools and the availability of treatment options. Still, many steps must be taken in order to improve cancer care; at the time of writing, chances for change are poor. One major issue blocking the provision of better care is the (free-of-charge) service of governmental institutions; although this may be helpful to many, it still needs to be studied and applied in well-planned protocols.

There are a few oncology hospitals in Iraq, and many oncology units, all affiliated with the Ministry of Health, are found in most governorates. The majority of cancer cases are treated in the capital of Baghdad, and fewer numbers are treated in other large cities such as Basra, Mosul, and Kurdistan. In the past few years, a few private-sector institutions have been established and have started providing cancer care, though the safety and efficacy of these services are questionable owing to the lack of quality control and supervision by higher authorities. Yet, many new advanced diagnostic tools, including cytogenetics, genetics, imaging, pathology, and other laboratory services are still missing or lack experts' interpretations. Positron emission tomography (PET) is now available in a few private sectors. There is a shortage of several new therapeutic interventions, including new chemotherapies and monoclonal antibodies, due to their high cost.

Radiotherapy is the standard treatment for many types of malignancies, but radiation machines are few in number in Iraq. Governmental machines are old and the new systems need well-trained technicians. The cost of private radiotherapy (available in a few centers) is expensive, and their standards are dubious. There is a 4- to 6-month waiting list for governmental services, whereas, in the private sector, immediate appointments are possible.

Surgical oncology is new and is limited to just a few surgeons who have practiced in this area for years. Most of the surgeries for oncology patients are performed by general surgeons, who may not immediately refer these cases to oncology centers. Sometimes patients initiate consultations only after experiencing a recurrence of tumors.

The Ministry of Health is struggling to overcome these challenges in cancer care and has recently established special committees and a program to send patients needing bone marrow transplantation or difficult surgeries to India, Lebanon, or Turkey.

With respect to pain management, Iraq has low opioid consumption, and current evidence has shown that pain management strategies and assessment of pain are suboptimal due to the shortage of medicines and inappropriate or limited regulations for their use and a highly restrictive approach. Another obstacle is the lack of training in analgesics prescriptions. Many preventive measures, such as strategies to control smoking, obesity, vaccinations for certain infections, and infection control policies, are nonexistent. All of these negative aspects, together with the insufficient number of multidisciplinary teams, have a negative impact on patients' quality of life.

To date, there are only limited data and studies in Iraq regarding the financial, social, and emotional burden on patients diagnosed with cancer and on their families. Generally, Iraq has inadequate resources for standard cancer care; this lack affects the country's mortality rate, end-of-life care, and hence, the quality of care offered to cancer patients. Screening programs can help to identify cancer earlier in order to increase the chances of cure and decrease the burden of terminal diseases. But these programs are mostly unavailable.

Palliative care incorporated with spiritual care is necessary, especially considering the significantly high cancer-related mortality rates in LMICs, which include most Islamic and Arabic countries such as Iraq. This care will help to reduce the burden of advanced disease on an already fragile health system.

Islamic Values and Beliefs Regarding Cancer Patients

The diagnosis of cancer often causes severe spiritual distress that affects the physical, mental, emotional, and social aspects of an individual's health. It might push the patients to question themselves about their faith. The reaction to cancer diagnosis is usually influenced by the patient's and family's beliefs and social and cultural backgrounds. Islam as a religion is interweaved with people's lives, including their manners and attitudes. Therefore, their professed faith intimately affects their reactions to stress, illness, and ways of coping in difficult times.

In Western and non-Islamic nations treating Islamic patients, delivering spiritual care and sometimes medical care requires an awareness of Islamic norms and beliefs, which can be obtained during an interview with the patient in the presence of a companion. Such interviews may include questions about their sexual and medical history, physical examination process, touch techniques, treatment types, sources of natural medicines, and issues of dietary restriction.

Although some Muslim women dress similarly to Western women, the majority dress more conservatively and usually cover their hair with a veil (hijab) and are more comfortable if the health care provider announces their arrival before entering the treatment room. They often prefer to be examined by a person of the same gender. Understanding these manners and values will help establish trust and enforce the relationship between the Muslim patient and the health care provider, providing a culturally competent relationship and religious-based care.

In Iraq and many other countries in the Middle East, South and Southeast Asia, and Africa, where Islam is the predominant religion, spiritual guidance based on the Islamic approach is thought to be effective in promoting good health and good coping mechanisms. Muslims' view of terminal illness as a test of faith stems from a saying of the Prophet Muhammad: "The greatest reward comes with the greatest trial. When Allah loves people, He tests them. Whoever accepts that wins His pleasure but whoever is discontent with that earns His wrath." This understanding of the nature of pain provides good coping strategies. Some Muslims attribute the pain of the illness to a form of punishment for past sins and believe that the pain will purify their souls before transitioning into the next world following death. They face their illnesses with patience and prayers. They read the Quran, along with their treatment plans, which may help lessen their anxiety and stress and give them hope about cure. "And when I am ill, it is He Who cures me"—*Surah Ash-Shu'ara* (The Poets), Chapter 26: verse 80.

The nuclear and extended family are usually the first to know about the disease, discuss treatment protocols, and make decisions regarding treatment. This might have a dual impact: a positive effect by reducing the stress and providing emotional support, and a negative effect by perhaps affecting the treatment plan and decisions about end-of-life care.

The belief that only God can know the circumstances of a death permits health professionals to continue avoiding speaking of death or incurability [11]. Patients with terminal diseases may insist on more active chemotherapy and may refuse palliative care, as they perceive palliative treatment to be equivalent to the end of life. Patients at advanced stages of their illness or their families may look for traditional or alternative therapies.

In Iraq, with all its ethnic diversities (mainly Shiite and Sunni), patients with cancer may seek help from religious clerics (the imam or sheik) who play an important role as either complementary or spiritual healer.

The Sunni school of thought advocates a practice called Roquia Sharia, through which a religious practitioner, having a very particular set of skills acquired over a long career, uses the Quran to cure diseases as they believe that the Quran has supernatural powers and can cure any illness.

With regard to the Shiite school of thought, people believe in the healing power of imam masooms (the masoom is a sinless person, never having committed any sinful act/the descendant of the Prophet Muhammad). They take their patients to the holy sites (the graves of imams) asking for cure or relief; this occurs mainly in the holy shrines of Karbala, Najaf, and Baghdad.

Why Spiritual Care?

Serious illness such as cancer may cause spiritual struggles and consequent crises. As a result, the patient may experience negative emotions encompassing shock, denial, anger, guilt, anxiety, depression, and loss of hope that influence their well-being and hampers a future comprehensive care plan. Spirituality and personal beliefs can create a positive mental status that helps the patient accept the diagnosis, feel better about themselves, and decrease the burden on the family and caregiver. Providing professional spiritual and culturally competent care helps the patient cope with their spiritual struggles and can result in reduced anxiety, depression, and anger; helps the patient adjust to the effects of cancer and side effects of treatment (better ability to cope); reduces the sense of feeling alone in the face of crisis and at a time of weakness; encourages the patient to find the strength to go on and enjoy life during cancer treatment; increases positive feelings, including optimism, feeling worthy, and beloved; improves quality of life, and helps to develop new perspectives on life issues.

At least 50% of patients favor discussing their religious or spiritual beliefs or concerns with their physician or other health professional [12]. A well-trained spiritual caregiver can provide a compassionate presence, promote active listening, and offer appropriate rituals and prayers based on the patient's individual beliefs and religion.

Barriers to Spiritual Care Provision in Iraq

In the Middle East, nearly one-half of hospital staff members say that they would like to provide spiritual care more often than they actually do [13]. To date, hospitals in Iraq do not provide structural spiritual care or have spiritual practice because there are many barriers to such care: notably, lack of knowledge in the area of spirituality; difficulty in defining spirituality; absence of clear guidelines for hospitals and health care professionals in providing spiritual care; lack of training and education on spiritual care; and nurses' and physicians' inadequate skills and competencies in providing such care.

Other barriers are related to patients' perceptions; the majority of patients are not even aware of the concept of spirituality. Some see it as a sensitive area and too personal to be addressed. Many patients fear death and prefer to deny it and so they avoid talking about this issue altogether. Even the family may not permit talk about death or terminal illness. The Iraqi individual is often shy and lacks the confidence to talk about their feelings and has insecurities that make the mission of providing spiritual-based care difficult. Aside from this, there is no designated, specific role for spiritual caregiving as a profession.

Conclusion

Cancers and chronic medical diseases are becoming a huge burden on the health system in countries with limited resources. Provision of appropriate, cultural-based models of care for cancer patients represents a big challenge worldwide. Spirituality has been recognized as an essential element for health and well-being, and it is crucial to the way cancer patients cope with their illness. Spirituality can create a more positive attitude toward cancer diagnosis and treatment. Every patient has their own spiritual needs based on religious beliefs and cultural background. Although the majority of research in spirituality has been conducted in Western countries, research on spirituality and cancer in the Middle East has increased in recent years. In Iraq, the main barriers to spiritual care provision are the lack of knowledge about it; the difficulty in defining spirituality; and the shortage of clear guidelines for hospitals and health care professionals for providing spiritual care.

References

1. Karagözoğlu B (ed.). Contribution of Muslim scholars to science and technology. In: *Science and Technology from Global and Historical Perspectives*. Cham, Switzerland: Springer pp. 137–184. 2017. doi.org/10.1007/978-3-319-52890-8_6
2. Chamsi-Pasha MA, Chamsi-Pasha H. Avicenna's contribution to cardiology. *Avicenna J Med*. 2014;4(1):9–12. doi:10.4103/2231-0770.127415
3. Soubani AO, Khan FA. The discovery of the pulmonary circulation revisited. *Ann Saudi Med*. 1995 Mar;15(2):185–186. doi: 10.5144/0256-4947.1995.185. PMID: 17587936
4. Martin-Araguz A, Bustamante-Martinez C, Fernandez-Armayor, Ajo V, Moreno-Martinez JM. Neuroscience in al-Andalus and its influence on medieval scholastic medicine, *Revista de neurología*. 2002;34(9):877–892.
5. Callahan R, Darzi A. Five policy levers to meet the value challenge in cancer care. *Health Aff*. 2015;34(9):1563–1568.
6. Kazdaglis GA, Arnaoutoglou C, Karypidis D, Memekidou G, Spanos G, Papadopoulos O. Disclosing the truth to terminal cancer patients: A discussion of ethical and cultural issues *East Medit Health J*. 2010;16(4):442–447.
7. Mansour EA, Pandaan IN, Gemeay EM, Al-Zayd AH, Alenize EK. Disclosure of cancer diagnosis to the patient: A cross-sectional assessment of public point-of-view in Saudi Arabia. *Arch Nurs Pract Care*. 2017;3(1):38–44.
8. National Cancer Institute. Spirituality in Cancer Care. 2009. Accessed from www through:http://www.cancer.gov/cancertopics/pdq/supportivecare/spirituality/Patient/page1.
9. Puchalski C, Ferrell B, Virani R, et al. Improving the quality of spiritual care as a dimension of palliative care: The report of the Consensus Conference. *J Palliat Med*. 2009;12:885–904.
10. Mottahari M. *Human in the Qur'an*. 8th ed. Qum: Sadra Pub, 1996:36.
11. Al-Shahri MZ. Islamic theology and the principles of palliative care. *Palliat Support Care*. 2016;14(6):635–640.
12. Pargament KI, Koenig HG, Tarakeshwar N, Hahn J. Religious struggle as a predictor of mortality among medically ill elderly patients: A two-year longitudinal study. *Arch Intern Med*, 2001;161(15):1881–1885.
13. Bar-Sela G, Schultz MJ, Elshamy K, et al. Training for awareness of one's own spirituality: A key factor in overcoming barriers to the provision of spiritual care to advanced cancer patients by doctors and nurses. *Palliat Support Care*. 2019 Jun;17(3):345–352.

33

The Impact of Latin American Cultural Values, Attitudes, and Preferences on Palliative Cancer Care

An Overview from Patients' and Families' Perspectives, Chile

Pamela Turrillas and Mariana Dittborn

"Regardless of the location,
at home or in the hospital as long as it happens by my side"
—*Brazilian caregiver* [1]

Palliative and End-of-Life Care

Latin America's demographic patterns of a progressively ageing population and high mortality associated with advanced chronic diseases have determined a growing need for palliative and end-of-life (PEoL) care delivery [2,3] as a regional priority for health care systems [4,5]. Approximately 20% of Latin Americans are expected to be older than 65 years of age by 2050 [6], and it is estimated that by 2030, 1.7 million cases of cancer will be diagnosed and more than one million cancer deaths will occur annually [7].

The development of PEoL care in the Latin American region is relatively recent, with incipient and progressive development having occurred after 1980 [8]. According to the Atlas of the Latin American Association of Palliative Care (ALCP) [8] and the Global Atlas of Palliative Care [9], PEoL care provision in the region is widely unequal, with 46% of existing PEoL care services serving just 10% of the population [9]. This disparate service provision is correlated with the differences within and across Latin American countries regarding size, urban-rural population, human development indexes, income indicators, poverty levels, and health care services development and resources [8,10]. Regional issues require adequate and contextualized planning from those responsible for public policies and the development of national health frameworks in order to provide good quality, respectful, and dignified care for those people living with advanced illness and approaching death, as well as their families [5,11].

According to the 2006 Declaration of Venice: Palliative Care Research in Developing Countries, research conducted in high-income countries is only partially beneficial and is not necessarily applicable to developing countries [12]. Differences in patients' demographic characteristics, illness trajectory, care setting, culture, and preferences give place to a wide range of end-of-life and illness experiences. These differences might eventually act as barriers or facilitators upon PEoL care access, use, and delivery [13]. Additionally, differences in PEoL care service models may lead to variations in understandings, attitudes, and preferences toward PEoL care [14]. For PEoL care to be effective and comprehensively delivered, it has to be grounded on the particular cultural context in which it is to be implemented [15–18].

The Latin American Cultural Context

PEoL care is a patient-centered model that seeks to improve the quality of life of patients and their families living with life-limiting illnesses [9] through a comprehensive and multidimensional assessment and management that includes, but is not limited to, pain and symptom control, psychosocial care, spiritual care, surrogate decision making and advance care planning and end-of-life medical decisions [9,13,19].

For PEoL care to be optimal, each individual's unique experiences, beliefs, and values should orient every single clinical encounter. Health care providers should ensure that these are at the center of care plans and decisions, and create the care environment that allows patients and caregivers to develop the knowledge, skills, and confidence to make informed decisions about their health care [15,20].

Understanding patients' values, beliefs, attitudes, and preferences is essential in shaping the care to be delivered to them. Research on PEoL care in Latin America has steadily increased over the last two decades. It is primarily focused on service provision and symptom control, but it also includes patients' and caregivers' attitudes and preferences toward PEoL care [21]. Furthermore, most widely known evidence-based literature on Latinx values and beliefs toward PEoL care comes from immigrant-focused studies. Acculturation—the process through which individuals adjust to a new culture [22]—and significant differences in service structures [14] might this evidence does not accurately represent the Latin American population in their countries of origin.

Organizational leaders and policymakers should promote research activity in the region, consider locally developed evidence, and work with civil society to integrate stakeholders' values, views, and experiences in the development of PEoL care policies and national frameworks [23].

Integrating Latinx Cultural Values into Palliative and End-of-Life Cancer Care

Traditional Latinx values such as *familismo*, respect, *personalismo*, religiosity, *fatalismo*, and *dignidad* play an important role in patients', caregivers', and communities' experiences and behaviors toward PEoL care. Acknowledgment of these values is essential to progress toward developing a culture-centered palliative care model for this population [16].

Familismo, Personalismo, and Respect

Family is a key cornerstone of a person's life, including well-being and care. *Familismo*, a traditional value acknowledged in Latin American culture, places emphasis on family loyalty and cohesion. There is a sense of connection and interdependence among family members which involves a broad network of support that may include not only first-degree relatives but also extended family members, friends, and neighbors [18,24].

Latin American family structure has undergone profound changes in recent decades. New and diverse forms of families, smaller sizes and female-headed households are continuously increasing in the region. These new structures are also highly variable within and across countries due to their association with socioeconomic factors [24]. Despite moving from a "male breadwinner model" to a "dual-earner model," the traditional patriarchal family structure and the female caregiver model persist, maintaining gender inequalities, among other factors, regarding access to paid work and thus perpetuating poverty [25]. Deficient provision of social protection in Latin America also contributes to the need for the family to protect its members by their own means [24].

Values such as solidarity and support are reciprocal among members of the family. Likewise, there is a common sense of duty or obligation in providing material and emotional support to members of the extended family [26]. Closely related, filial obligation is associated not only with loyalty among family members, but also with respect, or *respeto*, for the elders of the group, entailing a perception of relatives as behavioral and attitudinal referents. Under this collectivist worldview, the extended Latinx family plays a significant role in making important decisions together with or without the patients themselves, explaining why individuals might sacrifice their needs over the needs of the family [22].

Hence, the broadly accepted idea of autonomous decision making, which endorses self-determination to make informed decisions about medical care, needs to be balanced and understood within the context of cultural values. An individualistic approach might be perceived as contradictory to the prevailing family-centered values and the social meaning of individual competency [27]. Autonomy might be best understood from a relational perspective where decisions, including PEoL care decisions, affect and are affected by others [28].

In Latin America, hierarchical relationships are the prominent role model in family dynamics and in the communities in general. Respect for authority figures as well as a person' sociodemographic characteristics such as age, gender, and socioeconomic status determine the type of relationship between individuals [24]. This is also observed in relationships between health care professionals and patients and their families, in which professionals are perceived and regarded as an authority, whose judgments are strongly taken into account in the decision-making process [22]. Despite this traditional hierarchical social paradigm, Latin Americans' social role and public engagement have changed profoundly over the last two decades. Citizens across the region are increasingly demanding more rights and opportunities to actively participate in shaping the policies that affect their lives [29].

Additionally, Latin American patients and their families tend to develop personal and trusting relationships with health care professionals—*personalismo*—which encourages friendliness, appropriate physical contact, smooth communication, and cooperation [26]. Kindness, or *simpatía,* is also important in this interaction and reflects the clinician's ability to be polite and pleasant even in the face of stress [30]. On the other hand, patients and their family members expect respect to be reciprocal; lack of respect in the relationship, together with detachment and ineffective communication, might lead to the patient's dissatisfaction with care, nonadherence to treatment, and poor compliance with medical advice [1,31]. These values in relationships are built over time and require reciprocity. The clinician also shares self-disclosure around personal information, creating an environment of trust and confidence. Eventually, these values might be more important when selecting a practitioner than their professional credentials. However, this behavior may vary depending on patients' socioeconomic status [22].

Spirituality and Religiosity, *Fatalismo,* and *Dignidad*

Religion and spirituality are important principles in the lives of many Latin Americans. Beliefs and values associated with religion and spirituality are diverse, determined by the many dimensions of these aspects in the region due to an ethnic composition originating from multiple indigenous groups and a strong European and African influence [32]. Spirituality has a broader meaning than religion or faith, encompassing the subjective experiences of a deeper and more meaningful vision according to which people live and how they connect with the moment, with themselves, with others, with nature, and with the sacred dimension [33]. However, the terms *religion* and *spirituality* might still frequently be used interchangeably in the region [34].

Latin America represents almost 40% of the world's total Roman Catholic population; two-thirds of the Latinx people declare that religion is very important in their lives. In recent decades, however, identification with Catholicism has declined throughout the region, along with an increase in Protestant and nonreligious affiliations. Many Latin Americans, including Catholics and Protestants, report adopting beliefs and practices that are often associated with Afro-Caribbean, Afro-Brazilian, and indigenous religions such as the *"evil eye,"* witchcraft, and reincarnation. Religiosity and religious practices vary greatly within and between Latin American countries, and gender, age, and professed faith are factors that determine, for example, participation in religious services and frequency of prayer [32].

Latin Americans also commonly express *fatalismo,* the strong belief that uncertainty is inherent to life and one should accept each day coming with its own fate. This belief is manifested in the conviction that one should consider cancer as a death sentence or pain and illness as God's punishment [30]. Thus, when experiencing illness and suffering, patients and families will turn to spiritual practices and religious communities as sources of strength to face their sorrow [1].

Closely related to compassionate care is *dignidad*, which is associated with feeling worthy and valued, and being respected by others. At the end of life, patients may fear being treated inhumanely, feeling vulnerable by their physical appearance or functional decline associated with dependency on others. These concerns about the loss of autonomy in daily activities or in managing their own medication and, consequently, becoming a burden for their family caregivers, may impact a patient's sense of worthiness [18].

Attitudes and Preferences Regarding Palliative and End-of-Life Care

As cultural values form people's attitudes and behaviors toward health care, common practices in PEoL care, such as truth-telling, involvement in decision-making processes, and implementation of advance directives may vary among cultures [35,36]. However, considering the wide variability in traditions, socioeconomic status and PEoL care development in the region, inaccurate regional stereotypes and generalizations across or within countries should be avoided [21].

Mixed Understandings around PEoL Care and Pain Relief

As in other regions [37], Latin American patients and caregivers hold mixed understandings about PEoL care's scope and meaning. Although some consider it to be a model of care that is focused on quality of life and that includes patients and families as the unit of care [1,38–41], many still associate the concept of PEoL care with death [39] and abandonment [40–43], interpreting a referral to the palliative care team as neglect by the health care system.

Similarly, misunderstandings regarding pain relief and opioid use are common among patients, caregivers, and health care professionals. Pain is one of the most concerning symptoms for caregivers [44,45], who are proactive in looking for different means to alleviate their patient's suffering, including the use of popular remedies and rituals. However, some patients and caregivers would regard pain as part of the disease and therefore something that has to be borne [46,47]. At the same time, patients' awareness of pain relief as a right seems to be increasing [46,48], validating this symptom to be acknowledged, objectivated, communicated, and managed [46–48]. However, opiophobia is common among patients and caregivers [46,47,49], including fears that opioid use will lead to addiction or that it could hasten the patient's death. The belief that morphine is used as a last-resort medication and implies imminent death is acknowledged as an important barrier to pain management in the region [50,51].

Information and Decision-Making Processes

Considering *familismo* and the collectivistic view of Latino society, patients have traditionally been regarded as passive actors in the decision-making processes related to their health, leaving families with the responsibility of managing information and decisions [22,52,53]. However, it is important to note that recent studies conducted in the region suggest this might be not the case. Patients tend to have a general preference to be informed about their diagnosis and prognosis [45,48,54–57] and prefer to be involved in the decision-making processes, with or without sharing this information with their families—commonly referred to as active and passive decision-making styles [58,59]. As for caregivers, they tend to withhold information about diagnosis and prognosis from the patient, an attitude that is frequently based on fears that this will take away the patient's hope and trigger their further deterioration [42,47,55,60]. This attitude, together with a wider reluctance to openly discuss death and dying in society [47] and the lack of legal frameworks on advance directives and PEoL decisions in most Latin American countries [15] might operate as barriers against integrating patients' values and preferences in their care at the end of life.

Place of Care, Place of Death, and the Caregiver's Role

Meeting patients' preferences regarding place of care and place of death is considered a priority for the delivery of good quality PEoL care [61,62]. In a culture where family includes extended relations, friends, and neighbors, for many home is considered as a more comfortable and familiar place, allowing more autonomy and freedom for both patients and caregivers, and more flexibility to receive visits and support from relatives and friends [1,40,42,44,47,63]. For others, hospital is preferred because it is considered a sign of hope for cure and because it provides more intensive measures as well as a more reliable financial, emotional, and professional source of support for both patients and caregivers [1,42,47,54]. However, we ought to consider that, given the scarce development of home PEoL care services in the region, these preferences are likely to be determined not only by patients and caregivers' wishes but for access to good care in the preferred environment [64].

Caregivers, mostly women, are generally positive about taking the caregiver's role, driven by feelings of love, retribution, and reciprocity [41–43,45,47,65–67] and also considering it as a faith-based mission [39.42,67]. However, some caregivers will take this responsibility to fulfill their social obligation or filial duty [43,47,65,66] after a family agreement [65] or because of the lack of alternative means to provide care. Caregivers are generally enthusiastic and committed to their role, learning new skills to provide better care and looking for solutions to the problems they face [1,41–44,55,65,67,68]. However, many are overburdened and sacrifice themselves by neglecting their personal care and relationships. Feelings of uncertainty and fear are also common, especially when facing the active dying process and symptom exacerbation for those caring for their relatives at home [1,40,41–45,47,55,66,67]. Caregivers are emotionally and financially overburdened and feel frustrated and helpless because of the lack of support, knowledge, and skills needed to provide care and comfort to their relatives. In response, they ask for appropriate training, continuous professional support, and access to homecare services [40,44,45].

Spiritual Care and the Relationship with Clinicians

When facing advanced cancer and death, religious rituals and religious community support are sources of strength, comfort [69,70] and peace to patients and caregivers alike [1,47,54,55,65]. This includes an important role of the priest or religious leader during the illness and death experience. For many, faith is the motivation to devote themselves to their relative's care [41,48,55], and it is a source of both hope for cure and acceptance of God's will in the time and the context of death. In this sense, hope for cure and acceptance of death are commonly experienced simultaneously [43,71].

Spiritual pain is expressed in terms of "heartache" and "soul ache," which are healed with prayer and relationships with loved ones [72]. Although some might wish to address spiritual care by openly talking about God and faith as a source of hope and strength during the process, most patients and caregivers associate the spiritual dimension of their care with receiving dignified, humanized, and compassionate care, without necessarily addressing faith and religion issues explicitly with the health care team. Patients and caregivers appreciate cheerful and optimistic clinicians who support their hopes, and they also welcome being cared for by approachable, reliable, and compassionate professionals who take the time to listen to them, understand their suffering, and demonstrate genuine interest in helping them [40,42,48,54,68,73,74].

Final Considerations

Latin America's demographic changes have produced an increasing demand for appropriate care for those experiencing advanced illness and for their families. To respond to this demand, understanding cultural values, attitudes, and preferences toward PEoL care is pivotal in providing good quality care grounded within the context of local needs. The significant growth in regional research activity in this field shows the commitment to achieving a comprehensive understanding of patients' and families' needs, views, and experiences and encouraging further development of PEoL care services in Latin America. As described, traditional Latinx values continue to play an essential role in shaping PEoL care experiences. However, Latin American societies are undergoing a transformation process associated with sociodemographic and cultural changes that have an impact on people's PEoL care experiences, that is, a stronger demand for both active participation in public policies and individual health care decisions. Changes in the traditional family structure have an impact on the availability and disposition of relatives to undertake the informal caregiver role. Considering the views of patients, caregivers, and communities in national frameworks, training programs, and service development is essential if Latin American countries are to achieve universal health care coverage.

References

1. Pinheiro M, Demutti F, Martins P, Murillo De Oliveira Rafael C, Tupinambá U, De Lima S. Oncological patient in palliative care: the perspective of the family caregiver. *J Nurs UFPE line*. 2016;10(5):1749–1755. doi:10.5205/reuol.9003-78704-1-SM.1005201622

2. Mathers CD, Loncar D. Projections of global mortality and burden of disease from 2002 to 2030. *PLoS Med.* 2006;3(11):2011–2030. doi:10.1371/journal.pmed.0030442

3. Krakauer EL, Kwete X, Verguet S, et al. Palliative Care and Pain Control. In: Jamison DT, Gelband H, Horton S, et al., editors. Disease Control Priorities: Improving Health and Reducing Poverty. 3rd edition. Washington (DC): The International Bank for Reconstruction and Development / The World Bank; 2017 Nov 27. Chapter 12. Available from: https://www.ncbi.nlm.nih.gov/books/NBK525276/ doi: 10.1596/978-1-4648-0527-1_ch12

4. National Palliative and End of Life Partnership Care. *Ambitions for Palliative and End of Life Care: A National Framework for Local Action 2015–2020*; 2015. September 2015 Available online at http://endoflifecareambitions.org.uk/

5. Field MJ, Cassel CK. Approaching death: Improving care at the end of life. *Health Prog.* 2011;92(1):25.

6. Comisión Económica para América Latina y el Caribe (CEPAL). *Observatorio Demográfico, 2019.* Santiago; 2020.

7. Goss PE, Lee BL, Badovinac-Crnjevic T, et al. Planning cancer control in Latin America and the Caribbean. *Lancet Oncol.* 2013;14(5):391–436. doi:10.1016/S1470-2045(13)70048-2

8. Pastrana T, De Lima L, Pons JJ, Centeno C. *Atlas de Cuidados Paliativos En Latinoamérica-Edición Cartográfica.* 2013; Houston: IAHPC Press.

9. Connor SR, Sepulveda Bermedo MC. *Global Atlas of Palliative Care at the End of Life* Worldwide Hospice Palliative Care Alliance and World Health Organization, London UK, Geneva; 2014.

10. Pastrana T, Eisenchlas J, Centeno C, De Lima L. Status of palliative care in Latin America: Looking through the Latin America Atlas of palliative care. *Curr Opin Support Palliat Care.* 2013;7(4):411–416. doi:10.1097/SPC.0000000000000008

11. The General Medical Council. Treatment and care towards the end of life. 2010:10.

12. The European Association for Palliative Care, International Association for Hospice and Palliative Care. The Declaration of Venice: Palliative care research in developing countries. *J Pain Palliat Care Pharmacother.* 2007;21(1):31–33. doi:10.1080/J354v21n01

13. Mularski RA, Dy SM, Shugarman LR, et al. A systematic review of measures of end-of-life care and its outcomes. *Health Serv Res.* 2007;42(5):1848–1870. doi:10.1111/j.1475-6773.2007.00721.x

14. Cain CL, Surbone A, Elk R, Kagawa-Singer M. Culture and palliative care: Preferences, communication, meaning, and mutual decision making. *J Pain Symptom Manage.* 2018;55(5):1408–1419. doi:10.1016/j.jpainsymman.2018.01.007 Epub 2018 Jan 31. PMID: 29366913.

15. Soto-Perez-de-Celis E, Chavarri-Guerra Y, Pastrana T, Ruiz-Mendoza R, Bukowski A, Goss PE. End-of-life care in Latin America. *J Glob Oncol.* 2017;3(3):261–270. doi:10.1200/JGO.2016.005579

16. Steinberg S. Cultural and religious aspects of palliative care. *Int J Crit Illn Inj Sci.* 2011;1(2):154–156. doi:10.4103/2229-5151.84804

17. Clark D. Cultural considerations in planning palliative and end of life care. *Palliat Med.* 2012;26(3):195–196. doi:10.1177/0269216312440659

18. Adames HY, Chavez-Dueñas NY, Fuentes MA, Salas SP, Perez-Chavez JG. Integration of Latino/a cultural values into palliative health care: A culture centered model. *Palliat Support Care.* 2014;12(2):149–157. doi:10.1017/S147895151300028X

19. Blank RH. End-of-Life decision making across cultures. *J Law, Med Ethics.* 2011;39(2):201–214. doi:10.1111/j.1748-720X.2011.00589.x

20. Steinhauser K, Christakis N, Clipp E, et al. Preparing for the end of life: Preferences of patients, families, and other care providers. *J Pain Symptom Manage.* 2001;22(3):727–737.

21. Dittborn M, Turrillas P, Maddocks M, Leniz J. Attitudes and preferences towards palliative and end of life care in patients with advanced illness and their family caregivers in Latin

America: A mixed studies systematic review. *Palliative Medicine.* 2021;35(8):1434–1451. doi:10.1177/02692163211029514.

22. Del Rio N. The influence of Latino ethnocultural factors on decision making at the end of life: withholding and withdrawing artificial nutrition and hydration. *J Soc Work End Life Palliat Care.* 2010;6(3-4):125–149. doi:https://dx.doi.org/10.1080/15524256.2010.529009

23. World Health Assembly. WHA67.19 Strengthening of palliative care as a component of comprehensive care throughout the life course. *Sixty-seventh World Heal Assem.* 2014;(May):5. https://apps.who.int/iris/handle/10665/162863

24. Sunkel G. *El Papel de La Familia En La Protección Social En América Latina.* Santiago, Chile; 2006.

25. OECD. Gender inequality in unpaid work. In: *The Pursuit of Gender Equality: An Uphill Battle.* Paris: OECD Publishing; 2017.

26. Santiago-Rivera A. Latino values ad family transitions: Practical considerations for counseling. *Counsel Hum Dev.* 2003;35(6):1–12.

27. Elliott AC. Health care ethics: Cultural relativity of autonomy. *J Transcult Nurs.* 2001;12(4):326–330. doi:10.1177/104365960101200408

28. Gómez-Vírseda C, de Maeseneer Y, Gastmans C. Relational autonomy: What does it mean and how is it used in end-of-life care? A systematic review of argument-based ethics literature. *BMC Med Ethics.* 2019;20(1):76. doi:10.1186/s12910-019-0417-3

29. OECD, Cumbre Ministerial Virtual sobre inclusión social OCDE-America Latina y el Caribe. *Diálogo social inclusivo y participación ciudadana para mejorar la cohesión social y la identificación con las medidas de recuperación*; OECD Publishing; 2020.

30. Carteret M. Cultural Values of Latino Patients and Families. Dimension of Culture. https://www.dimensionsofculture.com/2011/03/cultural-values-of-latino-patients-and-families/ Accessed October 2020. https://healthyhispanicliving.com/healthcare_policy/personalized_care/cultural_values_of_latino_patients_and_families/

31. Flores G, Abreu M, Schwartz I, Hill M. The importance of language and culture in pediatric care: Case studies from the Latino community. *J Pediatr.* 2000;137(6):842–848. doi:https://doi.org/10.1067/mpd.2000.109150

32. Pew Research Center. *Religion in Latin America. Widespread Change in a Historically Catholic Region*; Washington, DC, 2014.

33. Puchalski CM, Vitillo R, Hull SK, Reller N. Improving the spiritual dimension of whole person care: Reaching national and international consensus. *J Palliat Med.* 2014;17(6):642–656. doi:10.1089/jpm.2014.9427

34. Thiengo PCS, Gomez A, Mercês M, et al. Spirituality and religiosity in health care: An integrative review. *Cogitare enferm.* 2019; e58692:24.

35. Kwak J, Haley WE. Current research findings on end-of-life decision making among racially or ethnically diverse groups. *The Gerontologist.* 2005;45(5):634–641.

36. Searight HR, Gafford J. Cultural diversity at the end of life: Issues and guidelines for family physicians. *Am Fam Physician.* 2005;71(3):515–522.

37. Patel P, Lyons L. Examining the knowledge, awareness, and perceptions of palliative care in the general public over time: A scoping literature review. *Am J Hosp Palliat Care.* 2020;37(6):481–487. doi:10.1177/1049909119885899

38. Cardona MJM, Herrera M del CZ. Necesidad de cuidados culturalmente congruentes en personas con enfermedad cardiovascular al final de la vida. *Enfermeria.* 2017;6(1):25–36.

39. Nunes M da G dos S, Rodrigues BMRD. Tratamento paliativo: Perspectiva da família. *Rev Enferm.* 2012;20(3):338–343.

40. Oliveira M do BP de, Souza NR de, Bushatsky M, Dâmaso BFR, Bezerra DM, Brito JA de. Oncological homecare: Family and caregiver perception of palliative care. *Esc Anna Nery - Rev Enferm.* 2017;21(2):1–6. doi:10.5935/1414-8145.20170030

41. de Andrade Ramalho MN, Da Silva LB, Mangueira SDO, Silva TC de L e, De Lucena CH, Pinto MB. Cuidados paliativos: percepção de familiares cuidadores de pessoas com câncer/ Palliative care: The perception of family caregivers of cancer patients. *Ciência, Cuid e Saúde.* 2018;17(2):1–7. doi:10.4025/cienccuidsaude.v17i2.39276

42. Oliveira SG, Quintana AM, Denardin-Budó M de L, et al. Representações sociais do cuidado de doentes terminais no domicílio: O olhar do cuidador familiar. *Aquichan.* 2016;16(3):359–369. doi:10.5294/aqui.2016.16.3.7

43. Marchi JA, de Paula CC, Girardon-Perlini NMO, Sales CA. Significado de ser-cuidador de familiar com câncer e dependente: Contribuições para a paliação. *Texto e Context Enferm.* 2016;25(1):1–8. doi:10.1590/0104-07072016007600014

44. Carrillo GM, Arias-Rojas M, Carreno SP, et al. Looking for control at the end of life through the bond: A grounded theory on the hospital discharge process in palliative care. *J Hosp Palliat Nurs.* 2018;20(3):296–303. doi:https://dx.doi.org/10.1097/NJH.0000000000000447

45. Rocío L, Rojas EA, González MC, Carreño S, Diana C, Gómez O. Experiences of patient-family caregiver dyads in palliative care during hospital-to-home transition process. *Int J Palliat Nurs.* 2017;23(7):332–339. doi:10.12968/ijpn.2017.23.7.332

46. Alonso JP. Treatment for cancer pain at the end of life: A case study in a palliative care service in the Autonomous City of Buenos Aires. *Salud Colect.* 2013;9(1):41–52. doi:https://dx.doi.org/10.1590/S1851-82652013000100004

47. Luxardo N, Brage E, Alvarado C. An examination of advanced cancer caregivers' support provided by staff interventions at hospices in Argentina. *ecancer.* 2012;6(1):1–10. doi:10.3332/ecancer.2012.281

48. Villas Boas de Carvalho M, Barbosa Merighi MA. O cuidar no processo de morrer na percepção de mulheres com câncer: uma atitude fenomenológica. *Rev latino-americana enfermagem.* 2005;13(6):951–959. doi:10.1590/s0104-11692005000600006

49. Jiménez AMC, González M, Ángel MCV, Krikorian A. Impacto familiar de la sedación paliativa en pacientes terminales desde la perspectiva del cuidador principal. *Psicooncologia.* 2016;13(2–3):351–365. doi:10.5209/PSIC.54441

50. Rico MA, Campos Kraychete D, Jreige Iskandar A, et al. Use of opioids in Latin America: The need of an evidence-based change. *Pain Med.* 2016;17(4):704–716. doi:10.1111/pme.12905

51. García CA, Santos Garcia JB, Rosario Berenguel Cook M del, et al. Undertreatment of pain and low use of opioids in Latin America. *Pain Manag.* 2018;8(3):181–196. doi:10.2217/pmt-2017-0043

52. Blackhall LJ, Frank G, Murphy ST, Michel V, Palmer JM, Azen SP. Ethnicity and attitudes towards life sustaining technology. *Soc Sci Med.* 1999;48(12):1779–1789.

53. Kreling B, Selsky C, Perret-Gentil M, Huerta EE, Mandelblatt JS, Coalition LACR. 'The worst thing about hospice is that they talk about death': Contrasting hospice decisions and experience among immigrant Central and South American Latinos with US-born white, non-Latino cancer caregivers. Banks S, Caicedo L, Canar J, et al. (eds). *Palliat Med.* 2010;24(4):427–434. doi:https://dx.doi.org/10.1177/0269216310366605

54. Galvão MIZ, Borges M da S, Pinho DLM. Comunicação interpessoal com pacientes oncológicos em cuidados paliativos TT—Interpersonal communication with oncological patients in palliative care. *Rev baiana enferm.* 2017;31(3):1–12. doi:10.18471/rbe.v31i3.22290

55. Inocenti A, Rodrigues IG, Miasso AI. Vivências e sentimentos do cuidador familiar do paciente oncológico em cuidados paliativos. Rev. Eletr. Enferm. [Internet]. 31º de dezembro de 2009 [citado 9º de outubro de 2021];11(4):858–865. Disponível em: https://revistas.ufg.br/fen/article/view/5197

56. Justo Roll I, Simms V, Harding R. Multidimensional problems among advanced cancer patients in Cuba: Awareness of diagnosis is associated with better patient

status. *J Pain Symptom Manag.* 2009;37(3):325–330. doi:https://dx.doi.org/10.1016/j.jpainsymman.2008.02.015

57. Palma A, Cartes F, Gonzalez M, et al. ¿Cuánta información desean recibir y cómo prefieren tomar sus decisiones pacientes con cáncer avanzado atendidos en una Unidad del Programa Nacional de Dolor y Cuidados Paliativos en Chile? [Information disclosure and decision making preferences of patien.] *Rev Med Chil.* 2014;142(1):48–54. doi:https://dx.doi.org/10.4067/S0034-98872014000100008

58. Yennurajalingam S, Rodrigues LF, Shamieh OM, et al. Decisional control preferences among patients with advanced cancer: An international multicenter cross-sectional survey. *Palliat Med.* 2018;32(4):870–880. doi:https://dx.doi.org/10.1177/0269216317747442

59. Yennurajalingam S, Parsons HA, Duarte ER, et al. Decisional control preferences of Hispanic patients with advanced cancer from the United States and Latin America. *J Pain Symptom Manag.* 2013;46(3):376–385. doi:https://dx.doi.org/10.1016/j.jpainsymman.2012.08.015

60. Allende-Pérez S., Cantú-quintanilla G., Verástegui-Avilés E. La trascendencia del Consentimiento Informado en bioética y la complejidad de informar al paciente terminal su pronóstico en la primera visita: visión del paciente y familiares en el Instituto Nacional de Cancerología. *Gac Mex Oncol.* 2013;12(4):244–249.

61. Gomes B, Calanzani N, Gysels M, Hall S, Higginson IJ. Heterogeneity and changes in preferences for dying at home: a systematic review. *BMC Palliat Care.* 2013;12(1):7. doi:10.1186/1472-684X-12-7

62. Gomes B, Higginson IJ, Calanzani N, et al. Preferences for place of death if faced with advanced cancer: A population survey in England, Flanders, Germany, Italy, the Netherlands, Portugal and Spain. *Ann Oncol Off J Eur Soc Med Oncol.* 2012;23(8):2006–2015. doi:10.1093/annonc/mdr602

63. Oliveira SG, Quintana AM, Budó M de LD, Kruse MHL, Beuter M. Home care and hospital assistance: Similarities and differences from the perspective of the family caregiver. *Texto e Context Enferm.* 2012;21(3):591–599. doi:10.1590/S0104-07072012000300014

64. Grunfeld E, Urquhart R, Mykhalovskiy E, Johnston G, Burge FI, Craig C. Toward population-based indicators of quality end-of-life care: Testing stakeholder agreement. *Cancer.* 2008;112(10):2301–2308. doi:10.1002/cncr.23428

65. Moraes e Silva CA, Acker JIBV. O cuidado paliativo domiciliar sob a ótica de familiares responsáveis pela pessoa portadora de neoplasia. *Rev Bras Enferm.* 2007;60(2):150–154. doi:10.1590/s0034-71672007000200005

66. Queiroz AHAB, Pontes RJS, Souza ÂMA e, Rodrigues TB. Percepção de familiares e profissionais de saúde sobre os cuidados no final da vida no âmbito da atenção primária à saúde,. *Ciênc saúde coletiva.* 2013;18(9):2615–2623.

67. Sena EL da S, de Carvalho PAL, Reis HFT, Rocha MB. Percepção de familiares sobre o cuidado à pessoa com câncer em estágio avançado. *Texto e Context Enferm.* 2011;20(4):774–781. doi:10.1590/S0104-07072011000400017

68. Silva MM, Moreira MC, Leite JL, Erdmann AL. Análise do Cuidado de Enfermagem e da Participação dos Familiares na Atenção Paliativa Oncológica. *Texto e Context Enferm.* 2012;21(3):658–666. doi:10.1590/S0104-07072012000300022

69. Delgado-Guay MO, Palma A, Duarte ER, et al. Spirituality, religiosity, spiritual pain, and quality of life among Latin American patients with advanced cancer (LAAdCa): A multicenter study. In: *2016 Palliative and Supportive Care in Oncology Symposium;* 2016;34:(26_suppl):246–246.

70. Delgado-Guay MO, Palma A, Duarte ER, et al. Spirituality, religiosity, spiritual pain, and quality of life among caregivers of Latin American patients with advanced cancer: A multicenter study. *J Clin Oncol.* 2016;34(26_Suppl):245. doi:10.1200/jco.2016.34.26_suppl.245

71. Oliveira SG, Quintana AM, Denardin-Budó M de L, Moraes N de A de, Lüdtke MF, Cassel PA. Internação domiciliar do paciente terminal: o olhar do cuidador familiar. *Rev Gaúcha Enferm.* 2012;33(3):104–110. doi:10.1590/s1983-14472012000300014

72. Delgado-Guay MO, McCollom S, Palma A, et al. Spirituality among Latino caregivers of patients with advanced cancer: A qualitative study. *J Clin Oncol.* 2017;35(31_Suppl):180. doi:10.1200/JCO.2017.35.31_suppl.180

73. Alonso JP. Cuidados paliativos: Entre la humanización y la medicalización del final de la vida. *Cienc e Saude Coletiva.* 2013;18(9):2541–2548. doi:10.1590/S1413-81232013000900008

74. Araújo MMT, da Silva MJP. Communication with patients in palliative care: favouring cheerfulness and optimism. *Rev da Esc Enferm.* 2007;41(4):668–674. doi:10.1590/s0080-62342007000400018

34

The Impact of Culture and Belief on Cancer Care in Costa Rica, Costa Rica

Ana Barrantes Ramírez and Isaías Salas Herrera

Colonial Times

With Christopher Columbus's discovery of America in 1492, the Spaniards arrived to the continent with new ideas; however, they also brought with them a series of diseases such as smallpox, typhoid fever, syphilis, measles, flu, dysentery, and malaria. The indigenous people did not have the immunity to defend themselves against these new diseases, which led to an even higher morbidity and mortality rate than that caused by the battles between the explorers and the native population [1]. All of these new vulnerabilities, along with the deplorable health conditions of the region's people, caused infectious contagious diseases to be extremely lethal and to spread rapidly, resulting in the death of thousands of indigenous people in those communities and territories [1].

Another important factor resulting from the cultural introduction of the Spanish people to the Americas, according to Ibarra (1998) was the socioeconomic impact of these diseases. The native communities dispersed, and the resulting loss of crops led to famine and death for these impoverished and starving populations. The indigenous groups relocated in order to seek better conditions for planting their crops and feeding themselves. This nomadic behavior led to the propagation of diseases to other communities, resulting in serious health repercussions [1].

Concerned with finding solutions to their health problems, the indigenous people adopted beliefs in the healing properties of medicinal plants, either by cultivating them on their own or finding them in the nearby mountains. These practices became very common in the 18th century.

The Role of Witchdoctors, Healers, and other Actors

Later on, doctors, midwives, and healers emerged, playing an important role in preventing the spread of disease in Costa Rica. The practice of folk medicine was performed by both men and women, especially the elderly, who were deemed wise. In 1805, the government of Tomás Acosta (1744–1821) introduced inoculations, improving the immunological conditions of the population. In this endeavor, Acosta had the support of a healer, who was responsible for educating and preparing those who distrusted this new method of healing to accept the vaccinations.

Several factors led to the eventual failure of inoculated vaccines: poor hygiene, malnutrition, the improvised healers' lack of medical knowledge, among others. The ineffectiveness of the inoculations reinforced the belief in and use of medicinal plants as an alternative method of treating disease [2].

In the 19th century, homes had large plots of land, making it easier to grow medicinal plants and reinforcing this practice. Families began to cultivate medicinal plants in order to control their illnesses; women working in the home started to grow medicinal herbs themselves. Older women practiced the professions of witchdoctors, traditional healers, and midwifery [2].

Costa Rica's Myths about Death and Disease

Healers and soothsayers continued offering treatments and solutions for health problems and for controlling diseases. They carried out practices such as divination, crystallomancy, tarot cards, gypsy flower, magic, evil, hypnotism, superstition, and witchcraft, all of which were not accepted and were widely criticized by communication outlets such as the *ECO Católico*, the unofficial weekly newspaper of the Catholic Church in Costa Rica sent to the whole country beginning in 1890. These practices were labeled as undesirable and were repudiated by the clergy [2].

Indigenous people believed that medicinal plants could cure disease. Esteban Núñez illustrated how aborigines used herbs and plants such as sahinillo (*Dieffenbachia oersteii*), cedron seeds (*Aloysia citrodora*), cacao (*Theobroma cacao*), fern leafs, and gavilana (*Neurolemma lobata*) to perform healing rituals [3].

Another figure who played a role in the management and control of disease from the 1800s onward was the witchdoctor who, without a formal education but with much experience in the management of diseases, used essences, plants, and pharmaceutical chemical products to help deal with diseases.

Religion and Spirituality

Spiritual experiences are no longer the exclusive domain of religious, holy. or mystical leaders; rather, they are now part of daily life for many people. Most Costa Ricans live a spiritual life, to some extent; for example, they believe in the Holy Trinity and the Virgin Mary, and according to Sedó Masís P, one of the most importants was "La Negrita de los Angeles," [4] but they do not attend mass or confession. Many seek alternative forms of spirituality such as prayer and processions, which are believed to prevent prevalent diseases, epidemics, and other social calamities thought to be divine retribution or punishments from the gods. To avoid them, one could resort to prayers and introspective walks [5].

Since the mid-20th century, Costa Ricans have believed that offering prayers, sacrifices, or rituals to saints could cure their illnesses and perform miracles. For example, many people pray for Dr. Moreno Cañas, a physician who died in 1938 as legend goes, advocated the ritual of leaving a glass of water at night near a napkin and a knife while praying; the next morning this water must be drunk by the sick person, and he will be healed [6].

The Beginning of Health Sciences

Trained health professionals Costa Ricans came back in 1838 to bring about changes in the approach to health care, such as the design of a social security system, while using the Catholic Church as a means of educating the public about new advances in the management of diseases. The country, aware of its health situation of Costa Rican population declining due to diseases (plagues) and there are no doctors to cure diseases, began to attach great importance to prevention and decided to send health professionals to different countries in Europe (Germany, France, Belgium, England, Italy, Switzerland) and Mexico. Their interest was in acquiring epidemiological knowledge that would help Costa Rica prevent infectious contagious diseases by establishing protocols and standards of care and developing new approaches and ways of organising the country's health care. Over time, however, they realized that prevention alone was insufficient; new medicaments were also required to better control diseases [7].

As the governing body, the Ministry of Health in 1927, established a national drug commission to devise a basic model for essential drugs, identified by the World Health Organization for developing countries such as ours. This commission would lead to better, more comprehensive management using a preventive and curative approach, with easily accessible essential drugs, including pain control drugs and cancer treatments (chemotherapy, radiotherapy, hormone therapy, immunotherapy and monoclonal antibodies) and treatment for cardiovascular diseases [7].

Medical management in Costa Rica incorporates spirituality as an essential component of disease management. The spiritual belief in a Supreme Being allows medical staff to control physical pain as if we were administering a potent opioid analgesic like morphine; therefore, it is necessary to promote spirituality as a complementary part of the total management of pain. The element of spirituality can help reduce opioid consumption, thus limiting the undesirable side effects of these drugs and reducing suffering during the final phase of life. As Costa Rica is primarily Christian, much can be achieved through spirituality, though this belief is continually declining with the new generation.

Beliefs about Cancer

Costa Rica has a social security system that provides universal health coverage through resources from the owner of the worker's company, the employee, and the government. This has allowed for the establishment of prevention programs and the alleviation of suffering for all who require and request it, with better access to services at all three levels of care: health care, medicine, and diagnostic means (including lab tests and governmental agencies).

Cancer is the second-leading cause of death in Costa Rica. According to data from the National Tumour Archive at the Ministry of Health in Costa Rica, on average, every two hours a family mourns a death due to cancer; 24 people are diagnosed with this disease daily. In 2018, cancer caused 1.3 million deaths and 3.7 million new cases in South and Central America [8].

Costa Ricans, like people the world over, experience a lot of fear when hearing the word "cancer." This fear explains why people delay medical check-ups; they do so in an attempt to avoid receiving bad news, thereby decreasing the chances of an early diagnosis of the disease. This cultural behavior is similar to that of people in other Latin American countries, and it is equally prevalent among men, women, and people of all ages. It is common for the patient to shy away from medical services and instead see a witchdoctor, healer, or shaman.

When Costa Ricans are diagnosed with cancer, they look for many healing options, including the use of natural medicines such as noni berries (*Marinda citrifolia*), soursop (*Annona muricata*), sabila (*Aloe vera*), homeopathy, floral therapy, potions prescribed by the witch doctor or shaman, or self-medication with nonpharmacological substances (e.g., blue scorpion venom), and also many people believe that cancer can be cure by spirituality [9].

Changes in diet are in line with religious beliefs, as are invocations of the spirits of people with a great spiritual heritage such as Dr. Moreno Cañas, Maritza, Sister María Romero; religious pilgrimages; and processions promising cures.

In their study of how beliefs influence cancer recovery, researchers discovered that certain behaviors and actions helped patients overcome disease. In 2017, Dr. Pablo Saz-Peiró wrote that Costa Ricans who survived cancer commonly possessed certain characteristics, such as having a career, staying active, being confident, optimistic, tolerant, intelligent, and self-sufficient, as well as being a perfectionist [10].

Recent research carried out by the Common Core State Standards (C.C.S.S) initiative has shown that relation of cancer to death is still deeply rooted within the population: seven out of ten people still associate cancer with death. This "doomsday" myth becomes part of the problem, as the fear of contracting cancer is so high that it can lead to delayed diagnosis and, consequently, to a poorer prognosis for survival. Thomas Meoño Martín, a specialist in family and community medicine at Costa Rica University, has stated that out of fear of a cancer diagnosis, people "wait to see if the body recovers and [so they] lose valuable time" [11]. As a result, to give people a better understanding of the disease and prepare them to combat it, the early symptoms of cancer are explained in detail in public educational forums.

As we already mention many costarican people have opted to deal with many illnesses by their own ways including magic, medicinal plants, religion, and others, also, the way how we learn to confront health problems was very interesting from the colonization by Spain to the actual world we live in, expanding over the continent and making other countries practice the same traditions. Many people have approved that beliefs can cure a problem even though science don't know how, but hope is the last thing ever lost.

References

1. Ibarra E. The epidemics of the Old World among the indigenous people of Costa Rica: Before the Spanish conquest, myth, or reality? (1502–1561). 1998. Retrieved 2020 from: https://dialnet.unirioja.es/servlet/articulo?codigo=2457941
2. Marín J. From healers to physicians. An approach to the social history of medicine in Costa Rica: 1800–1949. 1995. Recovered 2020 from: https://www.revistas.una.ac.cr/index.php/historia/article/view/10198

3. Nuñes E. Medicinal plants of Costa Rica and its folklore. 1975. Retrieved 2020 from: https://repositorios.cihac.fcs.ucr.ac.cr/cmelendez/bitstream/123456789/415/1/plantasmedicinalesdecostaricaysufolclore.pdf

4. Sedó Masís P. La Negrita de Los Angeles: Pilgrimages, promises, clothing and carpets ... expressions of faith in Costa Rica. Vice-Chancellor of Social Stock, University of Costa Rica. 2015:32. Consulted on August 4, 2019. Recovered from: http://www.kerwa.ucr.ac.cr/bitstream/handle/10669/29342/Virgen%20de%20los%20%C3%81ngeles.pdf?sequence=1&isAllowed=y

5. Fajardo G, Ferrer Y. Health control of communicable diseases in Hispano-America. 16th, 17th, and 18th century. 2003. Retrieved 2020 from: https://www.medigraphic.com/pdfs/gaceta/gm-2003/gm036l.pdf

6. Soto, M. Dr. Ricardo Moreno Cañas: "Holy Man" from the Costa Rican cultural imaginary. For: Soto Masis María Auxiliadora. 2018. Retrieved 2020 from: https://populardrama.wordpress.com/2018/12/01/dr-ricardo-moreno-canashombre-santo-del-imaginario-cultural-costarricense/

7. Jaramillo J. Medical evolution: Past, present, and future. 2001. Retrieved 2020 from: http://actamedica.medicos.cr/index.php/Acta_Medica/article/view/64/52

8. Quesada J. Cancer in Costa Rica: More than 5,000 deaths and 12,000 diagnoses. 2020. Retrieved 2020 from: https://www.crhoy.com/nacionales/cancer-en-costa-rica-mas-5-mil-muertes-y-12-mil-diagnosticos

9. National Cancer Institute. Spirituality in cancer treatment (PDQ®)—Version for health professionals. Washington, DC: 2017. 2021 NIH, website: https://www.cancer.gov/espanol/cancer/sobrellevar/dia-a-dia/fe-y-espiritualidad/espiritualidad-pro-pdq#_AboutThis_1

10. Saz-Peiró P. Psychotherapy, meditation, and cancer. 2017. Retrieved 2020 from: https://www.researchgate.net/publication/318635538_Psychotherapy_meditation_and_cancer

11. Bolaños B, Quesada S. Cancer deaths will double in Costa Rica. Are we ready? 2019. Retrieved 2020 from: https://semanariouniversidad.com/pais/las-muertes-por-cancer-se-duplicaran-en-costa-rica-estamos-preparados/

35

Reflections on Middle Eastern Cultural Perspectives in Cancer Care

Manal A. Al-Zadjali, Anna E. Brown, Warda A. Al Amri, Amal J. Al Balushi, Thamra S. Al Ghafri, and Nabiha S. Al Hasani

Introduction

Cancer is one of the leading causes of illness and death worldwide; in 2018, there were 18.1 million new cancer cases and 9.6 million deaths [1]. In the Middle East region alone, in the same year, there were 676,508 new cancer cases and 418,955 deaths from the disease [1]. Furthermore, it is projected that by 2040, there will be 27.5 million new cases of cancer each year, an increase of 61.7% from 2018 if current trends continue [2]. According to Silbermann and Hassan [3], beliefs surrounding the causes and significance of cancer are interconnected with culture. Therefore, health professionals should consider culture-specific beliefs as important determinants of the interpretation of cancer, its treatment, and likely outcomes related to the prevention and control of the disease [4].

This chapter provides a reflection on some of the cultural issues influencing cancer care in Middle Eastern countries. The Middle East extends from Morocco in the west to Iraq in the east, and from Lebanon and Syria in the north to Yemen in the south [5]. Although variations in culture exist among and within countries and national groups in this vast geographical area, they share core cultural values and beliefs. These cultural values play a significant role in decision making regarding cancer care, diagnosis, treatment and management [6], and health outcomes [7].

Culture and Cancer Care

Culture has been defined as a system of beliefs, values, and traditions that has been passed on across members of a society over generations [7]. Culture is designed to ensure the survival and well-being of members of a society and to provide them with common ways to find meaning and purpose throughout their lives [6]. It shapes peoples' emotional and physical reactions to cancer care [8]; hence, cultural factors must be studied extensively to ensure better quality of prevention, diagnosis, management, and palliative care.

Prevention

Despite the continuous advancements in detection and management, cancer remains a challenging threat to societies throughout the world. Individuals' health-seeking behaviors, in terms of prevention screening and perceptions of life, are often subjected to influences by several factors. Although late presentation is always linked to lack of knowledge and access to screening programs, there are other factors that are not often mentioned [9]. In the Middle East, these factors are related mainly to religion, spirituality, family values and dynamics, stigma, and social values.

Religion and Spiritual Needs

Although the terms *religion* and *spirituality* are often used interchangeably, they are not considered to be the same. For the purpose of this text, we define spirituality as "a dynamic and intrinsic aspect of humanity through which persons seek ultimate meaning, purpose, and transcendence, and experience relationship to self, family, others, community, society, nature, and the significant or sacred. Spirituality is expressed through beliefs, values, traditions, and practices" [10].

An individual's religion and spirituality have great influence on their health-seeking behavior and thus, on their decisions concerning screening and prevention. In the Middle East, Islam is the most common religion and it encourages preventive behavior. Islamic teachings prohibit certain habits and lifestyle-related behaviors that are deemed to be directly related to many malignancies, these teachings assert that obedience to these prohibitions will reduce the incidence of malignancies [11]. For instance, smoking, alcohol consumption, and homosexuality are prohibited. Likewise, perceptions guided by religious beliefs can influence screening practices and the decisions related to it. These prohibitions, in turn, can significantly affect the rate of mortality and morbidity, for early detection of cancer can increase survival rates [12].

In the Middle East, religion and social norms are difficult to separate. Whereas Islam dictates a conservative approach to matters related to medical or physical exposure, social norms can also play an important role in determining people's attitudes toward health care and its related aspects [3]. Furthermore, religious beliefs are often maintained even when an individual relocates from their country of origin. For instance, one study explored the practices of and barriers to breast and cervical cancer screening of 50 Arab Muslim Women (AMW) in southwestern Pennsylvania [13]. The study reported that 25% of the women felt that modesty and embarrassment were barriers to getting a mammogram: they could not expose their breast in front of strangers. But 72% reported that Islam allowed physical exposure when it was absolutely necessary. Similar results were reported from a study of adults in Oman that investigated barriers to seeking medical assistance; in that study, approximately 37.3% of the sample ($n = 999$) felt embarrassment in seeking medical help [12].

Family, Family Values, and Family Dynamics

In the Middle Eastern culture, the highest value is accorded to the family, which is considered to be the foundation of the community's prosperity. The role of the family in cancer prevention can be summarized as (1) willingness to access screening facilities, (2) awareness of risk factors and the impact of a family history of cancer, and (3) family dynamics that may influence relationships, behaviors, and well-being.

In many countries in the Middle East, promoting health and taking preventive actions presents many challenges; patients often resist access to cancer prevention/screening facilities due to misconceptions and feelings of embarrassment [14]. However, with increased awareness among women, these challenges can be reduced. Another challenge is that the dissemination of information regarding public health and cancer prevention is rarely geared toward the family as a whole. Families may struggle to find reliable information on cancer prevention, even though many of them do seek this information when a family member is diagnosed with cancer. Most families self-manage the considerable stress and weight of their caregiving responsibilities, which often constitutes a critical bond among patients, families, and clinicians [15].

In addition, people in many of these countries are not well informed regarding the risk factors for cancer, including obesity in women (which is highly prevalent in the Middle East) and their family's cancer history [16], for which there is no sustainable health reporting system. Future health plans may consider early screening and health education for families that have a high risk for cancer [17]. Family dynamics and relationships affect behaviors and well-being. In Middle Eastern culture, in order to raise awareness, it is vital to involve families as a unit. This measure will help facilitate decisions related to screening, choices for a healthy lifestyle, and management of conflicts during decision making.

Stigma and Social Values

There is stigma linked to the word "cancer," to the extent that many people in the Middle East refrain from even mentioning it by name [18]. This mindset can negatively impact public health efforts to reduce the burden of cancer on the broader society. Cancer stigma may not just affect cancer patients; families and communities may be equally affected. This might discourage people from engaging in cancer prevention or early detection. Various studies have found that negative beliefs about cancer are indeed associated with lower screening uptake, lower rates of self-examination, and higher health care avoidance for fear of having the illness and mental illnesses [19]. However, limited studies in the Middle East have systematically explored the stigma surrounding cancer. Reports on feelings of fear, social taboos, and guilt have occasionally been reported [20]. As Middle Eastern culture is family-oriented, every individual has a defined role in the family. For instance, women are obliged to fulfill multiple roles in their families, and these roles are greatly affected by their being screened or diagnosed. Additionally, cancer is linked with stigma, and once a person is screened and is diagnosed, their family and society might react negatively towards them. Therefore, they would rather suffer in silence than take preventative actions [9].

Diagnosis and Management

Early diagnosis and treatment is the key to a better prognosis in cancer care. Since the Middle East is a family-oriented culture, multiple factors can influence diagnosis and treatment, including: social views, nondisclosure, spiritual perspectives, complementary medicine, communication, and attitudes toward patients and health professionals.

Social Views
Extended families with close relationships are the norm in Middle Eastern cultures. Children usually live with their parents until they are married. Even when they move out, they remain in close contact with their families. The positions are reversed when parents age: children assume the role of caretaker as long as the parents are alive. In addition, they rely on each other during sickness and illness, thereby intensifying their relationship [3]. Therefore, the sickness of one individual influences the entire family.

This pattern can be seen when patients visit the health care facility for diagnosis or treatment; they are usually accompanied by a family member. However, it is not only the nuclear family who is involved in diagnosis and decision making, but the extended family members as well. In some Middle Eastern, North African, and South Asian societies, the family has the ultimate authority in the treatment decision making as the patient is interconnected with the entire family [21]. Although this might sound like a great support system during the management of the disease, it might have a negative impact on the care. In Oman, for instance, families' involvement in the decision making results in the patient's loss of autonomy, delay in treatment and, eventually, their chance of survival [22].

Nondisclosure
Many patients prefer not to seek medical advice or be diagnosed at all with cancer owing to their fear of becoming a burden. Subsequently, this reticence leads to a delay in diagnosis. In addition, as a family-oriented culture, the disease is usually disclosed not only to the patient but also to the family. In some instances, the families may request that the diagnosis not be revealed to the patient under the assumption that this will protect the patient psychologically. In contrast, once diagnosed, some patients tend to conceal their diagnosis from others, at least initially [23].

For many patients, being diagnosed with cancer is a sign of approaching death. Others consider it as a test from God, whereas some believe that it is a punishment for undisclosed past sins, uncontrolled anger, or social humiliation [23]. Others may ascribe it to an "Evil Eye" [18]. In addition, once they are diagnosed, patients usually feel more comfortable speaking to strangers due to the social stigma and the way cancer is perceived and framed by their close community [18]. All of these factors further complicate the disclosure process. Therefore, it is important to understand how the patient and family perceive the disease, and it is imperative that the sociocultural factors related to disclosure of information regarding diagnosis be thoroughly assessed.

Spiritual Perspectives
When diagnosed with cancer, one's spirituality is often challenged. However, belonging to a certain faith can enhance one's spirituality and may improve one's psychological well-being [24]. Being primarily Muslims, Middle Easterners believe in peace,

accepting pain and illness, seeking help and a peaceful death. For instance, Malaysian Muslim women diagnosed with breast cancer often accept their disease as a gift from God to forgive their sins and grant them a place in heaven. They value the disease as an awakening sign telling them to perceive life differently and enjoy it as never before. Also, it is regarded as a way to regain the strength to face life's difficulties more openly and optimistically [25]. A study aimed at investigating the burden of cancer care on the primary caregivers of Iranian patients with hematologic cancer showed that the spiritual health of the caregivers was at a high level [26]. Assessing the spiritual needs of patients and their caregivers is important in providing comprehensive care.

Complementary and Traditional Medicine

Complementary and traditional medicine (CTM) is commonly practiced in Middle Eastern countries. It is regarded as an alternative to conventional oncology care or as a complementary approach, with the purpose of providing maximum benefits from both natural and scientific treatment sources. CTM is most commonly used in Jordan, Saudi Arabia, Turkey, Israel, Morocco, and Iran [27]. Recently, there has been a surge toward integrating CTM with conventional supportive care. For example, a study conducted in Israel and the Palestinian Authority revealed that patients with cancer prefer the model of care in which the CTM is integrated with the goal of reducing many side effects of oncology treatment and improving quality of care. The complementary medicines used in this study included Arab herbs and traditional remedies [28]. CTM was used mainly for better survival/cure and quality of life, as shown by a regional survey of 339 health care providers from 16 Middle Eastern countries [29]. In addition, Arabic and Islamic traditional herbs were found to be a good source of complementary and alternative medicine in cancer management and were considered promising, with low toxicity and minimal side effects [30].

Often, patients diagnosed with cancer strongly adhere to and carefully comply with chemotherapy and other cancer treatment modalities, and yet still seek alternative medicines or traditional remedies. In many Middle Eastern countries, people use various traditional remedies along with the hospital's treatment plan. Although some traditional and complementary medicines can interact with the endogenous antioxidants that impair the efficacy of chemotherapy and oncology treatment, people continue to use them [31]. Because oncologists tend to discourage patients from using these alternative medicines, patients are less likely to disclose their use of them to their provider [31]. For instance, in Oman, many cancer patients increase their intake of turmeric without informing their doctor, and only after assessing their liver enzymes does the doctor realize that the patient has been using complementary medicine. In addition, some herbal formulas contain ingredients that negatively impact the patient's health and the progress of the disease, but patients continue to use them as they believe that, while herbs may not do any good, they will also not cause any harm.

In addition, therapies such as "Wasam," a traditional remedy used to treat several diseases including cancer, are widely used throughout the Middle East. Wasam basically involves the application of heated metal on different areas of the skin to contour the tumor [32]. However, this therapy has been found to cause more harm than good. For example, a retrospective study conducted in Oman to analyze the frequency of a locoregional spread in female breast cancer patients who received Wasam therapy revealed that the breast cancer patients with Wasam therapy showed higher and earlier locoregional metastasis compared to patients who did not have the treatment [32]. However, in many cases it is the family's decision instead of the patient's informed decision that holds sway.

Communication
Communicating with cancer patients is always a challenge. The life-threatening disease, the physical and psychological suffering, the complexity of information, along with the patient's emotions, are just some of the daily communication challenges in the cancer setting [33]. Not only that, in a dynamic cultural context which reflects how people interact, live, understand, and shape their behaviors, communication has variability. In societies such as those in the Middle East, which are characterized by multiple faiths, cultures, and different civilization backgrounds, it is essential that care providers demonstrate responsiveness and respect for the patients' health beliefs, practices, and cultural needs [33]. The care provider's attitude greatly affects how patients and communities view the diagnosis and treatment of cancer and improves how they relate to health care providers and health institutions generally.

Palliative Care

Palliative care is the most important aspect of people-centered health services, for it is the act of caring not only for the individuals suffering from life-threatening illnesses but for their families as well. It is all about working to improve their quality of life through the prevention and control of suffering, early detection, and assessment, diagnosis, and management of pain and other problems associated with their illness, whether physical, psychosocial, or spiritual [34]. Therefore, palliative care should start at the time of diagnosis. Unfortunately, as palliative care is often, in Middle Eastern cultures, linked with death and dying, its implementation faces several challenges including pain management and the many myths and taboos related to death.

Pain Management
Studies suggest that 30–40% of patients with early–stage cancer and 70–80% of patients receiving treatment or with advanced disease have inadequate pain control. This problem affects their quality of life and physical and psychological well-being [35]. In the Middle East, the majority of patients who are diagnosed with cancer present when the disease is at an advanced stage and there are low chances for cure; therefore, at this point, the only option is pain relief and palliative care [36]. However, cultural barriers to effective pain management exist, and these pose challenges to health professionals [35]. Among cultural barriers are different perceptions of pain and death and concerns about possible addiction to and abuse of pain medications, leading to inadequate prescribing by physicians and insufficient use by patients. Regulatory obstacles that govern the accessibility, use, and prescription of opioids, together with false beliefs and lack of knowledge, contribute to a situation where pain relief for palliative care in the Middle East has been designated as inadequate [35].

Taboos about Death and Dying

People often form their worldview of death based on their cultural background. Although most Middle Easterners are Muslim, there are both differences and similarities in their cultural backgrounds and lifestyles. This affects their beliefs and, consequently, the care delivered to them. Because of these cultural taboos about cancer, health care professionals often face difficult challenges when they are providing palliative care. Therefore, it is important to consider the myths and taboos that are related to cancer care and death. For instance, one myth in India and many other countries is that cancer is always painful and can cause death in a very short time [37] and that hospitalization can make the situation even worse [38,39]. Moreover, it is also thought that once a person is diagnosed with cancer, they can never regain health or return to normality [37,38,40].

In Islam, death is believed to be a beginning rather than an end, as life on earth is considered a journey and the destination is the hereafter. Therefore, Muslims live their lives knowing and accepting the idea that death is inevitable and one has no control over it [36]. Accepting their disease as "God's Will" may influence their approach to seeking prevention and treatment. In addition, pain is considered to be one of the manifestations of cancer, and people are encouraged to accept and live with it [36]. Middle Eastern cultural beliefs do not support active euthanasia or assisted suicide; instead, they advocate the use of life support when there is some hope of revival, but they may not accept artificial functioning of the organs if physical death is imminent. Despite their acceptance of death, Middle Easterners are often discouraged from grieving in front of the patient. However, once a patient dies, grieving loudly is acceptable [39]. Understanding the stigma, myths, and taboos can help design and improve the quality of care delivered and, ultimately, the cancer patient's quality of life.

Conclusion

The Middle East is often described as a region with multiple faiths and cultures. It is impossible to apply the lessons learned in Western cultures to the Middle East. The diversity of Middle Eastern culture obliges health care professionals to assess and study the culture as well as create policies that meet the needs of their individual patients. In such an environment, there is no one formula to suit all.

References

1. International Agency for Research on Cancer. Global cancer observatory: Cancer today; October 2018. https://gco.iarc.fr/today/data/factsheets/populations/900-world-fact-she ets.pdf. Accessed November 29, 2020.
2. Ferlay J, Colombet M, Soerjomataram I, et al. Estimating the global cancer incidence and mortality in 2018: GLOBOCAN sources and methods. *IJC*. 2018;144(8):1941–1953. doi: https://doi.org/10.1002/ijc.31937
3. Silbermann M, Hassan EA. Cultural perspectives in cancer care: Impact of Islamic traditions and practices in Middle Eastern countries. *J Pediatr Hematol Oncol*. 2011;33(Suppl 2):S81–S86.

4. Dardas LA, Simmons, LA. The stigma of mental illness in Arab families: A concept analysis. *J Psychiatr Ment Health Nurs*. 2015;22(9):668–679. doi: 10.1111/jpm.12237

5. Salim EL, Moore M, Al-Lawati JA, et al. Cancer epidemiology and control in the Arab world—past, present and future. *APJCP*. 2009;10(1):3–16.

6. Kagawa-Singer, M. Impact of culture on health outcomes. *J Pediatr Hematol Oncol*. 2011;33(Suppl 2):S90–S95. doi: 10.1097/MPH.0b013e318230dadb

7. Daher M. Cultural beliefs and values in cancer patients. *Ann Oncol*. 2012;23 (Suppl 3):66–69. doi: 10.1093/annonc/mds091

8. Silbermann M, Epner DE, Charalambous H, et al. Promoting new approaches for cancer care in the Middle East. *Ann Oncol*. 2013;23(Suppl 7):vii5–vii10. doi: 10.1093/annonc/mdt267

9. Elobaid Y, Tar-Ching Aw, Jennifer NWL, Hamid S, Grivna M. Breast cancer presentation delays among Arab and national women in the UAE: A qualitative study. *SSM Popul Health*. 2016;2:155–163. doi: http://dx.doi.org/10.1016/j.ssmph.2016.02.007

10. Puchalski CM, Vitillo R, Hull SK, Reller N. Improving the spiritual dimension of whole person care: Reaching national and international consensus. *J Palliat Med*. 2014;17(6):642–656. doi: 10.1089/jpm.2014.9427

11. Albar MA. Islamic teachings and cancer prevention. *J Family Community Med*. 1994;1(1):79–86.

12. Al Azri M, Al Maskari A, Al Matroushi S, et al. Awareness of cancer symptoms and barriers to seeking medical help among adult people attending primary care settings in Oman. *Health Serv Res Manage Epidemiol*. 2016;3:1–10. doi: 10.1177/2333392816673290

13. Salman K. Health beliefs and practices related to cancer screening among Arab Muslim women in an urban community. *Health Care Women Int*. 2012;33(1):45–74. doi: 10.1080/07399332.2011.610536

14. Fearon D, Hughes S. Brearley SG. Experiences of breast cancer in Arab countries. A thematic synthesis. *Qual Life Res*. 2020;29(2):313–324. doi: 10.1007/s11136-019-02328-0

15. Alananzeh IM, Kwok C, Ramjan L, Levesque JV, Everett B. Information needs of Arab cancer survivors and caregivers: A mixed methods study. *Collegian*. 2019;26:40–48. doi: https://doi.org/10.1016/j.colegn.2018.03.001

16. Charafeddine MA, Olson SH, Mukherji D, et al. Proportion of cancer in a Middle Eastern country attributable to established risk factors. *BMC Cancer*. 2017;17(1):337. doi: 10.1186/s12885-017-3304-7

17. Elkum N, Al-Tweigeri T, Ajarim D, Al-Zahrani A, Amer SM, Aboussekhra A. Obesity is a significant risk factor for breast cancer in Arab women. *BMC Cancer*. 2014;14:788. doi: 10.1186/1471-2407-14-788

18. Salem H, Nashif S. Psychosocial Aspects of female breast cancer in the Middle East and North Africa. *Int J Environ Res Public Health*. 2020;17(18):1–16. doi: 10.3390/ijerph17186802

19. Merhej R. Stigma on mental illness in the Arab world: Beyond the socio-cultural barriers. *Int J Hum Rights Healthc*. 2019;12(4):285–298. doi: https://doi.org/10.1108/IJHRH-03-2019-0025

20. Haddou Rahou B, El Rhazi K, Ouasmani F, et al. Quality of life in Arab women with breast cancer: A review of the literature. *Health Qual Life Outcomes*. 2016;14:64. doi: 10.1186/s12955-016-0468-9

21. Al-Bahri A, Al-Moundhri M, Al-Mandhari Z, Al-Azri M. The role of patients' families in treatment decision-making among adult cancer patients in the Sultanate of Oman. *Eur J Cancer Care*. 2018;27(3):e12845. doi: 10.1111/ecc.12845

22. Burney I. The trend to seek a second opinion abroad amongst cancer patients in Oman: Challenges and opportunities. *Sultan Qaboos Uni Med J*. 2009;9(3):260–263.

23. Fearon D, Hughes S, Brearley SG. Experiences of breast cancer in Arab countries. A thematic synthesis. *Qual Life Res.* 2020;29:313–324. doi: https://doi.org/10.1007/s11136-019-02328-0

24. Harandy TF, Ghofranipour F, Montazeri A, et al. Muslim breast cancer survivor spirituality: Coping strategy or health seeking behavior hindrance? *Health Care Women Int.* 2009;31(1):88–89. doi: https://doi.org/10.1080/07399330903104516

25. Ahmad F, Muhammad MB, Abdullah AA. Religion and spirituality in coping with advanced breast cancer: Perspectives from Malaysian Muslim women. *J Relig Health.* 2010;50(1):36–45. doi: 10.1007/s10943-010-9401-4

26. Abbasnezhad M, Rahmani A, Ghahramanian A, et al. Cancer care burden among primary family caregivers of Iranian hematologic cancer patients. *APJCP.* 2015;16(13):5499–5505. doi: http://dx.doi.org/10.7314/APJCP.2015.16.13.5499

27. Ben-Arye E, Samuels N, Daher M, et al. Integrating complementary and traditional practices in Middle-Eastern supportive cancer Care. *JNCI Monographs.* 2017;2017(52):11–17. doi: https://doi.org/10.1093/jncimonographs/lgx016

28. Ben-Arye E, Massalha E, Bar-Sela G. et al. Stepping from traditional to integrative medicine: Perspectives of Israeli-Arab patients on complementary medicine's role in cancer care. *Ann Oncol.* 2014;25(2):476–480. doi: 10.1093/annonc/mdt554

29. Ben-Arye E, Schiff E, Mutafoglu K, et al. Integration of complementary medicine in supportive cancer care: Survey of health-care providers' perspectives from 16 countries in *the Middle East. Support Care Cancer.* 2015;23(9):2605–2612. doi: 10.1007/s00520-015-2619-7

30. Ahmad R, Ahmad N, Naqvi AA, Shehzad A, Al-Ghamdi MS. Role of traditional Islamic and Arabic plants in cancer therapy. *J Tradit Complement Med.* 2017;7(2):195–204. doi: 10.1016/j.jtcme.2016.05.002

31. Gall A, Anderson K, Adams J, Matthews V, Garvey G. An exploration of healthcare providers' experiences and perspectives of traditional and complementary medicine usage and disclosure by Indigenous cancer patients. *BMC Complement Altern Med.* 2019;19(259):1–9. doi: https://doi.org/10.1186/s12906-019-2665-7

32. Al-Lawati T, Mehdi I, Al Bahrani B, Al-Harsi K, Al Rahbi S, Varvaras, D. Does alternative and traditional WASAM (Local cautery) therapy facilitate an early and more extensive locoregional metastasis of breast cancer? *Gulf J Oncology.* 2016;1(22):37–42.

33. Brown O, Ham-Baloyi T, Rooyen DR, Aldous C, Marais LC. Culturally competent patient-provider communication in the management of cancer: An integrative literature review. *Glob Health Action.* 2016;9:1–13. doi: http://dx.doi.org/10.3402/gha.v9.33208

34. World Health Organization (WHO). Palliative care; 2020. http://www.who.int/cancer/palliative/definition/en/. Accessed November 25, 2020.

35. Nasser SC, Nassif JG, Saad AH. Physicians' attitudes to clinical pain management and education: Survey from a Middle Eastern country. *Pain Res Manag.* 2016;2016:1–9. doi: https://doi.org/10.1155/2016/1358593

36. Silbermann M, Arnaout M, Daher M, et al. Palliative cancer care in Middle Eastern countries: Accomplishments and challenges. *Ann Oncol.* 2012;23(Suppl 3):iii15–iii28. doi:10.1093/annonc/mds084

37. Pankaj S, Nazneen S, Kumari A, et al. Myths and taboos: A major hindrance to cancer controls "inherited knowledge" a blessing or curse. Surgery after 21 cycles of chemotherapy "a surgeon's ordeal". *Ind J Gyn Oncol.* 2018;16(2):1–3. doi: https://doi.org/10.1007/s40944-017-0172-7

38. Sarki A, Roni BL. This disease is "not for hospital": Myths and misconceptions about cancers in Northern Nigeria. *JOGHR.* 2019;3:1–5. doi: 10.29392/joghr.3.e2019070

39. El-Kurd, M. Cultural diversity and caring for patients from the Middle East. Paper presented at PCQN Conference Call; September 2013. https://www.pcqn.org/wp-content/

uploads/2012/11/Sept-Call_Cultural-Diversity-and-Caring-For-Patients-From-Middle-East.pdf. Accessed November 25, 2020.

40. Shiri FH, Mohtashami J, Nasiri M, Manoochehri H, Rohani C. Stigma and related factors in Iranian people with cancer. *APJCP*. 2018;19(8):2285–2290. doi: 10.22034/APJCP.2018.19.8.2285

36

Spirituality, Culture, Traditions, and Other Beliefs Affecting Cancer Care, Uganda

Anne Merriman, Germans Natuhwera, and Eve Namisango

Introduction

"The Earth has entered an entirely new geological epoch: the Anthropocene, or the age of humans. It means that we are the first people to live in an age defined by human choice, in which the dominant risk to our survival is ourselves." [1]

Beliefs are almost as varied as the numbers populating our world today. Each country has its own history and experiences, resulting in specific cultural and other beliefs that affect its peoples' health. Within each tribe, family unit and individual, there are personal experiences affecting beliefs, values, norms, cultural practices, religions, and individual spirituality. However, there are other influential factors, such as the economy of a country and the way in which health professionals and clinicians who have professed their dedication to the Hippocratic oath talk to patients, with either curing, caring, or making money their priority. Meanwhile, in some countries, palliative care, which attends to all those in need and those who are suffering (taking into account the family's budget), is slow to be recognized as a specialty. Medical professionals can promote wrong beliefs, too! It is in palliative care that we probe the beliefs affecting patients' behaviors toward cancer care as we try to conform to their wishes while respecting their culture, values, norms. and religious beliefs.

Although this chapter draws mainly on A.M.'s own recall of living in seven countries and working with cancer patients for 56 years, the authors E.N. and G.N. have contributed their lived and patient experiences too, which are invaluable. Interviews with colleagues still working with cancer patients (in both active/curative and palliative medicine/care) in seven countries enable us to see the changes in these factors over time.

Why are there so many differences and so few commonalities in different countries? Perhaps it is because we all seek meaning in life. As Viktor Frankl observed in his 1946 memoir, *Man's Search for Meaning*, "often this search is only enunciated by the dying" [1].

This chapter was written in the COVID-19 era, during which the fear of sudden illness, and even death, in communities has been overwhelming. The belief that hospital care is the best care may well have contributed to the spread of the virus and to the death of health workers in the overpopulated, underserved hospitals. In most low- and middle-income countries (LMICs), a patient must have a family member in attendance at all times to carry out basic hygiene and daily functions. The exclusion of families from accompanying a patient and the additional burden on nursing staff have not only reduced basic nursing standards and hygiene, but have also caused severe psychological stress, both to the dying and to their families. Lockdown measures have certainly contributed to deaths from other causes, which are now neglected in many countries in favor of COVID-19 services and the associated public health preventive measures. This is an example of how conditions, changing with time, can affect the utilisation of cancer care and other services. This chapter covers countries from the highest to some of the lowest on the Human Development Index (HDI).

Country Highlights

The United Nations Development Programme's evaluation of the HDI (HDI 2020) gives us an idea of the economic status of our chosen countries. The HDI takes into account the economic development and education levels of each country.

We have studied three higher-income countries whose HDI (2020) ratings are as follows: Ireland: 2, Singapore: 11, and UK: 13. Malaysia is middle-HDI at 62. The LMICs are India: 131, Kenya: 145, Uganda: 159, and Nigeria: 161. We draw your attention to these statistics because the economy of each country and each family's finances are important factors in obtaining cancer treatment. These factors also affect the patients' choice of treatment, how soon they present, as well as if they present at all. Educational status is often linked to a family's financial situation. As we present the main area for this chapter, we would ask the reader to keep in mind their own country's economy as reflected in the HDI [2].

In 1986 [3], the World Health Organization (WHO), in its best-selling book *Cancer Pain Relief*, stated that curative services that were in line with those of developed countries would not be available to LMICs for generations. The WHO especially emphasised the need for pain and symptom control and the management of total pain as identified in palliative care. Since 1986, populations have increased dramatically, yet health services have not always proportionately expanded to keep up with the need. As a result, the percentages of those without treatment for cancer are growing. While cancer treatment is now available in the highest HDI countries, even for the poor, it can be delayed for the poorest and the underserved geographical localities. In nearly all low-resource countries, many poor patients cannot even consider cancer treatment, as the cost is so great and the services so very sparse and distant.

SINGAPORE: Singapore is one of the most highly developed countries in the world. The highest cause of death there is cancer (31%). The country has one of the best health and insurance systems to cover the poorest members of the population (although they may have to wait longer than their wealthier counterparts for the service). The small population of 5.5 million, is therefore, easier to govern and manage financially. The majority of Singaporeans are of Chinese origin: 74.3%; the rest are Malay 13.4%, Indian 0.9%, and other 3.2% (2018 EST) [4].

Singapore, originally part of the west Malay Peninsula, was occupied by the Malay. In the colonial era, the British imported Chinese and Indians into Malaysia to help build the railways and to work in the rubber plantations. Malay are still the majority group in East and West Malaysia, but Singapore is now dominated by people of Chinese origin. Each country of origin has its own varieties of customs, values, norms, religions, and beliefs. Singapore Island is small; land is scarce, so that the growing population lives mainly in high-rise flats. The country continues to claim land from the sea to cope with their increasing population and industries.

MALAYSIA: Malaysia has a total population of 32 million, but it is divided by the South China Sea into two landmasses: East and West Malaysia. The main ethnic groups are: Malay 62%, Chinese 20.6%, and Indian 6.2%. There are distinct differences in approach to life and work among the Malay, Indians, and Chinese. In 1983, when A.M. lived and worked in the early days of a new medical school, University Sains Malaysia (USM) in Penang, privileges were given to Malay professing the Muslim faith; 90% of medical students were Malay citizens and their education was free. This preference no longer holds: all ethnic groups are now treated equally. Life's meaning and values for the Malay are more philosophical, and as such, work and tasks are completed more slowly as meditating needs time, too.

INDIA: India's population is an astounding 1.3 billion. Indo-Aryans make up 72%, Dravidian 25%, and Mongoloid and other 3% (2000) [5]. More than 30 languages are spoken in India, most of which have their own alphabet. Each state has its own system of government and law, which makes cohesion very difficult. There is a huge gap between the rich and the poor. Development has been affected by major discrimination against women/girls and castes (see India: CIA Facts, 2020) [5].

UNITED KINGDOM: The UK is the leader of the British Empire, an empire that is rapidly declining. Its present population is 67 million. With the passage of Brexit, the fear has arisen that the remaining integral parts of the empire will declare independence, perhaps leaving just England in the UK. The UK has the best health care system in the world, the National Health System (NHS), created in 1948. The arrival of COVID-19 has put the NHS under a huge strain. Everything is free for children and the elderly and at a very affordable cost for the rest of the population. There are exemptions for chronic illnesses, cancer, disability, and some extreme social circumstances [6]. The system is funded primarily by tax-paying citizens who are taxed during their working lifetime. In addition to the NHS, there is a private health system and health insurance at a cost for the wealthier. With the arrival of many cultures that are now part of every community, followed by the more recent influx of refugees, the health system has had to adapt to many cultures and the needs of different religions.

IRELAND: Ireland is second in the HDI and is, therefore, considered one of the most developed countries in the world. Like Singapore, it has a small population (also 5 million) but its landmass is much larger than Singapore's, so the population is scattered except around the capital, Dublin. It rapidly moved up the HDI following the Celtic Tiger, a period of rapid economic growth fueled by foreign direct investment from the mid-1990s to the late 2000s. With free movement within the European Union, Ireland welcomed a workforce (the majority being Polish and Catholic) from the Continent, which improved most health services and increased tourism. For generations, the government was closely linked to and regulated by the Catholic Church. However, the prominence of the Catholic faith, as measured by attendance in churches, has greatly declined, as it has in other European countries. Nevertheless, on census forms, many still enter their religion as Catholic, even though most are now agnostic.

AFRICA: In most African LMICs, less than 50% have access to health services, and less than 5% of cancer patients have access to curative services. This is mainly because of cost limitations, resulting in the paucity of specialized cancer curative treatments, but also stemming from the affordability of the holistic approach found in traditional medicine.

KENYA: Kenya prided itself on being the most peaceful country in Africa until the 1990s when trouble commenced over presidential elections, ending in many deaths. This unrest occurred three times during the following 20 years. Kenya has the best private hospitals and up-to-date medical systems in East Africa, but the poorer of its citizens have little assistance when ill. The population totals 53.5 million, the majority of whom are indigenous. Indians, the second largest ethnic group in Kenya, have resided there for several generations, having been brought into Kenya to help with building the railways. Kenya has a long history of British occupation, when both good and dissolute times were had by the white population (documented in major films such as *White Mischief* and *Out of Africa*). However, the white population has diminished considerably since those times; the younger generation, who were educated abroad, have remained abroad, and the number of those remaining, being mostly in the older age groups, has dwindled considerably. Kenya has come into its own, but this independence has brought troubles, as explained earlier. Kenya is a beautiful country with a magnificent coastline, large safari parks, and lakes, and not surprisingly, tourism is a large source of the country's income, though it has diminished as a result of the pandemic.

UGANDA: Uganda's neighbors are Kenya, Tanzania, Congo, South Sudan, and Rwanda. Although many of these countries have suffered from unrest since 1986, Uganda has apparently maintained peace during these years. This is in stark contrast to the situation during the prior 20 years, which were fraught with fear and war in the North due to the cruelty of Kony rebels and the Ugandan army. Refugees from the proximal countries and more distant neighbors such as Somalia make up Uganda's total population. Thus, the refugee facilities have become stretched, and what is more alarming, the differing cultures and beliefs of people from the incoming countries have produced conflict and unrest in the camps. Uganda has had the same president since 1986. The rapidly growing population, now 46 million, has doubled in the last 30 years, and the number of 15-year-old and under in the population hovers around 48–50%. Although COVID-19 cases have spiked and are now flattening out, public health preventive measures such as severe lockdowns and the use of military force to ensure response to lockdown regulations have caused gun violence-associated deaths, worsened poverty and hunger levels, and disrupted access to health care, including cancer and palliative care services.

NIGERIA: Nigeria, with over 213 million people, boasts the largest population in Africa. With its enormous population, 250 ethnic groups, and 500 + indigenous languages, it is a complex country. Each geopolitical political zone (GPZ) has a university and medical school with at least one great medical service. However, each GPZ is the size of a small country with its own government structure responsible to the main government in the capital, Abuja. Religious differences played a major role in the Biafran War (1966–1970) and have continued to play a large role in these recent times of unrest. The biggest problem the country faces involves hostilities between the Muslim North and the Christian South.

Spirituality

In line with the existing evidence and the reality that the concept of spirituality differs from country to country [7], we must come to terms with a definition of our own, which is based on definitions from palliative care practitioners. We asked one clinician in each of six countries to describe what they believed to be the meaning of spirituality. Although the language and emphasis for different approaches varied, the common conclusion was that the spirit was as important for health as the body.

Following are some extracts from longer definitions of spirituality:

- Spirituality is the sum of a person's values, connections, meaning, and purpose of life. (R.G., India)
- Spirituality is that passion within people that is in search of meaningful purpose in life. It is exhibited in the way they express their passion, for example, Michael Jackson in music and Mother Teresa in prayer. Spirituality is made up of many segments, only one of which is religion. (Sr. G.T., Singapore)
- Spirituality is the framework for meaning in life. (Dr. E.Z., Malaysia)
- Spirituality is one's belief in a supreme being that is higher than themselves (either the almighty God or a human-made god). (Sr. S.N, Nigeria)
- Spirituality is what life is to me. However, my spirituality is very much intertwined with my religion. (Dr. Z.A, Kenya)
- Spirituality is the essence of our being. (Dr. M.M., UK)
- Spirituality is defined by the sense of connection to something bigger than us.
(Dr A.N., Ireland)

Like culture, spirituality also has great influence on our health care-seeking behaviors and choices. The most common reasons for not accessing cancer treatment include one's relationship with spirituality and preferred religion. In the African countries, among the segments for spirituality (the first four definitions above), religion is the biggest segment of all. This finding sometimes puts attendance at religious services higher than their attention to humanism and the value of a sinless life.

From time to time, cult religions arise and soon disappear, as they can do serious damage. In AM's time in Uganda, three cults have emerged, steering patients away from cancer treatment and other Western treatments. Hundreds of members of one cult were persuaded to commit mass suicide on the basis that the world was coming to an end in the year 2000. Followers therefore surrendered all their possessions to the cult leaders. The members committed mass suicide together in three different parts of the country. There have been reports of three cults; Atuhaire [8] has reported an earlier one.

The traditional religion in Africa was mainly Ubuntu, which originated with the Bantu. When the missionaries arrived, they of course brought with them new forms of religion and condemned traditional religions. They set strict rules binding new members to the churches, often rebuking the good as well as the evil. All traditional spiritual beliefs were considered witchcraft. Yet, Ubuntu values were expressed by their openness to all. These distinctions were explained by Nelson Mandela and Bishop Tutu. The teachings of Christ are more akin to the traditional Ubuntu than the selfishness that is so rampant in the modern world, which has affected many African countries today.

Religion dictates that members must obey certain regulations and practices [9]. These regulations and practices are mixed with myths and beliefs and, as such, we find, for example, that the daughters of Hindus are prohibited from becoming nurses because they may not handle excreta from patients. This prohibition has had a huge impact on health services in India. Christians who see nursing as a vocation are being called upon to fill the void. As a result of the increase in the number of born-again churches, with their declarations of healing miracles through prayer and faith healing, there is generalized failure of cancer patients to seek cancer care or they cease cancer treatment altogether. This is true for all countries in Africa.

In addition, common to many cultures is the relationship with our ancestors or gods, who must not be offended. The cause of cancer is often attributed to having offended a person living or dead. Sacrifices must be offered in atonement. Taoism demands prayer and incense to the ancestors on a daily basis, and, if this duty is neglected, it may lead to disease, including cancer. Taoists believe that the way to cure illness is not through medical treatment, but rather through sacrifices made to atone for one's neglect. The belief that cancer will be cured if one admits to their sins, repents, atones, and converts to another religion has left many to die without treatment and in guilty torment.

Traditional beliefs can be confusing and direct the spirit. The extreme types of healers, called witchdoctors, are found mainly in Africa, but they are also quietly emerging in other cultures. They use the spirit to persuade the vulnerable, the sick, and their relatives to take part in evil practices, even killing children for their organs in order to attain healing for very important persons (VIPs) in the community.

Notably, the other segments of the spirit may be neglected as the religious segment grows larger. These are mainly composed of and expressed by the persons we are, our history, our aims in life and our relationships. Many of these segments of spirituality will continue to change with time and situation.

Increasingly, in many countries today wealth has replaced compassion as the drive for further investigation and treatment of illnesses. Medics are asking for higher fees for seeing a patient, and many patients, rather than being examined, are simply advised, in order to save time and make more money for the caregiver. Treatment for cancer is controlled by what we can afford, our life experiences, and those we trust and from whom we take advice.

Culture and Traditions

We operationalize culture to refer to ideas, customs, and social behaviors of a particular people or society. Many of these aspects of culture are referred to as traditions when they are passed down from one generation to the next.

Culture produces values, norms and beliefs that affect cancer care [10]. Some are inherited from our countries of origin and others from local circumstances. In Africa, "West is best," and relatives who have gone abroad often advise unwisely. For example, the United States stresses the evils of addiction to opioids (of which morphine is one), and prescription drugs are publicly pronounced to be a prevalent cause of addiction. Of course, there are many social reasons why there are many addicts in the developed world, associated with the culture, social situation, individual history, and background that differ in every country. Oral morphine, in its cheapest form, relieves cancer pain and suffering among the millions who do not have access to any form of active cancer treatment, and most take such treatment too late. Hospice Africa Uganda and the other palliative care services in 90% of our districts have treated up to 60,000 Ugandan patients with oral morphine without causing addiction or diversion. and all structures are in place to protect the families and children. Yet, we have messages coming from the United States, where much different social circumstances contribute to addiction, trying to stifle the availability of morphine through the WHO, which has proven, and stated for many years, that morphine is the best and cheapest form of pain control. Thus, international pressure can interfere with cancer care.

These international messages are heard and enforce scaremongering among politicians who fear they may be accused of drug laundering. This combination of adhering to others and misguided cultural beliefs leaves cancer patients to suffer in excruciating pain. Reaction to advice depends on the trust in the person explaining medically and the patients' and families' embodiment of beliefs. Moreover, each ethnic group adheres to many different traditions. One common tradition is the influence of relatives and/or friends, especially when they come from a more developed country.

Singapore has three main ethnic groups, each of which has its own beliefs, traditional medicines, and cultures: Chinese, Indian and Malay. Taoism is the traditional Chinese religion and is most common among the older generation. Many of these adherents have since passed, so it is less prevalent now and has been overtaken by Buddhism. Chinese languages and writings stemmed from the part of China they came from. The most common language was Hokkien and is now being replaced by the coordinating new language, Mandarin, the official Chinese language worldwide.

The young Samsui women, imported for hard labour in the construction of Singapore in 1930s and '40s,[1] later became maids for the British Army and richer families in 1950–60. They are fondly remembered by the children of the British Army officials who were part of the British occupation of Singapore and Malaysia, which ended in the 1960s. Most remained unwed, preferring to work hard to send money home to their families in China. By the 1980s these ladies were already ageing; all were Taoist and struggled to marry their culture with the rapid economic and building developments in Singapore. Wearing their traditional dress, which they donned for their work as maids, they lived close to one another in high-rise apartments, separated from their families who were back in China. These women preferred and trusted their Chinese traditional medicine, rather than Western medicine. There are now very few Samsui ladies left in Singapore. However, Chinese traditional medicine is now becoming more popular worldwide, and some Westerners have abandoned conventional cancer treatments for traditional treatments.

Indians are primarily Hindu. But a fair number of them make a Christian subgroup. The main subgroup is made up of the Tamils from southern India. They have colorful traditions as well as their own religious festivals.

Malay are almost all Muslim and follow Muslim traditions regarding medical treatment and the care of ill men and women. In the Muslim tradition, there are stringent regulations on handling the body of the deceased. Primarily, the deceased must be buried within 24 hours of death.

> One of the most difficult traditions in India is the attitude toward women and the preferential power granted to men. Not surprisingly then, females are not brought to the doctor. Interviewing the elderly of India in 1982, I visited a grandmother who was minding an infant girl who was very ill with a high temperature. I asked her why she was not taking her to the clinic, and her immediate answer was, "they only have paracetamol there," which was true, as I had visited it. I offered to give her a prescription and to pay for an appropriate antibiotic for the child. Her answer was, "Let her die . . . she is a girl."

This way of thinking devalues and diminishes cancer referrals. Two streams of medical services operate in India: Western medicine and Ayurveda. The government recognizes both and allows them to work together side by side in clinics. The elderly, chronically ill, disabled, and cancer patients are seen by the Ayurveda specialists who have their own (and often effective) treatments. Children and those with acute infections attend the Western clinics. But oncology treatments are part of "Western medicine." The incidence of cancer far exceeds the number of treatment centers, and so many people are left with progressing cancer and suffer in pain, particularly women.

As a dowry is paid to the man by the bride's father for marrying his daughter, there is great temptation for a married man with a sick wife to let her die, get a new wife and be paid for it, too! This is comparable to A.M.'s experience in Kenya, when she visited the mother of five children in her 40s, who had breast cancer and was near the end of life. She was now alone. Her husband would not pay for any treatment as he was saving up for his next wife (in Africa the suitor buys his wife). This situation occurs in many African countries.

The tradition of Sati in India is no longer practiced. However, in 1983, when A.M. was based in Benares, the Holy City of Hinduism, she was told that, although it was against the law, in the past when a woman married she would promise to die on the funeral pyre of her husband. Some of the elderly widows favored this tradition and still practiced Sati. With this tradition in mind, when a woman was ill herself, all health priorities were for her husband. A woman made no plans to live as a widow, knowing she would die with her husband.

Traditions are basically beliefs or customs that have been handed down from one generation to another [11]. Many traditions are not written in any form but instead are handed down from generation to generation through oral communication, practice, and way of life. In many African countries, the body is buried either in the family compound or near to it, as the ancestors will be controlling the lives of future generations. This requirement, in itself, affects whether a seriously ill patient is taken to hospital or is kept at home. Poor families face a double whammy here in that if they have not completely paid the hospital bill, the body may not be released from the mortuary. Once they have the body, it is very costly to transport it home or to the village. This issue is particularly difficult for Muslims (who are found in every one of the seven countries), who must be buried within 24 hours of death, as dictated by the Muslim faith.

Traditionally, many believe that when a loved one dies, the spirit continues to control future generations [12]. Notably, even the dying person must reconcile with the ancestors before transitioning so that the ancestors can prepare an environment in which they can welcome and support the newly dead. The ancestors must be pleased with the deceased's life, and if they have been offended in any way, they must be appeased. Ancestor worship is still followed in many cultures. With a life-threatening illness such as cancer, retribution for past wrongdoings must be made to the offended ancestor(s) before death. In Africa, this act of retribution may mean traveling far from the cancer center to the family village where the ancestors are often buried. However, when burial is in a cemetery, this is usually closer to the home.

Other Beliefs

When addressing other beliefs, we must not forget the influence of belief in the efficacy of the treatment. We have all seen patients who believe that a certain herbal medicine or certain prayers will relieve their pain or cure them.

> I (and others) witnessed, in Nigeria, perfectly well young persons, come to the hospital demanding to be admitted because they were going to die, yet the doctors could not find anything wrong with them. The youths insist they have had a spell put on them by an enemy and that they will die. We witnessed that those who were admitted did die, while those who went home were not seen again.

With the arrival of the Internet some years ago, many patients now search for information and treatments on their own following diagnosis, and many believe what they find, keeping them from getting cancer treatment in their own countries. This is a worldwide phenomenon, and it first came to A.M.'s attention in Uganda in 1993 by a retired teacher who had early cancer of the prostate. After consulting the Internet and learning the possible complications and suffering expected, he attempted to take his own life.

Beliefs regarding the causes of cancer affect the choices made regarding care. The belief that illness is the result of a person having offended someone living or dead or a punishment from a higher power is common to several cultures. In order to cure this illness, atonement must be paid to the offended one who may be a person who is still alive, an ancestor or a god. The ancestor may demand special rituals, which are made known to the patient by a traditional healer or a medium. This consultation usually comes at a financial cost. Often, the patient will have to return to the place of the ancestors (their village) to make atonement, thus leaving treatment behind until they can return to the hospital, depending on the cost. This will often affect (delaying or disregarding) the preferred cancer treatment.

Most countries in Africa are at a great disadvantage, with more than 50% of their population not seeing a health worker. In a small pilot study conducted with the three most populous tribes in Uganda, the two main barriers to cancer care access were finances and information from relatives. A lot of discussion and advice is heard among relatives. Sadly, however, in most cases, the advice is confusing and contradicts preferred modern medicine. Both of these barriers counted as more than 90% of the reasons for not accepting

Table 36.1 Culture, Spirituality, Traditions, and Beliefs Affecting Cancer Care in Uganda

	Response rate % (*n*=30)
1. Beliefs about cause of cancer	
Infection and catching from other	66.7
I am bewitched	46.7
Heredity/genetics	30.0
I have offended God	23.3
Smoking and alcohol use	13.3
Consuming processed foods	6.7
Family planning use	6.7
I don't know	10
2. Types of medical advice and treatments available and commonly used in the communities	
Spiritual healing	80
Traditional herbal	76.7
Western (modern) medicine	76.7
Traditional witchcraft	23.3
3. Other barriers to cancer care access	
Cost	93.3
Long distance	53.3
Delays in referral system	50
Bad experience of preferred/or nonpreferred treatment	60
Advice from others (relatives, medical friends, traditional beliefs, spiritual advisors)	93.3
Stigma associated with cancer illness	10

Source: Survey of 30 cancer patients, key informants (religious and cultural/traditional leaders), and laypeople from communities in central, western, and southwestern Uganda: November 2020

medical treatment. The next most common beliefs linked to the causes of cancer were being bewitched (47%) and hereditary elements (30%), as shown in Table 36.1.

The most prevalent medical advice initially sought is spiritual healing and second is Western and traditional medicine. Most patients have already received traditional advice and treatment before approaching Western medicine. As mentioned earlier, culture, beliefs, and traditions are complex. These vary from place to place, from region to region (Table 36.2).

Examples of Quotes from the Interviews

- *Many patients give up when the various ways they have tried to find a cure fail. Personally, I have tried to use some herbal medicine when the cancer is still benign … boil and let the patient take half a litre three times daily for one month.* (Catholic priest)
- *After the failure of ordinary medication, many patients will embrace divine intervention because, traditionally, there is a strong belief that cancer is incurable.* (Protestant bishop)

Table 36.2 Forms of Advice and Treatments Commonly Used in Uganda, by Region

Type of advice/treatment	Response rate by region (%)
Traditional herbal	
Western	80
Central	70
Southwestern	80
Spiritual healing	
Western	80
Central	90
Southwestern	70
Modern (western) medicine	
Western	60
Central	90
Southwestern	80

Source: Survey on 30 cancer patients and community members; laypeople, religious, and traditional/cultural leaders in Uganda: November 2020

- *People tend to concentrate on spiritual treatment for cure, thus avoiding medical treatments which lead to the cancer advancing. Cost and long distances are also major prohibiting factors . . . many usually end up not accessing the treatment at all, and thus, dying due to poverty.* (cultural leader)
- *Many people tend to hide . . . they fear that once a biopsy is done, the result will be death.* (cancer prostate patient)

Some are afraid to go near a hospital because they have heard of, or seen, a cancer patient going into hospital and coming home in a box, therefore leading them to believe that hospitals may kill patients. But health professionals themselves are preventing pain control and access to cancer and palliative care. Most still do not understand palliative care as a specialty in pain control, management of symptoms, approach to quality of life, and a good death. A.M. found this in Europe as well as in LMICs. The best recognition and understanding was in Singapore. Yet, it has been proven scientifically, as well as by experience, that patients who receive palliative care along with curative therapy live longer with a better quality of life [13]. With improved quality of life, patients eat and sleep better. Palliative care can work better in Uganda than in the European countries where it is hindered by colleagues' ignorance of the modern proof that oral morphine does not give the " 'high" craved by addicts who have to "mainline" intravenously.

Finally

The following patient's story gives an idea of the complex interactions that different beliefs have with cancer treatment:

Charity (not her real name) is a 26-year-old female from a rural area in North West Uganda. She is a Protestant by faith. She came to our hospice with a confirmed diagnosis of choriocarcinoma. She reported developing abdominal pain and P/V discharge, the cause of which she attributed to a co-wife who stole her underpants and performed some witchcraft on it. She was advised and referred to a Uganda cancer institute, which she nonetheless declined, and instead, she went herbal.

In the tradition of polygamy, there is the common problem of rivalry among wives and the belief in witchcraft as a cause of cancer. As this patient believed that the cancer was caused by witchcraft, she was certain medical treatment would not help!

Conclusion

Cancer treatment is affected by spiritual beliefs, culture, traditions, other beliefs, and the economy of the country and of the patient and family. All of these elements are intertwined to define and make people who they are. As these fluctuate with time, the approach to cancer treatment often changes during a person's lifetime.

In today's world, when traveling, teaching, working ,or volunteering from North to South is so common, it is essential that the traveler, and especially the volunteer, understands and is prepared to learn more about spiritual beliefs, cultures, traditions, and other beliefs of the particular country they are visiting.

We must all be prepared to witness patients' varying responses to cancer treatments, which may be influenced by the health care professionals' belief in the efficacy of the treatment, as well as the strength of the patients' belief that the chosen treatment is the best treatment for their condition.

Acknowledgments

The authors wish to thank the many individuals who offered advice, as well as those who performed and assessed the questionnaires in Uganda: Bernadette Basemera, Betty Kasigwa, and Ndinawe John Bosco Kateera, together with the nurses of Mobile Hospice Mbarara, Hospice Kampala, and Little Hospice Hoima, the three sites of Hospice Africa in Uganda for the study of three local tribes. Also, we thank Hanif Kasozi for her Monitoring & Evaluation expertise.

Special gratitude is extended to the following for their assistance in answering questionnaires and for their time on phone calls, which brought us up to date on current factors affecting cancer care in each country:

Southeast Asia
India: M. R. Rajagopal, MD, Chairman, Pallium India, Director, Trivandrum Institute of Palliative Sciences (WHO Collaborating Centre for Training and Policy on Access to Pain Relief)

Singapore: Sr Geraldine Tan, Executive Director, St Joseph's Home and Hospice, Jurong

Malaysia: Dr. Ednin Hamzah, Chief Executive Officer, Hospis Malaysia

Africa

Kenya: Dr. Zipporah Ali, Palliative Care Physician, Executive Director of Kenya Hospices and Palliative Care Association

Nigeria: Sr Sylvia Ngozi, MMM, BA (DevStudies), Maynooth University, Ireland, Nurse Midwife, Matron of Family Health Centre/VVFCentre, Itam, Uyo, Akwa Idom State, Nigeria

Uganda: The authors and teams of Hospice Africa Uganda

Europe

Ireland. Aoife Nic Shamhrain, Irish GP, MB, BCH, BAO, MRCGP, FRACGP. DRCOG, Dip-MSK; and Dr. Darren Peter Doherty, MB, BCH, BAO, BSc, Irish NCHD
UK: Dr. Mike Merriman, FRCGP Partner and Trainer, Medical Centre, Kirby Primary Care Network, Merseyside

Stories from Different Countries

KENYA *(From A.M.: Shows how inborn beliefs carry throughout life, even among the highly qualified)*

<u>Story 1</u>: A principal of a college had breast cancer. She was seeing a traditional healer who told her not to accept surgery, chemo, or any other therapy. Upon examination, her swollen red breast was ready to burst. She declined any conventional treatment even though she was in severe pain. Counseling made no difference.

UGANDA *(From A.M.: We can put Western learning into the man, but we cannot take the culture out of the man!)*

<u>Story 2</u>: A young mother was dying of stage 4 HIV. We happened to be there when she started Cheyne Stokes breathing. We called her husband, newly returned from the West, having completed training in his specialty. The minute the pause came after a deep breath, he produced a piece of material and, pulling her head back, he tied it around her neck to stop her breathing further. Shocked, I yelled at him to stop, but he would not, saying this was his culture!

KERALA *(From Dr. Raja Gopal: This case indicates the situation in Kerala of husbands working abroad, as well as the fear of disfigurement overriding medical advice and the horrors of lockdown.)*

<u>Story 3</u>: She was a mother of two, with breast cancer. Husband working in the Gulf came home to her. Operation was recommended, but she refused, afraid of pain and disfigure-ment and, instead, sheopted for indigenous medicine. Two years on, with her husband unemployed and resources exhausted, she came to PC with secondaries in her lungs, fungating foul-smelling ulcer on breast, lymphedema arm, with infected lesions. While there, lockdown demanded quarantine on both sides of the border, so the family couldn't

reach her or her children. She died without a final hug of farewell to her children, leaving her husband a broken man. What emotional scars would the children grow up with?

MALAYSIA *(From Dr. Ednin Hamzah)*
(A.M.: The following cases indicate the problems with family pressure, especially husbands making decisions for their wives. The names have been changed. Case 5 involves hiding truth from patients.)

Story 4: Madam See, age 62, with advanced colon cancer lives with her husband but is cared for by her son and two daughters. Bone pain is controlled with morphine, and she is comfortable. Her oncologist advises oral chemo to reduce progression. She refuses as she does not want to burden her family. Her family feels that she is giving up, and so the medication is given to her anyway by her husband, who tells her that it's a supplement.

Story 5: Siti, 38, a university lecturer, was diagnosed with breast cancer. Mastectomy followed by chemotherapy was advised. She consulted her husband but later decided not to have the surgery as that would affect her relationship with her husband and her ability to care for her three children, aged 10–15. She understands, but relationships stand in her way.

SINGAPORE: *(From A.M.: Preferred belief due to denial and disbelief in the cause of pain, delayed treatment)*

Story 6: Chew Mary, 30, married Daniel on December 28, 1997. They honeymooned in Thailand, Chinese New Year 1988. She developed stomach pains in Thailand but thought it was due to spicy food. When she did not improve, she went to hospital back in Singapore and investigation showed cancer of stomach. Operation and chemo were only palliative. We looked after her, with Daniel, at home. She died a year and a day after marriage, on December 28, 1988. Daniel gave up his job and looked after her till the end. His grief lasted many years.

IRELAND *(From A.M.: The only story that touches on a common belief today; the belief that cures can be found on the Internet)*

Story 7: James, 42, recently married with no children, was diagnosed with non-gestational choriocarcinoma. Chemotherapy was recommended. On the Internet he found a keto diet and lost 20 kilos in 2 months. Too weak to continue with chemo, he was advised to get palliative care for quality of life. End-of-life care was further complicated by the patient's desire to fly overseas and attend an alternative cancer care clinic which he had researched online for a treatment based on high doses of Vitamin C, a ketogenic diet, and marijuana-derived products. This desire to continue alternative therapies and his belief in their efficacy further fueled denial of prognosis and poor recognition of current care needs. Goal setting at end of life was severely impacted, as well as relations with loved ones who did not share his belief in alternative therapy.

UK and IRELAND *(From A.M.: We can do better in Uganda!)*

<u>Story 8</u>: Personal experiences with friends and relatives throughout the past two years showed me that the promotion of stigma by some primary care doctors, oncologists, and other health professionals continues in the UK and Ireland. I saw oncologists and teams in both countries refusing to prescribe oral morphine or to honor requests from patients' relatives to refer them to palliative care until they were dying. Meanwhile, families suffered watching their loved ones in pain and suffering. The backlash is that the public believes that a referral to palliative care means they are dying. This is also seen in LMICs. It is sad to witness this in the countries where palliative care was first defined by Dame Cicely Saunders and promoted to the world since 1967.

Note

1 Samuel, D. S. *Singapore's heritage: Through places of historical interest,* 1991, p. 44. Singapore: Elixir Consultancy Service. (Call no.: RSING 959.57 SAM)

References

1. Viktor Frankl, *Man's Search for Meaning,* Beacon Press, 2006, ISBN 978-0807014264
2. Steiner A. *UNDP. Foreword to UNDP Human Development Report.* New York, NY/UNDP, 2020.
3. World Health Organization. *Pain Relief.* 1st ed. WHO Geneva, 1986.
4. CIA. *CIA Factsheet 2020: Singapore.* CIA World Fact Book, CIA, 2020.
5. CIA. *CIA Factsheet 2020: India.* 2020.
6. National Institutes of Health. *Who can get free prescriptions.* NHS, London; 2021. Available from: https://www.nhs.uk/nhs-services/prescriptions-and-pharmacies/who-can-get-free-prescriptions
7. Bedi M, Devins GM. Cultural considerations for South Asian women with breast cancer. *J Cancer Survivorship.* 2016;10(1):31–50.
8. Atuhaire P. *Uganda's Kanungu cult massacre that killed 700 followers.* By Patience Atuhaire, BBC News, Kanungu, London/BBC. Published 17 March 2020 [cited 2021 February 2021].
9. Simão T, Caldeira S, Campos De Carvalho E. The effect of prayer on patients' health: Systematic literature review. *Religions.* 2016;7(1):11.
10. Kahissay MH, Fenta TG, Boon H. Religion, spirits, human agents and healing: a conceptual understanding from a sociocultural study of Tehuledere Community, Northeastern Ethiopia. *J Relig Health.* 2020;59(2):946–960.
11. Merriam Webster Dictionary. 1828. https://www.merriam-webster.com/dictionary/tradition.
12. Ekore RI, Lanre-Abass B. African cultural concept of death and the idea of advance care directives. *Indian J Palliat Care,* 2016. 22(4):369–372.
13. Temel JS, et al. Early palliative care for patients with metastatic non-small-cell lung cancer. *N Engl J Med.* 2010;363(8):733–742.

37

Sociocultural Context and Its Impact on Communication, India

Naveen Salins and Srinagesh Simha

Introduction

Communication consists of verbal, non-verbal and written communication [1]. A skilled communication involves the ability to comprehend a concept, developing active assertions, valuing others' perspectives, and enabling a shared understanding [2]. The term *sociocultural* refers to beliefs, traditions, habits, and patterns prevailing in a social or cultural context [3]. Regional cultures, ethnicities, diverse languages, societal attitudes, and lifestyles underpin the fabric of sociocultural context [4]. Comprehension of this diversity in a multicultural society facilitates communication [5]. Moreover, the clinical voice literature alludes to speaker's voice function and communication to the sociocultural functioning [6]. This chapter explores the impact of sociocultural context in communication in a cancer and palliative care setting.

Impact of Sociocultural Context on Communication

It is vital to know the preferences of patients and family caregivers about disclosure of diagnosis and prognosis. It will avoid undermining patients and families and avoid rupture of the therapeutic alliance [7]. In patients and their families with life-limiting conditions, health-related communication like disclosure of diagnosis and prognosis is an intricate process and not just a mere handover of information. Therefore, disclosure without understanding the patient and family caregivers' viewpoints could adversely impact communication outcomes [8,9]. Although communication practices in high-income countries emphasize complete open disclosure of diagnosis, the majority of physicians practicing in Europe and Asia do not fully agree with this approach [10]. Italians are often not informed about their cancer diagnosis and the majority of them are unaware about their prognosis [11]. Although the Japanese prefer full disclosure of the diagnosis, they favor only partial disclosure of their prognosis. Not surprisingly, they are traumatized by the unexpected and unilateral disclosure of their prognosis by their health care providers. They prefer to remain uninformed of their prognosis, as they fear it will become a self-fulfilling prophecy [12]. As a result, Japanese physicians have adopted individualized communication approaches over a generic approach, while conveying information about diagnosis and prognosis [13]. The physicians in Tanzania choose a reflective, roundabout method for health-related communication instead of a direct approach [14].

The ethos of clinical practice in high-income countries emphasizes full disclosure of diagnosis and prognosis in a life-threatening situation, as it is ethically justified, upholds the principle of self-determination, and facilitates patients participation in treatment decision-making [15]. However, in societies and cultures where collective autonomy is in vogue, patients and their families make a collective decision and are responsible for the collective decision [16]. Therefore, the same principle of full-disclosure applicable in some cultures and societies may not be applicable to others [17]. Moreover, studies have shown that inappropriate disclosure could increase pain scores and poor physical and emotional functioning, and an insightful disclosure may reduce long-term emotional distress and improve physical health [18,19].

Health care providers often attribute patient and family reluctance to knowing the truth and the psychological indisposition of truth-telling as important impediments for disclosure [20]. Health care providers in India commonly believed that patients and families do not prefer to know about diagnosis and prognosis. These beliefs impacted physicians' communication practices and warranted a study to explore their ontology. The majority of the studies relating to communication of health-related information are conducted in high-income countries among Caucasian and some Asian populations [21–23]. The findings of these studies are uncritically accepted and adopted into clinical practice in other cultures, societies, and economies. The studies have shown that culturally appropriate and sensitive communication of diagnostic and prognostic information provides hope, improve recall of information, and enable patients and families to participate in decision making [24,25]. Moreover, it enables higher satisfaction and lower levels of anxiety and depression when information is communicated thoughtfully by the physicians [26]. Therefore, sociocultural competence among health care providers is imperative for effective communication.

A study has been conducted to discern the preferences and attitudes of patients and family caregivers upon disclosure of cancer diagnosis and prognosis in India [27]. Two hundred and fifty patients and an equal number of caregivers participated in the cross-sectional observational study, and all participants answered seven questions on diagnosis and four questions on prognosis. The majority of patients participating in this study preferred full disclosure of name of illness, seriousness of illness, treatment options, success of treatment, progress of treatment, how treatment works, side effects of treatment, future course of illness, future symptoms, future complications, and expected length of survival. Only a small proportion of caregivers preferred full disclosure of all these aspects of the disease. The patients felt that knowing diagnosis and prognosis may help them to be prepared, plan further treatment, anticipate complications, and plan for future and family. The caregivers felt that patients' knowledge of diagnosis and prognosis may negatively impact the future course of illness and that as a result, patients may experience stress, depression, and loss of hope and confidence [27]. The study revealed two important aspects of sociocultural impact on communication: (1) it debunked the myth among the Indian health care providers that patients and families in the Indian sociocultural context do not prefer to know about the diagnosis; and (2) it exposed the reluctance among the families about patients knowing their diagnosis and prognosis.

The health care provider's sociocultural beliefs and their understanding and expectations of the society could form presuppositions that develop into practice tendencies.

In low-income countries and in some cultures and societies, it is a common belief that the patient's informational needs are low and that the family caregivers often try to protect the patients from adverse health information [28]. Contrary to this belief, the above-mentioned study showed that patients preferred full disclosure of the diagnosis and prognosis [27]. The studies conducted worldwide in patients with cancer showed that patients wanted physician to be truthful about their prognosis, and they wanted to know the impact of illness on their daily lives and life expectancy [29–31]. Disclosure of prognosis influenced choosing treatment options and making treatment decision making [32]. However, it has to be done in a perceptive and culturally appropriate manner.

In traditional societies like India, the family is part of the illness experience, and so the illness is perceived as a malady of the family; this is in contrast to the Caucasian population where illness is seen primarily in terms of the individual [33]. In some cultures, family support is central to an individual's experience with cancer. It can enable unburdening of physical, social, and financial responsibilities, and it facilitates patients' ability to cope with the illness experience emotionally [34]. Direct rendition of Western culture's emphasis on autonomy, individual responsibility, and empowerment to other cultures could cause unwarranted burden or stress on the individuals and families [35]. In Eastern cultures, families like to guard their loved ones from adverse news, so that not allowing patients to know is often considered an act of love [36]. In Egypt, families feel that patients must be protected from adverse communications, be made dependent, and be nurtured and not involved in the decision making [37]. Therefore, culturally appropriate, individualized, and family-centric communication takes precedence over standard prescriptive communication [38].

Health care providers often perceive communicating diagnosis and prognosis as stressful. Often, it is due to lack of training and contextual understanding, which makes them avoid such communications [39]. Moreover, physician beliefs regarding outcomes of communications such as breaking bad news leading to distress, depression, and reduced life expectancy also hinder effective communication [40]. Moreover, constraints of time and discussions on medical treatment receive priority over communication [41]. This could lead to gaps in communication, which is often linked to treatment noncompliance, lack of rapport, and general dissatisfaction [42]. In certain Eastern cultures, the family members dictate the decision making, and the patients are often kept in the dark regarding their health information [43]. In India, a distinctive form of collusion exists between health care providers and family; the patient is aware of this collusion and accepts it [44].

Culture is an integrated pattern of human behavior, thought, communication, ways of interacting, roles and relationships, expected behaviors, beliefs, values, practices, and customs [45]. Cultural competency refers to awareness of one's own culture and worldview, having a positive attitude toward the cultural difference, possessing knowledge about cultural practices, and acquiring cross-cultural communication skills [46]. Across the trajectory of cancer, sociocultural aspects impact communication. As discussed earlier, during the early phase of illness it impacts attitudes toward disclosure of diagnosis and prognosis. However, this is not limited to the early phase of the trajectory; rather, it extends to all phases of the illness trajectory in cancer.

In the decompensation phase, communication often centers around beliefs about the cause and meaning of illness. These beliefs vary across countries and regions, and are largely shaped by religious traditions, with overtones of elements of culture [47]. Different religions support diverse views related to health, illness, and death. In India, Hinduism considers illness to be the consequence of one's past sins or karma [48]. Religious beliefs and cultural outlook can shape understanding of the origins of illness, particularly cancer. In many ethnicities, dietary causes are understood to be the primary cause of cancer, rather than genetic or biological factors. Among Caucasians, individuals are expected to fight nature and involve themselves in a struggle to fight cancer and recover. In Eastern cultures, individuals are expected to live in harmony with nature, with docility and fatalistic views being common. In many conventional societies, disease is considered God's punishment [48]. Health care providers should be able to address contradictory views and beliefs related to cancer during their communication to achieve shared decision making and common therapeutic goals [33]. The questions Kleinman [49] raises provide an excellent exploratory tool that can be used to explore the beliefs and meaning of illness:

1. What do you think caused this problem?
   It is asked to know what patients and families believe or perceive to be the cause of the illness.

2. Why do you think this problem started, and when did it start?
   It is to explore their hidden beliefs, myths, and misconceptions about why the patient developed cancer or any illness.

3. What do you think this problem does inside your body? How does it work?
   It is to understand the patient's and family's views about what the cancer or illness does to the body and its impact.

4. How severe is this problem? Will it have a short or long course?
   It is to explore the prognostic understanding of illness.

5. What kind of treatment do you think you should receive?
   It is to know the patient and family preferences about treatment or no treatment.

6. What are the most important results you hope to receive from this treatment?
   It is to know the expectation/outcome of the treatment.

7. What are the chief problems this illness has caused?
   It is to understand the symptoms or complications developed due to cancer/illness.

8. What do you fear most about the illness/problem?
   It is to find out what aspect of illness and its outcomes worries them the most.

In the dependency phase, communication often revolves around the meaning of pain and suffering. Every culture and social group has its own distinctive semantics of pain and suffering, its own multifaceted expressions by which ill or sad people make others aware of their distress. It is often signaled, both verbally and nonverbally, by a person in pain or distress, and these expressions and their behavior are usually colored by societal and cultural determinants [50]. It often depends on aspects such as whether the cultural values or the societal expectations support or undermine the display of emotions and verbal expression in response to pain. A few cultural groups expect an extravagant display of emotion in the presence of pain, but others value stoicism, restraint, and playing down the pain [51]. Some cultures believe that they should withstand pain bravely and serve as a role model, perhaps to improve their standing in life after death. A few believe that pain is a sign of progress and a road to recovery. Pain is also perceived as part of God's plan, a test of their faith, or as atonement for past sins [52]. In some cultures, people are very stoic regarding pain and may maintain a neutral facial expression despite experiencing severe pain. The Australian Aborigines do not consider pain to be a health problem, and the Nepalese seldom seek medical attention for pain [52]. Black and Hispanic patients are more likely to be undertreated for their pain across health settings, and stereotyped perceptions about race, ethnicities, and barriers in communication are the predominant reasons for undertreating pain [53]. It could lead to health practitioners misinterpreting an unwillingness to discuss appropriate pain management. In some cultures, and societies, patients and families also believe that the use of opioid pain medication is the equivalent of euthanasia. They also believe, falsely, that the use of opioids means death is imminent. Administration of opioids early in the development of pain will decrease options for treatment in the future. They may also refuse opioids due to fear of [54]. Learning about pain management, cultural competence, and sensitive communication enables effective pain management in people with life-limiting illness [52].

In the decline and terminal phase, communications pertain to sociocultural attitudes toward death and dying. Dame Cecily Saunders felt that finding meaning in suffering is a healthy process that could facilitate management of pain, symptoms, and distress. Sociocultural situatedness and culturally sensitive communication provide the key that opens the door to understanding the meaning of suffering, dying, and death [55]. People from Eastern cultures often request that providers not disclose a terminal diagnosis, for they want to avoid emotional suffering and preserve hope. Moreover, they feel that the impending death should be discussed with family first, who may or may not inform the patients. Few Christian and Muslim groups consider end-of-life care, and limitation of life-sustaining treatment contradicts their religious teachings. Buddhists do not prefer administration of drugs that cloud the mind near death. Taiwanese believe that it is a bad omen if one discusses impending death, and so they try to avoid discussing death [56]. African Americans are generally accepting of end-of-life care and death.

Every culture has its own views about the meaning and purpose of life, death, and what happens after death. These views determine their response to one's own death and the death of their loved ones. Some believe in a life after death, and some feel that the spirit of the deceased lives perpetually, influencing the lives of the family members. These beliefs have a strong sociocultural basis and often enable families to make meaning of death, comfort them, and help them to cope with their loss. Therefore, understanding the sociocultural context is vital during the dying and bereavement phases.

Before communicating with patient and family, it is important for health care providers to know how people approaching death are cared for, who is present, and what ceremonies are performed both before and after death. It is also important for them to understand how a person's body is handled after death and whether the body is buried or cremated. In some cultures, such as the Filipino and African American, grief is expressed loudly and publicly, and, in some cultures, it is expressed quietly and privately. It helps the health care providers to be prepared before communication. Knowing how long family members are expected to grieve and observe the mourning period will determine when a bereavement call or bereavement visit is performed [57].

Conclusion

Communication is vital in understanding sociocultural issues. "Two people with the same faith tradition and cultural upbringing may have different end-of-life issues that create pain, challenge, or distress. This may be because of the choices made in their lives and/or the circumstances that surround them" [56]. The ABCDE approach of exploring the sociocultural context can be a valuable tool in determining the influence of social and cultural factors before communicating.

- **Attitudes:** Attitudes toward diagnosis/prognosis, truth-telling, limitation of treatment, end-of-life care, dying
- **Belief:** Beliefs of family regarding treatment, suffering, meaning of death
- **Context:** Historical, political context, migrant, refugee, oppressed
- **Decision making:** Decision-making styles—individual, collective, or other
- **Environment:** Resources, local/community support

When practicing in an urban multicultural society, the cultural diversity of cancer patients is bound to increase, and cultural sensitivity and competence are therefore essential for professionals. Understanding the sociocultural context during communication improves therapeutic outcome and minimizes disparities in medical care. Cultural competence can be achieved by being aware of possible biases and prejudices related to culture and societal stereotyping. It also influences the understanding of ethical norms and principles, which has a strong sociocultural situatedness. It governs the inconsistency of truth-telling attitudes and practices worldwide, as well as the different roles of family in the information and decision-making process involving the cancer patient. It also plays a huge role in providing palliative care, care for the dying, and support to the family after the patient's death.

References

1. San-Valero P, Robles A, Ruano M, Martí N, Ch·fer A, Badia JD. Workshops of innovation in chemical engineering to train communication skills in science and technology. *Educ Chem Eng.* 2019;26:114–121.

2. Chung Y, Yoo J, Kim S-W, Lee H, Zeidler D. Enhancing students communication skills in the science classroom through socioscientific issues. *Int J Sci Math Educ*. 2014;14:1–27.

3. Ponterotto J. Qualitative research in multicultural psychology: Philosophical underpinnings, popular approaches, and ethical considerations. *Cult Divers Ethnic Minority Psychol*. 2010;16 4:581–589.

4. Clauss-Ehlers CS (ed). *Encyclopedia of cross-cultural school psychology*. Springer Science & Business Media, 2010.

5. Taufiq M, Rokhman F. Scientific communication skills profile of prospective science teachers based on sociocultural aspects. *J Pendidikan IPA Indonesia*. 2020;9(2):187–193.

6. Azul D, Hancock AB. Who or what has the capacity to influence voice production? Development of a transdisciplinary theoretical approach to clinical practice addressing voice and the communication of speaker socio-cultural positioning. *Int J Speech-Language Pathol*. 2020;22(5):559–570.

7. Rahman SA, Mahmud M, Mohamed AST, Rashid S, Bachok NA (eds). Disclosure of Cancer Diagnosis and Prognosis from Patients' Perspectives at Hospital Universiti Sains Malaysia (HUSM). In Proceedings of the Regional Conference on Statistical Sciences, 2010, pp. 256–263.

8. Alamri A. Cancer patients' desire for information: a study in a teaching hospital in Saudi Arabia. *Eastern Medit Health J = La revue de sante de la Mediterranee orientale = al-Majallah al-sihhiyah li-sharq al-mutawassit*. 2009;15 1:19–24.

9. Montazeri A, Tavoli A, Mohagheghi M, Roshan R, Tavoli Z. Disclosure of cancer diagnosis and quality of life in cancer patients: Should it be the same everywhere? *BMC Cancer*. 2008;9:39.

10. Mitchell JL. Cross-cultural issues in the disclosure of cancer. *Cancer Pract*. 1998;6 3:153–160.

11. Costantini M, Morasso G, Montella M, Borgia P, Cecioni R, Beccaro M, et al. Diagnosis and prognosis disclosure among cancer patients. Results from an Italian mortality follow-back survey. *Ann Oncol*. 2006;17 5:853–859.

12. Sato R, Beppu H, Iba N, Sawada A. The meaning of life prognosis disclosure for Japanese cancer patients: A qualitative study of patientì narratives. *Chronic Illness*. 2012;8:225–236.

13. Miyata H, Tachimori H, Takahashi M, Saito T, Kai I. Disclosure of cancer diagnosis and prognosis: A survey of the general public's attitudes toward doctors and family holding discretionary powers. *BMC Med Ethics*. 2004;5:7.

14. Harris JJ, Shao J, Sugarman J. Disclosure of cancer diagnosis and prognosis in Northern Tanzania. *Soc Sci Med*. 2003;56 5:905–913.

15. Gordon E, Daugherty C. *"Hitting You over the Head": Oncologists' Disclosure of Prognosis to Advanced Cancer Patients*. Hoboken, NJ: Wiley-Blackwell: Bioethics; 2003.

16. Kachanoff FJ, Kteily N, Khullar TH, Park H, Taylor D. Determining our destiny: Do restrictions to collective autonomy fuel collective action? *J Personal Soc Psychol*. 2019 September;119(3):600.

17. Hagerty R, Butow P, Ellis P, Lobb E, Pendlebury S, Leighl N, et al. Communicating with realism and hope: Incurable cancer patients' views on the disclosure of prognosis. *J Clin Oncol*. 2005;23 6:1278–1288.

18. Lheureux M, Raherison C, Vernejoux J, Nguyen L, Nocent C, Lara MTd, et al. Quality of life in lung cancer: Does disclosure of the diagnosis have an impact? *Lung Cancer*. 2004;43(2): 175–182.

19. Lieberman M. The role of insightful disclosure in outcomes for women in peeí directed breast cancer groups: A replication study. *Psychè Oncol*. 2007 October;16(10):961–964.

20. Shahidi J. Not telling the truth: Circumstances leading to concealment of diagnosis and prognosis from cancer patients. *Eur J Cancer Care*. 2010;19 5:589–593.

21. Jenkins V, Fallowfield L, Saul J. Information needs of patients with cancer: Results from a large study in UK cancer centres. *Br J Cancer*. 2001;84(1):48–51.
22. Kumar DM, Symonds R, Sundar S, Ibrahim K, Savelyich B, Miller E. Information needs of Asian and White British cancer patients and their families in Leicestershire: A cross-sectional survey. *Br J Cancer*. 2004;90:1474–1478.
23. Wang S, Chen C-H, Chen Y, Huang H-L. The attitude toward truth telling of cancer in Taiwan. *J Psychosom Res*. 2004;57 1:53–58.
24. Barnett M. Effect of breaking bad news on patients' perceptions of doctors. *J Royal Soc Med*. 2002 July;95(7):343–347.
25. Stoner M, Keampfer SH. Recalled life expectancy information, phase of illness and hope in cancer patients. *Res Nurs Health*. 1985;8 3:269–274.
26. Schofield P, Butow P, Thompson J, Tattersall M, Beeney LJ, Dunn S. Psychological responses of patients receiving a diagnosis of cancer. *Ann Oncol*. 2003;14 1:48–56.
27. Ghoshal A, Salins N, Damani A, et al. To tell or not to tell: Exploring the preferences and attitudes of patients and family caregivers on disclosure of a cancer-related diagnosis and prognosis. *J Glob Oncol*. 2019 November;5:1–2.
28. Laxmi S, Khan JA. Does the cancer patient want to know? Results from a study in an Indian tertiary cancer center. *South Asian J Cancer*. 2013;2:57–61.
29. Fried T, Bradley E, O Leary J. Prognosis communication in serious illness: Perceptions of older patients, caregivers, and clinicians. *J Am Geriatr Soc*. 2003 October;51(10):1398–1403.
30. Greisinger A, Lorimor R, Aday L, Winn R, Baile W. Terminally ill cancer patients. Their most important concerns. *Cancer Pract*. 1997;5 3:147–154.
31. Kutner J, Steiner J, Corbett K, Jahnigen D, Barton P. Information needs in terminal illness. *Soc Sci Med*. 1999;48(10):1341–1352.
32. Degner L, Kristjanson L, Bowman D, et al. Information needs and decisional preferences in women with breast cancer. *JAMA*. 1997;277 18:1485–1492.
33. Surbone A. Cultural aspects of communication in cancer care. *Support Care Cancer*. 2007;16:35–40.
34. Sk C. Exploration of concerns and role of psychosocial intervention in palliative care--a study from India. *Ann Acad Med Singapore*. 1994;23:256.
35. Ho A. Relational autonomy or undue pressure? Family's role in medical decision-making. *ScanJ Caring Sci*. 2008;22 1: 128–135.
36. Tse C, Chong A, Fok S. Breaking bad news: A Chinese perspective. *Palliat Med*. 2003;17:339–343.
37. Ali N, Khalil H, Yousef W. A comparison of American and Egyptian cancer patients' attitudes and unmet needs. *Cancer Nurs*. 1993;16(3):193–203.
38. Ballard-Reisch DS, Letner JA. Centering families in cancer communication research: acknowledging the impact of support, culture and process on client/provider communication in cancer management. *Patient Educ Couns*. 2003;50 1:61–66.
39. Ranjan P, Kumari A, Chakrawarty A. How can doctors improve their communication skills? *J Clin Diag Res*. 2015;9 3:JE01-4.
40. Ml S. Talking about cancer: How much is too much? *Br J Hosp Med*. 1987 July;38(1):56–58.
41. Holland J, Geary N, Marchini A, Tross S. An international survey of physician attitudes and practice in regard to revealing the diagnosis of cancer. *Cancer Invest*. 1987;5(2):151–154.
42. Kasteler J, Kane R, Olsen D, Thetford C. Issues underlying prevalence of "doctor-shopping" behavior. *J Health Soc Behav*. 1976;17(4):329–339.
43. Chaturvedi S. Ethical dilemmas in palliative care in traditional developing societies, with special reference to the Indian setting. *J Med Ethics*. 2008;34: 611–615.
44. Chaturvedi S, Loiselle C, Chandra P. Communication with relatives and collusion in palliative care: A cross-cultural perspective. *Indian J Palliat Care*. 2009;15:2–9.

45. Weech-Maldonado R, Dreachslin JL, Epane J, Gail J, Gupta S, Wainio JA. Hospital cultural competency as a systematic organizational intervention: Key findings from the national center for healthcare leadership diversity demonstration project. *Health* Care Manage Rev. 2018;43 1:30–41.
46. Jongen C, McCalman J, Bainbridge R. Health workforce cultural competency interventions: a systematic scoping review. *BMC Health Serv Res.* 2018 December;18(1):1–5.
47. Martsolf D. Cultural aspects of spirituality in cancer care. *Seminars in Oncol Nurs.* 1997;13(4):231–236.
48. Chaturvedi SK, Strohschein FJ, Saraf G, Loiselle CG. Communication in cancer care: psycho-social, interactional, and cultural issues. A general overview and the example of India. *Front Psychol.* 2014;5:1332.
49. Hsieh J-G, Hsu M, Wang Y-W. An anthropological approach to teach and evaluate cultural competence in medical students—the application of mini-ethnography in medical history taking. *Med Educ Online.* 2016;21:32561.
50. Helman C (ed). *Culture, Health and Illness.* 5th ed. CRC Press, 2007.
51. Peacock S, Patel S. Cultural influences on pain. *Rev Pain.* 2008;1(2):6–9.
52. Givler A, Maani-Fogelman PA. The importance of cultural competence in pain and palliative care. *StatPearls* [Internet]: StatPearls Publishing; 2020.
53. Bonham VL. Race, ethnicity, and pain treatment: Striving to understand the causes and solutions to the disparities in pain treatment. *J Law Med Ethics.* 2001;28:52–68.
54. Saini S, Bhatnagar S. Cancer pain management in developing countries. *Indian J Palliat Care.* 2016;22:373–377.
55. Martin EM, Barkley W, Jr. Improving cultural competence in end-of-life pain management. *Nursing2019.* 2016;46(1):32–41.
56. Lunn JS. Spiritual care in a multi-religious context. *J Pain Palliat Care Pharmacother.* 2003;17:153–166.
57. Leit, C, Pereira V, Maciel C. Exploring the communication of cultural perspectives in death-related interactive systems. In Proceedings of the XVI Brazilian Symposium on Human Factors in Computing Systems; 2017 October 23, pp. 1–10.

38

Emotional State, Spirituality, and Religion's Effect on the Acceptance of Cancer, Morocco

Asmaa El Azhari and Abdellatif Benider

Introduction

Across the world, cancer is one of the leading causes contributing to the increase of health-related suffering and is found to be associated with the highest number of deaths. For example, it is expected that in the year 2060, more than 16 million people per year will die of cancer (an increase of 109% between 2016 and 2060) and suffer from serious health-related illnesses (Figure 38.1) [1].

The association between cancer and death transforms the disease into a heavy burden on health systems and poses a real "terror" for health professionals and patients in terms of physical, mental, and spiritual suffering. For this reason, historically and still today in some cultures, cancer patients have not generally been informed of their diagnosis because it was believed that patient information was harmful and extremely stressful. With the progress of cancer treatments in the late 1970s, models of care evolved toward respecting patient autonomy and, as a consequence, informing them about their cancer diagnosis, raising new communication challenges for both patients and physicians [2].

Of all the conversations between doctors and patients, none is more important than the one in which the doctor must inform the patient of the diagnosis and/or prognosis of the disease [3]. As for physicians, announcing a cancer diagnosis continues to be a difficult task, constituting for many patients the first step toward establishing a relationship of trust and a doctor–patient alliance—that is, when the announcement phase is achieved in a gentle and fluid way for the patient and the attending physician. The quality of the bad news announcement also has a significant impact on patients [4]. In this sense, appropriately delivered bad news is associated with better emotional adjustment for the patient [3] and a better outlook on the disease.

Another crucial factor influencing the patient's acceptance of a cancer diagnosis is their current state of mind, which is, in part, determined by a complex mix of lifelong beliefs, perceptions, and expectations, and which helps to create and provide meaning to their life via religious traditions or via mediations, nature and/or art in the case of secular culture [5].

The religiosity and spirituality of each patient, often straddled, impact the way they accept, live, and adapt to the stressful situation that cancer presents. According to several experts, they can help the patient cope with the disease even when it is associated with the threat of imminent death [6].

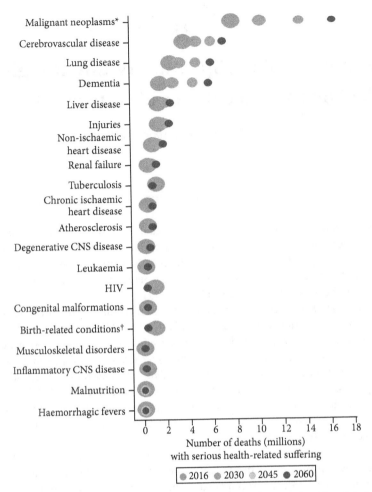

Figure 38.1 Health conditions driving the global burden of serious health-related suffering (2016–60)

Excluding leukemia; including birth trauma, low birthweight and premature birth[1]

The Impact of the Patient's Emotional State on the Illness Experience

You have cancer. Hope or frustration?

" … I had just turned forty and after several months of denial, I had finally convinced myself to have a breast biopsy. This morning, the doctor was going to tell me the results. He was calm and very serene and, as soon as he opened his mouth, I quickly felt enveloped by the warmth of his voice. Finally, the fateful word was *spoken and, contrary to what I expected, hope and deliverance took the place of the anguish that had paralyzed me for months."*

—*Cancer patient, 2020*

Buckman defines bad news as "any information that could drastically alter the patient's vision of his or her future, whether at the time of diagnosis or following the failure of the curative intention" [7].

There is no greater anxiety-provoking situation for a person, whether sick or not, than an uncertain future. And when the future is hopeless, patients, or any person for that matter, can no longer escape frustration, fear, sadness, and depression. Indeed, cancer is more terrifying when it compromises hope. At the time of diagnosis, and throughout the stages of the disease, the patient will be led over and over again to question the object of their deepest hope: getting well, a time without pain or a good death [5].

In many patients, this hope will be constantly nourished by their closest entourage, such as witnessing their children grow, or by the struggles they had to overcome throughout their lives, such as completing a personal project. However, some people (caregivers and patients' families) confuse denial with hope. In certain cultures, it is not uncommon to hear a doctor tell the family of a cancer patient in an advanced palliative situation: "the patient should not know the truth, he should be reassured, don't you see that he has hope?" The family adheres to this conspiracy of silence, as does the patient, even if the deterioration of the patient's general condition reveals a reality other than the lie used by the patient, his family, and his doctor in order to protect themselves. The patient's caregivers and entourage use false reassurances and lies as defense mechanisms, giving rise to false hopes that will keep the patient in denial. Denial is a psychoadaptive mechanism that might have some benefit for the patient in the beginning and allows them the time they need to assimilate what they are going through, but this dissimulation should not be extended in time as it might generate much anguish and psychological and spiritual distress for the patient when they realize the lack of coherence between their declining physical condition and the false hopes for recovery instilled by family and the caring environment.

Hope should not be based solely on the possibility of a cure, but also on deeper resources intrinsic to the patient that allow him to maintain, at any moment, a level of hope corresponding to every situation that arises, regardless of the prognosis. Even with the discontinuation of the specific cancer treatments, the patient will always have hope: the hope not to suffer. These patients have in common hope that is based fundamentally on faith [8]. For them, the faith will promote adjustment through hope and provide meaning to what is happening to them [9].

However, patients suffering from cancer have different levels and/or resources of hope. Levels vary from patient to patient and depend on several factors. From the moment a person receives a cancer diagnosis, they must face difficult challenges, questioning their life paths on all levels: physical, psychological, and spiritual; patients and their families will often feel confused and lost in their medical care process [8]. The level of hope that recently diagnosed cancer patients feel does not seem to be significantly influenced by the stage of their disease; however, age seems to be inversely proportional to the level of hope [10]. When patients get support from their medical care teams, this support, along with the treatments they receive, becomes an essential source of hope for them. On the other hand, extended, inefficient treatments and the degradation of the patient's physical condition threatens their ability to continue cultivating hope [11]. For these palliative cancer patients, faith seems to be their main source of hope [12]. As several studies have shown, one's intrinsic religious beliefs, family support, spiritual resources, as well as effective coping styles will allow them to move toward a positive psychosocial adjustment to the disease and the treatments [8] and toward keeping a higher level of hope and acceptance of the disease and, eventually, a reconciliation with life and death [11].

This positive force, hidden in the depths of our souls and directed toward the future, is the key to a better experience of the disease [13] and will be intimately linked to the inner peace experienced by everyone who endeavors to understand their own existence.

Spiritual Well-being before, during and after Cancer

Why me?

"Man is not destroyed by suffering; he is destroyed by suffering without meaning."
                                   —Victor Frankl (1984), *Man's Search for Meaning*

The way in which we look at our lives, values, and perception of meaning and purpose of life, illness, well-being, and death, constitute our spirituality [6]. This is a fundamental human phenomenon that helps create life's meaning and is characterized by values related to oneself, others, nature, life, and all that is considered as Ultimate; it is different from religion because it is experienced before one knows anything about religion. It may sometimes be part of an institutionalized religion, but not always [14].

According to the National Comprehensive Cancer Network (NCCN), spirituality is "the relationship people have with a force or a power beyond themselves that helps them feel connected and enriches their lives" [15]. This state of enrichment, personal growth, and spiritual well-being is not a constant throughout our lives. For some, a cancer diagnosis is an opportunity for profound introspection directed toward strengthening their spiritual well-being, and, for others, it is a source of a questioning that will cause them to doubt everything they have ever believed in, throwing them into intense spiritual distress.

Between one extreme and another, from well-being to spiritual distress, there are several stages, phases, and nuances specific to each patient. It is not a "black and white" situation for which a patient must be definitively classified, but rather a long path of contemplation meant to lead the patient toward a state of emotional balance, allowing them to cope with the disease and treatment regardless of the outcome.

This generic human characteristic [6] is at the heart of the experience of many cancer patients and their families. In the context of advanced disease, most patients have spiritual concerns and consider spiritual and religious peace and the absence of pain to be the most important factors affecting their well-being in the face of death. In the same context, there is an important association between the quality of life and the spirituality of patients who consider spiritual care to be an important part of the overall management of their cancer [16].

In addition, it has been shown that spiritual well-being preserves patients' quality of life and averts the desire for a hasty death despite severe physical symptoms. When appropriate spiritual care is provided to these patients, it allows them to overcome the negative impact that severe symptoms have on their quality of life and their desire to die [17]. In this sense, it can be very beneficial and interesting for caregivers to be able to measure spirituality and all its complexities by using the available scales for spiritual evaluation in order to meet the spiritual needs of patients and their families. However, this remains a difficult task, for there is still no consensus on how to adequately take it into account [5]. Indeed, for caregivers, the exact definition of what constitutes spirituality is uncertain, though we do know that spirituality correlates with quality of life, satisfaction with the care provided, and the decisions taken throughout a potentially life-threatening illness such as cancer [18].

According to the European Organization for Research and Treatment of Cancer (EORTC), quality of life (QOL) depends not only on the physical and psychosocial welfare of the patient and the extent to which they are satisfied with management of the disease, but also on their personal sense of fulfillment and well-being. According to the EORTC, QOL not only represents how the patient perceives the functional effects of the disease and its treatment, but also reflects how the patient feels about their position in life within the context of their cultural values. The patient's quality of life will increase as the gap between expectations and achievements decreases [19].

Indeed, as soon as a cancer patients enter the gates of the disease and its treatments, their overall and spiritual well-being will depend on their quality of life, that is, on how they perceive the evolution of their state of health in all its components, while maintaining their personal view of life. Before reaching this phase of life, characterized by the disease, people have already had many life experiences. Those dealing with cancer do not come from nowhere; they have always incorporated their ethereal and material environments that define quality of life, state of well-being, and basic spirituality, which cannot be separated from what will follow. A "core spirituality" or "a basic spiritual state" depends on a person's own history and life experience. This fundamental, individual spirituality provides serenity and peace for some, but for others it can have a burst of negative effects. For many cancer patients, this will play a very complex role in the acceptance of the cancer and influence patients' initial reaction to the diagnosis, while they are still naive of the stressful symptoms, treatments, and complications to come. This usual state of spirituality will then be challenged and can evolve in either one direction or another, in line with the evolution of the disease, in all aspects: physical, psychological, and social (Figure 38.2).

Some patients face spiritual distress when suffering uncontrollable pain, or from the financial burden or inability to pay for their treatments; others experience this distress even when everything is in order from a symptomatic and financial standpoint. Many patients express their feelings of peace and tranquility when they are satisfied with the control of their disease; others feel stoically at peace even if they are consumed by intense pain difficult to control.

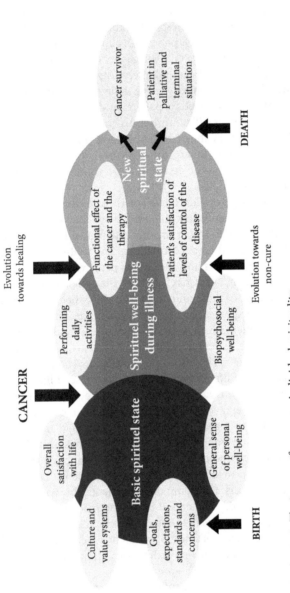

Figure 38.2 The impact of cancer on individual spirituality
Prior to a cancer diagnosis, patients have a basic individual spirituality that affects many aspects of QOL, such as the satisfaction that people express about life and the general feeling of personal well-being, how they perceive their position in life within their cultural context and value system, as well as their perception of their expectations and achievements of their goals in life [19]. Cancer, its symptoms and its treatments, impact patients' QOL, leading their spiritual well-being toward a new spiritual state that will determine the postdisease QOL for recovering patients, or the QOL for palliative patients facing death.

So what is this factor that influences and differentiates between the patients? Who defines their states of mind beyond the seriousness of the disease, the severity of the treatments, and the quality of care, as well as the adversities of life in general?

Religious Coping as an Adaptation Tool

My God does not forsake me!

"And (remember) Job, when He cried to his Lord: truly trouble has seized me, but thou art the Most Merciful of those who are Merciful. So We listened to him: We remove the distress that was on him, and We restored his people to him, and doubled their number, as a Grace from Ourselves, and a thing for commemoration, for all who serve Us."

—The Glorious Quran: 9:83–84

When all the cards are played and fate has been pronounced, can we escape it? It is clear that no one can flee their own destiny, but many patients use religion as a tool to adapt and come to terms with the cancer diagnosis, and sometimes they use it to escape the incurability of their disease. Through their faith in God, expressed via a religion, they will try to rise to levels of peace and tranquility that will allow them to breathe out the fear generated by their fateful situation.

The religiosity of each individual is defined by their religious affiliation and beliefs, as well as their participation in the rituals and activities of one of the traditional religions [6,20]. Religion is a mode of spirituality, but the two are not synonymous [6]. Religion and its practices are a means by which we, as believers, can channel and consolidate our relationship with God. Each one of us, through prayer, reading a verse from the Torah, the Bible, or the Quran, or even through fasting, try to be heard by God and receive God's mercy. The materialization of this divine acknowledgment and mercy is perceived and interpreted differently by each person depending on their situation, faith, wisdom, maturity, and spirituality. Prayer is one of the religious activities common to all monotheistic religions. Literature reviews of populations suffering pain show that prayer is the most important religious practice used to cope with pain; moreover, the worse the pain, the more frequent are the prayers [21]. However, the role of prayer in the relief of pain is not clear. Other researchers claim that religious coping behavior allows the patient to deal better with the disease and avoid depression and pain in a significant way [22]. Strengthening these behaviors improves the quality of life and health of patients suffering from chronic diseases [23].

In the case of cancer, patients are confronted with symptoms resulting from treatments as well as other symptoms that may be severe or even refractory, causing great suffering. For them, using religious coping can be very particular and, at the same time, complex. This particularity of religious coping depends on four key elements:

- The patient's basic spiritual state.
- The patient's quality of life and spiritual well-being while coping with cancer.
- The patient's expectations from religious coping, "*What do I expect from God?*".

- The patient's perception and interpretation of the "results" from utilizing an adaptation tool: *"Has God fulfilled my expectations?"*; *"How has God fulfilled my expectations?"*; *"Am I satisfied with His answers to my expectations?"* In short, the meaning that the patient gives to the negative or positive events that will follow one another throughout their illness.

The interaction of these elements will define two types of religious coping: a positive religious coping, in which the patient manages negative events by strongly believing in the unconditional support from God; and a negative religious adaptation, in which the patient constantly experiences insecurity and denial in their relationship with God, thinking they were abandoned and/or punished by God [22], as it was God who inflicted the disease upon them.

Hence, for some cancer patients and their families, faith is the most important factor influencing their decision making after the recommendations of their treating physicians [24]. Thus, positive religious concepts can be a means of support for specific cancer treatments [25] and are associated with better quality of life and spiritual well-being during the advanced stages of the disease [5]. In addition, it has been shown that there is a significant negative correlation between the perception of pain and positive religious coping [22].

Positive religious coping can exist even during the most stressful situations a cancer patient can go through. It is not conditioned by the absence of negative events, but rather by faith. Many patients will not pray to God in order to ask Him to cure them or relieve their symptoms, but to give them the strength to endure adversity and preserve their integrity, even when faced with the most persistent symptoms and the most challenging situations. They will pray for God to lead them toward unconditional acceptance of the disease, even though it is the source of their extreme suffering. This mechanism of adaptation is used, for example, in Islam, where Muslims believe that every soul is only able to endure what it can with the help of Allah, as expressed in the following Quranic verse: *"On no soul doth Allah place a burden greater than it can bear. It gets every good that it earns, and it suffers every ill that it earns. (Pray:) Our Lord! Condemn us not if we forget or fall into error; Lord! Lay not on us a burden that which Thou didst lay on those before us; Lord! Lay not on us a greater burden than we have strength to bear. Blot out our sins, and grant us forgiveness. Have mercy on us. Thou art our Protector; Help us against those who stand against faith"* [26].

Muslim patients, through religious coping, do not perceive their disease as a punishment. On the contrary, they feel privileged to have to go through it since, in their perception, it purifies them from all their sins, thus allowing them to reach paradise; it is a sign of God's love for them. Moreover, religious resources help a patient adapt to the most unfortunate prognosis and to accept one's own death [27]. Indeed, in Arab-Muslim culture, dying cancer patients are considered martyrs. Death is no longer distressing for these patients but becomes their liberation, as expressed in the following Quranic verse: *"Who say, when afflicted with calamity: 'To Allah we belong, and to Him is our return'. They are those on whom (descend) blessings from their Lord, and Mercy. And they are the ones that receive guidance"* [28].

For believers, the practices of monotheistic religions play a crucial role in their perception and acceptance of all aspects of their lives, including disease, suffering, and death. From the moment of the diagnosis, they stick to the principle of trusting in God (the tenet of reliance) who is capable of healing, if He wishes, even the incurable [29]. This principle, referred to in Arabic as *tawakkul*, is not only used by Islamic patients and their families but also by the caretaking environment. *"Trust in God"* or *"Everything is in God's hands"* are often the answers doctors give their patients when asked about their prognosis. However, in order to make healthy use of it and not mislead the patient into false hopes or confusion, it is important while using religious resources to keep the patient informed about their disease. In turn, through a positive religious coping, the patient will be able to surrender to God in order to find meaning in what they are going through.

Conclusion

Cancer and its consequences bring about a devastating experience for patients and their families. It can shake the faith of the strongest believers and be the source of doubt, leading them to question the meaning of existence. However, building spiritual well-being, fundamental for a better quality of life, is possible. When patients are well informed about their illness and perceive that their disease is well controlled and cared for at all levels, they feel *"protected"* from stressful events that could disturb their tranquility. As illness and symptoms progress, faith is a fundamental tool to maintain hope, for whatever reason.

References

1. Harding, R, Sleeman KE, et al. The escalating global burden of serious health-related suffering: Projections to 2060 by world regions, age groups, and health conditions. *Lancet Glob Health.* 2019;7:e883–892.
2. Gorniewicz J, et al. Breaking bad news to patients with cancer: A randomized control trial of a brief communication skills training module incorporating the stories and preferences of actual patients. *Patient Couns.* 2016, http://dx.doi. org/10.1016/j.pec.2016.11.008
3. Ptacek JT, Ptacek JJ. Patients 'perceptions of receiving bad news about cancer. *OJC* 19 2001; 4160–4164. doi: http://dx.doi.org/10.1200/JCO.2001.19.21.4160
4. P. Von Blanckenburg F, Hofmann M, et al. Assessing patient's preferences for breaking bad news according to the protocol: the MABBAN scale. *Patient Couns.* 2020;103:623–1629.
5. Peteet JR, Balboni MJ. Spirituality and religion in oncology. *CA Cancer J Clin.* 2013;63:280–289.
6. Qasem Ahmed W. Spiritual care at the end of life: Western views and Islamic perspectives. *Int J Human Health Sci.* 2018;2(2):65–67.
7. Buckman A. Breaking bad news: why is it still so difficult, *Br. Med. J.* 288 1984;1597–1599.
8. Weaver AJ, Flannelly KJ. The role of religion/spirituality for cancer patients and their caregivers. *Southern Med J.* 2004; 97(2):1210–1214.

9. Moadel A, Morgan C, Fatone A, et al. Seeking meaning and hope: self-reported spiritual and existential needs among an ethnically diverse cancer patient population. *Psychooncology.* 1999; 8:378–385.

10. Duggleby W, Ghosh S, Cooper D, Dwernychuk L. Hope in newly diagnosed cancer patients. *JPSM.* 2013; 46(5):661–670.

11. Chi GC. Hope in patients with cancer. *Oncol Nurs Forum.* 2007;34(2):415–424.

12. Ballard A, et al. A comparison of the level of hope in patients with newly diagnosed and recurrent cancer. *Oncol Nurs Forum.* 1997;24(5):899–904.

13. Van Dongen E. "I wish a happy end." Hope in the lives of chronic schizophrenic patients. *Anthropol Med.* 1998; 5:169–192.

14. Bjarnason D. Concept analysis of religiosity. *Home Health Care Manag Pract.* 2007;19(5), 350–355.

15. https://www.nccn.org/patients/resources/life_with_cancer/spirituality.aspx (accessed 27 November 2020)

16. Winkelman WD, Lauderdale K, Balboni MJ, et al. The relationship of spiritual concerns to the quality of life of advanced cancer patients: preliminary findings. *J Palliat Med.* 2011;2:1022–1028.

17. Wang YC, Linen CC. Spiritual well-being may reduce the negative impacts of cancer symptoms on the quality of life and the desire for hastened death in terminally ill cancer patients. *Cancer Nurs.* 2016; 39(4):43–50.

18. Richardson P. Assessment and implementation of spirituality and religiosity in cancer care: Effects on patient outcomes. *Clin J Oncol Nurs.* 2012;16 (4):150-155.

19. https://qol.eortc.org (accessed 29 November 2020)

20. Bjarnason D. Concept analysis of religiosity. *Home Health Care Manag Pract.* 2007;19(5):350–355.

21. Koenig HG. Religion and medicine IV: Religion, physical health, and clinical implications. *Int J Psychiatry Med.* 2001;31(3):321–336.

22. Goudarzian AH, Jafari A, Beik S, Nesami MB. Are religious coping and bread perception related together? Assessment in Iranian cancer patients. *J Relig Health.* 2017. doi 10.1007%2Fs10943-017-0471-4

23. Taheri-Kharameh Z, Saeid Y, Ebadi A. The relationship between religious coping styles and quality of life in patients with coronary artery disease. *Iranian J Cardiovasc Nurs.* 2013; 2(1):24–32.

24. White V. Cancer as part of the journey: The role of spirituality in the decision to decline conventional prostate cancer treatment and to use complementary and alternative medicine. *Integr Cancer Ther.* 2006;117–122.

25. Tatsumura Y, Maskarinec G, Shumay DM, Kakai H. Religious and spiritual resources, CAM, and conventional treatment in the lives of cancer patients. *Alt Ther Health Med.* 2003; 9(3):64.

26. *The Glorious Quran*: 2. 286.

27. Alcorn SR, Balboni MJ, Prigerson HG, et al. 'If God wanted me yesterday, I wouldn't be here today' Religious and spiritual themes in patients' experiences of advanced cancer. *J Palliat Med.* 2010;13:581–588.

28. *The Glorious Quran*: 2:156–157.

29. Al-Shahri Z. Islamic theology and the principles of palliative care. *Palliat Support Care.* 2016;14(6):635–640.

39

Breast Cancer Survivorship in Nigeria

The Experience of Survivors and Need for Development of Supportive Care, Nigeria & UK

Eme Asuquo, Omolola Salako, Therese Mbangsi, Kate Absolom, Bassey Ebenso, Kehinde Okunade, Temitope Adeleke, and *Matthew J. Allsop*

Breast Cancer Survivorship Care in Nigeria

In sub-Saharan Africa (SSA), breast cancer is the primary cause of cancer morbidity and the second-most common cause of cancer mortality [1]. Incidence rates of cancer in SSA are some of the lowest in the world, yet it has high mortality rates relative to other regions, indicative of poorer survival outcomes [2]. In SSA, cancer incidence and mortality are both projected to continue to rise in the coming decades [3,4]. Poor survival rates from breast cancer have been attributed to multiple factors, including the unavailability and unaffordability of treatment and factors influencing late-stage presentation and engagement with treatments (e.g., poor diagnosis, stigmatization, fear of disfigurement, and the influence of traditional and spiritual healers) [5–8]. In Nigeria, the most populous country in SSA, breast cancer is the most common type of cancer, representing around 22.7% of all new cancer cases and 38.7% of all cancer diagnoses in women. Incidence rates range from 36.3 to 50.2/100,000 and, similar to wider regional trends, is increasing [4,9–11].

The health care pathway, as experienced by breast cancer patients, is characterized in three stages [12]: discovery, examination, and follow-up (including technical and informational needs for the types of treatments) and survivorship. The latter stage has been an evolving, and now distinct, phase along the cancer care continuum in terms of health care and research in high-income settings such as the United States [13]. For high-income countries, there are a variety of survivorship care models; however, there is little evidence regarding their effectiveness. Furthermore, the lack of clarity concerning optimal timeframes for monitoring patients and the intensity of care that health professionals should be trained in and deliver, act as barriers to their wider development [14]. Health systems in low-resource settings have limited capacity to provide access to quality, long-term health care for the growing number of cancer survivors [14]. For example, the inadequate access to health systems' services and resources in low- and middle-income countries (LMICs) such as Nigeria hinder the capacity to provide ongoing evaluation and support, including reassurance about the effectiveness of treatments and remission. Furthermore, limited attention has been given to the needs of people undergoing cancer treatment and those who survive cancer and to the development and adaptation of supportive services and programs in SSA, with a lack of integration into standard care [15,16].

The broad definition of the term *survivorship* includes people who have been diagnosed with cancer, are currently living with it, or have not had any recurrence of cancer for a defined period of time [17]. There are a growing number of people, worldwide, who are living with treatable but incurable breast cancers (such as secondary and advanced breast cancers) Innovative treatments, typically in the high-income countries, are extending the life expectancy of many patients and are creating new challenges in providing appropriate monitoring and supportive care [18]. There has been limited research to determine the needs and preferences of women with breast cancer at each stage of the disease, as reflected in the above definition, to guide the development of supportive interventions. Emerging literature from the SSA region highlights the fact that breast cancer survivors report treatment-induced long-term complications [15]. This can include both physical (e.g., shoulder pain and disability, lymphedema, increased susceptibility to cardiovascular diseases, chemotherapy-induced menopause and infertility, cognitive impairment, infertility, sexual dysfunction, secondary cancer) and psychosocial components (e.g., fear of disease recurrence and death, anxiety, depression, altered body image, loss in sense of femininity following mastectomy, and relationship breakdown) [15,19–21]. Furthermore, spirituality, faith and religion have a crucial role to play when coping with a breast cancer diagnosis and adapting to life with cancer, especially in its advanced stages [22–30].

Given limited resources, determining how best to improve the quality of breast cancer care for those undergoing and moving beyond treatment is a public health challenge [31,32]. Meeting the physical, emotional, and social concerns of women during the breast cancer survivorship period is more difficult in LMICs than in high-resource settings [33,34]. While emerging evidence exists across SSA, in Nigeria there is a need to begin to understand the experiences of breast cancer survivors in order to identify targets for the development of locally appropriate service development and advocacy efforts.

In this chapter, we present narrative accounts of breast cancer survivors, detailing their experiences from diagnosis to the present and exploring their culture and beliefs pertaining to living with cancer. The narratives were derived from a panel discussion hosted by Sebeccly Cancer Care and Support Centre, a nongovernmental organization based in Lagos, Nigeria, dedicated to supporting women living with breast cancer. In November 2020, a focus group discussion facilitated by Sebeccly staff and the research team was conducted via Zoom with three women from diverse ethnic and social backgrounds currently undergoing treatment or who had completed treatment for primary breast cancer in the last 12 months. Topics for discussion included participants' experiences of initial symptoms, access to health care, and living with cancer, with the focus group facilitated by members of the team (E.A., O.S.). The participants were approached by the Sebeccly team one week prior to the meeting and were provided with the topic guide and information about the panel. Those who opted to participate attended in person at the Sebeccly offices in Lagos, where social distancing measures were in place. Participants were set up individually in separate rooms, each with a video-enabled mobile phone device to participate in the discussion. The panel was recorded and a transcript created; the Framework Method [35] was used to inductively and deductively structure and organize the discussion.

Experiences of Breast Cancer Survivors in Nigeria

Three main themes arose from discussions with the participants: (1) detection and treatment of cancer; (2) sources of support; and (3) cultural and societal aspects of survivorship. Content from the focus group has been synthesized in Figure 39.1, providing an overview of the experiences of participants, from diagnosis to the present day.

Living with Breast Cancer

Detection and Treatment

All participants noticed a lump in their breast before diagnosis, and only one of the survivors whose mother had died of breast cancer had been examining her breast monthly and undergoing annual clinical screening.

> "I always check my breast every month and yearly as my mother died of breast cancer." (Participant 2)

Participants reported a process of denial before seeking medical care, even after they had started their treatment, with one of the participants visiting multiple hospitals and traditional medicine practitioners in an attempt to obtain alternative treatments.

> "... when I told my friends I had cancer, they told me it was a spiritual attack and so I went looking for alternative treatments and to different churches looking for a cure. I didn't get treatment for 3 years." (Participant 3)

Furthermore, delays in accessing care were related to fear and concerns around the prospect of needing a mastectomy and what life would be like living with one breast.

> "I went from hospital to hospital in different states for about 5 months to find out if I could treat the cancer without cutting off my breast, until my doctor told me the earlier I start treatment the better my chances of surviving this cancer." (Participant 1)

The emotional impact of the diagnosis was immediate and devastating to participants, with no expectations of a positive outcome.

> "I immediately became afraid and felt all my dreams with my children and husband were shattered. I remembered what had happened to my mother who did not go to the hospital, but was drinking holy water and praying until the cancer burst and she eventually died." (Participant 2)

Throughout diagnosis and before and after treatment, faith and religion recurred as a means of coping and a source of support for living with their condition. However,

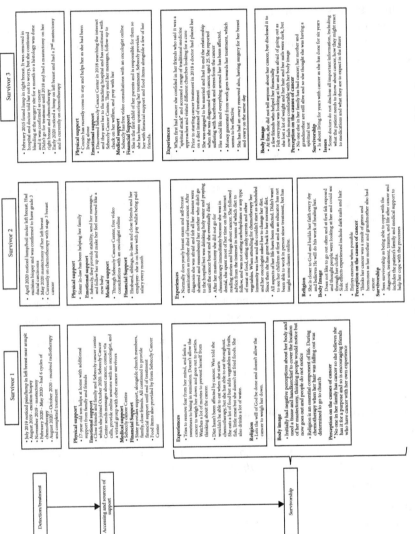

Detection/treatment

Accessing and sources of support

Survivorship

Survivor 1

- July 2019 noticed pain/lump in left breast near armpit
- August 2019 – excision biopsy
- November 2019 – mastectomy
- February 2020 – May 2020 – had 6 cycles of chemotherapy
- August 2020 – October 2020 – received radiotherapy and completed treatment

Physical support
- 17-year-old son helps at home with additional support from family and friends

Emotional support
- Close friends and family and Sebecely cancer center which she joined October 2020. Sebecely Cancer Center sends messages about cancer, contact via calls, provide online sessions with an oncologist, and a virtual group with other cancer survivors

Medical support
- Sebecely Cancer Centre

Financial Support
- Sister provides support, alongside church members, family, close friends. All continued to provide financial support until end of treatment
- Food items also provided by from Sebecely Cancer Center

Experiences
- Tries to remove fear from her mind, and feels a reluctance to being in remission. Doesn't allow the cancer to weigh her down and goes out to parties. Watches a lot of movies to prevent herself from thinking about the cancer.
- Diet hasn't been affected by cancer. Was told she wouldn't be able to eat when she started chemotherapy, but she has been able to eat throughout. She eats a lot of food but adds vegetables and fruits, fish, little meat but she doesn't eat fried foods. She also drinks a lot of water.

Religion
- Lets the will of God be done and doesn't allow the cancer to weigh her down.

Body Image
- Initially had negative perceptions about her body and used a tissue and handkerchief to cover the location of her mastectomy, thinking people would notice but now goes out freely, thinking people do not notice

Perception on the causes of cancer
- Religion is an essential component of life. During chemotherapy when her hair was falling out was determined to go to church
- No one in her family has cancer so she believes she has it for a purpose and so is encouraging friends who have cancer with her own experience

Survivor 2

- April 2020 noticed lump/boil under left breast. Had excision biopsy and was confirmed to have grade 3 ductal carcinoma
- May 2020 mastectomy of her left breast
- Currently on chemotherapy with stage 3 breast cancer

Physical support
- Sister in-law has been helping her family

Emotional support
- They provide stability, send her messages, and follow her up and make her feel nurtured like a new baby

Medical support
- Through Sebecely Cancer Center (free video consultations with an oncologist online

Financial Support
- Husband, siblings, in-laws and close friends and her employer: she is on leave with pay whilst being paid salary every month

Experiences
- Normally does yearly breast exam and self-breast examination as mother died of breast cancer. After diagnosis she was afraid and felt all her dreams were shattered and remembered her mother who didn't go to the hospital but was drinking holy water and praying until the cancer burst and she eventually died.
- After her mastectomy she did not go for chemotherapy immediately because she was in denial, she spent most of her time on the internet reading stories and blogs about cancer. She followed advice from the internet in terms of which diet to follow, and was not eating carbohydrates or any type of meat or food, eating only carrots and other vegetables. When attending for chemotherapy her immunity was low and she couldn't start as scheduled and her oncologist asked her to change her normal diet. Since then she has gone back to her normal diet.
- All aspects of her life have been affected. Didn't want to see her children at first and as an educator has not been able to work in-person since treatment, but has taught some classes online.

Religion
- She is closer to God and builds her faith every day and believes He will do his work of healing her.

Body Image
- Does not like to go out often and at first felt exposed and thought people were looking at her and could see through her clothes.
- Side effects experienced include dark nails and hair loss.
- Enjoys exercise when possible.

Perception on the causes of cancer
- Thinks her cancer was a result of genes and hormones as her mother and grandmother also had cancer

Survivorship
- Sees survivorship as being able to cope with the diagnosis, treatment, trauma, and life after cancer and includes the patient's family and medical support to help her cope with the processes

Survivor 3

- February 2015 found lump in right breast. It was removed in hospital and doctor told her not to worry, but she continued bleeding at the surgery site for a month so a histology was done and it was confirmed as cancer
- Didn't go for treatment until 2018 and had a mastectomy on her right breast and chemotherapy
- Early 2020 noticed a lump on left breast and had a 2nd mastectomy and is currently on chemotherapy

Physical support
- Cousin has recently come to stay and helps her as she had been living alone

Emotional support
- Discovered Sebecely Cancer Center in 2018 searching the internet and they sent her to the teaching hospital and has continued with Sebecely Cancer Center. They send her messages, follow-up to check on her welfare, and pray with her

Medical support
- Sebecely has free video consultations with an oncologist online

Financial Support
- She is the first child of her parents and is responsible for them so she has been sponsoring her treatment. Sebecely provides her with financial support and food items alongside a few of her friends.

Experiences
- When first had cancer she confided in her friends who said it was a "spiritual attack" and accessed a range of traditional medicine approaches and visited different churches looking for a cure
- Prior to starting cancer treatment in 2018 a doctor had placed her on a diet instead of treatment
- She was engaged to be married and had to end the relationship when she was diagnosed with cancer, aged 25. She reported suffering with heartbreak and stress from the cancer
- Her social life and everything around her has been affected.
- Money generated from work goes towards her treatment, which seems to be effective
- She has had an ovary removed also, having surgery for her breast and ovary on the same day

Body Image
- At first, did not tell anyone about her cancer, but disclosed it to a few friends who helped her financially
- Felt everyone was looking at her and was afraid of going out as she lost a lot of weight and her hair and her nails were dark, but now feels more comfortable with her body image

Perception on the causes of cancer
- No one else in her family has had cancer, her mother and grandmother are still alive and so she thought she was having a spiritual test

Survivorship
- Is about living for years with cancer as she has done for six years

Issues
- Some doctors do not disclose all important information, including what the patient needs to know about cancer, how they might react to medications and what they are to expect in the future

Figure 39.1 An overview of content and themes derived from discussions with participants

there was one account of the issue of faith delaying or leading to abandonment of treatment.

"*After my mastectomy, I had someone tell me that I should just have faith and believe that all is gone, so I didn't immediately go for chemotherapy. I spent most of my days on the Internet looking for a cure, as I felt hopeless, until my husband and I agreed that since we have started the medical path we should just continue on it and support it with our faith.*" (Participant 2)

Sources of Support

Emotional support from family was provided for all participants, during and after treatment. Some participants received support from their husbands, children, extended family, friends, and work.

"*I get support from my 17-year-old son, who helps me do everything at home, and from family, friends, and my office*" (Participant 1)

"*My sister-in-law helps me take care of the home*". (Participant 2)

Family members or friends were often accompanying participants when participants received their initial diagnosis and when they were undergoing treatment.

"*I went with my younger brother for my breast scan and then with a family friend to get another breast scan for a second opinion.*" (Participant 2)

However, the diagnosis of cancer for Participant 3 led to the breakdown and end of the relationship with her fiancé.

Financial support came from a range of sources for two participants, including the participants themselves, friends, charities, their church, and employers.

"*… my bosses in the office are very supportive and give me money anytime I call on them and my church members and close friends who have continued to give me money until I finished my treatment.*" (Participant 1)

"*I have support from my husband, siblings, in-laws and close friends and my office gave me leave with pay. They have been paying my salary every month since I started treatment, for about 8 months.*" (Participant 2)

One participant funded their own treatment costs, supplemented by support from Sebeccly Cancer Center.

"*I am the first child of my parents and am responsible for them, so I have been sponsoring my treatment on my own. Sebeccly provides me with financial support, food items, as do a few of my friends … at first I did not tell anyone but decided to tell a few friends when I needed financial help and they have helped me financially.*" (Participant 3)

All participants reported receiving support from Sebeccly Cancer Care and Support Centre, an organization they discovered online, or from Sebeccly staff who would attend outpatient and hospital clinics to identify women who might benefit from their patient assistance program. Sebeccly provides patient education, treatment support at partner hospitals, and coping resources such as support groups, recovery care products, and navigation services. Weekly check-in calls and messages are sent to women, including the participants, to check on their welfare, pray with them, and provide clarity and information to address concerns. They also provide food and welfare services.

Experiences of Survivorship

All the participants expressed a belief in God, with the experience of living with cancer strengthening their faith and outlook.

> "I have removed fear from my mind, so my journey has been sweet. I let the will of God be done, I don't allow the cancer to weigh me down. I go out, go to parties and not many people know I have cancer." (Participant 1)

However, her prior experience of seeing her mother live with and die from breast cancer led Participant 2 to ensure that medical support was sought rather than relying on religion alone.

> "I did not allow my religious beliefs to prevent taking the necessary medical steps, as that was what happened to my mum - don't worry, don't go anywhere, we will be praying for you, you will be drinking holy water. So, when I called my siblings, they told me that we should act immediately, since we already knew what's up." (Participant 2)

The participants' beliefs surrounding the cause of their cancer varied. One participant thought the cause was genetic due to her family history of cancer, as her mother and grandmother both had cancer. Another felt cancer was sent as a test from God. And one participant, now in remission, thought cancer had been sent with a purpose, which included supporting friends and others who have also been diagnosed with cancer.

All participants did not want to spend time around others or in social situations shortly after treatment. This was partly a consequence of the physical effects of treatment (e.g., removal of breast, weight loss, loss of hair, and dark nails). All participants felt cancer had affected their lives in multiple ways. For example, the collapse of a relationship (Participant 3), and feeling as though other people would look at them, or could see through their clothes, and know they had undergone surgery.

All participants had their own sense of the meaning of survivorship and what it entails, such as the ability to cope with a diagnosis, treatment, trauma, and life after cancer. Participant 3 felt that survivorship was about being able to endure life living with cancer, which she had been experiencing for six years.

Discussion

The current evidence base underpinning breast cancer survivorship in Nigeria, and SSA in general, is lacking, providing little guidance on how best to develop supportive cancer care services in the region. We present insights into the lives of three women with breast cancer who self-identified and are referred to as cancer survivors by the services supporting them. The women avoided diagnosis and treatments at different stages, due to factors relating to finances as well as multiple mixed internal and external messages about the best course of action. When participants did seek to engage with services, their experiences involved the complex navigation of fragmented medical services, while being influenced by culturally accepted ideas of how to seek and achieve cure or manage cancer. Their diverse experiences and reflections on living with breast cancer at different stages of the cancer care continuum highlight the multitude of factors influencing engagement and sustaining interaction with care, including those relating to culture and beliefs, and the broad sources of support. Survivorship is understood as actively enduring life and living with cancer, as well as life following the completion of cancer treatment.

The experiences of the participants aligned with the sparse literature describing sociocultural factors influencing interaction with health services at earlier stages of the disease trajectory. A recent study from Nigeria [36] found religion to be a prominent factor, having positive, negative, and existential effects on breast cancer perceptions, alongside the influence of family and traditional beliefs. The role of religion was evident in the narratives of the participants, with cancer being seen as the will of God as well as being a means for strengthening faith and healing. While one participant ascribed the cause of cancer to genetic and familial history, the role of cancer as a spiritual test was also noted. Cancer arising through a spiritual cause or curse, or as an act of God, is a common attitude in women with breast cancer in the neighboring country of Ghana [37]. In Nigeria, women with breast cancer may attribute the cause of breast cancer to evil spirits, curses, or being promiscuous [38], requiring a spiritual solution for a cure.

The role and influence of family and the wider community can be central to decision making regarding health issues. One of the three participants outlined receiving financial support from her husband, extended family, and friends. Husbands have been identified as a primary source of comfort, financial support, and involvement in decision making concerning access to breast cancer screening services in Nigeria [38]. The few women who felt their husbands did not influence their decision to access cancer screening were gainfully employed and were financially independent [38]. Concerns arose about others' perceptions, particularly following a mastectomy. Participants reported heightened awareness of how others would perceive them, with one participant feeling that people could see the site of their mastectomy through their clothes. This perception, alongside reservations about telling others about their diagnosis, may have been influenced by the enduring stigma associated with cancer. Globally, cancer continues to be laden with social stigma, such as it is contagious, a fatal disease, and a punishment [39]. Previous research on social stigma in Nigeria highlights the notion that the ways people react to illness or disease are strongly linked to broader social and cultural processes [40]. Without a better understanding of the cultural conceptualizations of cancer, the sources and underlying drivers of stigma and discrimination will remain problematic and may be a barrier to developing effective responses [40].

A critical element to address is the lack of financial support to undergo diagnostic testing, treatments, monitoring, and follow-up care for breast cancer and increasing the equity in access to care. Due to inadequate health funding in SSA, breast cancer survivors report increased financial constraints caused by high out-of-pocket payments for treatment, resulting in debt and loss of assets [41]. Consequently, follow-up care for breast cancer becomes financially challenging [41]. Funding for health care remains a common issue for both breast cancer survivors and their caregivers, despite not being reflected in current frameworks of priorities for breast cancer survivorship in LMICs [15]. Reducing human suffering and mortality is key to safeguarding the rights of those living with breast cancer, and it is imperative to invest in breast cancer care as well as early detection in order to improve survival rates and economic productivity [42–44]. One recommended approach, highlighted from research in both Kenya and Nigeria, is for breast cancer survivors to engage in political advocacy and push for governmental commitment toward breast cancer control and insurance schemes to subsidize high treatment costs and workforce training [45–49]. It is strongly recommended that the issue of breast cancer survivorship be prioritized with other urgent health concerns in SSA and that collaboration is supported across governments, oncology experts, civil societies, and international donor agencies affiliated with breast cancer [47–49].

There is a particular need for established supportive care, rehabilitation, and surveillance services in SSA to enhance survival outcomes and quality of life [13]. Breast cancer survivors are at risk of disease recurrence and treatment complications; hence, they should be monitored for early detection and management [50]. Participants reported discovering Sebeccly Cancer Care and Support Centre through Internet searching or by meeting a staff member in an outpatient department. Accounts did not convey a clear pathway or referral process to identify the necessary support for patients with breast cancer. Emerging from the limited literature in the SSA region are approaches that may have usefulness in Nigeria. One intervention approach that could address fragmented care is navigation services through which a person (a navigator) engages with a patient to determine barriers to care and provides information to improve access to all components of the health system, not just primary care [51]. In the context of low- and middle-income settings, there is evidence that this approach can improve screening rates, postoperative complications, and patient retention [52]. A recent pilot study within oncology care has suggested that online patient navigator tools may be feasible and have utility in Nigeria [53]. However, there is currently no integration of navigation services across the three tiers of primary health care: general hospitals and medical centers, tertiary health institutions, and private practices.

Alongside developing coordination of services and support, there is scope to develop patient-level approaches for improving survivorship care. Participants reported confusion and uncertainty about the cause of their cancer and gaps in understanding their disease. Limited studies have examined the provision of evidence-based psychosocial interventions and self-management strategies that inform and educate breast cancer survivors on improving quality of life and well-being in SSA [54]. Based on participant accounts, there may be scope to explore these types of approaches to increase information provision and self-management, particularly around causes and effects of cancer and treatments, diet, and exercise. Promotion of both healthy eating and exercise has been shown to enhance emotional, physical, and cognitive functions [55–57]. In order to enable a wider range of support, there is a need to address the significant gap in availability and access to psycho-oncologists, which is critical to providing effective psychosocial care to survivors [58–59].

In conjunction with developing patient-level approaches, additional stakeholders need to be considered. Caregivers play a critical role in supporting patients, as outlined by participants. While not reflected well in the existing literature on breast cancer survivorship in SSA, the World Health Organization policy on palliative care recommends including the well-being of caregivers as an integral entity in the care of people living with cancer [60]. Developing survivorship care for patients should also consider, wherever possible, the ability to support known problems of caregivers, such as receiving insufficient information on breast cancer symptom management, financial constraints, fear of death, and depression [61–63]. It is critical for employers, too, to support patients during survivorship, finding ways to accommodate breast cancer survivors through flexible working hours, risk assessments, job reassignments, and rehabilitation for long-term complications; these approaches are known to have enhanced work productivity in the United States, Spain, and Holland [41,64,65]. Further support is needed for breast cancer survivors with physically demanding jobs who report a low quality of life [42,64,65]. Across low- and middle-income countries, the burden of breast cancer results in lost productivity and tax revenues, causing a detrimental effect on nations' economies [66]. The feasibility and effective implementation of these approaches needs to be assessed in the context of a country like Nigeria, where the informal economy accounts for as much as 83% of the nonagricultural labor force [67]. Furthermore, employers should extend health insurance plans to cover treatment costs. However, only about 5% of Nigerians have health insurance; 70% of the population still finance their health care through out-of-pocket expenditure [68].

Conclusion

Survivorship care for women with breast cancer in Nigeria is underdeveloped, with a limited evidence base to inform the progression of supportive services. We provide insight into the wide-ranging factors that influence the experience of women with breast cancer and their interaction with health services in Nigeria. Cultural factors and beliefs, including those relating to religion, spiritual causes of cancer, and perceived beliefs of others regarding cancer are evident. It is acknowledged that there are few opportunities for survivorship in LMICs at this time [69], although efforts to influence policy, develop resources, and bring together national oncology organizations may support increases in capacity in this context. For example, nongovernmental organizations such as Sebeccly Cancer Care are developing innovative approaches to survivorship care, including online resources, peer mentors, and networks, grounded in extensive experience supporting women with breast cancer at all stages of the disease trajectory. There is an urgent need to develop the evidence base underpinning cancer care in Nigeria, but increasing commitments are being made to develop nationally acceptable guidelines and policies for quality services for all cancer survivors under a strategic framework for hospice and palliative care. This offers the promise of an environment in which survivorship care can be developed as part of wider efforts to increase the reach and quality of oncology care in the country.

References

1. Parkin DM, Bray F, Ferlay J, Jemal A. Cancer in Africa 2012. *Cancer Epidemiol Biomarkers Prev.* 2014;23(6):953–966.
2. Joko-Fru WY, Miranda-Filho A, Soerjomataram I, et al. Breast cancer survival in sub-Saharan Africa by age, stage at diagnosis and human development index: A population-based registry study. *Int J Cancer.* 2020;146(5):1208–1218.
3. Black E, Richmond, R. Improving early detection of breast cancer in sub-Saharan Africa: Why mammography may not be the way forward. *Glob Health.* 2019;15:3.
4. Pace LE, Shulman LN. Breast cancer in sub-Saharan Africa: Challenges and opportunities to reduce mortality. *The Oncologist.* 2016;21(6):739–744.
5. Allemani C, Matsuda T, Di Carlo V, et al. Global surveillance of trends in cancer survival: Analysis of individual records for 37,513,025 patients diagnosed with one of 18 cancers during 2000–2014 from 322 population-based registries in 71 countries (CONCORD-3). *The Lancet.* 2018;391(10125):1023–1075.
6. Foerster M, Anderson BO, McKenzie F, et al. Inequities in breast cancer treatment in sub-Saharan Africa: Findings from a prospective multi-country observational study. *Breast Cancer Res.* 2019;21(1);93.
7. McCormack V, McKenzie F, Foerster M, et al. Breast cancer survival and survival gap apportionment in sub-Saharan Africa (ABC-DO): A prospective cohort study. *Lancet Glob Health.* 2020;8(9):e1203–e12.
8. Carlson RW, Scavone JL, Koh WJ, et al. NCCN framework for resource stratification: A framework for providing and improving global quality oncology care. *J Natl Compr Canc Netw.* 2016;14(8):961–969.
9. Coleman M, Quaresma M, Berrino F, et al. Cancer survival in five continents: A worldwide population-based study (CONCORD). *Lancet Oncol.* 2008;9:730–756.
10. Youlden DR, Cramb SM, Dunn NAM, Muller JM, Pyke CM, Baade PD. The descriptive epidemiology of female breast cancer: An international comparison of screening, incidence, survival and mortality. *Cancer Epidemiol.* 2012;36(3):237–248.
11. Foerster M, Anderson, BO, McKenzie F, et al. Inequities in breast cancer treatment in sub-Saharan Africa: Findings from a prospective multi-country observational study. *Breast Cancer Res.* 2019;21:93.
12. Cherif E, Martin-Verdier E, Rochette C. Investigating the healthcare pathway through patients' experience and profiles: Implications for breast cancer healthcare providers. *BMC Health Serv Res.* 2020;20(1):735.
13. Nekhlyudov L, Ganz PA, Arora NK, Rowland JH. Going beyond being lost in transition: A Decade of progress in cancer survivorship. *J Clin Oncol.* 017;35(18):1978–1981.
14. Jones J, Howell D, Grunfeld E. *Cancer survivorship: A local and global issue in cancer control. The Lancet Glob Health.* 2018;6:S19.
15. Ganz P YC, Gralow J, Distelhorst S, et al. Supportive care after curative treatment for breast cancer (survivorship care): Resource allocations in low- and middle-income countries. A Breast Health Global Initiative 2013 consensus statement. *Breast.* 2013;22(5):606–615.

16. Mutebi M, Edge J. Stigma, survivorship and solutions: Addressing the challenges of living with breast cancer in low-resource areas. *South African Med J.* 2014;104(5):383–385.

17. Hodgkinson KBP, Hobbs K, Wain G. After cancer. The unmet supportive care needs of survivors and their partners. *J Psychosoc Oncol.* 2007;25(4):89–104.

18. Cardoso F, Costa A, Norton L, et al. ESO-ESMO 2nd international consensus guidelines for advanced breast cancer (ABC2)†. *Ann Oncol.* 2014;25(10):1871–1888.

19. Lema VM. Sexual dysfunction in premenopausal women treated for breast cancer - Implications for their clinical care. *Afr J Reprod Health.* 2016;20(2):122–128.

20. Odigie C, Dawotola A, Margaritoni M. Psychosocial effects of mastectomy on married African women in northwestern Nigeria. *Psychooncology.* 2010;19(8):893–897.

21. Smit A CB, Roomaney R, Bradshaw M, Swartz L. Women's stories of living with breast cancer: A systematic review and meta-synthesis of qualitative evidence. *Soc Sci Med.* 2019;222: 231–245.

22. Mandizadza EJR, Chidarikire SA Phenomenological study into the role of spirituality and religiousness in the mental health of people with cancer in Zimbabwe. *J Spirituality Ment Health.* 2016;18(2):145–161.

23. Adam A, Koranteng F. Availability, accessibility, and impact of social support on breast cancer treatment among breast cancer patients in Kumasi, Ghana: A qualitative study. *PLoS one.* 2020;15(4):e0231691.

24. Wigginton B, Farmer K, Kapambwe S, Fitzgerald L, Reeves MM, Lawler SP. Death, contagion and shame: The potential of cancer survivors' advocacy in Zambia. *Health Care Women Int.* 2018;39(5):507–521.

25. Wanchai A, Stewart BR, Armer JM. Experiences and management of breast cancer-related lymphoedema: A comparison between South Africa and the United States of America. *Int Nurs Rev.* 2012;59(1):117–124.

26. Meacham E, Orem J, Nakigudde G, Zujewski JA, Rao D. Exploring stigma as a barrier to cancer service engagement with breast cancer survivors in Kampala, Uganda. *Psychooncology.* 2016;25(10):1206–1211.

27. Karikari NA, Boateng W. Socio-cultural interpretations of breast cancer among female patients at the cape coast teaching hospital, Ghana. *Ghana Soc Sci J.* 2018;15(2):143–160.

28. Ogunkorode A, Holtslander L, Ferguson L, Maree JE, Anonson J, Ramsden VR. Seeking divine intervention to manage the advanced stages of breast cancer in southwestern Nigeria. *Cancer Nurs.* 2020; 44(3):E163–E169.

29. Obrist M, Osei-Bonsu E, Awuah B, et al. Factors related to incomplete treatment of breast cancer in Kumasi, Ghana. *Breast.* 2014;23(6):821–828.

30. Mwaka AD, Mangi SP, Okuku FM. Use of traditional and complementary medicines by cancer patients at a national cancer referral facility in a low-income country. *Eur J Cancer Care.* 2019;28(6):e13158.

31. Tompkins C, Scanlon K SE, Ream E, Harding S, Armes J. Survivorship care and support following treatment for breast cancer: A multi-ethniccomparative qualitative study of women's experiences. *BMC Health Serv Res.* (2016);16:401

32. Tompkins C, Scanlon K, Scott E, Ream E, Harding S, Armes J. Survivorship care and support following treatment for breast cancer: A multi-ethnic comparative qualitative study of women's experiences. *BMC Health Serv Res.* 2016;16(1):401.

33. Pennery E, Mallet J. A preliminary study of patients' perceptions of routine follow-up after treatment for breast cancer. *Eur J Oncol Nurs.* 2000;4(3):138–145; discussion 46–47.

34. Forouzanfar MH, Afshin A, Alexander LT, et al. Global, regional, and national comparative risk assessment of 79 behavioural, environmental and occupational, and metabolic risks or clusters of risks, 1990–2015: a systematic analysis for the Global Burden of Disease Study 2015. *The Lancet.* 2016;388(10053):1659–1724.

35. Gale NK, Heath G, Cameron E, Rashid S, Redwood S. Using the framework method for the analysis of qualitative data in multi-disciplinary health research. *BMC Med Res Methodol.* 2013;13(1):117.

36. Elewonibi B, BeLue R. The influence of socio-cultural factors on breast cancer screening behaviors in Lagos, Nigeria. *Ethn Health.* 2019;24(5):544–559.

37. Opoku SY, Benwell, M, Yarney J. Knowledge, attitudes, beliefs, behaviour and breast cancer screening practices in Ghana, West Africa. *PAMJ.* 2012;11:28.

38. Elewonibi B, BeLue R. The influence of socio-cultural factors on breast cancer screening behaviors in Lagos, Nigeria. Ethnicity & Health. 2019;24(5):544–559.

39. Daher M. Cultural beliefs and values in cancer patients. *Ann Oncol.*2012;23 (Suppl 3):66–69.

40. Ebenso B, Newell J, Emmel N, Adeyemi G, Ola B. Changing stigmatisation of leprosy: An exploratory, qualitative life course study in Western Nigeria. *BMJ Glob Health.* 2019;4(2):e001250.

41. Subramanian S, Gakunga R, Jones M, et al. Financial barriers related to breast cancer screening and treatment: A cross-sectional survey of women in Kenya. *J Cancer Pol.* 2019;22;100206

42. Quinlan E, Maclean R, Hack T, et al. Breast cancer survivorship and work disability. *J Disab Pol Stud.* 2011;22(1):18–27.

43. Ginsburg O. Breast and cervical cancer control in low and middle-income countries: Human rights meet sound health policy. *J Cancer Pol.* 2013;1(3–4):e35–e41.

44. World Health Organization. Innovative Care for Chronic Conditions, building blocks for action: Global report. 2002 [Available from: https://www.who.int/chp/knowledge/publi cations/icccglobalreport.pdf?ua=1].

45. Errico KM, Rowden D. Experiences of breast cancer survivor-advocates and advocates in countries with limited resources: A shared journey in breast cancer advocacy. *The Breast J.* 2006;12:S111–S6.

46. Dvaladze A, Kizub DA, Cabanes A, et al. Breast cancer patient advocacy: A qualitative study of the challenges and opportunities for civil society organizations in low-income and middle-income countries. *Cancer.* 2020;126:2439–2447.

47. Yip CH, Taib NA. Challenges in the management of breast cancer in low-and middle-income countries. *Future Oncol.* 2012;8(12):1575–1583.

48. Azenha G, Bass LP, Caleffi M, et al. The role of breast cancer civil society in different resource settings. *The Breast.* 2011;20:S81–S7.

49. Morhason-Bello IO, Odedina F, Rebbeck TR, et al. Challenges and opportunities in cancer control in Africa: A perspective from the African Organisation for Research and Training in Cancer. *The Lancet Oncol.* 2013;14(4):e142–e51.

50. Thompson HS, Littles M, Jacob S, Coker C. Post-treatment breast cancer surveillance and follow-up care experiences of breast cancer survivors of African descent: An exploratory qualitative study. *Cancer Nurs.* 2006;29(6):478–487.

51. Peart A, Lewis V, Brown T, Russell G. Patient navigators facilitating access to primary care: A scoping review. *BMJ Open.* 2018;8(3):e019252.

52. Dalton M, Holzman E, Erwin E, et al. Patient navigation services for cancer care in low-and middle-income countries: A scoping review. *PloS one.* 2019;14(10):e0223537-e.

53. Chidebe RCW, Pratt-Chapman ML. Oncology patient navigation training: Results of a pilot study in Nigeria. *J Cancer Educ.* 2021 Jan;7;1–7.

54. Oluka OC, Shi YY, Nie SF, Sun Y. Boosting cancer survival in Nigeria: Self-management strategies. *APJCP.* 2014;15(1):335–341.

55. Crookes DM, Shelton RC, Tehranifar P, et al. Social networks and social support for healthy eating among Latina breast cancer survivors: Implications for social and behavioral interventions. *J Cancer Survivorship.* 2016;10(2):291–301.

56. Mohammadi S, Sulaiman S, Koon PB, Amani R, Hosseini SM. Impact of healthy eating practices and physical activity on quality of life among breast cancer survivors. *APJCP*. 2013;14(1):481–487.

57. Yaw YH, Shariff ZM, Kandiah M, et al. Diet and physical activity in relation to weight change among breast cancer patients. *APJCP*. 2014;15(1):39–44.

58. Van Oers HM, Schlebusch L. Anxiety and the patient with breast cancer: A review of current research and practice. *South Afr Family Pract*. 2013;55(6):525–529.

59. Clegg-Lamptey J, Dakubo J, Attobra Y. Psychosocial aspects of breast cancer treatment in Accra, Ghana. *East African Med J*. 2009;86(7):348–353.

60. Gomes B, Higginson IJ. Evidence on home palliative care: Charting past, present, and future at the Cicely Saunders Institute—WHO Collaborating Centre for Palliative Care, Policy and Rehabilitation. *Progr Palliat Care*. 2013;21(4):204–213.

61. Wang T, Molassiotis A, Chung BPM, Tan JY. Unmet care needs of advanced cancer patients and their informal caregivers: a systematic review. *BMC Palliat Care*. 2018;17(1):96.

62. Ekiran M, Fajemilehin B. Psychosocial burdens of family care-giving to breast cancer survivors at two university teaching hospitals, in Lagos, Nigeria. *Nigerian Q J Hosp Med*. 2014;24(1):71–75.

63. Osse BH, Vernooij-Dassen MJ, Schadé E, Grol RP. Problems experienced by the informal caregivers of cancer patients and their needs for support. *Cancer Nurs*. 2006;29(5):378–388.

64. Main DS, Nowels CT, Cavender TA, Etschmaier M, Steiner JF. A qualitative study of work and work return in cancer survivors. *Psychooncology*, 2005;14(11):992–1004.

65. Hoving JL, Broekhuizen ML, Frings-Dresen M. Return to work of breast cancer survivors: A systematic review of intervention studies. *BMC Cancer*. 2009;9(1):117.

66. Ginsburg O, Rostich AF, Conteh L, Mutebi M, Paskett ED, Subramanian S. Breast cancer disparities among women in low- and middle-income countries. *Curr Breast Cancer Rept*. 2018;10(3):179–186.

67. Office of the National Security Adviser. Policy Brief: Violent radicalisation in northern Nigeria: Economy & Society. Abuja, Nigeria: Office of the National Security Adviser; 2015.

68. Alawode GO, Adewole DA. Assessment of the design and implementation challenges of the National Health Insurance Scheme in Nigeria: A qualitative study among sub-national level actors, healthcare and insurance providers. *BMC Public Health*. 2021;21(1):124.

69. Truant TL, Fitch MI, O'Leary C, Stewart J. Global perspectives on cancer survivorship: From lost in transition to leading into the future. *Can Oncol Nurs J*. 2017;27(3):287–294.

40

Impact of Culture and Beliefs in Brain Tumor Patients' Care in Indonesia, Indonesia

Tiara Aninditha, Feranindhya Agiananda, and Henry Riyanto Sofyan

Introduction

Cancer is a highly debilitating disease, causing distress among those afflicted with it and their loved ones. Studies in Indonesia show the relationship between the impact of cancer and one's mental well-being. Cancer patients suffer from the stigma of negative public perception and experience fear and shame because of it [1]. Many have a low quality of life (QOL) and suffer from anxiety and depression [2]. The perception of cancer differs greatly from country to country. Asians, particularly Indonesians, consider cancer a dangerous, deadly, and incurable disease and hold that undergoing cancer treatment causes physical, emotional, and financial losses. They tend to believe that once they are diagnosed with cancer, they won't live long and will die in the near future. Some Asians also believe that it is their fate, aligned with God's will, and the only thing they can do is to accept as well as surrender to this condition. They believe that healing comes only from God, not from their medical treatment [3].

Among brain tumor patients, QOL is significantly decreased owing to neurological signs and symptoms [4]. Brain tumor patients have also shown psychological distress, with as many as 68.6% suffering from depression (7.9–90% of cases [5]) and anxiety (29-60% of cases [6]) due to the imminent loss of functional status, occupation, and individual freedoms. This condition worsens during the course of therapy, which can be aggressive and cause many adverse side effects [7]. The diagnosis of a brain tumor is a shocking, stressful event and is considered to be the most terrifying diagnosis of all malignancies due to its symptoms, which include significant decline in physical and cognitive function, and to its poor prognosis. Most patients are initially unable to accept their condition and need great emotional support and companionship from their loved ones and family members in order to overcome their condition [8].

Cancer Beliefs of Indonesian Brain Tumor Patients

Indonesia is one of the largest countries in Southeast Asia, with a large population and multiple ethnic groups. The diverse sociodemographic characteristics, sociocultural beliefs, perceptions regarding diseases, influence from significant others, and the accessibility and availability of medical services and their related costs, particularly in rural areas, contribute to the pattern of health-related behaviors in Indonesian people [9].

Indonesian cancer patients often seek medical help while in its later stages, which leads to poor treatment outcomes. Most patients do not adhere to therapy due to patient-related factors such as a lack of awareness/knowledge, their own cancer beliefs, their treatment beliefs; treatment-related factors such as financial burden, emotional burden and side effects of the treatment; patient/health care provider relationships, and factors such as a one-way/paternalistic communication style and an unmet need for information; social and economic factors, and health care system-related factors such as severity of symptoms and level of disability [3]. In Indonesia, a majority of brain tumor patients are admitted to hospital only when their condition worsens; Prior to seeking medical help, 69.2% of patients receive a Karnofsky Performance Scale (KPS) of <70, which indicates the severity of the disease and an inability to perform their daily activities. As many as 63.3% of patients present with hemiparesis (a complete paralysis of half of the body), and 30.9% experience a decrease in cognitive awareness [10].

A common phenomenon in brain tumor patients is their struggle to maintain a balance of hope with the reality of the illness, as the prognosis and illness trajectories are often not fully known. They have to face great uncertainty, particularly with regard to their medical treatment, as compared to other illnesses [11]. A study conducted in Java, the most populated island in Indonesia, shows that health on that island is defined by the ability to complete daily activities, and as long as the Javanese are not hindered in their daily activities, they consider themselves to be healthy. This perspective also plays an important role in the delay of cancer diagnosis and treatment in Indonesia [12].

Most Indonesians imagine and believe that cancer treatment and cancer care is terrifying and closely related to surgery. Surgery is conceptualized as a frightening procedure with awful operating tools. Their misperceptions about cancer care, coupled with false beliefs about the disease itself, make them more likely to delay their treatment. Also, they do not have enough information regarding the disease, and, consequently, they tend to be unaware of their actual condition. Indonesians prefer to adhere to traditional medicine as an alternative treatment, as it is considered to be less invasive and able to improve the symptoms as well as cure the patient [3].

An additional consideration is that the long duration of cancer treatment causes financial and emotional burdens. The uncertainty of the treatment outcome often results in cancer patients losing the hope of recovering from the disease. Chemotherapy as one of the cancer treatments may cause a variety of side effects, including pain, fatigue, nausea, dizziness, loss of appetite, sleep disturbance, and hair loss. These side effects can be debilitating for most patients and may cause them to skip their treatment schedule. In summary, three aspects of treatment may predetermine an Indonesian cancer patient's negative attitude toward health care (i.e., seeking medical treatment at a later phase of the disease): (1) financial burden; (2) emotional burden; and (3) side effects of treatment [3]. One case report from Indonesia was that of a 21-year-old girl who was diagnosed with a brain tumor and decided not to undergo any further cancer therapies. The only procedure she agreed to was the installation of a ventriculo-peritoneal shunt that would lower her intracranial pressure. She did not undergo any specific treatment related to her condition, even though she suffered from many symptoms, including total memory loss, severe headaches, and blurred vision. A decision to delay, or even refuse, therapy is not a surprising one, as the majority of Indonesian people have strong religious beliefs shaped by its culture. They believe that God is in control and that everything happens according to God's plan. On the other hand, it is common for Indonesians to use religion/spirituality as one of the coping tools for overcoming distress. This shows that the roles of both religion and culture equally determine Indonesians' health-behavior [13].

Aside from the patient's beliefs, the communication style between doctors and patients in Indonesia (as well as in many other regions throughout Asia) is different from that in Western countries. Western medicine encourages clear and open communication using a style of partnership consultation in which both parties actively engage in conversation and share information during consultation. In contrast, in Indonesia, there is a gap between the information desired by patients and the information offered by health providers. The dominant role of health providers, coupled with the educational gaps between doctors and patients, complicates matters even more, creating a barrier in implementing a desirable partnership style. Recent studies conducted in Yogyakarta in Central Java show that many factors contribute to the paternalistic or one-way doctor–patient communication style, including the doctors' sense of superiority due to the educational gap between doctor and patient [14,15].

Furthermore, cultural aspects of Indonesian people, such as conflict avoidance and respect for people of higher status, including health providers, discourage patients from taking an active role in doctor–patient communication. This kind of passive behavior stems from their culture and prevailing norms. Indonesians tend to follow conventional models of patient–doctor relationships, in which patients are supposed to be passive and show respect to doctors. They are reluctant to talk about their need for information because they fear taking up the health provider's time and think that the doctors will undervalue their questions or request for information. Indonesians' tendency to preserve *rukun*, or social harmony, causes them to avoid conflict. They often use ambiguous, indirect, and affectively neutral kinds of communication in order to develop a harmonious relationship. This cultural issue therefore hinders patients from mentioning their confusion and/or disagreement with the health providers, as well as precludes them from building a two-way communication. This issue, which has been a challenge for both Indonesian health care providers and patients, must be dealt with immediately in order to reduce the discrepancies between the desired and practiced communication styles, as well as the delivery of optimal health care [16,17].

Indonesian Culture and Breaking Bad News

Bad news is commonly linked to serious and life-threatening conditions, including death, end-of-life care, cancer, and acute critical condition. On the other hand, with other conditions such as a chronic or disabling disease, the need to implement a painful or demanding treatment is also considered to be bad news. Another definition of bad news is any information regarding health care practices where there is a potential threat to one's mental and physical well-being, a feeling of hopelessness and a change in previous lifestyle [18]. The amount of information received by patients varies between countries, based on their cultural background. The dilemma between telling the truth or nondisclosure due to different patients' preferences must be considered prior to giving information to the patients and their relatives. Culture shapes one's understanding of a disease, and morbidity and death have enormous effects on how people perceive the principles of autonomy and nonmaleficence (i.e., first, do no harm). In addition, culture also determines the communication patterns that are very important for building patient–physician relationships [19].

From recent studies, attitudes and responses regarding the delivery of bad news varies, depending on one's cultural background. Most countries in Asia have strong paternal views, and protecting patients' emotional well-being seems to be a priority. The main reason for not giving the patient full and complete information is to maintain the patient's hope. This is considered to benefit their health condition more than just knowing the truth. For Asian patients, including Indonesians, breaking bad news straightforwardly is considered uncaring, impolite, and rude. They prefer to hear the bad news indirectly, which creates ambiguity and the possibility of hope. "You have widespread cancer" or "this cancer is incurable" is too harsh for Asian people to hear, whereas people in Western cultures actually prefer a direct statement like this [20].

In Asia, and, in this case, Indonesia, a family member is considered to be part of a family unit and the patient's decisions and actions (including further medical decisions) require family consent; a patient's decision has to be discussed and agreed upon by other family members. In the Batak and Minangkabau tribes, which are 2 of the 10 largest tribes in Indonesia, the role of extended families in making decisions regarding the patients' further treatment plan is considered to be very important. In order to determine which treatment the patient will undergo, all family members, including extended family members, often discuss this matter together. Conversely, in West Sumatra, the wife's family is considered to be more responsible than the husband's family and are entitled to make decisions within the family.

More traditionally, Javanese men are considered to have the role of the head of family and are responsible for making decisions for the family. The men place their family at the center of their lives with the instilled values of *tentrem* (peace), *hangat* (emotional warmth), and *kasih sayang* (unconditional love and giving). They also fully believe in the proverb *"mangan ora mangan waton kumpul"* (that is, even if there is no food to eat, being together is the most important thing) [21–24].

The role and the main principle of the family is to give psychosocial support and to provide encouragement and empathy to the patient. This really describes Indonesian family culture, where the family feels a strong responsibility to care for their family members suffering from a disease. In contrast to Indonesian culture, Western culture requires its people to solve their problems, on their own, and they have fewer discussions with their families regarding their condition. Apart from the complexities of decision making within an Indonesian family, Indonesian culture has some positive aspects and advantages: for example, they have a very strong bond and support system when facing problems and difficult situations; these are unlikely to be found in Western countries [24]. There are three types of family involvement when making decisions: (1) the patient and the family have equal roles, (2) the patient asks their family to decide, or (3) the family takes over all matters related to decision making without considering patients' preferences. Nonmaleficence remains the primary reason for not disclosing bad news to patients, so as to prevent any psychosocial burden. Imparting information regarding serious conditions directly to the patient is considered to be a harmful act. The principle of nonmaleficence should be prioritized as, in their community, it is not common to talk about death [21,22].

The uniqueness of Indonesian culture could increase psychological distress, such as anxiety and depression, in brain tumor patients. The most stressful moment occurs during the diagnosis process [25], which is very difficult for both the doctors and the patients. In addition, cancer treatment involving surgery followed by radiotherapy, or a combined treatment of surgery, radiation, and chemotherapy, causes significant pressure, which can be closely related to physical and psychological distress. To prevent such distress, adaptive coping strategies should be developed for patients with cancer in order to minimize the cause of stressors [26].

Most Indonesian people with cancer use religion as a coping mechanism, and there are both positive and negative coping methods. Positive coping is when they can build support based on their spirituality, and negative coping is when they have spiritual struggle and doubt [27]. A previous study of cancer patients in Surabaya, Indonesia, showed a significant correlation between negative religious coping methods and higher serum cortisol levels and symptoms of anxiety. Likewise, individuals with good, positive religious coping skills showed lower serum cortisol levels and fewer symptoms of anxiety [28,29]. Another study showed that cancer patients who use positive religious coping methods were more likely to have greater emotional well-being and showed fewer signs of distress, confusion, and depression. On the contrary, those who distanced themselves from God were more likely to have a less emotional well-being [26,30].

Multidisciplinary Management and Its Challenges When Treating Brain Tumor Patients in Indonesia

The comprehensive management of brain tumor patients is quite challenging. These challenges affect several areas of a patient's life, such as motor dysfunction, verbal communication barriers, physical weakness, and incontinence. Family members also have to adapt to the degenerative conditions of the patient, including their physical and cognitive capacity, personality, and changes in mood [31,32]. It seems very beneficial to do early detection of the psychosocial, emotional, and physical symptoms of cancer patients, which will increase the chances of positive outcomes of treatment and increase the rate of survival. One study showed that ignoring psychological symptoms in cancer patients leads to many unfavorable consequences, including diminished quality of life, reduced threshold of pain, refusal of treatment, communication difficulties, increased risk of suicide, longer hospitalization, and reduced expectation of survival [33]. Indonesian culture complicates these matters even more, as a stigma is still firmly attached to people who seek help from mental health professionals; they often become victims of injustice and abuse by the public [34].

A study in Bali, Indonesia, concluded that Indonesian people being treated by mental health professionals suffer two forms of stigma: public stigma (stigma coming from society) and self-stigma (stigma coming from the sufferer and their own family). Those who seek help from mental health professionals are considered to be weak and not religious enough to overcome problems. Moreover, Indonesian people also believe that mental illness is a form of punishment from God for sins they committed in the past and is perceived as a cursed illness. To conclude, mental illness is understood as a weakness of faith, or so-called *imaan*; the belief is that the devil or black magic is the cause of illness and that mental illness is a punishment for the patients' past sins [34,35].

Data obtained from a study conducted in East Java, Indonesia, showed that a patient's mental health significantly correlates with the stigma toward that patient, causing punitive social measures, including social exclusion and discrimination, not only toward the patient but toward the entire family as well. This unpleasant experience leaves them reluctant to seek psychological treatment. In order to avoid these perceived stigmas, most family members of mentally ill patients prefer to seek treatment from traditional or alternative healers, including Kiyai or ulama, chaplains, dukuns (shamans), and Chinese healers, rather than undergo professional treatment. Families often hide or ignore the patients' mental condition and avoid going to a mental health care facility due to their embarrassment. Consequently, many who need this treatment are not taken for help [36].

Conclusion

Culture and belief may negatively impact Indonesian brain tumor patients and their care, and delay diagnosis and therapy, affecting the prognosis for patients and their health-seeking behavior. Therefore, this potential impact should be considered by health care professionals when communicating any diagnosis, treatment, and prognosis in order to prevent a communication gap between health-care professionals and the patient's family. On the other hand, Indonesian culture is positively impacted by the strong support system provided by the family that alleviates patient burden during such stressful situations.

References

1. Solikhah S, Matahari R, Utami FP, Handayani L, Marwati TA. Breast cancer stigma among Indonesian women: a case study of breast cancer patients. *BMC Women's Health.* 2020;20(1):116–21.
2. Setyowibowo H, Purba FD, Hunfeld JAM, et al. Quality of life and health status of Indonesian women with breast cancer symptoms before the definitive diagnosis: A comparison with Indonesian women in general. *PLoS one.* 2018;13(7):e0200966.
3. Iskandarsyah A, de Klerk C, Suardi D, Soemitro M, Sadarjoen S, Passchier J. Psychosocial and cultural reasons for delay in seeking help and nonadherence to treatment in Indonesian women with breast cancer: a qualitative study. *Health Psychol.* 2014;33(3):214–221. doi:10.1037/a0031060
4. Taphoorn MJ, Sizoo EM, Bottomley A. Review on quality of life issues in patients with primary brain tumors. *Oncologist.* 2010;15(6):618–626.
5. Sitorus JJR, Agiananda F, Aninditha T, Wiguna T, Lukman PR. Distress in brain tumor patients and its related factors. *Neurona.* 2017;34(2):91–96.

6. Liu R, Page M, Solheim K, Fox S, Chang SM. Quality of life in adults with brain tumors: Current knowledge and future directions. *Neuro Oncol.* 2009;11(3):330–339.
7. Randazzo D, Peters KB. Psychosocial distress and its effects on the health-related quality of life of primary brain tumor patients. *CNS Oncol.* 2016;5(4):241–249.
8. Vierhout M, Daniels M, Mazzotta P, Vlahos J, Mason W, Bernstein M. The views of patients with brain cancer about palliative care: A qualitative study. *Curr Oncol.* 2017;24(6):374. doi:10.3747/co.24.3712
9. Widayanti A, Green J, Heydon S, Norris P. Health-seeking behavior of people in Indonesia: A narrative review. *J Epidemiol Glob Health.* 2020;10(1):6. doi:10.2991/jegh.k.200102.001
10. Laila MN, Andriani R, Sofyan HR, Aninditha T. Factors influencing performance status in patients with intracranial tumor at Cipto Mangunkusumo General Hospital. *Neurona.* 2019;37(1):1–6.
11. Philip J, Collins A, Brand C, et al. Health care professionals' perspectives of living and dying with primary malignant glioma: Implications for a unique cancer trajectory. *Palliat Support Care.* 2013;13(6):1519–1527. doi:10.1017/s1478951513000576
12. Fles R, Bos A, Supriyati, et al. The role of Indonesian patients' health behaviors in delaying the diagnosis of nasopharyngeal carcinoma. *BMC Public Health.* 2017;17(1): 510–8. doi:10.1186/s12889-017-4429-y
13. C Teo, I Teo, C Beng Im-Teo. Recovery from brain cancer through strong faith in God and herbal therapy: An ethnographic case study and structured interview. *Internet J Family Pract.* 2006;5(1):1–6.
14. Claramita M, Susilo A, Kharismayekti M, Dalen J, Vleuten C. Introducing a partnership doctor-patient communication guide for teachers in the culturally hierarchical context of Indonesia. *Educ for Health.* 2013;26(3):147. doi:10.4103/1357-6283.125989
15. Claramita M, Nugraheni M, van Dalen J, van der Vleuten C. Doctor–patient communication in Southeast Asia: A different culture? *Adv Health Sci Educ.* 2012;18(1):15–31. doi:10.1007/s10459-012-9352-5
16. Kim Y, Kols A, Bonnin C, Richardson P, Roter D. Client communication behaviors with health care providers in Indonesia. *Patient Educ Couns.* 2001;45(1):59–68. doi:10.1016/s0738-3991(01)00144-6
17. Kim Y, Putjuk F, Basuki E, Kols A. Increasing patient participation in reproductive health consultations: An evaluation of "Smart Patient" coaching in Indonesia. *Patient Educ Couns.* 2003;50(2):113–122. doi:10.1016/s0738-3991(02)00193-3
18. Payan E, Montoya D, Vargas J, Velez M, Castano A, Krikorian A. Barriers and facilitating communication skills for breaking bad news: From the specialists' practice perspective. *Colomb Med.* 2009; 40(2):158–166.
19. Kagawa-Singer M, Blackhall L. Negotiating cross-cultural issues at the end of life. *JAMA.* 2001;286(23):2993–3001. doi:10.1001/jama.286.23.2993
20. Barclay J, Blackhall L, Tulsky J. Communication strategies and cultural issues in the delivery of bad news. *J Palliat Med.* 2007;10(4):958–977. doi:10.1089/jpm.2007.9929
21. Tse C, Chong A, Fok S. Breaking bad news: A Chinese perspective. *Palliat Med.* 2003;17(4):339–343. doi:10.1191/0269216303pm751oa
22. Arbabi M, Rozdar A, Taher M, et al. Patients' preference to hear cancer diagnosis. *Iran J Psychiatry.* 2020;9(1):8–13.
23. Subandi M. Family expressed emotion in a Javanese cultural context. *Cult Med Psych.* 2011;35(3):331–346. doi:10.1007/s11013-011-9220-4
24. Effendy C, Vissers K, Tejawinata S, Vernooij-Dassen M, Engels Y. Dealing with symptoms and issues of hospitalized patients with cancer in Indonesia: The role of families, nurses and physicians. *Pain Pract.* 2014;15(5):441–446. doi:10.1111/papr.12203

25. Chirico A, Lucidi F, Merluzzi T, et al. A meta-analytic review of the relationship of cancer coping self-efficacy with distress and quality of life. *Oncotarget.* 2017;8(22):36800–36811. doi:10.18632/oncotarget.15758

26. Nuwa M, Kusnanto, Utami S. The influence of age and coping mechanism on the resilience of cancer patients undergo chemotherapy. *The 9th Int Nursing Conference.* 2018. 28–36.

27. Ahmad F, Binti Muhammad M, Abdullah A. Religion and spirituality in coping with advanced breast cancer: Perspectives from Malaysian Muslim women. *J Relig Health.* 2010;50(1):36–45. doi:10.1007/s10943-010-9401-4

28. Sawitri B, Soetjipto, Ishardyanto H. Religious coping associated with serum cortisol and anxiety symptoms on late-stage breast cancer patients. *Eurasia J Biosci.* 2020;14:1807–1811.

29. Nuraini T, Andrijono A, Irawaty D, Umar J, Gayatri D. Spirituality-focused palliative care to improve Indonesian breast cancer patient comfort. *Indian J Palliat Care.* 2018;24(2):196. doi:10.4103/ijpc.ijpc_5_18

30. Hills J, Paice J, Cameron J, Shott S. Spirituality and distress in palliative care consultation. *J Palliat Med.* 2005;8(4): 782–788.

31. Ganefianty A, Kariasa I, McAllister S, et al. Quality of life of primary brain tumor patients before and 3 months after discharge from a hospital in Bandung, Indonesia. *Makara J Health Res.* 2019;23(1):25–31. doi:10.7454/msk.v23i1.10147

32. Caruso R, Breitbart W. Mental health care in oncology. Contemporary perspective on the psychosocial burden of cancer and evidence-based interventions. *Epidemiol Psychiatr Sci.* 2020;29:1–4. doi:10.1017/s2045796019000866

33. McFarland D, Holland J. The management of psychological issues in oncology. *Clin Adv Hematol Oncol.* 2016;14(12):999–1009.

34. Putro B. Mental health problem in Indonesia in public stigma and self-stigma practices. *Int Conf Cult Stud.* 2018;1(1):151–155.

35. Wahyuni S, Suttharangsee W, Nukaew. Religious belief in mental illness and its influences on seeking treatment: Indonesian patients' perspectives. *Songklanagarind J Nurs.* 2017;37: 60–68.

36. Subu M, Elliott J, Holmes D. Persistent taboo understanding mental illness and stigma among Indonesian adults through grounded theory. *Asian J Pharm Nurs Med Sci.* 2017;5(1):1–11.

41

The Contribution of Spiritual, Religious, and Customary Heritage to the Personalization of Modern Oncology in Multiethnic Societies of Developing Countries

The Model of Montenegro, Montenegro

Nada Cicmil-Sarić, Milena Raspopović, and Damira Murić

Introduction

The word "culture" refers to the overall social heritage of a group of people; that is, to the learned patterns of thought, feelings, and actions of a group, community or society, as well as expressing those patterns in material objects. Anthropologists consider culture to be a defining feature of the genus *Homo* [1]. Although religion and spirituality often go hand in hand, they certainly need to be specifically considered, defined, and set. Religion can be defined as "belief in God or gods that require worship, and this is usually expressed through behavior and rituals" or "a particular system of belief, worship and the like, which generally includes a code of ethics" [2]. Spirituality could be termed a "trait or factual spirituality, a non-physical state" or a "dominant spiritual character expressed by way of thinking, lifestyle and the like; spiritual inclination or note" [2]. Religion could be a format for spirituality. It is a format that allows the expression of spirituality as its perhaps most important content. Spirituality is food and medicine for the human soul. Faith or disbelief in a god or deity is a matter of human choice, and it is shaped and acquired throughout life, as is our character. On the other hand, spirituality is our innate essence, which, similar to temperament, we bring to this world at birth. Therefore, in terms of religious or nonreligious affiliation, the inhabitants of the planet Earth differ. When it comes to spirituality and its meaning for humans, about our spiritual needs, feelings, and vulnerability of the soul, all people are, regardless of religious affiliation, if not the same, then very similar. If different religions can sometimes be obstacles to one another and cause misunderstanding or disagreement, spirituality is a common denominator for believers of all religions, as well as for atheists and agnostics.

When we look at energy circles, we see that the degree of their importance grows from individual to general and universal: energy of survival, energy of species maintenance, energy of belonging to a small group, energy of belonging to a large group, energy of flora and fauna, energy of space, energy of spirituality, and energy of a universal god. The energy of belonging to a larger group, which includes, among other things, religion, represents the fourth energy level, while the energy of spirituality is the one that makes us human beings of a much higher level: The energy of spirituality in these eight steps occupies a very high, seventh place.

For many people, interest in spirituality and religion arises only when they or a family member becomes ill. Atheists exist in all countries and religious groups today. The importance of the presence of spirituality and belief for atheists in a state of serious illness requires special criteria for consideration. Yet, it cannot go unnoticed that great communal and personal calamities, illnesses, and suffering almost regularly lead to an intensified expression of the need for spirituality through the religious personalization of God. A young 28-year-old woman who was being treated for a malignant disease once told me the following: "I didn't even know about God until I got sick."

If spirituality is the driving force and if religion is a form that facilitates and mediates its expression, then customs, habits, and symbols are their product and their outward manifestation. Different cultures also nurture different ways of experiencing death and one's own illness as well as the illness of a family member. The roots of this are established in the religions to which the inhabitants of the planet Earth belong. Numerous customs and habits follow the religious affiliations and understandings of certain ethnic groups. Heaven, hell, resurrection, previous lives, funeral customs, and even the manner and colors of clothing that symbolize mourning, vary. During several decades of working in oncology practice, I have often seen, and still see in the sick rooms, various types of objects that symbolize faith: icons, candles, rosaries, religious records, amulets. It is obvious that people have a need for these symbols to be close to them in order for them to feel safe, protected, to feel that they are not alone, to be understood. On the other hand, when it comes to illness, there are many similarities in behavior and customs in different cultures: illness as a temptation and a challenge, compassion for the sick, different forms of support, visits to the sick, faith and hope for a good outcome, and so on, are just some of the common denominators for members of different social communities in this domain. Generally speaking, the vast majority of patients, regardless of their religious affiliations, want to have as many visits as possible and as many supportive people around them as possible. Although the modes of realization differ in various cultures, the motives are similar; the paths leading to their realization may have different courses, but the goals they lead to are the same [3].

Personalized Medicine and Personalized Oncological Approach: From a Holistic Approach, through a Personalized Path to Individual Application of Medical Care

Patients suffering from the same type of malignant disease usually have a very different final therapeutic outcome. Certainly, the biological factors, the stage of the disease, and the characteristics of the tumor itself are of great importance, as well as the timely, appropriate treatment and monitoring of the patient. In doing so, we must always keep in mind that it is the same disease, but each patient is a different host for it, both physically and culturally. Viewed from a holistic perspective, it is necessary to pay attention to the spiritual well-being of patients, given the existential nature of many issues related to the diagnosis and type of cancer.

Personalized medicine is a synonym for the phrase "the right medicine, for the right patient at the right time." However, the patient brings all their individual dimensions into this in the broadest, holistic sense of the word. Therefore, the ultimate goal of personalized medicine, and even oncology, is to individualize this personalization, according not only to the need, but also the measure and cut of each individual. Accomplishing this trend would be a guarantee for the most successful treatment. In countries where there is a holistic, biopsychosocial model and approach from the very beginning until the end of a malignant disease, not only in palliative care, but also the overall outcome of treatment, the quality of treatment, and life expectancy are improved [4,5].

Although there is no sign of equality between religion and spirituality, for a large number of patients, contact with religious professionals would strengthen spirituality and facilitate its recognition and expression in the right way. How can we ensure the constant and active presence of Catholic and Orthodox priests, imams, rabbis, and other spiritual leaders during the treatment of the sick? Viewed in this way, this spiritual treatment could be considered one of the forms of targeted therapy in medicine or oncology [6].

Montenegrin Society Yesterday and Today

Montenegro is a developing country, not only in terms of economic progress but in its cultural and spiritual development. Montenegro is beginning to accept the diversity of all individuals: those who are similar to themselves and those who are not. Estimates provided in 2011 by the Central Intelligence Agency (CIA) in Montenegro indicate the following religious composition [7]:

- Orthodox 72.1%
- Muslims 19.1% (Sunnis)
- Catholics 3.4% (mostly Roman Catholics)
- Atheists 1.2%
- Other 1.5%
- Unspecified 2.6%

In the former Yugoslavia, state atheism was part of official state policy during the rule of the Communist Party of Yugoslavia from 1945 to 1990. From the late 1980s, the number of believers within Yugoslavia, and later throughout the successor states, increased spectacularly. While the number of atheists was estimated at 31.6% in 1987, in 2002, only 2.7% of the total population of the successor states of Yugoslavia and Montenegro declared themselves to be atheists or nonbelievers [8]. These facts undoubtedly show that the power of belief and spirituality is steadfast and indestructible.

The level of education and social status, as well as the ethnic group, is of great importance in the treatment of cancer patients. The growing multiculturalism of developing countries, including Montenegro, day by day, more and more, is as much a treasure as it is a challenge. Over time, developed countries have understood, accepted, overcome, and transformed ethnic, religious, customary, and racial differences into a kind of economic nation. Developing countries do not have the privilege of functioning as a rich state union, so they often still stumble upon relict or revived remnants of the past. Developing societies often threaten to become societies of rich individuals and numerous poor. When it comes to a disease, even a malignant one, the sufferer, together with the disease of the body and mind, brings in a whole range of their cultural achievements and social and economic aspects [9]. Belief and practice of magic, alternative methods of treatment (which is not uncommon worldwide and in Montenegro), refusal of certain interventions and means of treatment (especially surgery, psychological counseling, and transfusions), and feelings of injustice or discrimination due to an inability to obtain expensive medical services will certainly contribute to a poor final outcome for a cancer patient. Lately, clinicians have increasingly noticed a positive flow in patients who have regular conversations with psychologists. Previously, this type of assistance was almost exclusively refused: "It is not enough that I am sick, but now they declare me crazy."

What malignant patients in Montenegro have in common are malignant disease, suffering, desire, hope and faith in healing, the need for understanding, and the presence of those who are emotionally close to the patient and are ready to provide protection, support, and assistance. There is a common desire for reconciliation, forgiveness, preservation of dignity, and spiritual salvation. Also common are the same accommodation conditions, specific oncological and palliative symptomatic treatment and care. What differs is that each sick patient is a unique and irreplicable individual in time and space, in their experience in terms of trust, scope of commitment, quality and content of services provided by the medical professional, and health system of their country. In this context, a highly personalized approach—biological, social, legislative, ethical, psychological, customary and spiritual—is an essential condition without which the best possible outcome in both palliative and curative terms cannot occur [10].

People in the Balkans and in Montenegro, regardless of religious affiliation, have traditionally been taught that they should suffer and keep feelings to themselves, that the external manifestation of feelings is an expression of weakness, and that such a prototype is a reflection of a positive, strong person. For Balkan people, sharing emotions with others, asking for help and support, crying, are characteristics expressing weakness and shame. Openness to spiritual persons or, in the absence of spiritual representatives, to the medical psychologist, represents a new age for Balkans and even Montenegrins in this domain. Opening up to a medical psychologist is a step toward spiritual enlightenment and, when a spiritual care team (SCT) is established, an increasing number of people suffering from malignant diseases find meaning in the fight for health and life and do not surrender to fate.

Oncology institutions in Montenegro have been functioning on the basis of multidisciplinary teams (MDTs) for more than two decades. Professional clergy are not involved in the work of these teams, and the country does not have spiritual care teams. The spirit of unity of "brothers and sisters in need" could be strengthened within the MDT and SCT [11]. This is especially true when it comes to the Balkan mentality, where malignant disease is still partly perceived as a stigma: people consider themselves stigmatized, the community pities them instead of showing compassion, many individuals have all the best recipes for the life of another person, in this case the patient, and at the same time they, have great disorder and dissatisfaction in their own lives. A person's sovereign right to privacy when they are at an extremely vulnerable moment, when they are seriously ill, is endangered. This social attitude results in the patient withdrawing and avoiding social communications and gatherings, which, in turn, significantly reduces their quality of life and limits their ability to transmit emotions and receive true information and advice.

Altogether, this has a negative effect on the final therapeutic outcome of the patient. Three years ago, several employees with many years of experience in oncology, had the idea to create a space in our oncology facility in Podgorica where patients could stay, think in peace, socialize during hospitalization, and have access to literature that would help strengthen their spirituality. The idea was not realized because the management of the clinical center, though initially showing understanding and support, finally estimated that the social situation was still not mature enough for this model of organizing spiritual support for the sick [12]. It is very important that there is a certain optimal approach to psychosocial help that leads to the well-being of cancer patients, as well as their families. Also, health psychologists working with oncology patients try to understand the nature of the individual, their health and psychological problems, and work on reducing stress. Physicians in clinical practice feel this "relaxation" of the patient and the positive impact of the work of psychologists on the patient and their relatives. I (Nada Cicmil-Sarić) recognized two facts in this area in my own practice where an assessment of the patient did not prove to be correct: it happened to me personally; I did not recognize the moment when the patient became too emotionally attached to the doctor. Second, I originally assessed that the patient was coping very well with his illness and that the condition was well tolerated, but my assessment proved to be incorrect. This clearly illustrates and emphasizes the importance of the work of a medical psychologist in an oncology MDT.

The Role of the Medical Psychologist in Working with Oncology Patients

Spiritual methodologies that our psychologists use when working with oncology patients enable the individual's transformation through awareness and the integration of repressed emotions, which changes both their environment and personal destiny. We are aware of what we know and what we don't know, but there are things we don't know we don't know until we expose ourselves to them. As C. G. Jung has observed, "the mind exposed to a new idea never returns to its original form." "Until the unconscious comes to the place of the conscious, it will guide our lives [13]."

One technique that psychologists use in working with oncology patients is the PEAT (Primordial Energy of Activations and Transcendence) methodology, which belongs to the areas of applied psychological and spiritual technologies. PEAT methods were developed by psychologist Živorad Mihajlović Slavinski [14]. The goals of meridian therapies, alternative psychodisciplines that have been developed in the last 10 years, are to eliminate unwanted emotional, psychological, and physical states, and in some methodologies such as PEAT, to expand consciousness and spiritual maturity and development [15].

Traumatic experiences during peoples' lives leave certain emotional charges in the following four elements: images, thoughts, emotions, and bodily sensations, thus producing a state of illness. That is where the presence of spirituality comes into play because the being itself must have a deeper quantum origin, with significant psychosomatic and transpersonal implications.

Our psychologists approach the patient as an energetic being suffering from a malignant disease. The patients are guided to a specific awareness so that they accept their situation, and this, of course, works on the problem that led to that state of physical disease, which has actually been caused by a spiritual block. PEAT techniques bring a person to the realization of dual emotions (which we call primordial polarities) and the charges that exist in it, and spiral processes, through exercises, lead to their integration or neutralization of the same. After the exercises, patients already feel the benefit of the process and relief. By integrating polarity, we enter a state of Oneness and accelerate our spiritual development. By further applying deep PEAT, we increasingly recognize Oneness as our essence and gradually free consciousness from the dual perception of self and world. In other words, we gain wholeness and freedom, which is the essence of spiritual evolution. The cause of our distorted perception of ourselves and the world is charged by our repressed thoughts and emotions.

The Relationship between Psychology and Spirituality, Our Experiences, and Considerations

The relationship between psychology, on the one hand, and spirituality and religion, on the other, is quite complex. While some view that there are no points of contact between them (primarily empirically and methodologically), there are also authors from the domain of psychology who emphasize the importance of spirituality for the development of humans and the maintenance of their mental health. Thus, Jung saw spirituality as an integral part of the self and considered it the basis for human development [13,16]. Spirituality here represents the need to integrate experience, for wholeness. In his theory, Frankl deals with spirituality in light of the search for the meaning of life. He argued that religion can have a beneficial effect on the mental state and mental balance, although this is not its primary intention [17]. If we look at the spirituality of our patients in Frankl's way, we will see that recognition that their life has meaning and purpose unequivocally helps patients cope with malignancy.

It is not surprising when we witness patients in prayer, while receiving chemotherapy, placing icons next to them or reading spiritual literature during hospitalization. Psychologist's task is to validate someone's beliefs and religious feelings, whatever they may be, and to direct them in order to overcome difficulties as successfully as possible. Petar Jeknić in his book *Memento Mori* emphasizes the importance of spirituality in successfully overcoming the fear of dying [18] According to Jeknić, the essence of spirituality is peace, in the "here and now," regardless of health or some other condition. The goal of spirituality is to encourage and support the patient in overcoming hopelessness, without creating a false hope that will only become an additional burden to the patient. Awakening a person's spiritual capacities reduces the intensity of the fear of dying.

If we approach patients from the angle of rational-emotional behavioral psychotherapy—whose basic postulate is that how we think about events affects our emotions and behaviors about those events as well as our further thinking—then it is extremely important for us to know what meaning our patients attach to what is happening to them, in light of their beliefs [19]. How one will assess the impact of cancer depends on the core belief system about oneself, others, and the world at large and, of course, on the specific beliefs about disease and treatment that are part of that system [20]. Two people who find themselves in the same or similar situation, depending on their beliefs, can have completely different reactions to the disease and its course. Thus, in practice, we often meet patients who are extremely depressed and anxious, influenced by the belief that malignancy should not happen to them, that they should not suffer, that they should not die, and so on. At the same time, we also meet patients who are in an equally difficult situation and develop more adequate emotions such as worry, sadness, and regret, which are a reflection of a more flexible way of thinking, accepting mortality, acknowledging that the situation is not going in the desired direction, and the like.

Spirituality, religion, and culture certainly influence the formation of our beliefs and our practices, showing that people who have nurtured their own spirituality in some way can traverse this path more easily, starting with learning about malignant disease, through treatment and, in some cases, the return of disease and, eventually, death. We will distance ourselves from the conclusion that spirituality always results in more successful coping strategies, although there are results that support this observation, explaining the link between well-being and spirituality by the mediating role of social connection and experiencing the purpose of living [21]. It should be added that practices derived from spiritual-religious frameworks such as meditation, which have been used in mindfulness and relaxation techniques, have been shown to be effective in overcoming mental and somatic difficulties in our patients, as well as in the general population, which is increasingly accepting these methods.

Health psychologists, in their work with oncology patients, also apply various techniques aimed at making patients better tolerate the course of treatment, as well as to strengthen them mentally. One approach to this work is to develop support groups through workshops, during which attention is paid to patients' spiritual well-being, given the existential nature of many issues related to the diagnosis and type of cancer. Many patients are religious, so elements of spirituality permeate through psychological treatments. Spirituality can have a huge impact on a person's health and enhance recovery from trauma and illness, including cancer. Throughout the history of humankind, spirituality and religion have played a major role in the treatment of various physical and mental illnesses. Cancer is one of the most devastating diseases because it affects the physical, emotional, psychological, and spiritual well-being. A growing body of scientific literature supports the concept that spirituality can have a significant impact during cancer treatment, and we believe it should be integrated with conventional medicine to treat this complex disease [14].

Conclusion

What do we have today in Montenegro in the field of general cultural personalization and individualization in the treatment of patients with malignant disease, and what are the plans, needs, and perspectives? What has an effect on the good or bad outcome of each individual cancer patient? The fact is that not all patients need spiritual care. Most sufferers of severe, life-threatening diseases and malignancies express the need for spiritual care. Atheists or nonbelievers who have acute illnesses or diseases with a good prognosis may not need spiritual care. No patient should be imposed upon or be offered spiritual care without a prior careful assessment of their spiritual condition. Modern oncology has great promise, but the path from the mind of science to the heart of the patient's spirituality is long: the path is always the same, but the traveler can get lost on it. How can we help the sick so that this does not happen? Montenegrin oncology today offers the following:

1. MDTs for cancer patients
2. Medical psychologists in MDTs and practices
3. Transferral of the authority and role of the doctor in the psychological domain to a qualified medical psychologist
4. A medical psychologist to help destigmatize the patient with personalized work, with each patient helping to break down prejudices, sharing emotions, and "dosing" expectations and hopes as a means of psychological and spiritual recovery in order to encourage patients to fight and not leave their outcome to fate
5. The work of medical psychologists, individualized to each patient, as a link to achieving continuous contact between the patient and a competent clergyman
6. The opening of Montenegrin citizens of all religions to faith for success and meaning in the fight for health
7. Help for medical workers, family members, and others who visit the patient
8. A large presence of acceptance regarding diversity and the freedom to wear religious symbols and conduct processes and ceremonies as an expression of cultural personalization

Plans, Needs, and Perspectives

1. To work on recognizing and improving spirituality and the need for spiritual care for each individual cancer patient
2. To work on recognizing the spirituality of medical workers who care for the patient, their experience in this field and organized training and education in this area
3. To work on the formation of the SCT (patient + family + clergyman + nurse + medical psychologist + oncologist and other medical staff involved in patient care), establishing continual communication between the oncology patient and the institution's spiritual leader and to trust in inpatient and outpatient services
4. To develop even greater trust among the patients, doctors, medical psychologists, and the state health institutions

5. To introduce new systems and methods of application of health insurance and to implement decentralization of the current monopolistic position of the Health Insurance Fund of Montenegro

6. To work on creating a greater social product that would provide more material resources for health care so that no patient will feel disenfranchised, abandoned, powerless, or discriminated against

7. To further improve the balance, homogenization, and social justice in society with the priority goal of preventing selective justice, the worst form of injustice in the field of health care

Finally, another memory comes back to me (Nada Cicmil-Sarić) from my clinical practice: A patient once said to me, "Doctor, you don't know how much I like coming for checkups at your place." Honestly, I was surprised and confused; I wasn't sure I understood well what the man was telling me. He added: "Your name is Nada (hope), and that gives me strength and confidence that everything will be fine with me."

Confirmation that the saying is correct. "Hope dies last."

Does hope ever die at all?

References

1. Available on sh.wikipedia.org ›wiki
2. Available on www.gotquestions.org> Serbian
3. Silbermann M. *Cancer Care in Countries and Societies in Transition: Individualized Care in Focus*. New York: Springer Nature; 2016.
4. Christian JC, Brown, CG. Perspective: Balancing personalized medicine and personalized care. *Acad Med*. 2013 Mar;88(3):309–313.
5. Richardson P. Spirituality, religion and palliative care. *APM*. July 2014;3(3):150–159.
6. Koenig HG. The spiritual care team: Enabling the practice of whole person medicine. *Religions*. 2014;5:1161–1174.
7. CIA The World Factbook—Central Intelligence Agency—Field listing: Religions. January 2020.
8. www.tacno.net> beograd> feuilleton. 2002.
9. Brothers KB, Rothstein MA. Ethical, legal and social implications of incorporating personalized medicine into healthcare. *Per Med*. 2015;12(1):43–51.
10. Silbermann M, Arnaout M, Daher S, et al. Palliative cancer care in Middle Eastern countries: Accomplishments and challenges. *Ann Oncol*. April 2012;23(Suppl 3):15–28.
11. VandeCreek L, Burton L. Professional chaplaincy: Its role and importance in Healthcare. A White Paper. 2001.
12. Baldacchino D. Spiritual care in a hospital setting. Fifth bi-annual international student conference, Spiritual Care and Health Professions: Context and Practice. 2010.
13. Jung, CG. *Modern man in search of a soul*. New York: Harcourt, Brace; 1933.
14. Slavinski, ŽM. *Transcendence*, Belgrade: Živorad Mihajlović and Jadranka Stilin Mihajlović, Publishers; 2010.
15. Raković, D & Slavinski, ŽM. Meridijanske terapije i psihosomatske implikacije. In: Jovičić, S & Sovilj, M. (eds.). *Govor i jezik: interdisciplinarna istraživanja srpskog jezika II*. Belgrade: IEFPG; 2008: 23–25.

16. Mack ML. Understanding spirituality in counseling psychology: Considerations for research, training, and practice. *Couns Values*. 1994;39(1):15–31.

17. Frankl VE. *The Unconscious God: Psychotherapy and Theology*. New York: Simon and Schuster; 1975.

18. Jeknić P. *Memento mori*. Čačak: Legenda; 2017.

19. Walen SR. DiGiuseppe R, Dryden W. A *Practitioner's Guide to Rational-Emotive Therapy*, 2nd ed. Oxford: Oxford University Press; 1992.

20. Moorey S. Cognitive therapy. In: Holland JC., Breitbart, WS., Jacobsen, PB., Lederberg, M. S., Loscalzo MJ., McCorkle R. (eds.). *Psycho-oncology*, 2nd ed. Oxford: Oxford University Press; 2010:402–407.

21. Joseph S, Linley P, Maltby, J. Positive psychology, religion, and spirituality. *Mental Health, Relig Culture*. 2006;9(3):209–212.

42

Differences in Attitudes toward Advanced Cancer Care Planning through the Scope of Culture, Israel

Gil Bar-Sela and Inbal Mitnik

Introduction

During the past few decades, significant technological progress has been made in Western medicine, prolonging people's lives and enabling them to overcome many life-threatening conditions [1,2]. This progress has led to a growing need to define and develop end-of-life (EOL) care in order to ensure that people live well during their final stages of life and allow them to die with dignity [1–4].

The process of Advance Care Planning (ACP) was designed to improve decision making regarding EOL care and to help plan for it in accordance with patients' preferences, values, and goals [3–7]. The process aims to promote patients' active participation in the decision-making process and increase their sense of control and autonomy [4,8–10], particularly in cases that may present future mental and/or physical deterioration [9,11,12].

Ideally, ACP is meant to be a gradual and continuous process [5,13–14]. EOL discussions should be designed to clarify the patient's understanding of their medical state and the treatment options available to them [1,14]. During these conversations, it is important that patients have the opportunity to share their concerns regarding the dying process and to define their goals and expectations regarding EOL care [1,7].

In this process of review and discussion, the ACP should include two additional components: the first is the completion of advance directives (ADs)—written statements that document the patient's preferences regarding possible future medical decisions [5–7]. ADs are intended to ensure that, in the event they become incompetent and unable to express their wishes, patients are treated according to their preferences [8,9,15]. The second part is the assignment of a durable power of attorney (DPOA) for health care—the process by which patients nominate a designated surrogate who will make decisions for them, based on their preferences, if they become incompetent [16,17].

These two parts are closely related and, ideally, both of them should be completed. First, DPOAs are essential for unforeseen occurrences not already mentioned in the ADs, which may have been decided upon at an earlier time and under different circumstances and may not reflect the patient's wishes about a specific situation [9,18–20]. In addition, ADs were found to be very important for family members, particularly for the designated surrogate, to better understand the patient's preferences and to make decisions accordingly [20,21].

Advance Care Planning is not a generalized plan, for many factors influence individuals' needs and preferences regarding EOL care, such as race, age, diagnosis, and location of care. The process can be either *disease-specific* with discussions tailored to the patients' functional decline, which may differ between various medical conditions (e.g., sharp functional decline in advanced stages of cancer or a more gradual decline with other conditions) or *location-based,* which is usually included in the routine care of chronic-care populations with a higher prevalence of ADs, such as nursing homes or hospices [14].

Benefits of Advance Care Planning

The goal of ACP is to promote a realistic understanding of the situation and a sense of control among patients, empowering them by helping them to define their preferences and ensuring that the best medical decisions will be made for them [4,7,22]. For example, it was found that most patients wish for comfort at their EOL and prefer to avoid unnecessary, life-prolonging procedures [9,23].

This process may also strengthen the interactions between patients and their caregivers; open discussions increase patients' trust and satisfaction and promote the feeling that their concerns and values are being addressed [24,25].

The Advance Care Planning process has also been shown to give a greater sense of hope. Despite common concerns among health care professionals and family members, hope is related not only to prognosis, but also to the possibility of finding future treatments consistent with patients' preferences and values. The process may assist in redefining the patients' expectations and hopes regarding the future [24].

In addition, ACP has been found to promote quality of EOL care [3]. For example, a study of advanced cancer patients and their caregivers demonstrated that productive EOL discussions were associated with less aggressive medical care, such as lower rates of ventilation, resuscitation, and ICU admission. More aggressive medical care was associated with lower quality of life and higher risk of major depressive disorders in bereaved caregivers. In addition, patients who completed EOL discussions enrolled in hospice services earlier, resulting in better quality of life for both patients and caregivers [26]. Another study affirmed that patients who engaged in the process of ACP experienced improved EOL care, such as earlier use of hospice services and fewer cases of death at hospitals [7].

Challenges in Advance Care Planning

Several studies have documented the various barriers and challenges that arise during the ACP process and EOL discussions when patients and family members acknowledge the severity of the disease and the limitations of the medical treatment. They must cope with the harsh truth regarding their mortality and deal with the uncurtailed instability of the situation [14,27]. In some cases, these discussions may be highly distressing and anxiety-provoking for them. Hence, the process requires a degree of familiarity between physician and patient in order to recognize the patient's emotional resources, willingness and readiness to talk about it, and the right timing to do so [27,28].

In addition, studies have demonstrated the difficulty staff members experience in discussing such a complex issue and dealing with the emotional reactions of patients and family members [27]. This may be particularly difficult given the lack of proper resources, such as training for physicians in breaking bad news and adequate time for properly and gradually completing the process, as needed [14,29,30].

Studies have further demonstrated dilemmas concerning the process itself. First, there are questions regarding the appropriate timing to raise the issue: in earlier stages of the medical care or in advanced stages of the disease [9,23]. Second, dilemmas arise regarding the person who is responsible for relaying the information. It was found that physicians waited for patients to initiate the discussion, while patients felt it was the physician's role [22]. These issues cannot be clarified by protocol but rather depend on the ability to recognize the patient's needs and abilities and to discuss the issue openly. In addition, the need to nominate a close relative in the process of DPOA was found to be significantly challenging for patients, as it raised issues of trust in their close relationships [31].

Moreover, the process involves complicated and long forms written in formal legal language that a layperson might not understand without professional assistance [1,29,30]. Hence, instead of empowering patients and increasing their sense of control and autonomy, it forces them to depend on expert medical and legal knowledge rather than on their own understating and perceptions [1].

Finally, the encounter between the objective technical world of medicine and the subjective emotional world of the patient may be challenging when dealing with these sensitive issues [1]. Medicine is perceived as a rational and goal-oriented process in which words may be exchanged without establishing communication. However, many patients view ACP as a process of communication that aims to prepare them for death and dying by sharing their thoughts and concerns [1].

Cultural and Ethnic Aspects of Advance Care Planning

In the context of globalization and migration, people with different cultural and ethnic backgrounds interact with each other often. In these interactions, cultural aspects may become increasingly important and should be taken into consideration [32]. In the medical setting, the cultural perspective may be highly significant and may influence essential aspects of medical care [32–34]. This is especially applicable in EOL care, as people face limitations to cure and need to make difficult decisions regarding treatment choices. This situation may lead them to turn to their traditional practices and values in order to gain strength and help them to make decisions [33,35].

Cultural conceptions were found to be pertinent in the understanding of health, illness, and dying. Beliefs regarding what is considered a "good death" or "good health" may influence the definition of the appropriate medical practice, the physician's duties, the role of family and society [1,36], as well as attitudes toward palliative care and understanding its goals and services [32].

Attitudes toward Pain and Illness

Understanding pain and illness and their meaning to one's existence varies among cultures. For example, in the Latinx tradition, pain is perceived as a form of punishment from a spiritual power and people are expected to endure pain as a test of their personal strength [33]. Hence, patients from this culture may be more likely to underreport pain [33]. In the Hindu tradition, illness is attributed to bad karma, and suffering is perceived as a compensation for sins committed in a former life [37]. Sadly, critically ill patients may therefore be stigmatized rather than treated empathetically, and they may be expected to accept the suffering and acknowledge its goal [37–39].

Preferences Regarding Medical Care at EOL

In the Latinx culture, dying is perceived as natural and beyond human control, where a person's fate is in the hands of God. Hence, it is less acceptable to take aggressive action at the end of life, and this belief may be associated with later bereavement reactions [33]. In the Korean tradition, the values of devotion and respect for the elderly ("filial piety") may influence EOL preferences by the tendency to provide life-sustaining treatment and to prolong the elder's life [40]. Similarly, the same value may influence Korean physicians, who may focus on maintaining the consciousness and cognitive abilities of patients as a way of showing their respect for dying patients and their families [40]. Ethnic minorities in the Netherlands were found to perceive 'curative care' appropriate at EOL and may therefore feel uncomfortable with the concept of palliative care as presented by the medical establishment [32]. Likewise, it was demonstrated that African Americans prefer more aggressive care at EOL and have spiritual beliefs that may conflict with the goals of palliative care [41].

Euthanasia

In Judaism, with its perspective on the religious value of the sanctity of life, the view on EOL care is restrictive as doctors must persuade patients to accept life-supporting medical treatment and may not respect patients' wishes to withdraw it [36]. Similarly, Islamic law (Shari'a law) also views life as sacred and accordingly prohibits euthanasia [42]. In the Netherlands, euthanasia is legal and acceptable, owing to that nation's cultural and social values regarding the concept of "good care" and the perception of the procedure as an expression of self-determination [32,43]. In Germany, the term *euthanasia* is considered taboo, as it is related to the medical procedures carried out during the Nazi regime. The more common term is *medical assistance in dying*. Despite respecting the cultural value of a patient's autonomy, its active form is illegal as it involves a second person, which harms others [43].

Hospice

The concept of hospice originated in the United Kingdom and is now common world-wide. However, in traditional Spain, this type of setting for EOL care may contradict certain cultural concepts regarding the expected role of the family in times of illness and dying [44]. In addition, it has been found that African Americans have a more negative attitude toward hospice care than others. This may be attributed to issues of trust and difficulties in accepting the palliative concepts of care [41].

Patient's Autonomy and Disclosure

In some Mediterranean countries, such as Spain and Italy, the legal and moral obligation to openly discuss the medical situation with the patient does not fit the central role of the family, particularly in EOL care, as the patient becomes less involved and less active [32]. In addition, the emphasis on awareness contradicts the traditional Spanish ideas about "good death." Hence, in reality, many conversations are held outside the presence of the patient, with partial or nondisclosure within families regardless of patients' requests (thereby creating "a conspiracy of silence") [32]. In Israel, until the 1980s, the medical system was characterized by physician authoritarianism, and most patients were not involved in medical decision making [36]. However, the emergence of the patient's rights movement, along with the increasing dissatisfaction of patients, have led to legal and social changes emphasizing patients' autonomy, such as the enactment of the Patients' Rights Law in 1996 [45] or the 2004 ruling regarding a patient's right to be given personal medical information [36]. In Norway, with its cultural respect for privacy in addition to a strong taboo associated with death, various studies have demonstrated a general reluctance among health care professionals to openly discuss EOL issues [32]. In Japanese culture, unawareness of impending death and *Pokkuri* (sudden death) are considered to be part of "good death." Accordingly, allowing health care professionals to make decisions on behalf of the patient, rather than self-determination, is very common and widely accepted. Health care workers are allowed, and even encouraged, to ask for the family's advice before disclosing information regarding malignancy to patients. However, it should be noted that recent studies have demonstrated that this tendency is becoming less prevalent as Japanese physicians continue to perceive patient autonomy more positively [40]. In the Vietnamese tradition, patients see health care professionals as experts, and it is highly unlikely that they will question a doctor's orders or express their preferences regarding the treatment [46,47]. In Chinese culture, the common belief is that spoken words may become a reality [48]. This may lead to a reluctance to talk about EOL care or to acknowledge the impending mortality [33]. Patients may prefer an indirect means of communication regarding EOL, such as talking about other patients who use ACP and avoiding words such as "death" and "terminal illness" [33]. Among Mexican Americans, health care professionals are perceived to be the main decision makers regarding their medical care, and patients are therefore less involved and less active in the process [21].

Advance Directives

The cultural differences in the patient's autonomy can also be reflected in their attitudes toward advance directives (ADs). For example, Islamic law does not recognize living wills and ADs, as it is believed that only Allah can make decisions on life and death [39–42]. Among Latinx and Cambodian minorities in the United States, most patients believe that the inevitability of dying makes the discussion of ADs futile, leading to a low prevalence of AD discussions among these populations [49]. In addition, various studies have shown that African Americans were less likely than white people to have completed ADs, partly due to their discomfort discussing death and a conception that those who believe in God do not have to plan their EOL care [42,50].

Patterns in Sharing Medical Information

Cultural differences were found to determine who should be involved in the medical discussions and the decision-making process. For example, Native Americans may want their community leaders to be informed regarding their medical situation and to be involved in the decision-making process. African Americans may prefer that medical conversations be directed toward the oldest member of the family, typically the male [33]. Cambodian minorities in the United States tend to want the immediate family to be involved, while among Latinx patients, a more extended family structure is involved in the process [33,39].

Conclusion

In a multiculture society, it is highly important and challenging to provide appropriate EOL care that takes into consideration the individual's life experiences, beliefs, and perceptions regarding health, illness, and care [33,41].

In order to provide culturally sensitive EOL care, health care programs should acknowledge cultural variance and provide suitable services. For example, it was found that palliative care consultation intervention integrated with consideration of cultural aspects significantly reduces the disparity between white people and African Americans in completing Ads [50]. In addition, palliative care programs that combine curative life-prolonging therapies have increased the number of African American hospice enrollees. These programs take the preferences of this population into consideration and promote their trust in this type of setting [51].

There is a need for culturally sensitive research on contextual factors, acknowledging individual preferences concerning EOL communication and investigating these issues accordingly [52].

In addition, health care professionals should increase their knowledge regarding cultural practices, along with the understanding that such practices may differ among individuals, even those from the same tradition. They should be trained to recognize different cultural values and beliefs and to communicate about these issues without stereotyping [33,35]. Health care professionals should also consider their own cultural constructs, which have been found to influence the interaction as well [33,40,52].

The need for culturally sensitive care is especially important in hospitals located in heterogeneous populations where encounters between multicultural staff members and patients are more likely to occur. In these areas, people in key positions should participate in programs that facilitate knowledge regarding common cultural perceptions of health and illness in their community.

References

1. Shalev C, Reclaiming the patient's voice and spirit in dying: An insight from Israel. *Bioethics.* 2010;24(3):134–144.
2. Singer PA, Bowman KW. Quality care at the end of life. *BMJ.* 2002;324:1291. doi: https://doi.org/10.1136/bmj.324.7349.1291
3. Mullick A, Martin J. An introduction to Advance Care Planning: Practice at the frontline. In: Thomas K, Lobo B, Detering K (eds). *Advanced Care Planning in End of Life Care.* 2nd ed. Oxford: Oxford University Press; 2018:26–35.
4. Detering KM, Hancock AD, Reade MC, Silvester W. The impact of advance care planning on end of life care in elderly patients: randomized controlled trial. *BMJ.* 2010;340:1–9. doi: https://doi.org/10.1136/bmj.c1345
5. Sudore RL, Fried TR. Redefining the "planning" in advance care planning: Preparing for end-of-life decision making. *Ann Intern Med.* 2010;153:256–261.
6. Van Wijmen MP, Rurup ML, Pasman HR, Kaspers PJ, Onwuteaka-Philipsen BD. Advance directives in The Netherlands: An empirical contribution to the exploration of a cross-cultural perspective on advance directives. *Bioethics.* 2010;24:118–126. doi: 10.1111/j.1467-8519.2009.01788.x
7. Bischoff KE, Sudore R, Miao Y, Boscardin WJ, Smith AK. Advance Care Planning and the quality of end-of-life care in older adults. *J Am Geriatr Soc.* 2013;61(2):209–214. doi: 10.1111/jgs.12105
8. Quill TE. Perspectives on care at the close of life. Initiating end-of-life discussions with seriously ill patients: addressing the "elephant in the room". *JAMA.* 2000;284:2502–2507.
9. Silveira MJ, Kim SY, Langa KM. Advance directives and outcomes of surrogate decision making before death. *N Engl J Med.* 2010; 362:1211–1218.
10. Raskin W, Harle I, Hopman WM, Booth CM. Prognosis, treatment benefit and goals of care: What do oncologists discuss with patients who have incurable cancer? *Clin Oncol.* 2016;28:209–214. doi: 10.1016/j.clon.2015.11.011
11. The Support Investigators: A controlled trial to improve care for seriously ill hospitalized patients. The study to understand prognoses and preferences for outcomes and risks of treatments (SUPPORT). *JAMA.* 1995;274:1591–1598.
12. Kelly B, Rid A, Wendler D. Systematic review: individuals' goals for surrogate decision-making. *J Am Geriatr Soc.* 2012; 60:884–895. doi: 10.1111/j.1532-5415.2012.03937.x
13. Henry C, Seymour J. *Advance Care Planning: A Guide for Health and Social Care Staff.* London: Department of Health; 2007.
14. Waldrop DP, Meeker MA. Communication and advanced care planning in palliative and end-of-life care. *Nurs Outlook.* 2012; 60:365–369.
15. Brown BA. The history of advance directives: a literature review. *J Gerontol Nurs.* 2003;29:4–14.

16. Buchanan AE, Brock DW. Deciding for Others: The Ethics of Surrogate Decision Making. Cambridge: Cambridge University Press; 1989.

17. Beauchamp TL, Childress JF. *Principles of Biomedical Ethics*. 6th ed. New York: Oxford University Press; 2009.

18. Chambers CV, Diamond JJ, Perkel RL, Lasch LA. Relationship of advance directives to hospital charges in a Medicare population. *Arch Intern Med.* 1994;154:541–547.

19. Weeks WB, Kofoed LL, Wallace AE, Welch HG. Advance directives and the cost of terminal hospitalization. *Arch Intern Med.* 1994;154:2077–2083.

20. Shalowitz D, Garrett-Mayer E, Wendler D. The accuracy of surrogate decision-makers: A systematic review. *Arch Intern Med.* 2006;166:493–497.

21. Wendler D, Rid A. The effect on surrogates of making treatment decisions for others. *Ann Intern Med.* 2011;154(5):336–346.

22. Tierney WM, Dexter PR, Gramelspacher GP, Perkins AJ, Zhou XH, Wolinsky FD. The effect of discussions about advance directives on patients' satisfaction with primary care. *J Gen Intern Med.* 2001;16(1):32–40. doi: 10.1111/j.1525-1497.2001.00215.x

23. Bar-Sela G, Bagon S, Mitnik I, et al. The perception of Israeli oncology staff members regarding advance care planning. *Support Care Cancer* 2020; 28(9):4183–4191. doi: 10.1007/s00520-019-05253-7

24. Davison SN, Simpson C. Hope and advance care planning in patients with end stage renal disease: Qualitative interview study. *BMJ.* 2006;333(7574):886. doi:10.1136/bmj.38965.626250.55

25. Newton J, Clark R, Ahlquist P. Evaluation of the introduction of an advanced care plan into multiple palliative care. *Int J Palliat Nurs.* 2009;15(11):554–561.

26. Wright AA, Zhang B, Ray A, et al. Associations between End-of-Life discussions, patient mental health, medical care near death, and caregiver bereavement adjustment. *JAMA.* 2008;300:1665–1673. doi: 10.1001/jama.300.14.1665

27. Larson DG, Tobin DR. End-of-life conversations: evolving practice and theory. *JAMA.* 2000;284:1573–1578. doi:10.1001/jama.284.12.1573

28. Guo Y. Palmer JL, Bianty J, Konzen B, Shin K, Bruera E. Advance directives and do-not-resuscitate orders in patients with cancer with metastatic spinal cord compression: advanced care planning implications. *J Palliat Med.* 2010;13:513–517. doi: 10.1089/jpm.2009.0376

29. Bentur N. The attitudes of physicians toward the new "Dying Patient Act" enacted in Israel. *Am J Hos Pall Med.* 2008;25:361–365. doi: 10.1177/1049909108319266

30. Ein-Gal Y, Schwarzman P. Advanced medical directives—from vision to reality. *Israeli Family Pract.* 2012;167 (In Hebrew). As retrieved from: http://www.medicalmedia.co.il/publications/ArticleDetails.aspx?artid=4988&sheetid=342

31. Bar-Sela G, Bagon S, Mitnik I, et al. The perception and attitudes of Israeli cancer patients regarding advance care planning. J. of Geriatric Oncology. 2021; 12(8):1181–1185.

32. Gysels M, Evans N, Meñaca A., 2012 Culture and end of life care: A scoping exercise in seven European countries. *PLoS one.* 2012;7(4):e34188.

33. Weiner L, McConnell DG, Latella L, Ludi E. Cultural and religious considerations in pediatric palliative care. *Palliat Support Care.* 2013; 11(1):47–67. doi:10.1017/S1478951511001027

34. Contro N, Davies B, Larson J, Sourkes B. Away from home: Experiences of Mexican American families in pediatric palliative care. *J Soc Work End Life Palliat Care.* 2010;6:185–204.

35. Zager BS, Yancy M. A call to improve practice concerning cultural sensitivity in advance directives: A review of the literature. *Worldviews Evid Based Nurs.* 2011;8(4):202–211.

36. Schicktanz S, Raz A, Shalev C. The cultural context of patient's autonomy and doctor's duty: passive euthanasia and advance directives in Germany and Israel. *Med Health Care and Philos.* 2010;13:363–369.

37. Mazanec P, Tyler MK. Cultural considerations in end-of-life care: How ethnicity, age, and spirituality affect decisions when death is imminent. *AJN*. 2003;103(3):50–58.

38. Whitman SM. Pain and suffering as viewed by the Hindu religion. *J Pain*. 2007;8:607–613.

39. Steinberg SM. Cultural and religious aspects of palliative care. *Int J Crit Illn Inj Sci*. 2011;(2):154–156.

40. Morita T, Oyama Y, Cheng S. Palliative care physicians' attitudes toward patient autonomy and a good death in East Asian countries. *J Pain Symptom Manage*. 2015;50(2):190–199. doi: 10.1016/j.jpainsymman.2015.02.020

41. Johnson KS, Kuchibhatla M, Tulsky JA. What explains racial differences in the use of advance directives and attitudes toward hospice care? *J Am Geriatr Soc*. 2008;56(10):953–958.

42. Babgi A. Legal issues in end-of-life care: perspectives from Saudi Arabia and the United States. *Am J Hosp Palliat Care*. 2009;26:119–127.

43. Horn, R. Euthanasia and end-of-life practices in France and Germany. A comparative study. *Med Health Care Philos*. 2013;16;197–209.

44. Nunez Olarte JM, Guillen DG. Cultural issues and ethical dilemmas in palliative and end-of-life care in Spain. *Cancer Control*. 2001; 8:46–54.

45. The Patient's Rights Law, 1996 (In Hebrew), as retrieved from: https://www.nevo.co.il/law_html/law01/133_001.htm

46. Dell ML. Spiritual and religious considerations for the practicing pediatric oncologist. In: Wiener L. Pao M. Kazak AE, et al. (eds). *Quick Reference for Pediatric Oncology Clinicians: The Psychiatric and Psychological Dimensions of Pediatric Cancer Symptom Management*. Charlottesville, VA: American Psychosocial Oncology Society; 2009:268–272.

47. Campbell A. Spiritual care for sick children of five world faiths. *Paediatr Nurs* 2006;18:22–25.

48. Searight R, Gafford J. Cultural diversity at the end of life: Issues and guidelines for family physicians. *Am Fam Physician* 2005;71(3):515–522.

49. Cohen MJ, McCannon JB, Edgman-Levitan S, Kormos WA. Attitudes toward advance care directives in two diverse settings. *J Palliat Med*. 2010;13:1427–1432.

50. Zaide GB, Pekmezaris R, Nouryan CN, Mir TP. Ethnicity, race, and advance directives in an inpatient palliative care consultation service. *Palliat Support Care*. 2013;11 (1):5–11.

51. Casarett D, Abrahm J. Patients with cancer referred to hospice versus a bridge program: Patient characteristics, needs for care, and survival. *J Clin Oncol*. 2001;19:2057–2063.

52. Gysels M, Evans N, Menaca A. et al. Culture is a priority for research in end-of-life care in Europe: A research agenda. *J Pain Symptom Manage*. 2012;44(2):285–294. doi: 10.1016/j.jpainsymman.2011.09.013

43

Ugandan Culture

Spiritual Guidance in Caring for Cancer Patients, Uganda

Emmanuel B. K. Luyirika

Introduction

The cultural aspects of a society incorporate customary beliefs, language, religion, cuisine, social habits and norms, music, arts, and more. In contrast, spirituality is that which affects the human spirit or soul, as opposed to material or physical components or matters relating to religion or religious beliefs. In many circumstances, cultural and spiritual dimensions can be intertwined, influenced by exposure to information, formal and informal education, as well as access to financial and other resources.

The World Health Organization's (WHO) definition of palliative care [1] and the World Health Assembly's (WHA) resolution of 2014 [2] envisage the inclusion of physical, social, spiritual, and psychological approaches when caring for patients in need of palliative care, whether due to cancer or any other life-threatening diseases. Any cancer care approach must embrace the biological and psychosocial components that patients face in order to achieve the best possible outcome.

Spiritual and Cultural Diversity in Uganda

Uganda is a religiously diverse nation, with Christianity the most widely professed faith. According to the 2014 census, over 84%, of the population is Christian (Protestants, Roman Catholics and others), about 14 percent are Muslim, and the remainder follow traditional African religions or do not ascribe to any particular faith. Religious teachings greatly influence culture and how people understand and experience illnesses, including cancer.

Uganda has a very strong cultural heritage. Many of its regions have kingdoms, including Buganda, Busoga, Bunyoro, and Toro. The Uganda culture encompasses more than 50 African ethnic groups, as well as a small population of Europeans, Asians, and Arabs.

Beliefs regarding health care in Uganda range from those who believe they can be healed solely by prayer without stepping into a hospital to those who see the hospital or Western medicine as solutions provided by God for managing diseases. It is important to bear in mind that, in some cases, the distinction between culture and religion is so thin in Uganda that the two are often fused.

Approaches to Cancer Care

One of the oldest specialist cancer care programs on the African continent, established in 1967, is the Uganda Cancer Institute, a public medical care facility that provides modern cancer treatment modalities.

It is very common for Ugandans to seek other curative options before, during, and after their enrolment in the cancer care program, such as traditional or alternative healers, spiritual healers (especially within the Pentecostal movement, some of whom insist that prayer alone or undergoing specific church rituals is sufficient), but also other spiritual healers who complement the hospital-based care.

Often, patients do not disclose to their doctor the other interventions they have undergone, including ingesting traditional medicines and herbs whose doses and contents may not be known to either the patient or the attending doctor.

The Ugandan Context

Aside from the Uganda Cancer Institute, Uganda has plans to build regional cancer centers in Mbarara, Gulu, Arua, and Mbale in order to make cancer treatment modalities, including chemotherapy, surgery, and radiotherapy, more widely available.

According to GLOBOCAN 2020 [3], an online database providing estimates of cancer incidence and mortality in 185 countries for 36 types of cancer, Uganda's population of 45,741,000 million is estimated to have had 34,008 new cancer cases, 22,992 cancer deaths, and 62,548 prevalent cases (5-year) with 50% ≤ 15 years and 70% ≤ 30 years. GLOBOCAN's 2020 cancer statistics report for Uganda estimated that the most prevalent cancers for both men and women are cancer of the cervix, Kaposi sarcoma, breast cancer, prostate cancer, and Non-Hodgkin's lymphoma.

By gender, the most common cancers for males are Kaposi sarcoma, prostate, esophageal, liver, and non-Hodgkin's lymphoma; and for females, cervix, breast, Kaposi sarcoma, non-Hodgkin's lymphoma, and esophageal. The risk of dying from cancer in Uganda before the age of 75 years is 12%.

In a 2020 study by Jatho, Bikaitwoha, and Mugisha [4] on socioculturally mediated factors and lower levels of education as main influencers of functional cervical cancer literacy among women in Mayuge in eastern Uganda, they found that the majority of the women (96.8%) had limited cervical cancer literacy, with a mean score of 42%. Those who had completed a primary education or lower (OR = 3.91; p = 0.044) were more likely to have limited cervical cancer literacy. The study also found that the women had limited decisional, social, and financial support from their male partners, with overall low locus of control. Furthermore, most of the women (92.3%) were not aware of available cervical cancer services and had no intention to undergo screening (52.5%).

The Jatho et al. study concluded that the women had little cervical cancer literacy aside from oral health literacy, and that this oral health literacy was highest among women with a lower level of education. Among the women with an overall low locus of control scores, overall literacy seemed to be largely influenced by sociocultural constructs characterized by insufficient decisional, social, and personal resources.

The women in the study demonstrated scant knowledge of the services available in their community and showed low intention to screen. The study recommended a multistrategy cervical health empowerment program to improve cervical health literacy through oral dissemination of information.

In another study on breast cancer beliefs as potential targets for breast cancer awareness efforts to decrease late-stage presentation in Uganda [5], a total of 401 Ugandan women were surveyed; most of them had less than a primary school education and received medical care at community health centers. The majority of these women either believed in, or were unsure about, cultural explanatory models for developing breast cancer (> 82%), and the majority listed these beliefs as the primary causes of breast cancer (69%). By comparison, ≤ 45% of women believed in scientific explanatory risks for developing breast cancer. Although most believed that regular screening and early detection (88% and 80%, respectively) would find breast cancer at an early stage when it is easier to treat, they simultaneously held fatalistic attitudes toward their own detection efforts, including the belief or uncertainty that a cure would be impossible once they self-detected a lump (54%). Individual beliefs were largely independent of demographic factors. The study concluded that misconceptions about breast cancer risks and the benefits of early detection are widespread in Uganda and must be addressed in future efforts to increase breast cancer awareness. The study further stated that, until screening programs are put in place, most breast cancer will be self-detected and unless addressed by future awareness efforts, the high frequency of fatalistic attitudes held by women regarding their own detection efforts will continue to be deleterious to early detection of breast cancer in sub-Saharan countries like Uganda.

In a study by Isabirye, Mbonye, and Kwagala (2020) [6], overall cervical cancer screening uptake in central Uganda was found to be low, although the study further indicated that women from wealthier backgrounds, who had been sensitized by health workers and had more knowledge about cervical cancer and cancer screening, had greater odds of having ever been screened compared with their counterparts. The study concluded that endeavors to increase cancer screening should address the disparities in access to resources and information.

A study by Mwaka et al. in 2014 [7] concluded that two main factors promote the use of traditional medicines: (1) the multitude of barriers to biomedical facilities, such as unavailable medicines, unaffordable medical costs, the high cost of transport to facilities, long waiting times at facilities, absenteeism of health workers, discrimination and disrespect by some health workers, fear of embarrassment when diagnosed with some diseases, and language barriers; and (2) erroneous beliefs about the intrinsic efficacy and effectiveness of traditional medicines for many illnesses, the greater confidentiality afforded at traditional medicine practices due to fewer people in attendance at any one time compared to crowded modern medical practices, and the cheap cost and convenient methods of payment for traditional medicines.

Guidance on Approaching Cancer Patients

Understanding the Religious and Spiritual Dimensions

When providing cancer services to patients in Uganda, health care providers need to be aware of patients' religious and spiritual beliefs, for these beliefs affect uptake and adherence to treatment information and modalities. Patients often find themselves in situations where the scientific biomedical information they get from cancer facilities competes with what they know from their spiritual leaders, who may just recommend curative measures such as prayer or rituals. Working in conjunction with patients' spiritual care providers as support for better care is key.

The Population's Level of Education

The level of education that a patient has attained may, in a way, determine the amount of information and resources the patient can access; the higher the level of education, the more improved the chances are of understanding the information related by the care teams and, in turn, the rate of adherence to treatment. All efforts must be made to ensure that cancer care and treatment information is packaged properly and appropriately to meet the patients' needs, irrespective of their level of education.

Health Literacy Packages about Specific Cancers

Certain actions required for the proper management of specific cancers may infringe upon one's beliefs or cultural values. Surgical excision of an organ or amputation may have very serious spiritual and cultural repercussions for patients and should be properly and comprehensively addressed. Loss of a breast, testicle, penis, eye, or limb due to cancer has implications beyond curing the cancer, affecting one's cultural and spiritual position in society. In such cases, patients and their families need to receive more support to access patient user devices and prostheses and enable them to harmonize the biomedical choices and decisions with their spiritual and cultural stands, ensuring holistic care and healing.

Access to Resources and Information

The diagnosis of cancer comes at a huge cost to patients and their families, with an impact beyond the index patient, most evident in countries where patients have limited resources and have no access to universal health coverage schemes for cancer. A 2015 editorial in the *Daily Monitor* [8] chronicled the economic challenges of cancer patients, which leave families impoverished. This calls for sensitivity on the part of health care providers of cancer care services, as well as governmental agencies, to expedite access to universal health coverage for cancer patients.

Addressing Barriers to Accessing Services

Several barriers exist to cancer care, which call for a national cancer program that will address these challenges, beyond just providing treatment modalities. By the time people contract cancer and seek care, their resources are not adequate to overcome challenges on their own.

Beliefs about Traditional Medicines

To ensure a successful approach, cancer care providers should also be aware of the existence of strong beliefs about traditional medicines, which are often not disclosed by patients unless they are tactfully addressed.

Conclusion

As efforts are made to improve cancer care outcomes, patients' diverse spiritual and cultural beliefs must be recognized, and available methods must be utilized in order to improve access and adherence to treatment modalities and regimens.

References

1. Gwyther L, Krakauer EL. WPCA policy statement on defining palliative care. (WHO Palliative Care Definition). London: Worldwide Palliative Care Alliance; 2011. http://www. thewhpca.org/resources/item/definging-palliative-care. Accessed March 17, 2018.
2. Strengthening of Palliative Care as a Component of Comprehensive Care Throughout the Life Course, 2014 Sixty-Seventh World Health Assembly WHA67.19. 2014. https://apps. who.int/gb/ebwha/pdf_files/WHA67/A67_R19-en.pdf?ua=1
3. Globocan. Summary statistics, Uganda Fact Sheet. International Agency for Research on Cancer and World Health Organization; 2020, 1–2.
4. Jatho A, Bikaitwoha ME, Mugisha NM. Socio-culturally mediated factors and lower level of education are the main influencers of functional cervical cancer literacy among women in Mayuge, Eastern Uganda. *Ecancermedicalscience*. January 2020;14:1004. doi: 10.3332/ ecancer.2020.1004. eCollection 2020
5. Scheel JR, Molina Y, Anderson BO, et al. 2018. Breast cancer beliefs as potential targets for breast cancer awareness efforts to decrease late-stage presentation in Uganda. *J Glob Oncol*. 2018;4(4):1–9. Published online July 1, 2017 https://www.ncbi.nlm.nih.gov/pmc/articles/ PMC6180808/ Accessed February 22, 2021.
6. Isabirye A, Mbonye MK, Kwagala B. Predictors of cervical cancer screening uptake in two districts of Central Uganda. December 3, 2020. https://doi.org/10.1371/journal.pone.0243 281. Accessed February 22, 2021.
7. Mwaka AD, Okello ES, Orach CG. Barriers to biomedical care and use of traditional medicines for treatment of cervical cancer: An exploratory qualitative study in northern Uganda. First published June 13, 2014. https://doi.org/10.1111/ecc.12211. Accessed February 22, 2021.
8. *Daily Monitor* Editorial. The economic burden of cancer. Published October 13, 2015. https://www.monitor.co.ug/uganda/magazines/healthy-living/the-economic-burden-of-cancer-1627140. Accessed February 22, 2021.

44

Cultural-Spiritual Guidance in Caring for Cancer Patients in the Dominican Republic, Dominican Republic

Wendy C. Gómez García and Marleni R. Torres Núñez

Introduction

The Dominican Republic is an island-sharing country in the heart of the Caribbean Sea, with a population of approximately 10.5 million people and distinguished by a large number of cultural and psychoemotional features linked to the melting pot of races and customs that make up the local ethnicity. It has a mixture of Hispanic, African, and indigenous traditions depicting the diversity of beliefs, myths, taboos, practices, and methods typical of the Dominican people.

The origins of the Dominican Republic and the Caribbean region are characterized by migrations dating back to the 15th century, with the arrival of Caribbean Indians from the northern regions of South America as well as the arrival of Europeans—mainly Spanish, but also Portuguese, English, French, Dutch, and Danish—and the forced migration of black Africans who were then sold as slaves [1]. Other economic migrations included people from Arab countries in the 19th century and the migratory flow of neighboring Haitians, which increased in the 19th and 20th centuries. Thus, three important origins of identity in the Dominican Republic can be highlighted: pre-Columbian, Hispanic, and African. These movements brought with them myriad customs, languages, and religious and cultural beliefs, forming the ideological diversity of the people of this nation.

The Dominican Republic shares the island of Hispaniola with Haiti and is the second largest nation in the Caribbean, after Cuba. Because of its strategic location in the geographic center of the Caribbean, every important event has an impact on its soil. The physiological effects of disease and health issues on the Dominican people are influenced by their psychosocial-cultural history, making it essential to understand the various races, customs, ideologies regarding medical paternalism (medicine centered on doctors), socioeconomic levels, educational levels, and more.

Background

In 1494, after the arrival of the Spanish to the Americas, the settlement of La Hispaniola was founded, with Isabela as the capital city [2].

In 1503, the Hospital San Nicolás de Bari was built on the same land as the Chapel of Our Lady of Altagracia, at the request of King Fernando and Queen Isabel of Spain in order to provide assistance to economically disadvantaged Christians and indigenous people. The hospital, established by the Spanish during the 16th century, followed the medical model of Humorism, or the four humors of Hippocratic medicine [3]. Between the four humors was considered to be the correct or harmonious state of the body, and disease was considered to be an irregularity. For example, the person who had a tumor, from this medical point of view, had experienced a disturbance in the balance of their four humors [4].

In Spain at the beginning of the 17th century, the experimental medicine model began to develop in which cancer was understood as a local or regional disease related to ganglia and tumors. For example, doctors began treating breast cancer by removing breast tissue, the surrounding ganglia, and the pectoralis major. In the 18th century, the Hospital San Nicolás de Bari, which focused on the health of soldiers and the military, adopted the experimental model. The hospital began treating cancer-suggestive diseases such as tumors, masses, or nodules with surgery and radiotherapy around the middle of the 20th century [5].

Medicine during the era of Rafael Leónidas Trujillo Molina, the dictator who ruled the Dominican Republic for more than 30 years from 1930 until his assassination in 1961, was practiced in a peculiar way: a kind of family doctor visited the patient at home. Patients were taken to hospitals in "berths" because there were no transport facilities in this largely rural country; there was no culture of going to a health center, and doctors dared not demand from, criticize, or denounce the dictatorial regime of the time in any way. By 1960, the Dominican Republic was an eminently rural society. It had 44 hospitals, 136 clinics, one orphanage, 14 shelters, one mental hospital, and two medical laboratories. The public health system had just 60 doctors, 68 assimilated nurses, 35 practitioners, and 26 dentists [6].

Cancer in the Dominican Republic

To understand the history of cancer in the Dominican Republic, it is important to recognize the country's pioneers of oncology: Dr. Alberto Paiewonsky was a Dominican radiologist and radiotherapist who studied in the United States and England and was the first dean of the Medical School of the Universidad Autónoma de Santo Domingo (UASD, Autonomous University of Santo Domingo). In 1940, he joined the Padre Billini Hospital and, together with Dr. José Sobá, Minister of Public Health and a member of the Dominican Academy of Medicine, initiated the first oncological patient care facility in the country. They then coordinated with Dr. Heriberto Pieter, a Dominican oncologist who graduated from a medical school in France, and established the Institute of Oncology, Milagros de la Caridad, in Santo Domingo. Therefore, the work of the Instituto del Cancer (Institute of Cancer) began at the Padre Billini Hospital in September 1942 and was later officially incorporated in 1943 by executive decree. In turn, the foundation of the Dominican League Against Cancer was consolidated in 1942, consisting of well-known doctors from the Dominican Republic [7,8].

Since its inception, the Institute of Oncology, Milagros de la Caridad, has focused on education, early detection, prevention, and treatment of cancer. In 1972, its name was changed to the Dr. Heriberto Pieter Oncological Institute, in honor of the academic-humanitarian work carried out by its founding physician, Dr. Pieter [9–11].

On August 15, 2012, the National Cancer Institute, Rosa Emilia Sánchez Pérez de Tavares (INCART) opened his doors, classified as a third-level hospital. This classification corresponds to that of a highly specialized hospital dedicated to cancer, decentralized, with autonomous management. The category of institute is accorded based on the teaching, research, and regulation capacities of the practice of oncology in the Dominican Republic. INCART it's a complete institution where adults or children patients can find high level technology treatments regarding chemotherapy, radiation, diagnostics elements, between others; it belongs to government health system.

As part of the history of local academic societies, founded in 1982, the Dominican Society of Hematology and Oncology brought Dominican hematologists and oncologists together to fight cancer in the different branches of medicine and the subspecialization of haemato-oncology [12].

On October 14, 1998, the first meeting of a group of distinguished Dominican hematologists was held in order to share and strengthen knowledge of the field and to form the Dominican Society of Hematology. After several additional meetings, on February 22, 1999, all hematology specialists throughout the country were called to the premises of the then Dominican Medical Society promoted by Dr. Iván Sánchez Rhus. The Dominican Society of Hematology was formed with a group of selected Dominican hematologist leaders on the field [13].

In the field of pediatric oncology, there are currently six units in the country that provide care for childhood cancer. The unit with the largest number of pediatric patients is at the Dr. Robert Reid Cabral Children's Hospital, in the capital city of Santo Domingo. **University and governmental hospital** dedicated to the care of children from birth to 18 years of age. Free care is provided to all patients regardless of race, origin, migration record, or social security status. Approximately 100 new pediatric oncology cases are diagnosed each year, and since 2004 they have received support from the Friends Against Childhood Cancer Foundation (FACCI), and academic and logistic counseling from the St. Jude's Children's Research Hospital. Also, INCART Pediatric Center with same vision of patient center care offer holistic treatment to children and their families through clinical, psychosocial, emotional, and palliative support from the time of diagnosis, regardless of whether a cure exists, and are given timely access to chemotherapeutic drugs. In Dominican Republic a proposal for early childhood national strategic plan is currently in the planning stage, aiming to ensure that all children with suspected or diagnosed oncological diseases benefit from immediate clinical and comprehensive support through early detection, timely treatment, and surveillance interventions [14–16].

Religion and Spirituality

Religion plays a decisive role in the detection, treatment, and even prognosis of cancer. In the Dominican Republic, patients seek protection and support from natural (herbal) treatments, healing ritual, and the intervention of their pastor or priest.

The spiritual dimension of religion and its connection to the cause of disease and healing practices should be recognized and understood by health professionals. It is recommended that health care workers initially discern the patient's religious background so that it can be used favorably as support during treatment.

The religions throughout the country include Roman Catholics (57%), who believe in the existence of a God that can be contacted through intermediaries such as the church, the Virgin Mary, and the saints; evangelical Protestant Christians (25%), who in contrast to the Catholics reject the use of all kinds of religious images and focus on a direct relationship with the Creator; Seventh Day Adventists, the Jehovah's Witnesses, the Church of Jesus Christ of Latter-day Saints (Mormons) (less than 5%); and non-evangelical Protestants who believe on a direct relationship with God, atheists (who doesn't recognize a God as a creator of humanity), and others [17]. An undetermined number of the population practice voodoo and Afro-Caribbean rites such as Santería ("The Way of the Saints"), which usually does not conflict with the same individual's Christian self-designation and is based on a belief in a magical/religious syncretism that combines the basic concepts of the Christian faith with African beliefs. This constitutes a logical-metaphysical system that supports itself in faith [18]. It is of utmost importance to understand that in the Dominican Republic the thinking is that spirituality affects the perception of disease, causality, and healing methods. One palpable example is spiritism, a movement based on the belief that departed people souls can interact with the living, also with the traditional practice of popular healing-hand-touch used by at least one-third of the Catholic population in the Caribbean [19].

Spiritism, Santería, witches, and healers are all similar in terms of their impact on beliefs regarding the cause of the disease, treatment techniques, and diagnostic classifications. For example, healers consult saints to determine which herbs, roots, and different naturist cures to use. Witches also heal by expelling possessive spirits that sometimes take over an individual. The spiritist may be part of the medical team by creating a comprehensive approach to the treatment for cancer patients. A 2007 NHIS study reported that 28.2% of Dominicans use folk/traditional healers as a treatment option [20].

For many Dominicans, the support of healers, combined with traditional Roman Catholic prayer practices, allows them to confront the disease within the family unit and reaffirm the will of God ("If that is my fate, then so be it!"). These beliefs often present a barrier to physicians' confidence in patients and their level of independence in making decisions regarding their treatment; this could negatively impact the search of a cure.

In many cases, patients affected by cancer-related illnesses go to "healers" with the hope that they can help them through prayers and rites; but at the same time, they also go to the oncologist doctor because they understand that doctors are the most professionally appropriate person to help them. This is why some health professionals cover the walls of their clinics with a number of diplomas and certifications, trying to reassure their grades and knowledge level to patients and families, to instill faith in patients, an essential emotional need that must be satisfied.

Economic Factors

Cancer is without question one of the main causes of mortality and morbidity. The Dominican Republic is classified by the World Bank as a "middle-income" country.

In high-income countries, cancer receives considerable public attention. In middle-income countries, and especially in low-income countries, however, cancer receives less public attention than other diseases, such as diseases with an infectious etiology, which have historically been considered a priority [21].

In 2016, 1.8% of the country's gross domestic product (GDP) was spent on public health. This percentage was among the lowest in the Caribbean, surpassed only by Haiti, St. Kitts and Nevis, Jamaica, and Grenada. There is no fixed percentage or monetary amount designated for cancer prevention, detection, or treatment [22].

Inevitably, cancer will continue to attract more attention in the country. Given that the economic plan is to reduce poverty and expand the middle class, adopting the health care policies of high-income countries, where a rise in chronic diseases such as cancer is expected, will therefore result in a change in the current approach to the disease [23].

Cultural and Religious Factors Regarding Cancer

The Dominican Republic has been characterized by the religious, cultural, and socioeconomic aspects that have always been nuanced by the island's own history, as well as the mixture of races, the Spanish conquest, the Haitian occupation, the American intervention, liberal governments, and dictatorships in its recent past (Trujillo, 1930–1961). Since the Spanish conquest, the Catholic religion has permeated the narrative of medical paternalism in the area of health care. Patients wish to understand the therapeutic options available to them and participate in the decision making, but ultimately they prefer that their doctors make decisions regarding their health problems [24].

Since the arrival of the Spanish, and during the establishment of the Republic, the Dominican psychosocial cultural sphere has been closely linked to the clergy, especially the predominant Catholic clergy. The public health of the country has also been influenced by religion, conditioning this to a cultural concept of receiving free care, treatment, and health protection as a donation, a fact that does not escape patients diagnosed with cancer. The faithful and parishioners affected by these ills go to pastors for emotional cathartic rituals of "glorification" and exorcism of the ongoing disease. "Ensalmo," a prayer that is usually accompanied by a procedure or application of remedies, is said to have magical powers to heal the sick. Magical/religious rituals are performed, sometimes accompanied by prayers, and applications of alternative or naturopathic medicine endeavor to cure diseases [25,26].

Similarly and closely linked to the African American roots of the Dominican, as we have already mentioned, when patients are diagnosed with a catastrophic, chronic, and severe disease, sometimes they tend to think about the presence of spiritual and religious malignancy (disease secondary to evil presences or illness recognized as a divine punishment). Thus, among the main consultations carried out, they are often found attending the Santero, sorcerer, or spiritualist, looking for answers and healing. It is important to understand that the different religious denominations of the Dominican people are integrated into their daily life by filling emotional and intellectual voids; they provide an explanation for events, situations, and diseases and offer psychological healing and a sense of divine response that brings peace of mind and balance.

Culture, religion, and socioeconomic circumstances inevitably have an impact on cancer patients and their families, whether at the time the patient begins to present symptoms or upon diagnosis of the disease. Parents begin to question what they did wrong or what sin they committed that caused their child to be sick; or parents begin to blame each other for the cause of the cancer, based on certain behaviors or actions of their past, which can lead among other things to domestic violence, gender-based violence, alcoholism, infidelities, and vices. It is common to find refuge and explanation in the diagnosis and prognosis of the case by repeatedly reciting the phrase "Everything is in the hands of God" or "God has the last word," usually attributing good forecasts to divinity and undesirable developments to the failure of the health system, medical technology, or a delay in the timely care of the health care team. Such bad outcomes are also often associated with some kind of divine punishment or parental guilt.

Families often experience great compassion when faced with the high probability of not finding a cure, and they pray for divine intervention to find answers to a poor prognosis in their own or their children's treatment for cancer. Importantly, there is a direct correlation between the family's socio-academic status and the level of acceptance of the disease. Generally, in lower educational and cultural areas. there is greater acceptance of the disease by incorporating divine justification. In contrast, people with higher academic degrees or social status exhibit a higher rate of denial and search for scientific answers to oncological diagnoses.

The Dominican Republic, as part of Latin America, finds it very difficult to respond to the increase in morbidity and mortality caused by oncological diseases, mainly in advanced stages, and faces many challenges such as the inequitable distribution of health resources, lack of training, and limited diagnostic and supportive services.

The Dominican population , like Latin American populations generally, has to deal with a high incidence of risk factors such as hypertension, increased environmental pollution, a diet low in fruits and vegetables, and a high body mass index, which are the main causes of chronic diseases such as cardiovascular diseases and cancer in adults [27].

Conclusion

The Dominican Republic comprises a mixture of indigenous, Spanish, and African cultures, religions, and traditions. These components directly affect the perception, prevention, diagnosis, and management of diseases such as cancer. Spiritual beliefs range from the Santería, voodoo, and healers to Catholicism, the saints, and the church; each and every one of these plays a decisive role in discussions of disease.

When all the elements that lead to a feeling of stigma are analyzed and added to the customs and sociocultural beliefs of the Dominican people, the delay in seeking early intervention or denying the possible malignancy of the disease, unfortunately, creates a scenario of patients arriving late to timely care; their disease is usually at stage III-IV (metastatic disease). For this reason, it is expected that, in the near future, national cancer care programs will be created, starting from suspected oncological disease to early diagnosis, protocolized treatment, follow-up to side effects, and comprehensive palliative intervention for adults and children. Family customs, faith, and beliefs must always be taken into account and respected, and far from being rejected, these values must be integrated into the psychoemotional vision of treatment and used as holistic supplements that contribute to the emotional support of patients throughout the disease process.

References

1. Díaz JM, Sevilla MD. *Study on Cultural and Folk Manifestations for Artisanal Production in the Dominican Republic*. Santo Domingo: UNESCO: Dominican Institute for Integral Development; 2005.

2. Moya-Pons F. *The Dominican Republic: A National History*. 3rd ed. Princeton, NJ: Markus Wiener Publishers; 2010.

3. Cook DJ, Mulrow C, Haynes R. Systematic reviews: Synthesis of best evidence for clinical decisions. *Ann Intern Med*. 1997 Mar 1;126(5):376–380.

4. Fisher, Robert and Dybicz, Phillip. The Place of Historical Research in Social Work. *Journal of Sociology & Social Welfare*. 1999;26(3):105–124. Available at: https://scholarworks.wmich.edu/jssw/vol26/iss3/7.

5. Aranda E, Benavides M, Casas A, Felip E, Garrido M, Rifá J. Libro Blanco de la Oncología Médica en España. Madrid, Spain: Spanish Society of Medical Oncology (SEOM); Dossier 2007 (17–40 p.). Available at: https://periodicooficial.jalisco.gob.mx/sites/periodicooficial.jalisco.gob.mx/files/libro_blanco_de_la_oncologia_medica_en_espana-_ramon_colomer.pdf

6. De León V. Trujillo built emblematic hospitals. *Listin Diario*. May 31, 2911. Retrieved August 25, 2020, from https://listindiario.com/la-republica/2011/05/31/190260/trujillo-construyo-emblematicos-hospitales

7. Sección Agenda. Necrológicas: José Soba, cancerólogo. El País (ed). August 16, 1985. From https://elpais.com/diario/1985/08/17/agenda/493077602_850215.html

8. Stern H. August 11, 2018. Dr. Alberto Paiewonsky. *Resumen de Salud*. Retrieved 2020 from https://www.resumendesalud.net/157-articulos/12351-dr-alberto-paiewonsky

9. Dominican League Against Cancer. 2019. Retrieved 2020 from http://iohp.org/historia-iohp

10. ECANCER. November 22, 2014. Retrieved 2020 from ECANCER: https://ecancer.org/es/video/3313-breve-historia-de-las-ejecutorias-de-la-liga-dominicana-contra-el-cancer

11. Ciencia. Medicina. Oncologia. 2020. Biografía del Dr. Heriberto Pieter. Apprenderly (free study documents site). Recovered in 2020: https://aprenderly.com/doc/3128768/biograf%C3%ADa-dr.-heriberto-pieter

12. Sección Salud. April 20, 2015. Oncologists provide details of two scientific events. *Listin Diario*. Retrieved October 14, 2020, from https://listindiario.com/las-sociales/2015/04/20/363999/oncologos-ofrecen-detalles-de-dos-eventos-cientificos

13. SODOHEM. Our Story. Hematologia SD (ed.). 2019. Retrieved October 13, 2020, from https://programacasa2.net/sodohem/?page_id=2

14. Dr. Robert Reid Cabral Children's Hospital. Cabral HI (ed). 2020. Retrieved October 5, 2020, from http://www.hirrc.gov.do/index.php/sobre-nosotros/historia

15. Fundación Amigos Contra el Cáncer Infantil 2020. *Quiénes Somos*. FACCI. Retrieved September 20, 2020, from: https://www.facci.org.do/sobre-nosotros

16. *Listin Diario*. Technicians submit a proposal for a national strategic plan to reduce child cancer. September 26, 2020. Retrieved September 29, 2020, from https://listindiario.com/la-republica/2020/09/26/636733/tecnicos-entregan-propuesta-de-plan-estrategico-nacional-para-reducir-cancer-infantil

17. United States Department of State. 2017. https://do.usembassy.gov/wp-content/uploads/sites/281/Dominican-Republic-2017-International-Religious-Freedom-Report-English.pdf. Retrieved August 2020, from https://do.usembassy.gov/wp-content/uploads/sites/281/Dominican-Republic-2017-International-Religious-Freedom-Report-English.pdf

18. López-De Fede A, Haeussler-Fiore D. CIRRIE. Retrieved September 15, 2020, from Center for International Rehabilitation Research Information and Exchange: http://cirrie-sphhp.webapps.buffalo.edu/culture/monographs/domrep.php

19. Schmidt B. The power of the spirits: The formation of identity based on Puerto Rican Spiritism. *Revista de estudos da Religiao*. Año 6; vol. 1, (2), 2006:127–154. From https://www.researchgate.net/publication/26470707_The_Power_of_the_Spirits_The_Formation_of_Identity_based_on_Puerto_Rican_Spiritism

20. Rosario AM. Santeria as an informal psychosocial support among latinas living with cancer. Florida International University (ed.). November 17, 2014. doi:10.25148/etd.FI14110744

21. The World Bank. The World Bank in Dominican Republic. May 13, 2020. Retrieved September 25, 2020, from https://www.worldbank.org/en/country/dominicanrepublic/overview

22. Ministry of Economy, Planning and Development. 2020. Recovered October 1, 2020 from the Ministry of Economy, Planning and Development: https://mepyd.gob.do/wp-content/uploads/drive/UEPESC/Serie%20Informe%20Pais%20Republica%20Dominicana%20Y%20El%20Caribe/Republica%20Dominicana.pdf

23. Sloan F, Gelband H. *Cancer Control Opportunities in Low- and Middle-Income Countries*. Washington, DC: The National Academies Press. 2007 (69–105) https://doi.org/10.17226/11797. Retrieved October 3, 2020, from https://www.nap.edu/read/11797/chapter/1

24. Campos, J. The role of the doctor changed from "father" to partner. 2019. Listin Diario. Retrieved October 2, 2020, from https://listindiario.com/la-vida/2019/12/17/596056/el-rol-del-medico-cambio-de-padre-a-companero

25. López-Sierra HE. Cultural diversity and spiritual/religious health care of patients with cancer at the Dominican Republic. *Asia Pacific J Oncol Nurs*, 6(2):130–136. doi:10.4103/apjon.apjon_70_18

26. Enter PL. Healing by the word in the old age. Madrid: ANTHROPOS; 2005. Retrieved 2020 from https://www.torrossa.com/en/resources/an/4651173

27. Planning for cancer control in Latin America and the Caribbean—Lancet Oncology Commission. *The Lancet of Oncology*. 2013;14:391–436. Recovered October 10, 2020 from https://www.thelancet.com/pb/assets/raw/Lancet//pdfs/tlo-commission/tlo-commission-series-spanish.pdf

45

Jamaican Cultural and Spiritual Guidance in Caring for Cancer Patients, Jamaica

Dingle Spence, Kari Brown, Steven Smith, Dorothy Grant, and David Picking

Introduction

Jamaica is a small island nation in the Caribbean with a population of 2.8 million and a rich cultural heritage informed historically by colonialism. The Jamaican culture and societal norms of today have evolved over centuries and are the result of a melding of many traditions, cultures, and belief systems [1]. These include the traditions of enslaved African peoples that melded with those of European colonists and with the culture and traditions of indentured laborers and early commercial settlers who came principally from China, India, Syria, and Lebanon. As is typical of humanity the world over, cultural idiosyncrasies affect nearly every aspect of life, including attitudes and beliefs concerning illness and health.

Jamaica's health services operate through a largely free public system governed by the Ministry of Health and Wellness (MOHW) and are supplemented by the private sector (particularly for primary care). Cancer is the second leading cause of death, responsible for approximately 20% of all deaths [1]. The MOHW aims to reduce cancer incidence and mortality through developing its National Strategy and Action Plan [2], which includes the goal of ensuring that patients with advanced cancer receive support for psychosocial and spiritual concerns, although no formal guidelines for delivering this type of care currently exist.

While there may not be complete acceptance of health care professionals, nor formal guidelines for them, the general population continues to integrate cultural healing traditions and beliefs into their own care (albeit frequently without the assistance or even understanding of their health care providers). These cultural practices span the gamut from the use of traditional herbal medicines, folk beliefs that may modify people's attitude toward their health and dietary concerns to popular religious and spiritual traditions. These factors can modify care in positive but also, at times, negative ways. The following sections expand on some of these medicinal, cultural, and spiritual factors as they relate to Jamaican people and their care within the health system.

Cultural Factors Modifying Medical and Cancer Care in Jamaica

Traditional medicine (TM) in Jamaica is rooted in tradition and embedded in a broader cultural context of beliefs, practices, and worldviews that influence the use of plant-, animal- and mineral-based medicines, spiritual practices, and perceptions of health, disease and illness [3–6].

The traditional knowledge (TK) of Jamaica has been influenced by the coexistence of several cultures following the collision of the New and Old Worlds, colonization, chattel slavery, and indentured labor. The result is a unique cultural mix of African, Indigenous, European, and Asian ancestry [7–9].

Prior to the European colonization, from 1494, the Taíno, an indigenous Arawak people, established a highly developed culture in Jamaica in which the use of plants for religious ceremonies, rituals, and as medicines appears to have been well established [10–13]. While the subsequent Spanish colonization (1509–1606) led to their almost complete annihilation, evidence exists for the intermarriage among Taíno, free Africans, and escaped enslaved Africans, as well as the formation of Maroon communities within the mountainous interior and the development of a strong traditional knowledge and reliance on traditional medicine [14,15].

During the transatlantic slave trade, practitioners of African traditional medicine (ATM), who were among those forcefully transported to the island, are reported to have been skilled in the use of medicinal plants, bone setting, midwifery, spiritual healing, divination, and incantation [12,16–18]. Several forms of TM are deeply rooted in African religious practices, such as healing and spiritual protection [12]. Obeah, one of the oldest systems of belief in the Caribbean, involves spells and magic and healing practices that utilize plants, minerals, and animal material. Obeah, which today is seen mostly as a malicious form of black magic or witchcraft used to cause harm, continues to be criminalized under the Obeah Act, introduced as a colonial law to suppress Afro-Jamaican resistance following one of the largest slave rebellions in 1760 [19–21].

Contemporary Jamaica effectively has two health care systems, Western biomedicine and traditional medicine, with a significant proportion of the population continuing to rely on TM [12]. Many Jamaicans seek a diagnosis from a medical doctor but then follow treatment combining pharmaceutical drugs and self-medication with plant-based medicines. If the complaint is not resolved, they will often then visit traditional healers, including natural practitioners such as herbalists or bush doctors, nannas or lay midwives, or spiritual healers such as healers linked to Revivalism (mother and balm yard healers), church healers, psychic mothers and revealers, or occult healers such as Obeah and science men and women and sorcerers [9–12].

Rates of self-medication with plant-based medicines are high, with 73% of Jamaicans reporting their use on a regular basis [22]. Medicinal plant use is reported across a spectrum of health conditions, both self-limiting and chronic, including those with the highest mortality rates in Jamaica: cancer, cardiovascular disease, and diabetes [9,23]. Similarly, high levels of medicinal plant use are reported by patients receiving orthodox treatment for hypertension (79%) and diabetes (83%) [24]. While patient use of medicinal plants is high, conversely, physician awareness of such use is low, averaging 16% across a number of surveys [22,24–26].

The most common preparations of medicinal plants are decoctions (actively boiled) or infusions (steeped in boiled water) of dried or fresh plant material, used for specific health conditions, for general well-being, or for spiritual problems [27,28]. Root tonics represent another commonly consumed form of plant medicine, prepared as deep decoctions from predominantly wild-crafted forest species. Reported health benefits include improved sexual function in both men and women, as a general tonic to improve and maintain health and treatment of specific illnesses [9,29].

Traditional Medicine in Cancer Care

A survey of outpatients attending the oncology and urology clinics at the University Hospital of the West Indies (UHWI) reported 80% prevalence for medicinal plant use for the prevention and treatment of cancer, with soursop (*Annona muricata*) and guinea henweed (*Petiveria alliacea*; see Figure 45.1) being the most reported species. Among medicinal plant users, 89% stated that medicinal plants served a critical purpose in their cancer treatment, with the reasons cited being traditional use (37%), availability (33%), and efficacy (25%). Use was independent of education and income level, and 50% sourced information from friends and other cancer patients. Prevalence of concomitant use with prescription drugs on the same day was 75%, with 71% of these patients believing that there was no harm in taking both together. Only 15% of cancer patients using medicinal plants discussed their use with their doctor,

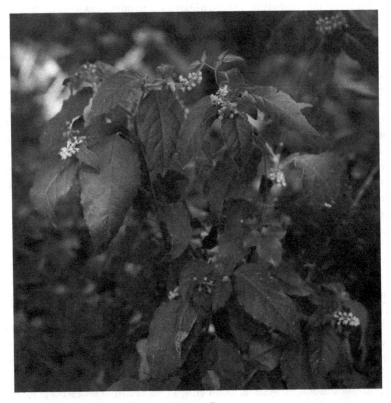

Figure 45.1 *Petiveria alliacea* (Guinea henweed)

Table 45.1 Ten Locally Available Botanical Species with Reported Anticancer Properties (Listed Alphabetically) [12,26,28,30–46]

Botanical species	Family	Local name	Native/Exotic (NA/EX)
Allium sativum	Amaryllidaceae	Garlic	EX
Annona muricata	Annonaceae	Soursop	EX
Cannabis sativa	Cannabaceae	Ganja	EX
Momordica charantia	Cucurbitaceae	Cerasee	EX
Morinda citrifolia	Rubiaceae	Noni	EX
Moringa oleifera	Moringaceae	Moringa	EX
Petiveria alliacea	Petiveriaceae	Guinea henweed	NA
Stachytarpheta jamaicensis	Verbenaceae	Vervain, vervine	NA
Curcuma longa	Zingiberaceae	Turmeric	EX
Zingiber officinale	Zingiberaceae	Ginger	EX

citing the doctors' lack of interest and refusal to engage in discussions about alternative treatment options [26].

A number of contemporary Jamaican publications cite information about locally available plants with reported anticancer properties; examples of 10 such plants are listed in Table 45.1 [12,26,28,30–36].

Table 45.2 details published research for five of the medicinal plants listed in Table 45.1. Most of the research on soursop (*Annona muricata*), guinea henweed (*Petiveria alliacea*) [26] and moringa (*Moringa oleifera*; see Figure 45.2) comprise predominantly in vitro and in vivo studies and indicate potential anticancer and chemopreventive properties. One case study cites that, with the use of soursop leaf tea together with capecitabine, a patient with metastatic breast cancer, previously refractory to multiple chemotherapy treatments, achieved stable disease for more than five years [37]. Results for the other two plants, ganja (*Cannabis sativa*) and turmeric (*Curcuma longa*), are cited in published case studies, clinical studies, systematic reviews, and meta-analyses. Results for ganja report promising early indications for the effective use of cannabinoids in the treatment of glioblastoma [38,39], adjunctive treatment for chemotherapy-induced nausea and vomiting (CINV), and alleviation of cancer/neuropathic pain in advanced cancer and paraneoplastic night sweats [40–43]. Results for turmeric and its key constituent, curcumin, provide evidence for clinically significant effects in patients with colorectal cancer [44], advanced pancreatic cancer [45], and localized prostate cancer [46], for safe and effective reduction of inflammation and pain in breast cancer patients [47] and adjunctive treatment for chemotherapy-induced hand–foot syndrome [48]. Positive results are also reported in clinical studies for feasibility, safety, and tolerability of combined curcumin and gemcitabine in gemcitabine-resistant pancreatic cancer [49,50], curcumin and docetaxel in advanced and metastatic breast cancer [51], and curcumin with FOLFOX[1] chemotherapy in metastatic colorectal cancer [52].

Table 45.2 Overview of Published Research Detailing Anticancer, Chemopreventive, Chemoprotective, and Adjunctive Treatment Properties for Five of the Medicinal Plants Listed in Table 45.1

Botanical species [local/common name]	Plant part used/ Phytochemical	Anticancer properties	Type of Research	Ref.
Annona muricata[*] [Soursop/ graviola]	Leaf, ethyl acetate extract	Apoptosis - A549 lung cancer cells	in vitro	[63]
	Leaf, ethyl acetate extract	Apoptosis - HCT-116 & HT-29 colon cancer cells	in vitro	[64]
	Leaf aqueous extract	Antiproliferative - BPH-1 cells & prostate size reduction	in vitro/in vivo	[65]
	Leaf & stem, DMSO extract	Antitumorigenic - pancreatic cell lines FG/COL0357 & CD18/HPAF	in vitro/in vivo	[66]
	Fruit, acetone extract	EGFR expression downregulation - breast cancer cell lines & xenografts	in vitro/in vivo	[67]
	Acetogenins	Cytotoxic - liver cancer cell lines, Hep G_2 and 2,2,15	in vitro	[68]
	Leaf, ethanol extract	Chemopreventive - skin tumour growth in ICR mice	in vivo/in vitro	[69]
	Leaf, aqueous extract	Metastatic breast cancer - 5 years stable disease in combination with capecitabine.	Case study	[37]
Cannabis sativa [Ganja]	Cannabinoids	Cytotoxic - glioma. 34 preclinical studies and one phase I/II clinical study indicating promising results	Systematic review	[38]
	Whole-plant extract (THC-CBD)	Glioma - phase 2 proof of concept study in 21 patients reports positive results [not published]	Clinical study	[39]
	Cannabinoids	Cannabinoids associated with improvements in CINV	Systematic review/ meta-analysis	[40]
	Cannabis-based medications	23 RCTs (1975–1991) indicate cannabis-based medications may be useful for treating refractory CINV	Cochrane review	[41]
	THC and/or CBD	Clinical studies (1975—2014) report evidence for medical cannabis reducing chronic or neuropathic pain in advanced cancer	Review of clinical studies	[42]

Table 45.2 Continued

Botanical species [local/common name]	Plant part used/ Phytochemical	Anticancer properties	Type of Research	Ref.
	Cannabinoids	Moderate level of evidence for cannabinoids alleviating cancer pain	Systematic review/meta-analysis	[40]
	Dronabinol (cannabinoid)	Successful management of persistent symptomatic paraneoplastic night sweats in five patients with advanced cancer	Case studies	[43]
Curcuma longa* [Turmeric]	Curcumin	Improved weight loss, reduced TNF-α serum levels, increased apoptosis, upregulated p53 expression, modulated apoptosis-related Bax and Bcl-2 molecules in colorectal cancer patients.	Clinical study	[44]
	Curcumin	Clinically relevant bioactivity reported in advanced pancreatic cancer patients	Clinical study	[45]
	Turmeric rhizome extract	Reduced incidence and severity of capecitabine (Xeloda) induced hand–foot syndrome	Clinical study	[48]
	Turmeric, broccoli, pomegranate whole-fruit powders, green tea extract, whole-food supplement	Significant short-term favorable effect on percentage rise in PSA in men with localized prostate cancer	Clinical study	[46]
	Curcumin	Combination chemotherapy with gemcitabine in patients with pancreatic cancer	Clinical study	[49, 50]
	Curcumin	Combination chemotherapy with docetaxel in patients with advanced and metastatic breast cancer	Clinical study	[51]
		Combination chemotherapy with FOLFOX in patients with metastatic colorectal cancer	Clinical study	[52]
	Curcumin, omega-3 fatty acid, hydroxytyrosol supplement	Reduction of C-Reactive protein (CRP) and decrease in pain scores in early-stage breast cancer patients receiving adjuvant hormonal therapy	Clinical study	[47]

Continued

Table 45.2 Continued

Botanical species [local/common name]	Plant part used/ Phytochemical	Anticancer properties	Type of Research	Ref.
Moringa oleifera[*] [Moringa]	Leaf & bark, ethanol extracts	Anticancer - HCT-8 colorectal and MDA-MB-231 breast cancer cell lines	in vitro	[70]
	Leaf, aqueous extract	Cytotoxic - pancreatic cell lines, Pnac-1, p34, COLO 357 and increased cytotoxic effect of chemotherapy (cisplatin) - Panc-1 cell line	in vitro	[71]
	Leaf, aqueous extract	Antiproliferation and apoptosis - squamous cell carcinoma KB cell line	in vitro	[72]
	Leaf, cold aqueous extract	Antiproliferative - A549, NCI-H23 lung, H358 non-small cell lung cancer, MCF-7 breast, A431 epidermoid carcinoma, HT1080 fibrosarcoma cell lines	in vitro	[73]
	Leaf, aqueous extract	Antiproliferative - A549 lung cancer cell line	in vitro	[74]
	Pod, aqueous extract	Chemopreventive - colon carcinogenesis model in male ICR mice	in vivo	[75]
	Leaf, methanol extract	Anticancer - Jab1 cervical cancer cell line	in vitro	[76]
	Leaf, methanol extract	Apoptosis - PC-3 prostate cancer cell line	in vitro	[77]
	Leaf, methanol extract	Apoptosis - A2058 metastatic melanoma cell lines	in vitro	[78]
	Leaf and seed residue, ethanol extract	Chemopreventive - breast cancer model, cytotoxic to MCF-7 breast cancer cell line and MDMA-MB-231 xenograft breast tumour mice	in vitro & in vivo	[79]
	Leaf, aqueous extract	Moringa plus radiation inhibited PANC-1 cell survival and antiproliferative against PANC-1 cells in nude mice.	in vitro & in vivo	[76]
	Leaf, aqueous extracts	Apoptosis in EAC, Ehrlich ascites carcinoma and HEp-2 laryngeal carcinoma cell lines and breast adenocarcinoma model in Balb/c mice	in vitro & in vivo	[80]
	Leaf, dried - feed	Chemoprevention in AOM/ DSS induced colorectal carcinogenesis in CD-1 mice	in vivo	[81]

Table 45.2 Continued

Botanical species [local/common name]	Plant part used/ Phytochemical	Anticancer properties	Type of Research	Ref.
Petiveria alliacea[*] [Guinea henweed/ anamu]	Leaf & stem, ethyl acetate fraction	Apoptosis in breast adenocarcinoma in vitro and tumor regression in vivo	in vitro & in vivo	[82]
	Leaf & stem, ethanol extract, ethyl acetate fraction	Cytotoxic - epithelial breast cancer cell lines / decrease tumor growth in vivo	in vitro & in vivo	[83]
	Leaf & stem, ethanol extract, ethyl acetate fraction	Cytotoxic - antitumour agent against A375 melanoma, K562 leukemia cell lines	in vitro	[84]
	Leaf & stem, ethanol extract, ethyl acetate fraction	Apoptosis via mitochondrial-dependent pathway & downregulation of HSP70	in vitro	[85]
	Dibenzyl trisulphide (DTS)	Microtubule-disrupting effect - SH-SY5Y neuroblastoma cell line	in vitro	[86]
	Dibenzyl trisulphide (DTS)	Cytotoxic/antiproliferation - SH-SY5Y neuroblastoma cell line	in vitro	[87]

[*] Use reported by outpatients attending the oncology and urology clinics at the UHWI [26].

The reported levels of discussion between patient and physician, averaging 16% [22,24–26] for both cancer patients and medicinal plant users are, in general, worryingly low. In comparison, 49% of cancer patients using medicinal plants in neighboring Trinidad reported discussing it with their doctor [53]. An earlier survey reported that 60% of physicians in Trinidad believe medicinal plant use can be beneficial to health, but the same survey reported low (15%) physician knowledge about this treatment modality [54].

High levels of medicinal plant use among Jamaicans, in general [22,24,25]. and among cancer patients, in particular [26], place great pressure on oncologists and health care professionals to educate themselves on the complex nature of these biologically active agents, their traditional and proven uses, potential benefits, and possible adverse effects and interactions with pharmaceutical drugs and other treatment protocols. Adverse drug reactions (ADRs) resulting from drug–drug interactions are well known and reported [55], while ADRs resulting from medicinal plant–drug interactions are not as well researched. This is particularly problematic in Jamaica and the wider Caribbean, where fewer plants have been investigated to date [55–57]. However, a growing number of evidence-based resources are available for Jamaican health care professionals and patients, providing greater opportunities for informed dialogue and safer integration of medicinal plant use in a clinical setting [28,58–62].

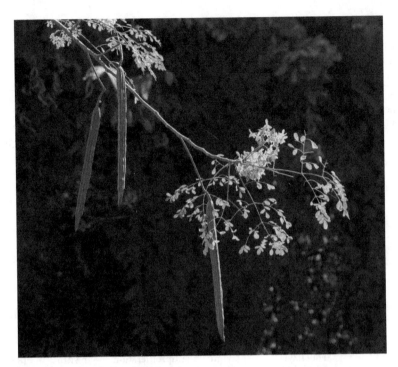

Figure 45.2. *Moringa oleifera* (Moringa)

Impact of Diet on Cancer Care

Diet, which is heavily influenced by culture, has become a well-recognized risk factor for certain cancers, particularly cancer of the gastrointestinal tract. For example, diets rich in salted, smoked, and pickled foods have been linked to the development of gastric cancer (which is especially common in Japan, China, and parts of South America), while diets low in fiber and high in red meat and fat (common in Western countries) have been linked to the development of colorectal cancer [88]. Although certain Jamaican dishes are accepted nationwide as cultural standards (such as the ackee and salt-fish national dish), it is difficult to define a typical Jamaican diet, as it varies significantly with socioeconomic status, geographical location, and other factors such as traditional and familial values. While keeping in mind that other important risk factors exist, it is worth noting that colorectal and gastric cancers are the third and fourth most common cancers, respectively, in Jamaican males (in fact, mirroring the trend worldwide) [89].

Prostate cancer is the most common cancer in Jamaica and also has the highest mortality rate [89,90]. Diet has emerged as a potential risk factor: a case-control study found increased odds of prostate cancer in Jamaican men consuming a high-carbohydrate diet (rice, pasta, sugar-sweetened beverages, and sweet baked foods) compared to those with a low-carbohydrate diet [91]. In that study, diets principally rich in vegetables/legumes, meats, or fast food were not found to be associated with prostate cancer risk. Indeed, diets rich in foods with a high glycaemic index such as refined sugars (e.g., white flour) are thought to contribute to tumorigenesis [92]. A subsequent investigation found that a pro-inflammatory diet (consisting of high amounts of red meat and sugar-sweetened soft drinks with low amounts of anti-inflammatory food groups such as fruits, vegetables, and whole grains) was associated with an increased risk of prostate cancer [93]. Furthermore, a study of Jamaican men suggested that the omega-6 fatty acid linoleic acid (found in the locally consumed ackee fruit) may be associated with higher Gleason scores on prostate biopsy [94], though subsequent studies have obscured the meaningfulness of this association [95,96]. As prostate cancer is the most common cancer diagnosed in men globally, insights into potential preventive factors, such as modifying dietary intake, may not only be highly consequential, but also generalizable to a broad subsection of men worldwide.

The potential benefits of dietary modification are often of paramount concern to Jamaicans with a recent cancer diagnosis. Many of these individuals are interested in the way in which certain dietary modifications might contribute to treating their illness. While collection of definitive evidence is ongoing, various epidemiological, observational, and preclinical studies suggest there are anticancer effects in numerous products, ranging from green tea, pomegranate juice, and berries to mushrooms and cruciform and carotenoid-containing vegetables [92]. Many dietary adjustments are both low risk and affordable, and it would be advantageous (particularly in low- and middle-income countries) for health policymakers and stakeholders to adapt and implement clear guidelines for the public on dietary choices, even as the wider medical community gradually adapts itself to such measures.

Cultural Attitudes and Beliefs in Cancer Care

Cultural attitudes and beliefs not only give root to the traditions mentioned in earlier sections, but also affect the approach of Jamaican people to preventive screening programs, of which uptake has reportedly been suboptimal for major cancers in Jamaica [97,98]. Studies analyzing sociocultural attitudes contributing to decreased screening have identified some major contributors: fear of painful procedures in breast [99] and cervical [100] cancers and discomfort/embarrassment associated with the digital rectal exams for prostate examination [101,102]. Fortunately, such attitudes and fears are likely mutable when intentionally addressed and culturally directed. One study conducted through a series of focus groups with Jamaican women found that culturally targeted fear appeal messaging had the potential to increase acceptability and uptake of a cervical self-sampling kit [100]. The importance of romantic/sexual partners in providing encouragement and dispelling fear and stigma related to cancer diagnosis and treatment should also not be understated. This preceding literature highlights the value of culture-targeted community health promotion and educational interventions [103–105], which ought to be carried out alongside improvement in health system-related issues (such as infrastructure and health provider referrals) [99–106]. Such an approach is likely to ensure the highest uptake of already existing cancer screening programs.

Religious and Spiritual Factors Modifying Cancer Care in Jamaica

The fabric of everyday life in Jamaica is interwoven with both religious and spiritual practices, at all levels of society. In Jamaica, it is common practice to pray or engage in some type of religious devotional exercise before embarking on almost any public or private activity, from the opening of parliament to the start of business meetings, school gatherings, football matches, meal times, and other secular events.

Christianity is the most widely practiced religion in Jamaica, accounting for the majority of religious affiliations reported among the population (Protestant: 64.8%, Roman Catholic: 2.2%, and Jehovah's Witness: 1.9%). Conversely, Jamaica's indigenous Rastafari movement is practiced by 1.1% of the population, while 21.3% report no religious affiliation [107].

It is, therefore, not unusual for patients to bring their particular faith or religious beliefs to the fore, in line with their health experience. Health care practitioners should be prepared to recognize, acknowledge, and help address religious and spiritual needs whenever they may arise, or to recognize them and make the appropriate referral to a spiritual care provider. It is quite common for patients diagnosed with end-stage cancers to invoke the will of God and to acknowledge that Jesus said, "It is not the healthy who need a doctor, but the sick" [108]. They accept that God works through people to get His work done in the world, and this includes doctors and nurses. He gave their skills to them, and He has also enabled researchers to discover new ways to treat some of the maladies that affect our bodies, with the end result being God's will [109].

A growing body of research indicates that the use of religious resources, strategies, and orientations for managing problematic life events and situations is widespread [110]. Regardless of the patient's ethnic, religious, or cultural background, a diagnosis of cancer invariably elicits existential and spiritual concerns, and people can become acutely aware of their own vulnerability to disease and suffering. Given the strong connection to faith and religion in Jamaica, it is critical to explore how religious concerns impact people's lives, including the use of strategies specifically related to coping with a cancer diagnosis.

Role of Religion and Spiritual Practices in Cancer Care in Jamaica

An initial response to a diagnosis of cancer may include feelings of depression, anguish, despair, anger, and nonacceptance or denial of the situation. With time, some people become more accepting of their situation, and their religious alignments and strategies become a robust component of their coping repertoire. Some even see cancer as a life-changer. This is often referred to as the "enlightenment" of cancer, or the "gift" of cancer [111].

Patients respond to a cancer diagnosis in different ways and may be concerned that God is punishing them or that they are being "taught a lesson." Such patients may feel abandoned, and even angry with God, as they process this difficult diagnosis and often unfavorable prognosis. On the contrary, there are also those patients with cancer who believe that the disease is the result of an Obeah spell or curse, and so they refuse conventional medical interventions as they would not be considered effective in this situation.

Whatever the reaction to the initial cancer diagnosis, patients will often state that their ultimate priority is to regain good health. Many of them also express the desire to live longer for the sake of their families or to accomplish a lifelong dream for themselves. Prayer has been a widely cited coping strategy for patients grappling with the discordance caused by the realities of a cancer diagnosis. Some researchers and clinicians have likened private prayer to a "spiritual treatment modality," a "spiritual self-care modality" or a form of complementary and alternative therapy [112–114]. The Jamaican context is no different, as prayer is considered a "go-to" treatment option.

Furthermore, some patients' understanding and interpretation of the suffering narratives in the Bible serve as a useful coping strategy. They believe that being afflicted by cancer is their personal suffering, and it is a way of participating in God's work; as one hymn suggests, Jesus cannot suffer alone and all the world go free [115]. Other reported religious coping practices, include rituals such as fasting, religious writings, lighting candles, and listening to inspirational music. Active engagement with religious communities can provide essential connections and support resources for patients and loved ones.

Spiritual Assessment Tool

Clinicians in the Jamaican setting have reported that a patient's strong religious views may make it difficult to engage patients and to provide appropriate spiritual care and support, as the patient and family may be steeped in their own dogmatic theological beliefs, which can act as a barrier to any intervention. In order to improve this aspect of care, a Jamaican hospital chaplain working at a dedicated public institution for cancer care developed the 3C's Spiritual Assessment Tool (Dorothy Grant, personal communication, 2016). It uses relatively neutral language and minimizes the use of specific religious terms such as faith, grace, and sin.

The 3C's Spiritual Assessment Tool appears in Box 45.1. Part 1 focuses on spiritual screening and has three important areas: crisis, connections, and care options. Part 2 is evaluative and processes the value of the intervention and method; it ascertains patients' assessment of the care received.

Although the chaplain's distinct role, as part of the health care team, is to engage with patients about their spiritual beliefs and needs and to explore appropriate interventions and strategies that provide support and direction (see Box 45.2), physicians and nurses can also screen and address spiritual issues using the 3C's spiritual history tool.

Summary, Recommendations, and Conclusions

Jamaica's geographic location and place in modern history have made the country a nest for the development of rich and diversely informed cultural traditions, attitudes, and beliefs. These inevitably and intimately impact the public's approach to

Box 45.1

Part 1

What is the **Crisis** being experienced?	What or who are your **Connections?**	What should be considered in your **Care Options?**
• Isolation • Fear • Grief • Loss of faith • Concerns with meaning • Isolation • Guilt • Hopelessness • Conflict • Ritual needs • Concerns about death	• Family • Spouse • Children • God • Community • Sacred texts • Religious ritual • Dress rituals • Dance rituals • Cultural practices	• Medical procedures • Ethical consideration • Cultural practices • Religious prohibition • Patient Autonomy issues • Decision-making markers

Part 2: Was the care compassionate? Was the care collaborative? What care gates were opened?

Compassionate Care Was your care compassionate?	Collaborative Care Was your care collaborative?	Care Gates What resources became accessible to you?
• Dignity • Communicative • Sensitive • Caring • Presence • Listening	• Referral • Family meetings • Medical consults • Interdisciplinary team • Ethical decisions	• Communication • Hope • Partnership • Comfort • God as healer • Peace (God, environment)

their own health and, specifically, to cancer care. This unique cultural admixture has led to the development of a strong traditional knowledge base and reliance on traditional medicine, which continues today in Jamaican society, with reported high rates of medicinal plant self-medication among patients with cancer. Many of these traditional medicines have been scientifically appraised (in Jamaica and elsewhere), with varying levels of evidence, and show promise in their anticancer properties and ability to reduce side effects associated with cancer treatment. The potential for interactions with conventional pharmaceuticals varies according to the specific plant and the method of extraction, and while in vitro and in vivo studies have provided preliminary evidence in some cases, more well-designed clinical studies are imperative to shed further light on this area. This is especially true in countries like Jamaica, where a substantial proportion of the population self-medicates, often without the knowledge and support of their physicians. Further studies to gain a better understanding of physicians' perspectives would also be enlightening.

As Jamaica maintains its membership in the World Health Organization, which has recognized spirituality as a dimension of care and advocates for complementary

---

Box 45.2 Using the Chaplaincy Taxonomy to Develop a Spiritual Care Plan (SCP) [116] for Ava

Ava is a 23-year-old woman diagnosed with vulvar cancer, with severe pelvic pain, itchiness, and bleeding from the vulva. She is a final year college student, a Catholic, and an active youth leader. Ava has four younger siblings and is engaged to be married to her fiancée, Robert. She cries incessantly and asks, 'Why me?' She is angry with God that her life is coming to an end so abruptly. She is distressed and does not want to share her feelings with her loved ones.

Crisis: Anger, abandonment, fear of poor health, lack of self-worth

Intended Effect (IE)	Method (M)	Intervention (I)
Promote a sense of peace	Explore the nature of God	Communicate patient's needs/concerns to others
Faith affirmation	Encourage end-of-life review	Ask guided questions about faith and spiritual beliefs and incorporate the related needs in the plan of care
Exploring hope	Discuss concerns	Provide grief resources

---

and alternative medicine (CAM) as an important health resource, the hope is that the country will bring physician education closer to the foreground of health care and seek to move toward a truly integrative medicine approach, especially in cancer care [117]. The introduction of a short undergraduate course in CAM and integrative medicine approaches would go a long way in bridging the gap between public practices and physicians' knowledge and awareness. The need for professionally trained hospital chaplains to deliver the care is also paramount.

Public education, through culturally relevant promotional messaging, has shown potential benefits of increasing screening uptake in Jamaica [100]. Public education around diet and nutrition, with specific emphasis on the role that a proinflammatory diet might play in the development of a new cancer, is vitally important, as is information on the importance of an integrative approach, as opposed to an alternative medicine-only approach.

Finally, the critical role of spirituality and/or religion in the lives of cancer patients, especially in a country such as Jamaica with its weighty ties between religion and culture, is undeniable. Spiritual support can help with coping and adequate adjustment, existential concerns, and bringing patients to a place of acceptance and peace. These positive effects are more prominent than the potentially negative role some spiritual beliefs can play, for instance, in those patients who deny lifesaving care due to beliefs in Obeah.

A truly integrated and holistic approach to cancer care would undoubtedly be beneficial to, and appreciated by, the general public served by health workers. For this approach to be effective, the care itself must not only be integrative, but the approach of health care providers should also be multidisciplinary, integrated, and mutually collaborative, with the ultimate goal of supporting healing and relieving suffering.

Note

1   Chemotherapy regimen comprised of Folinic acid (leucovorin) "FOL," Fluorouracil (5-FU) "F," and Oxaliplatin (Eloxatin) "OX."

References

1. Pan American Health Organization. *Health in the Americas+, 2017 Edition. Summary: Regional Outlook and Country Profiles.* 2017.
2. Ministry of Health. Strategic Plan an Action Plan for the Prevention and Control of Cancer in Jamaica 2013–2018. Accessed December 21, 2020. https://www.iccp-portal.org/plans/strategic-plan-and-action-plan-prevention-and-control-cancer-jamaica-2013-2018
3. Vandebroek I, Reyes-García V, de Albuquerque UP, Bussmann R, Pieroni A. Local knowledge: who cares? *J Ethnobiol Ethnomed.* November 2011;7:35. doi:10.1186/1746-4269-7-35
4. Aginam O. Beyond shamanism: The relevance of African traditional medicine in global health policy. *Med Law.* June 2007;26(2):191–201.
5. Sillitoe P. Developing together with indigenous knowledge: Mini review. *CAB Reviews.* 2017;12(33):1–4.
6. WHO. Traditional Medicine Strategy 2014–2023. World Health Organization. Accessed November 30, 2020, https://www.who.int/publications/i/item/9789241506096
7. Hall SD. Créolité and the process of creolization. In: Rodriguez EG, Tate SA (eds). *Creolizing Europe: Legacies and Transformations.* Liverpool: Liverpool University Press; 2015:12–25.
8. Picking D, Vandebroek I. Traditional and local knowledge systems in the Caribbean: Jamaica as a case study. In: Katerere D, Applequist W, Aboyade O, Togo C (eds). *Traditional and Indigenous Knowledge Systems in the Modern Era: A Natural and Applied Science Perspective.* Boca Raton, FL: CRC Press; 2019:chap 5.
9. Picking D, Delgoda R, Vandebroek I. Traditional knowledge systems and the role of traditional medicine in Jamaica. *CAB Reviews.* 2019;14:1–13. doi:10.1079/PAVSNNR201914045
10. Lloyd W. Letters from the West Indies, during a visit in the autumn of MDCCCXXXVI, and the spring of MDCCCXXXVII. London: Darton & Harvey; 1839.
11. Atkinson LG. The exploitation and transformation of Jamaica's natural vegetation. In: Atkinson L, (ed). *The Earliest Inhabitants: The Dynamics of the Jamaican Taíno.* Kingston: University of the West Indies Press; 2006:97–112.
12. Payne-Jackson AA, M. *Jamaican Folk Medicine: A Source of Healing.* Kingston: University of the West Indies Press; 2004.
13. Rouse I. *The Taíno: Rise and Decline of the People who Greeted Columbus.* New Haven, CT: Yale University Press; 1992.
14. Agorsah EK (ed.). *Maroon Heritage: Archeological Ethnographic and Historical Perspectives.* Kingston: Canoe Press, University of the West Indies; 1994: 210.
15. Hart R. *Slaves Who Abolished Slavery: Volume 2 – Blacks in Rebellion* Institute of Social and Economic Research. Kingston: University of the West Indies; 2002: 1–32.
16. Deason ML, Salas A, Newman SP, Macaulay VA, St AMEY, Pitsiladis YP. Interdisciplinary approach to the demography of Jamaica. *BMC Evol Biol.* February 23 2012;12:24. doi:10.1186/1471-2148-12-24
17. Franco JL. The slave trade in the Caribbean and Latin America. In: UNESCO (ed). *The African Slave Trade From the Fifteenth to the Nineteenth Century.* UNESCO; 1978:88–100.
18. Senior O. *Encyclopedia of Jamaican Heritage.* Kingston: Twin Guinep Publishers Ltd.; 2003.
19. Paton D. Obeah histories. Accessed November 30, 2020, https://obeahhistories.org

20. Fernandez-Olmos M, Paravisini-Gebert L. *Creole Religions in the Caribbean: An Introduction from Vodou and Santería to Obeah and Espiritismo*. 2nd ed. New York: New York University Press; 2011.

21. O'Neal E. *Obeah, Race and Racism: Caribbean Witchcraft in the English Imagination*. Kingston: University of the West Indies Press; 2020: 1–9.

22. Picking D, Younger N, Mitchell S, Delgoda R. The prevalence of herbal medicine home use and concomitant use with pharmaceutical medicines in Jamaica. *J Ethnopharmacol*. September2011;137(1):305–311. doi:10.1016/j.jep.2011.05.025

23. WHO. Noncommunicable Diseases (NCD) Country Profiles: 2018. World Health Organization (WHO). Accessed November 30, 2020, https://www.who.int/publications/i/item/ncd-country-profiles-2018

24. Delgoda R, Younger N, Barrett C, Braithwaite J, Davis D. The prevalence of herbs use in conjunction with conventional medicines in Jamaica. *Complement Ther Med*. February 2010;18(1):13–20. doi:10.1016/j.ctim.2010.01.002

25. Delgoda R, Ellington C, Barrett S, Gordon N, Clarke N, Younger N. The practice of polypharmacy involving herbal and prescription medicines in the treatment of diabetes mellitus, hypertension and gastrointestinal disorders in Jamaica. *West Indian Med J*. December 2004;53(6):400–405.

26. Foster K, Younger N, Aiken W, Brady-West D, Delgoda R. Reliance on medicinal plant therapy among cancer patients in Jamaica. *Cancer Causes Control*. Nov 2017;28(11):1349–1356. doi:10.1007/s10552-017-0924-9

27. Picking D, Delgoda R, Younger N, Germosén-Robineau L, Boulogne I, Mitchell S. TRAMIL Ethnomedicinal survey in Jamaica. *J Ethnopharmacol*. July 2015;169:314–327. doi:10.1016/j.jep.2015.04.027

28. Vandebroek I, Picking D. Popular medicinal plants in Portland and Kingston, Jamaica. *Advances in Economic Botany*. Cham, Switzerland: Springer International Publishing; 2020.

29. Mitchell SA. The Jamaican root tonics: A botanical reference. *Focus on Alt Complement Ther*. 2011;16(4):271–280. doi:https://doi.org/10.1111/j.2042-7166.2011.01124.x

30. Riley J, Riley M, Riley P. *In My Backyard: Powerful Herbs and Foods of the Caribbean. Part 1*. Saint Mary, Jamaica: Riley Publications; 2014.

31. Riley J, Riley M, Riley P. *In My Backyard: Powerful Herbs and Foods of the Caribbean. Part 2*. Saint Mary, Jamaica: Lifeboat Publications; 2016.

32. Harris I. *Healing herbs of Jamaica*. Royal Palm Beach, FL: AhHa Press Inc; 2011.

33. Austin S, Thomas M, Harris L, Henry LG. *Medicinal Plants of Portland, Jamaica*. 2nd ed. CIEER Inc; 2009.

34. Warner M. *Herbal Plants of Jamaica*. Oxford: Macmillan Education; 2007.

35. Picking D, Delgoda R, Younger N, Germosén-Robineau L, Boulogne I, Mitchell S. TRAMIL ethnomedicinal survey in Jamaica. *J Ethnopharmacol*. 2015;doi:10.1016/j.jep.2015.04.027

36. Lowe H, Payne-Jackson A, Beckstrom-Sternberg SM, Duke J. *Jamaica's Ethnomedicine: Its Potential in the Healthcare System*. 2nd ed. Kingston: Pelican Publishers; 2001.

37. Hansra D, Silva O, Mehta A, Ahn E. Patient with metastatic breast cancer achieves stable disease for 5 years on graviola and xeloda after progressing on multiple lines of therapy. *Adv Breast Cancer Res*. 2014;3:84–87. doi:10.4236/abcr.2014.33012

38. Rocha FC, Dos Santos Júnior JG, Stefano SC, da Silveira DX. Systematic review of the literature on clinical and experimental trials on the antitumor effects of cannabinoids in gliomas. *J Neurooncol*. January 2014;116(1):11–24. doi:10.1007/s11060-013-1277-1

39. Pharmaceuticals GW. GW Pharmaceuticals Achieves Positive Results in Phase 2 Proof of Concept Study in Glioma Globe Newswire. February 07, 2017. Accessed January 12, 2021, https://www.globenewswire.com/news-release/2017/02/07/914583/0/en/GW-Pharmaceuticals-Achieves-Positive-Results-in-Phase-2-Proof-of-Concept-Study-in-Glioma.html

40. Whiting PF, Wolff RF, Deshpande S, et al. Cannabinoids for medical use: A systematic review and meta-analysis. *JAMA*. June 23-30 2015;313(24):2456–2473. doi:10.1001/jama.2015.6358

41. Smith LA, Azariah F, Lavender VT, Stoner NS, Bettiol S. Cannabinoids for nausea and vomiting in adults with cancer receiving chemotherapy. *Cochrane Database Syst Rev*. November 2015;(11):CD009464. doi:10.1002/14651858.CD009464.pub2

42. Blake A, Wan BA, Malek L, et al. A selective review of medical cannabis in cancer pain management. *Ann Palliat Med*. December 2017;6(Suppl 2):S215–S222. doi:10.21037/apm.2017.08.05

43. Carr C, Vertelney H, Fronk J, Trieu S. Dronabinol for the treatment of paraneoplastic night sweats in cancer patients: A report of five cases. *J Palliat Med*. 10 2019;22(10):1221–1223. doi:10.1089/jpm.2018.0551

44. He ZY, Shi CB, Wen H, Li FL, Wang BL, Wang J. Upregulation of p53 expression in patients with colorectal cancer by administration of curcumin. *Cancer Invest*. March 2011;29(3):208–213. doi:10.3109/07357907.2010.550592

45. Dhillon N, Aggarwal BB, Newman RA, et al. Phase II trial of curcumin in patients with advanced pancreatic cancer. *Clin Cancer Res*. July 2008;14(14):4491–4499. doi:10.1158/1078-0432.CCR-08-0024

46. Thomas R, Williams M, Sharma H, Chaudry A, Bellamy P. A double-blind, placebo-controlled randomised trial evaluating the effect of a polyphenol-rich whole food supplement on PSA progression in men with prostate cancer—the U.K. NCRN Pomi-T study. *Prostate Cancer Prostatic Dis*. June 2014;17(2):180–186. doi:10.1038/pcan.2014.6

47. Martínez N, Herrera M, Frías L, et al. A combination of hydroxytyrosol, omega-3 fatty acids and curcumin improves pain and inflammation among early stage breast cancer patients receiving adjuvant hormonal therapy: Results of a pilot study. *Clin Transl Oncol*. April 2019;21(4):489–498. doi:10.1007/s12094-018-1950-0

48. Scontre VA, Martins JC, de Melo Sette CV, et al. Curcuma longa (Turmeric) for prevention of capecitabine-induced hand–foot syndrome: A pilot study. *J Diet Suppl*. September 2018;15(5):606–612. doi:10.1080/19390211.2017.1366387

49. Epelbaum R, Schaffer M, Vizel B, Badmaev V, Bar-Sela G. Curcumin and gemcitabine in patients with advanced pancreatic cancer. *Nutr Cancer*. 2010;62(8):1137–1141. doi:10.1080/01635581.2010.513802

50. Kanai M, Yoshimura K, Asada M, et al. A phase I/II study of gemcitabine-based chemotherapy plus curcumin for patients with gemcitabine-resistant pancreatic cancer. *Cancer Chemother Pharmacol*. July 2011;68(1):157–164. doi:10.1007/s00280-010-1470-2

51. Bayet-Robert M, Kwiatkowski F, Leheurteur M, et al. Phase I dose escalation trial of docetaxel plus curcumin in patients with advanced and metastatic breast cancer. *Cancer Biol Ther*. January 2010;9(1):8–14. doi:10.4161/cbt.9.1.10392

52. Howells LM, Iwuji COO, Irving GRB, et al. Curcumin combined with FOLFOX chemotherapy is safe and tolerable in patients with metastatic colorectal cancer in a randomized Phase IIa Trial. *J Nutr*. July 2019;149(7):1133–1139. doi:10.1093/jn/nxz029

53. Clement YN, Mahase V, Jagroop A, et al. Herbal remedies and functional foods used by cancer patients attending specialty oncology clinics in Trinidad. *BMC Complement Alt Med*. October 2016;16(1):399. doi:10.1186/s12906-016-1380-x

54. Clement YN, Williams AF, Khan K, et al. A gap between acceptance and knowledge of herbal remedies by physicians: The need for educational intervention. *BMC Complement Alt Med*. November 2005;5:20. doi:10.1186/1472-6882-5-20

55. Delgoda R, Westlake AC. Herbal interactions involving cytochrome p450 enzymes: A mini review. *Toxicol Rev*. 2004;23(4):239–249. doi:10.2165/00139709-200423040-00004

56. Cohall DH, Griffiths A, Scantlebury-Manning T, Fraser HS, Carrington CM. Drug-herb interaction: database of medicinal plants of the Caribbean, their indications, toxicities and possible interactions with conventional medication. *West Indian Med J*. October 2010;59(5):503–508.

57. Picking D. The contemporary use of medicinal plants in Jamaica and assessment of potential medicinal plant-drug interactions of select plants. PhD. The University of the West Indies; 2014: 1–35.

58. Delgoda R, Picking D. *Potential Drug Interactions for Commonly Used Medicinal Plants and Foods in Jamaica. Handbook for Healthcare Professionals*. Natural Products Institute, The University of the West Indies; 2015: 1–23.

59. NMCD. The Natural Medicines Comprehensive Database. Accessed January 22, 2021, https://naturalmedicines.therapeuticresearch.com

60. NCCIH. National Center for Complementary and Integrative Health. Accessed January 22,/2021, https://www.nccih.nih.gov

61. TRAMIL. Traditional Medicines in the Islands Network. January 22, 2021, http://www.tramil.net

62. MSKCC. Memorial Sloan Kettering Cancer Center's about Herbs database. Accessed December 1, 2020, https://www.mskcc.org/cancer-care/diagnosis-treatment/symptom-management/integrative-medicine/herbs

63. Moghadamtousi SZ, Kadir HA, Paydar M, Rouhollahi E, Karimian H. Annona muricata leaves induced apoptosis in A549 cells through mitochondrial-mediated pathway and involvement of NF-κB. *BMC Complement Alt Med*. August 2014;14:299. doi:10.1186/1472-6882-14-299

64. Zorofchian Moghadamtousi S, Karimian H, Rouhollahi E, Paydar M, Fadaeinasab M, Abdul Kadir H. Annona muricata leaves induce G_1 cell cycle arrest and apoptosis through mitochondria-mediated pathway in human HCT-116 and HT-29 colon cancer cells. *J Ethnopharmacol*. October 2014;156:277–289. doi:10.1016/j.jep.2014.08.011

65. Asare GA, Afriyie D, Ngala RA, et al. Antiproliferative activity of aqueous leaf extract of *Annona muricata L.* on the prostate, BPH-1 cells, and some target genes. *Integr Cancer Ther*. Jan 2015;14(1):65–74. doi:10.1177/1534735414550019

66. Torres MP, Rachagani S, Purohit V, et al. Graviola: A novel promising natural-derived drug that inhibits tumorigenicity and metastasis of pancreatic cancer cells in vitro and in vivo through altering cell metabolism. *Cancer Lett*. October 2012;323(1):29–40. doi:10.1016/j.canlet.2012.03.031

67. Dai Y, Hogan S, Schmelz EM, Ju YH, Canning C, Zhou K. Selective growth inhibition of human breast cancer cells by graviola fruit extract in vitro and in vivo involving downregulation of EGFR expression. *Nutr Cancer*. 2011;63(5):795–801. doi:10.1080/01635581.2011.563027

68. Liaw CC, Chang FR, Lin CY, et al. New cytotoxic monotetrahydrofuran annonaceous acetogenins from *Annona muricata. J Nat Prod*. April 2002;65(4):470–475. doi:10.1021/np0105578

69. Hamizah S, Roslida AH, Fezah O, Tan KL, Tor YS, Tan CI. Chemopreventive potential of *Annona muricata L* leaves on chemically-induced skin papillomagenesis in mice. *APJP*. 2012;13(6):2533–2539. doi:10.7314/apjcp.2012.13.6.2533

70. Al-Asmari AK, Albalawi SM, Athar MT, Khan AQ, Al-Shahrani H, Islam M. *Moringa oleifera* as an anti-cancer agent against breast and colorectal cancer cell lines. *PLoS one*. 2015;10(8):e0135814. doi:10.1371/journal.pone.0135814

71. Berkovich L, Earon G, Ron I, Rimmon A, Vexler A, Lev-Ari S. *Moringa Oleifera* aqueous leaf extract down-regulates nuclear factor-kappaB and increases cytotoxic effect of

chemotherapy in pancreatic cancer cells. *BMC Complement Alt Med.* August 2013;13:212. doi:10.1186/1472-6882-13-212

72. Sreelatha S, Jeyachitra A, Padma PR. Antiproliferation and induction of apoptosis by Moringa oleifera leaf extract on human cancer cells. *Food Chem Toxicol.* June 2011;49(6):1270–5. doi:10.1016/j.fct.2011.03.006

73. Jung IL. Soluble extract from *Moringa oleifera* leaves with a new anticancer activity. *PLoS one.* 2014;9(4):e95492. doi:10.1371/journal.pone.0095492

74. Tiloke C, Phulukdaree A, Chuturgoon AA. The antiproliferative effect of *Moringa oleifera* crude aqueous leaf extract on cancerous human alveolar epithelial cells. *BMC Complement Alt Med.* 2013/09/16 2013;13(1):226. doi:10.1186/1472-6882-13-226

75. Budda S, Butryee C, Tuntipopipat S, et al. Suppressive effects of *Moringa oleifera Lam* pod against mouse colon carcinogenesis induced by azoxymethane and dextran sodium sulfate. *APJCP* 2011;12(12):3221–3228.

76. Hagoel L, Vexler A, Kalich-Philosoph L, et al. Combined effect of *Moringa oleifera* Cells. *Integr Cancer Ther.* January2019–December 2019;18:1534735419828829. doi:10.1177/1534735419828829

77. Khan F, Pandey P, Ahmad V, Upadhyay TK. *Moringa oleifera* methanolic leaves extract induces apoptosis and G0/G1 cell cycle arrest via downregulation of hedgehog signaling pathway in human prostate PC-3 cancer cells. *J Food Biochem.* August 2020;44(8):e13338. doi:10.1111/jfbc.13338

78. Do BH, Nguyen TPT, Ho NQC, Le TL, Hoang NS, Doan CC. Mitochondria-mediated Caspase-dependent and Caspase-independent apoptosis induced by aqueous extract from *Moringa oleifera* leaves in human melanoma cells. *Mol Biol Rep.* May 2020;47(5):3675–3689. doi:10.1007/s11033-020-05462-y

79. Lim WF, Mohamad Yusof MI, Teh LK, Salleh MZ. Significant decreased expressions of CaN, VEGF, SLC39A6 and SFRP1 in MDA-MB-231 Xenograft breast tumor mice treated with. *Nutrients.* September 2020;12(10)doi:10.3390/nu12102993

80. Barhoi D, Upadhaya P, Barbhuiya SN, Giri A, Giri S. Aqueous extract of *Moringa oleifera* exhibit potential anticancer activity and can be used as a possible cancer therapeutic agent: A study involving in vitro and in vivo approach. *J Am Coll Nutr.* March 19 2020:1–16. doi:10.1080/07315724.2020.1735572

81. Cuellar-Nuñez ML, Luzardo-Ocampo I, Campos-Vega R, Gallegos-Corona MA, González de Mejía E, Loarca-Piña G. Physicochemical and nutraceutical properties of moringa (*Moringa oleifera*) leaves and their effects in an in vivo AOM/DSS-induced colorectal carcinogenesis model. *Food Res Int.* March 2018;105:159–168. doi:10.1016/j.foodres.2017.11.004

82. Hernández JF, Urueña CP, Cifuentes MC, et al. A *Petiveria alliacea* standardized fraction induces breast adenocarcinoma cell death by modulating glycolytic metabolism. *J Ethnopharmacol.* May 2014;153(3):641–649. doi:10.1016/j.jep.2014.03.013

83. Hernández JF, Urueña CP, Sandoval TA, et al. A cytotoxic *Petiveria alliacea* dry extract induces ATP depletion and decreases β-F1-ATPase expression in breast cancer cells and promotes survival in tumor-bearing mice. *Revista Brasileira de Farmacognosia.* 2017/05/01/ 2017;27(3):306–314. doi:https://doi.org/10.1016/j.bjp.2016.09.008

84. Urueña C, Cifuentes C, Castañeda D, et al. *Petiveria alliacea* extracts uses multiple mechanisms to inhibit growth of human and mouse tumoral cells. *BMC Complement Alt Med.* 2008;8(1):60. doi:10.1186/1472-6882-8-60

85. Cifuentes MC, Castañeda DM, Urueña CP, Fiorentino S. A fraction from *Petiveria alliacea* induces apoptosis via a mitochondria-dependent pathway and regulates HSP70 expression. *Universitas Scientiarum.* 2009;14:125–134.

86. Rösner H, Williams LAD, Jung A, Kraus W. Disassembly of microtubules and inhibition of neurite outgrowth, neuroblastoma cell proliferation, and MAP kinase tyrosine dephosphorylation by dibenzyl trisulphide. *Biochimica et Biophysica Acta (BBA)—Molec Cell Res.* 2001;1540(2):166–177. doi:https://doi.org/10.1016/S0167-4889(01)00129-X

87. Williams LA, Rösner H, Möller W, Conrad J, Nkurunziza JP, Kraus. In vitro anti-proliferation/cytotoxic activity of sixty natural products on the human SH-SY5Y neuroblastoma cells with specific reference to dibenzyl trisulphide. *West Indian Med J.* September 2004;53(4):208–219.

88. *Davidson's Principles and Practice of Medicine.* 21st Edition ed. Churchill Livingstone Elsevier; 2010.

89. Ferlay J, Ervik M, Lam F, et al. Global Cancer Observatory: Cancer Today. Lyon, France: International Agency for Research on Cancer. Accessed December 6, 2020. https://gco.iarc.fr/today

90. Gibson TN, Hanchard B, Waugh N, McNaughton D. Age-specific incidence of cancer in Kingston and St. Andrew, Jamaica, 2003–2007. *West Indian Med J.* October 2010;59(5):456–464.

91. Jackson M, Tulloch-Reid M, Walker S, et al. Dietary patterns as predictors of prostate cancer in Jamaican men. *Nutrition and Cancer.* 2013;65(3):367–374. doi:10.1080/01635581.2013.757631

92. Servan-Schreiber D. *Anticancer: A New Way of Life.* New York: Viking Penguin; 2008.

93. Shivappa N, Jackson MD, Bennett F, Hébert JR. Increased Dietary Inflammatory Index (DII) is associated with increased risk of prostate cancer in Jamaican men. *Nutr Cancer.* 2015;67(6):941–948. doi:10.1080/01635581.2015.1062117

94. Ritch CR, Wan RL, Stephens LB, et al. Dietary fatty acids correlate with prostate cancer biopsy grade and volume in Jamaican men. *J Urol.* 2007;177(1):97–101; discussion 101. doi:10.1016/j.juro.2006.08.105

95. Zhao Z, Reinstatler L, Klaassen Z, et al. The association of fatty acid levels and gleason grade among men undergoing radical prostatectomy. *PLoS one.* 2016;11(11):e0166594. doi:10.1371/journal.pone.0166594

96. Figiel S, Pinault M, Domingo I, et al. Fatty acid profile in peri-prostatic adipose tissue and prostate cancer aggressiveness in African-Caribbean and Caucasian patients. *Eur J Cancer.* March 2018;91:107–115. doi:10.1016/j.ejca.2017.12.017

97. Duncan JP, Weir P, Strachan S, Tulloch-Reid M. Opportunities for reducing morbidity and mortality due to leading cancers in a developing country. *J Public Health* (Oxford, England). 2015;37(4):688–690. doi:10.1093/pubmed/fdu109

98. Pan American Health Organization. Women's Cancer and Comprehensive Care in the Caribbean Situation and Challenges. Accessed January 16, 2021. https://www.paho.org/hq/dmdocuments/2016/NLC-Womens-Cancer-Report--2.pdf

99. Soares D, Walters N, Frankson M, Kirlew K, Reid M. Sociocultural deterrents to mammographic screening in Jamaica. *West Indian Med J.* January 2009;58(1)

100. McFarlane SJ, Morgan SE. Evaluating culturally-targeted fear appeal messages for HPV self-sampling among Jamaican women: A qualitative formative research study. *Health Commun.* 2020:1–14. doi:10.1080/10410236.2020.1723047

101. Bourne PA. Rural male health workers in Western Jamaica: Knowledge, attitudes and practices toward prostate cancer screening. *N Am J Med Sci.* 2010;2(1):11–17. doi:10.4297/najms.2010.111

102. McNaughton, Aiken W, McGrowder D. Factors affecting prostate cancer screening behaviour in a discrete population of doctors at the University Hospital of the West Indies, Jamaica. *APJCP.* 2011;12(5)

103. Anakwenze C, Coronado-Interis E, Aung M, Jolly P. A theory-based intervention to improve breast cancer awareness and screening in Jamaica. *Prev Sci: The Official Journal of the Society for Prevention Research.* May 2015;16(4)doi:10.1007/s11121-014-0529-4

104. Interis EC, Anakwenze C, Aung M, Jolly P. Increasing cervical cancer awareness and screening in Jamaica: Effectiveness of a theory-based educational intervention. *Int J Environ Res Public Health.* 2015;13(1): doi:10.3390/ijerph13010053

105. Capanna C, Chujutalli R, Murray S, Lwin K, Aung M, Jolly P. Prostate cancer educational intervention among men in western Jamaica. *Prev Med Rpts.* 2015 2015;2doi:10.1016/j.pmedr.2015.09.008

106. Bessler P, Aung M, Jolly P. Factors affecting uptake of cervical cancer screening among clinic attendees in Trelawny, Jamaica. *Cancer Control: J Moffitt Cancer Center.* October 2007;14(4): doi:10.1177/107327480701400410

107. Jamaica Religions - Demographics. Index Mundi. Updated November 27, 2020. https://www.indexmundi.com/jamaica/religions.html

108. *The Holy Bible, New International Version.* Mark 2:17. YouVersion; 2021.

109. *The Holy Bible, New International Version.* Matthew 6:10. YouVersion; 2021.

110. HG K, KI P, J N. Religious coping and health status in medically ill hospitalized older adults. *J Nerv Ment Dis.* September 1998;186(9): doi:10.1097/00005053-199809000-00001

111. Andrew W. Kneier PDRJS, D.Min. Cancer: Religion and Spirituality. https://med.stanford.edu/survivingcancer/cancer-sources-of-support/cancer-religion-spirituality-help.html

112. Hughes CE. Prayer and Healing: A Case Study. Research-article. https://doiorg/101177/089801019701500310. 2016-06-24 2016;doi:10.1177_089801019701500310

113. KS D, AL H. The prevalence of prayer as a spiritual self-care modality in elders. *J Holist Nurs: Official journal of the American Holistic Nurses' Association.* December 2000;18(4): doi:10.1177/089801010001800405

114. Bell RA, Suerken C, Quandt SA, Grzywacz JG, Lang W, Arcury TA. Prayer for health among U.S. adults: The 2002 National Health Interview Survey. Research-article. http://dxdoiorg/101177/1533210105285445. 2016-09-02 2016;doi:10.1177_1533210105285445

115. Shepherd Thomas AG. Must Jesus bear the cross alone. 1735.

116. Kevin M, Marilyn BJD. Chaplaincy Taxonomy User's Guide. Advocate Health Care. http://dev.spiritualcareassociation.org/docs/resources/taxonomy_white_paper/users_guide_chaplaincy_taxonomy.pdf

117. Organization WH. Traditional, Complementary and Integrative Medicine. https://www.who.int/health-topics/traditional-complementary-and-integrative-medicine#tab=tab_1

46

Indian Cultural-Spiritual Guidance in Caring for Cancer Patients, India

Aanchal Satija and Sushma Bhatnagar

Introduction

Spirituality is the basic facet of human existence and is a broader construct than religion. Religion, a set of beliefs and rituals in relation to a higher/divine being or God, is merely an expression of spirituality. Contrarily, spirituality embraces one's purpose in life, hunt for meaning, experience of the transcendent, and connectedness with self and others [1]. Although spirituality is usually recognized as a significant constituent of holistic care, existing definitions of spirituality in health care tend to be vague or extremely encompassing. If we go by existing definitions, almost all social, psychological, and ethical issues can be interpreted within the category of spirituality [2]. A consensus definition of spirituality in palliative care has been crafted by a group of interdisciplinary experts consisting of health care and spiritual care providers. They define spirituality as "the aspect of humanity that refers to the way individuals seek and express meaning and purpose and the way they experience their connectedness to the moment, to self, to others, to nature, and to the significant or sacred" [3].

There is growing recognition of the biopsychosocial-spiritual model of health care and its relevance to cancer patients or terminally ill patients [4,5]. Right from the diagnosis of a life-threatening disease like cancer, patients are confronted with myriad information often provoking questions relating to the purpose or meaning of life and to finding peace and hope [1]. The suffering of cancer patients is not limited to physical symptoms and psychosocial concerns; rather, they experience a plethora of spiritual challenges as well. Patients are often seen to be in pronounced spiritual distress, giving rise to questions such as "Why has this illness happened only to me?". They may wonder why they are suffering, whether faith in God can still have a place in their lives, and what will happen after death. Some might be angry at God, while others may seek forgiveness for their mistakes. They may feel hopeless, lonely, or guilty for some wrongdoing. Such concerns are usually addressed by multidisciplinary palliative care teams [1,6].

The acceptance of spiritual care as inherent to holistic patient management has been established with the rapidly increasing literature and formation of global networks, centers, and taskforces dedicated to spiritual guidance within both health care at large and palliative care in particular [7]. The revised definition of palliative care, presented by the International Association for Hospice and Palliative Care (IAHPC) [8], mentions identification, assessment, and treatment of spiritual problems for patients with serious illnesses such as cancer and the related suffering incurred. Both international and national organizations, that is, the World Health Organization (WHO) [9], the American Society of Clinical Oncology (ASCO) [10], the European Association for Palliative Care (EAPC) [11], the National Institute for Health and Care Excellence (NICE) [12], the Indian Council of Medical Research (ICMR) [13], and the Indian Association of Palliative Care (IAPC) [14] have also acknowledged the need to address spiritual issues for patients suffering with life-threatening diseases. Studies have demonstrated the association between spiritual well-being and quality of life and coping with physical or emotional issues arising from cancer [15,16]. Nonetheless, it has been found that nurses and physicians feel uncomfortable and ill prepared to provide spiritual care because of ambiguity and uncertainty about its definition and ways to address the spiritual needs of patients [2].

Dynamic and reciprocal connection is observed among the issues of culture, religion, and spirituality [17]. The concept of spirituality varies across cultures. India is a vast country with diverse religious, cultural, and spiritual backgrounds. Western guidance for spiritual care may not be applicable here [7,18]. Hence, to address the spiritual concerns of patients suffering with life-threatening conditions in India, there is need to understand the beliefs, practices, and rituals they follow. The purpose of this chapter is to provide evidence-based guidance for spiritual care for cancer patients in India.

Understanding Spirituality in an Indian Context

Findings on spirituality have often resulted from studies that focus primarily on quality of life or psychosocial concerns. Chaturvedi [19] identified spiritual concerns as an aspect of quality of life in Indian cancer patients via interviewing patients, their relatives, and even health care professionals, based on items such as peace of mind, satisfaction with religious activities and spiritual tasks, self-esteem or self-respect, happiness with family/relatives, and satisfaction with daily functioning. The majority of respondents considered their level of satisfaction with religious activities (like keeping fasts, visiting temples, chanting *mantras*, singing *bhajans* (religious songs), and performing *pujas* (rites), satisfaction with spiritual tasks (like *dhyana* (concentration), meditation, and yoga) and, above all, peace of mind to be very important. While exploring the psychosocial challenges faced by cancer patients, Pahwa et al. [20] demonstrated in their interview-based study that illness was a consequence of bad *karma* or sins performed in a previous life and that, by seeking forgiveness from God, they could be liberated. Spiritual healing at end of life primarily connected spirituality with a belief in *karma*.

Additionally, spirituality has been identified as an essential coping mechanism for Indian cancer patients. In a study conducted on postoperative head and neck cancer patients, Jagannathan and Juvva [21] demonstrated coping strategies adopted by these patients and their relation to illness and sociodemographic characteristics. Commonly used spiritual methods of coping were meditation, prayer and embracing a positive outlook. On the whole, female patients (45.5%) chose prayer and meditation to cope with treatment-related side effects, while males preferred to take medications. Also, patients with higher income (37.1%) preferred the route of medication/treatment, while patients with lower income (35.6%) chose to pray and meditate.

Very few empirical studies have focused on spirituality. Banerjee et al. [22] conducted an interviewer-administered, questionnaire-based study to determine how yoga modulates radiation-induced genotoxic stress and psychological stress. Sixty-eight breast cancer patients receiving radiotherapy were initially recruited for the study. Of the 58 who completed the study, 35 received the intervention, that is, yoga, which included meditation, *asanas* (postures), and *pranayama* (breathing exercises). The intervention group showed significantly lower scores for stress, anxiety, and depression compared to the control group. The integrated yoga approach helped in achieving the relaxation response that subsequently reduced stress in patients. Selman and Higginson [23] observed the effect of yoga as a complementary therapy in palliative care settings in London and New Delhi. The experiences of patients, carers, teachers, and assistants were observed, and it was concluded that patients were happier, more peaceful, and felt less worried; had better digestion and higher levels of energy. Indian respondents reported that yoga improved their spiritual health and helped them to connect better with the divine. Kandasamy et al. [24] correlated various physical and psychological symptoms like distress, depression, and anxiety with spiritual well-being in advanced cancer patients using the Functional Assessment of Chronic Illness Therapy (FACIT) spiritual well-being questionnaire. Significant correlations were seen between physical and psychological signs (e.g., dry mouth, loss of appetite, drowsiness, symptom distress, fatigue, sadness, and memory disturbance) and spiritual well-being. A negative correlation for depression and anxiety was observed, while positive correlation was seen with various domains of quality of life. To assess spiritual concerns, Simha et al. [25] interviewed 10 cancer patients admitted in hospice. A list with relevant spiritual themes was made based on the available literature. The most common concerns related to spirituality were faith in God, the benefit of *puja*, acceptance of one's situation, concerns about the future, belief in *karma*, the concept of rebirth, and the question, "Why me?" It was also affirmed that most of the patients considered spirituality and religion to be synonymous terms. Lewis et al. [26] assessed the correlation between spiritual well-being and fatigue with 200 cancer patients undergoing active treatment, using the FACIT spiritual well-being and fatigue questionnaire. They found that the symptom of fatigue was inversely associated with spiritual well-being; higher spiritual well-being was observed for females, while patients with gastrointestinal and head and neck malignancies and advanced disease status reported lower spiritual well-being.

In a systematic review conducted on spirituality for Indian terminally ill patients, Gielen et al. [7] described three dimensions of spirituality: relational, existential, and values. The relational dimension described the aspect of social connectedness with surrounding people like caregivers, friends or family, and even God or a Supreme Being. The relationship with a Supreme power, illustrated through religious practices or rituals, helps patients cope with their disease stress. Feelings like guilt, loneliness, and anger dominated when such connectedness was not established. The existential dimension ("Why me?") corresponds to the search for the meaning of life and helps in acceptance of disease. Concerns about family and faith in religion or God are two main values often affected when a patient suffers with terminal illness. It was clarified that religion was not a distinct factor, but it played a vital role in the above-mentioned spiritual dimensions.

It is evident that research on spiritual care for cancer patients has not yet gained sufficient attention in India. This may be because of the rich cultural diversity, varied perceptions of rituals, religion, and spirituality by local communities and the lack of a culturally appropriate and validated questionnaire for assessing spiritual needs. To bridge this gap, a few studies focusing exclusively on spiritual challenges faced by cancer patients were performed at a tertiary cancer hospital in New Delhi, North India.

Experiences at the Tertiary Cancer Center in Delhi

Culturally appropriate, valid, and reliable assessment questionnaires are necessary for evaluating spiritual distress and providing spiritual care [17]. Recognizing the distinct and diverse cultural and religious beliefs of the Indian population, we developed a 36-item questionnaire to identify spiritual concerns of cancer patients in India. This questionnaire demonstrated acceptable psychometric properties and revealed four factors, three of which—"shifting moral and religious values," "support from a religious relationship," and "existential blame"—corresponded to the relational, existential, and values dimensions of spirituality [7,27]. The fourth factor was "spiritual trust," which included items concerning fear/worries about self/family in the future [27]. Based on the 36-item spirituality assessment questionnaire [27], we have now developed a condensed Spirituality Distress Scale for Indian palliative care patients. The final scale consists of 16 items, including common existential issues such as loneliness, wondering why, forgiveness, and fear of the future and specific items of spiritual relevance to terminally ill patients in India like pain as *puja*, *karma*, and punishments for past sins or wrongdoing. The scale has also demonstrated strong internal consistency, convergent validity, and test–retest reliability. It is an effective and easy-to-use tool to evaluate spiritual distress among Hindi-speaking palliative care patients in India [28]. In another study conducted on cancer patients in India, anger was seen as a common sign of spiritual distress. Patients expressed more anger toward themselves rather than to God or a Supreme power. More than half of the patients were angry at themselves, considered their disease a punishment for wrongdoing, a sequelae of their *karma*, punishment from the divine, or as their fate. The study further revealed that, despite the illness, most of the patients (46%) trusted in God and the future, nearly 36% clung to divine support despite intense existential concerns, and only a small group of patients (17%) was spiritually distressed [18]. It was inferred from these studies that women experienced less spiritual trust than men. They expressed more anger, considered disease as their fate, and were more concerned about the future of their families [18,29]. The association between severe pain and spiritual distress was also observed, indicating the relationship between spirituality and physical pain, or spirituality as a means of coping with physical pain [18,27].

Pain is the most common and dreadful symptom affecting cancer patients during various stages of the disease trajectory and significantly affects their quality of life [30]. "Total pain," as described by Cicely Saunders, has physical, social, emotional, and spiritual dimensions, and the contribution of each aspect varies from individual to individual [6]. To date, many multidimensional instruments have been developed to measure and assess the impact of pain on patients' lives, such as the McGill Pain Questionnaire (MPQ), the Brief Pain Inventory (BPI), and the Pain Control in Palliative Care Questionnaire (PC-PCQ) [31], but none of these instruments includes all components of total pain. There is currently no universally accepted tool to assess "total pain" in cancer patients. We have developed and validated an 18-item Total Pain Scale consisting of four subscales (physical pain, psychological pain, social pain, and spiritual pain) for use with Indian cancer patients. The four subscales demonstrated good construct validity with the European Organization for Research and Treatment of Cancer (EORTC) quality of life and FACIT spiritual well-being questionnaires. According to the Total Pain Scale, physical pain contributed to only 32% of total pain while psychological, social, and spiritual aspects contributed to 25%, 26%, and 17% of total pain, respectively. It clearly highlighted the notion that pain due to psychosocial and spiritual concerns is considerably higher than physical pain from the disease itself. Hence, it is imperative to also address nonphysical challenges faced by patients. (S. P. Singh, Ph.D., unpublished data, February 2020).

Implications for Providing Spiritual Care for Cancer Patients in India

Currently, there are no national guidelines for providing spiritual care to cancer patients in India. The following recommendations are consequential to the authors' aforementioned research (refer to the earlier section Experiences at the Tertiary Cancer Center in Delhi) and experience in the field of assessing and managing spiritual distress in cancer patients. A two-tiered approach (see Figure 46.1) is recommended for spiritual history-taking.

The spiritual pain of patients at overcrowded oncology clinics can be quickly screened via a four-item spiritual subscale of the Total Pain Scale. The presence and

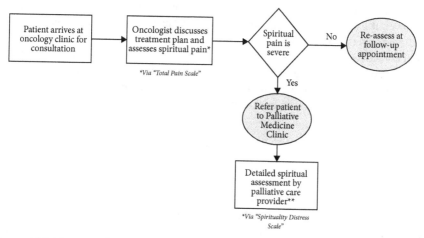

Figure 46.1 Two-tiered Approach for Spiritual Assessment

level of spiritual pain should be documented in patients' medical records and assessed at every follow-up visit as spiritual issues are dynamic and can change during the course of the disease trajectory. Patients who express severe spiritual pain should be referred to a palliative medicine clinic. Palliative care providers should take a detailed spiritual assessment in a comfortable, private room using the 16-item Spirituality Distress Scale. This tool can facilitate identifying, exploring, and acknowledging individual spiritual needs. This should be followed by a dialogue between the care-provider and patient, focusing on what aspects of life are meaningful to their religious beliefs, relationship with God or Supreme power, *karma* philosophy, and any other practice that may derive comfort. It is noteworthy that religious or spiritual beliefs are not consistent throughout all of India. Although there are regional variations in the traditions or beliefs to which people adhere, the spiritual doctrines of *atma* or soul (i.e., the inner eternal self), *karma* (i.e., the principle of cause and effect), and *mukti or moksha* (i.e., the liberation from the cycle of birth and death), are accepted by most Indian ethnicities [32]. Thus, the tools Total Pain Scale and Spirituality Distress Scale may be translated into regional languages and tested in other parts of India for the assessment of the spiritual needs of cancer patients.

It is often noted that physicians are reluctant to talk about spiritual issues with patients, and even patients are uncomfortable initiating a dialogue regarding their spiritual needs [33,34]. Spiritual history-taking requires the patient to share sensitive and personal information. It is important that the physicians and nurses are educated and trained for thoughtful conversation with the patients. Workshops or training programs focused on attaining the skills needed for difficult communications are thus recommended for nursing and medical undergraduate and postgraduate students.

Identifying the spiritual issues that are bothering the patient should be followed by an endeavor to resolve the spiritual distress. The latter is often difficult in an Indian scenario due to the absence of designated, trained spiritual advisors in the palliative care team. The clinician or nurse may suggest that the patient consult a spiritual or religious community according to their beliefs. It has been observed that spiritual interventions can significantly improve quality of life and spiritual well-being [35]. However, it is not clear if the spiritual interventions practiced in the Western world would be effective to a similar extent for Indian patients. Religion and spirituality are often considered synonymous by patients in India [7]; hence, they may prefer culturally adapted interventions such as religious activities (e.g., *puja*), meditation, or yoga. It is time for researchers and frontline palliative care members to jointly design robust scientific studies testing the effect of these interventions on Indian patients' well-being.

Conclusion

Spiritual crisis can be more troublesome when one is suffering with a life-threatening illness like cancer, and it impacts the patient's ability to cope with the disease and a declining quality of life. The extent to which spiritual care can improve a patient's outcome still needs to be researched. Due to the limited understanding of diverse, prevalent spiritual and religious beliefs and the emotional sensitivity of spiritual communications, health care professionals are reluctant to discuss patients' spiritual needs. It is essential to integrate spiritual care into oncology care and provide holistic treatment to the patient. For this purpose, routine assessment of spiritual distress via assessment tools developed specifically for Indian patients is recommended. To break the professional silence, physicians and nurses should be educated and trained to participate in spiritual discussions. Additionally, spiritual care interventions in oncology services in India are still fragmented; thus, it is recommended that culturally appropriate interventions be tested and that their effect on patients' lives be characterized. These recommendations are based on the authors' experience in North India; however, India is a land of spiritual diversity and, therefore, the assessment tools and interventions should be adapted according to the regional variations. Given the importance of spirituality in oncology care, there is an earnest need to develop consensus-based national guidelines to assess and manage spiritual distress associated with disease-related suffering.

References

1. Puchalski CM, King SDW, Ferrell BR. Spiritual considerations. *Hematol Oncol Clin North Am.* 2018;32:505–517.
2. Gielen J. Why does spirituality matter in end of life care? In: Das R, Nayak S (eds). *Concepts of Palliative Care.* Cuttack: A. K. Mishra Publishers; 2014:72–80.
3. Puchalski C, Ferrell B, Virani R, et al. Improving the quality of spiritual care as a dimension of palliative care: the report of the Consensus Conference. *J Palliat Med.* 2009;12:885–904.
4. Sulmasy DP. A biopsychosocial-spiritual model for the care of patients at the end of life. *The Gerontologist.* 2002;42:24–33.
5. Ben-Arye E, Bar-Sela G, Frenkel M, Kuten A, Hermoni D. Is a biopsychosocial-spiritual approach relevant to cancer treatment? A study of patients and oncology staff members on issues of complementary medicine and spirituality. *Support Care Cancer.* 2006;14:147–152.
6. Satija A, Singh SP, Kashyap K, Bhatnagar S. Management of total cancer pain: A case of young adult. *Indian J Palliat Care.* 2014;20:153–156.
7. Gielen J, Bhatnagar S, Chaturvedi SK. Spirituality as an ethical challenge in Indian palliative care: A systematic review. *Palliat Support Care.* 2016;14:561–582.
8. Radbruch L, Lima LD, Knaul F, et al. Redefining palliative care—A new consensus-based definition. *J Pain Symptom Manage.* 2020;60:754–764.
9. Pain relief and Palliative Care. In: *National Cancer Control Programmes: Policies and Managerial Guidelines.* 2nd ed. World Health Organization; 2002:83–91.
10. Osman H, Shrestha S, Temin S, et al. Palliative care in the global setting: ASCO Resource-Stratified Practice Guideline. *J Glob Oncol.* 2018;4:1–24.
11. Best M, Leget C, Goodhead A, Paal P. An EAPC white paper on multi-disciplinary education for spiritual care in palliative care. *BMC Palliat Care.* 2020;19:9.
12. End of life care for adults- Quality standard [QS13]. National Institute for Health and Care Excellence. 28 November 2011. https://www.nice.org.uk/guidance/qs13 Accessed December 13, 2020.

13. *Definition of Terms Used in Limitation of Treatment and Providing Palliative Care at End of Life.* Indian Council of Medical Research; 2018.

14. Definitions of Terms—I A P C. 2018. https://www.palliativecare.in/definitions-of-terms/ Accessed December 13, 2020.

15. Bai M, Lazenby M. A systematic review of associations between spiritual well-being and quality of life at the scale and factor levels in studies among patients with cancer. *J Palliat Med.* 2015;18:286-298.

16. Agarwal K, Fortune L, Heintzman JC, Kelly LL. Spiritual experiences of long-term meditation practitioners diagnosed with breast cancer: An interpretative phenomenological analysis pilot study. *J Relig Health.* 2020;59:2364-2380.

17. Lee Y-H. Spiritual care for cancer patients. *Asia-Pac J Oncol Nurs.* 2019;6:101-103.

18. Gielen J, Bhatnagar S, Chaturvedi SK. Prevalence and nature of spiritual distress among palliative care patients in India. *J Relig Health.* 2017;56:530-544.

19. Chaturvedi S. What's important for quality of life to Indians— in relation to cancer. *Indian J Palliat Care.* 2003;9:62-70.

20. Pahwa M, Babu N, Bhatnagar S. Fighting cancer is half the battle … living life is the other half. *J Cancer Res Ther.* 2005;1:98-102.

21. Jagannathan A, Juvva S. Life after cancer in India: Coping with side effects and cancer pain. *J Psychosoc Oncol.* 2009;27:344-360.

22. Banerjee B, Vadiraj HS, Ram A, et al. Effects of an integrated yoga program in modulating psychological stress and radiation-induced genotoxic stress in breast cancer patients undergoing radiotherapy. *Integr Cancer Ther.* 2007;6:242-250.

23. Selman L, Higginson IJ. "A softening of edges": A comparison of yoga classes at palliative care services in New Delhi and London. *Int J Palliat Nurs.* 2010;16:548-554.

24. Kandasamy A, Chaturvedi SK, Desai G. Spirituality, distress, depression, anxiety, and quality of life in patients with advanced cancer. *Indian J Cancer.* 2011;48:55-59.

25. Simha S, Noble S, Chaturvedi SK. Spiritual concerns in Hindu cancer patients undergoing palliative care: a qualitative study. *Indian J Palliat Care.* 2013;19:99-105.

26. Lewis S, Salins N, Rao MR, Kadam A. Spiritual well-being and its influence on fatigue in patients undergoing active cancer directed treatment: a correlational study. *J Cancer Res Ther.* 2014;10:676-680.

27. Bhatnagar S, Noble S, Chaturvedi SK, Gielen J. Development and psychometric assessment of a spirituality questionnaire for Indian palliative care patients. *Indian J Palliat Care.* 2016;22:9-18.

28. Bora S, Dutta K. IAPCON 2020: Conference Proceedings. *Indian J Palliat Care.* 2020;26:159-163.

29. Bhatnagar S, Gielen J, Satija A, Singh SP, Noble S, Chaturvedi SK. Signs of spiritual distress and its implications for practice in Indian palliative care. *Indian J Palliat Care.* 2017;23:306-311.

30. Satija A, Singh V, Singh SP, Mishra S, Bhatnagar S. The impact of pain on quality of life of patients with advanced cancer. *Indian J Palliat Care.* 2016;22:201.

31. Hjermstad MJ, Gibbins J, Haugen DF, et al. Pain assessment tools in palliative care: An urgent need for consensus. *Palliat Med.* 2008;22:895-903.

32. Inbadas H. Indian philosophical foundations of spirituality at the end of life. *Mortality Abingdon.* 2018;23:320-333.

33. Lucchetti G, Ramakrishnan P, Karimah A, et al. Spirituality, religiosity, and health: A comparison of physicians' attitudes in Brazil, India, and Indonesia. *Int J Behav Med.* 2016;23:63-70.

34. Chacko R, Anand JR, Rajan A, John S, Jeyaseelan V. End-of-life care perspectives of patients and health professionals in an Indian health-care setting. *Int J Palliat Nurs.* 2014;20:557–564.
35. Xing L, Guo X, Bai L, Qian J, Chen J. Are spiritual interventions beneficial to patients with cancer? A meta-analysis of randomized controlled trials following PRISMA. *Medicine* (Baltimore). 2018;97:e11948.

Index

For the benefit of digital users, indexed terms that span two pages (e.g., 52–53) may, on occasion, appear on only one of those pages.

Note: Tables, figures, and boxes are indicated by *t, f,* and *b* following the page number.

Abu Al-Qasim Al-Zahrawi, famed Islamic physician, 331
acceptance of cancer, effect of emotional state, spirituality, and religion on, 391, 399
    hope and, 393–94
    impact of cancer on individual spirituality, 396*f*
    impact of emotional state on illness experience, 392–94
    religious coping as adaptation tool, 397–99
    spiritual well-being before, during, and after cancer, 394–96
adjustment disorders, definition and treatment, 78
advance care planning, cultural influences on, 432–33
    advance directives, 437
    attitudes toward pain and illness, 435
    benefits of advance care planning, 433
    challenges in advance care planning, 433–34
    end-of-life medical care, 435
    ethnic aspects, 434–38
    euthanasia, 435
    hospice care, 436
    patient autonomy, 436
    sharing medical information, 437–38
advanced cancer care, spiritual and religious impacts on, 163–64, 169–70
    Australian patients and caregivers, spiritual well-being and views, 164–67
    implications for care, 168–69
    importance of spirituality or religion, 164–65
    pastoral care, 166
    and religious affiliation, 165
    role of hospitals in supporting spiritual or religious requirements, 166–67
    spiritual requirements and concerns, 165–66

advance directives, cultural preferences and aspects, 437
Africa
    cancer mortality in, 296
    racial and religious groups in, 295–96
    traditional religions and faith healing in, 297–99
    See also pain care, in French-speaking African countries
"Agony of Christianity" (de Unamuno), 195
Alberti, F. B., 100–1
American Medical Association Code of Ethics, from mid-19th century, 47
analgesics, access to in French-speaking African countries, 309–11, 315–16
    barriers to pain care, 311–15, 312*t*
    and education and skills training in palliative care, 314–15
    influence of beliefs and culture on pain management, 313–14
    main barriers to access, 311, 312*t*
    opioid consumption, 310*f*, 311–13
    opioid use, and training in palliative care, 314–15
    opioid use, fear of, 314
    opioid use, policies and regulations for, 315
anorexia, control in palliative care, 321
anxiety
    assessment of, 79–81
    definition of, 78–79
    management of, 81–82
    nonpharmacological intervention, 81–82
    pharmacological intervention, 81
    and unmanaged psychological disorders, 77
art therapy, and coping with grief, 88–89
assessment
    of anxiety and depression, 79–81
    of spirituality, 175–78, 176*t*
    in whole-person approach to care, 3–6

attributed dignity, 133
Australia
  Spiritual and Religious Impacts
    on Advanced Cancer Care in
    Australia, 163–72
Australian patients and caregivers, spiritual
    well-being and views, 164–67
  implications for care, 168–69
  importance of spirituality or religion, 164–65
  pastoral care, 166
  qualitative interview findings, 167
  and religious affiliation, 165
  role of hospitals in supporting spiritual or
    religious requirements, 166–67
  spiritual requirements and
    concerns, 165–66
autonomy-based ethical cultures, 150
Avicenna, Islamic physician, 331
Ayurvedic medicine, 236f, 236

beliefs and culture, impact on cancer care in
    Costa Rica
  beliefs about cancer, 354–55
  colonial times, 352
  medical management, 354
  myths about death and disease, 353
  religion and spirituality, 353
  witchdoctors and traditional healers, role
    of, 352–53
beliefs and culture, impact on cancer care in
    Iran, 215, 222–23
  during course of disease, 217–18
  in end-of-life care and death, 218–19
  four stages of palliative care, 215–16
  at onset of disease, 216–17
  pain management, 217–18
  prevention, screening, and early
    diagnosis, 216
  spiritual and religious beliefs, 221–22
  traditional medicine, role of, 219–21
beliefs and culture, impact on care of brain-
    tumor patients in Indonesia, 414, 419
  beliefs of Indonesian brain-tumor
    patients, 414–16
  diagnosis, truthful disclosure of, 416–18
  multidisciplinary management, challenges
    of, 418–19
  religion as coping mechanism, 418
beliefs and culture, influence on pain
    management, 313–14

bereavement
  in Hinduism, 237
  in Iranian culture, 219
Bhagayad Gita, 229–30
biofield therapies, and holistic care, 38
Biography of Loneliness (Alberti), 100–1
biopsychosocial-spiritual model, 4t, 8
  assessment and, 3–6
  compassionate gaze, 7
  treatment and, 6–7, 7t
blooming dignity, 133
Book of Job, compassion and, 190–93
brain-tumor patients, impact of culture and
    beliefs on care in Indonesia, 414, 419
  beliefs of Indonesian brain-tumor
    patients, 414–16
  diagnosis, truthful disclosure of, 416–18
  multidisciplinary management, challenges
    of, 418–19
  religion as coping mechanism, 418
breast cancer, in Ugandan context, 443
breast cancer, living with, 403–6
  detection and treatment, 403–5
  experiences of survivorship, 406
  support systems, 405–6
breast cancer, psychosocial aspects of, 302, 307
  communication issues, 304–7
  cultural variations on health and
    medicine, 302
  and perceptions of illness, 303–4
  and Turkish culture, 303
breast cancer survivorship, in Nigeria, 401–
    3, 409–10
  detection and treatment, 403–5
  experiences of survivorship, 406
  narrative accounts of survivors, 403, 404f
  support systems, 405–6
  wider context of, 407–9
burnout, phenomenon of, 94
Burns, David, 192

Cacioppo, J., 101
cancer, finding meaning in coping with, 157
  cultural competency, and care in health
    and disease, 149–50
  ethical cultures, autonomy-based vs.
    family-centered, 150
  and the Filipino family, 152–57
  global cancer burden, 148
  hospice care, 151–52

oncology, meaning-making in, 149
pain management, Filipino attitudes
    toward, 153–54
religiosity and spirituality in Philippine
    culture, 150–52, 156
spousal caregiving, 154–57
cancer, prevalence in Iran, 215
cancer care, cultural influences on, 296
cancer care, spiritual and religious impacts
    on, 163–64, 169–70
    Australian patients and caregivers,
        spiritual well-being and views, 164–67
    implications for care, 168–69
    importance of spirituality or
        religion, 164–65
    pastoral care, 166
    and religious affiliation, 165
    role of hospitals in supporting spiritual or
        religious requirements, 166–67
    spiritual requirements and
        concerns, 165–66
Cancer Pain Relief (WHO), 368
cancer patients
    and barriers to addressing psycho-social
        needs, 262–64
    guidance on approaching, 443–45
    unique challenges for, 34–36
care, cultural and spiritual influences in
    India, 475–76, 480–81
    implications for providing spiritual
        care, 479–80
    patient experiences, 478–79
    spiritual assessment, 479f
    spirituality in Indian context, 476–78
care, cultural and spiritual influences in
    Jamaica, 454, 465–67
    attitudes and beliefs regarding care, 463
    cultural factors modifying care, 454–63,
        456f, 457t, 458t, 462f
    diet, 462–63
    religious and spiritual factors modifying
        care, 464–65
    Spiritual Assessment Tool, 465, 466b
    spiritual care plan, 466b
care, cultural and spiritual influences in the
    Dominican Republic, 451–52
    cultural history and religious
        factors, 450–51
    economic factors, 449–50
    historical background, 446–47

and practice of oncology, 447–48
religion and spirituality, 448–49
care, cultural influences in Uganda, 441, 445
    approaches to cancer care, 442
    guidance on approaching cancer
        patients, 443–45
    spiritual and cultural diversity, 441
    Ugandan context, 442–43
care, cultural influences on, 296
caregiving
    attitudes and preferences in Latin
        America, 345
    in Iranian culture, 218
    spousal, 154–57
caring, at the culture and spirituality
    interface, 22–23, 29
    future research, 28–29
cervical cancer, in Ugandan context, 443
chaplain visits
    experiences in advanced cancer care, 166
    role of chaplains in spiritual care, 198–99
    as spiritual intervention, 178
children, providing psychosocial-spiritual
    support to, 57, 61
    discussing diagnosis, 57–58
    end-of-life care and palliative care, 61
    psychosocial status of families, 58–60
    traditional attitudes, 60
Chile
    The Impact of Latin American Cultural
        Values, Attitudes, and Preferences on
        Palliative Cancer Care, 340–51
China
    Caring at the Culture and Spirituality
        Interface, 22–31
    The Impact of Chinese Culture and Faith
        in Cancer Care, 240–47
    palliative care in, 23–24
Chinese culture and faith, impact of, 240
    decision-making, and families, 243–45
    family role in spiritual care, 241–42
    filial piety, 241
    providing diagnosis information, 242–43
    spiritual care, 245–46
    withholding diagnosis information, 240–41
Chochinov, H. M., 134f
Christianity, and psychosocial-spiritual
    healing, 297
cognitive-behavioral therapy, and holistic
    care, 38

communication
    and Middle Eastern cultural perspectives
        in cancer care, 362
    in palliative care, 323
    and psychosocial aspects of illness, 304–7
communication, and sociocultural context,
        382, 387
    ABCDE approach to exploring, 387
    death, discussion of, 386–87
    in decline and terminal phase, 386–87
    in decompensation phase, 385
    in dependency phase, 385–86
    diagnosis, disclosure of, 382–84
    family-centric communication, 384
communication, physician-patient
    in advanced cancer, 47–52
    and barriers to addressing psycho-social
        and emotional needs, 264
    compassionate truth-telling, 52–
        54, 331–33
    education to further skills in, 265
    gender and culture as barriers to, 216–17
    Indonesian brain-tumor patients, 416
    at onset of disease, 216
    in pediatric cancer, 57–58
compassion
    as a common language, 189–90
    examples of, 187–89
compassion and mindfulness practices for
        patients, 125–26, 129
    clinical practices and
        competencies, 128–29
    compassion-focused therapy (CFT), 126,
        127, 128–29
    transcultural and transreligious
        processes, 126–29
compassionate gaze, and whole-person
        approach to care, 7
compassion fatigue, 94–95
complementary therapies
    and cancer outcomes, 254
    disclosure of use, 253–54
    future research directions, 254–55
    and Middle Eastern cultural perspectives
        in cancer care, 361–62
    miracle drugs, 326
    reasons for use, 253
    use in Iran, 219–21
    use in low-to-middle-income
        countries, 252

constipation, control in palliative
    care, 321–22
Costa Rica
    The Impact of Culture and Belief on
        Cancer Care in Costa Rica, 352–56
Costa Rica, impact of culture and belief on
        cancer care
    beliefs about cancer, 354–55
    colonial times, 352
    medical management, 354
    myths about death and disease, 353
    religion and spirituality, 353
    witchdoctors and traditional healers, role
        of, 352–53
coughing, control in palliative care, 321
COVID-19 pandemic
    availability of family members
        during, 367–68
    enhancing patient dignity during,
        135, 137t
creative-arts-based therapies, and holistic
    care, 38
cultural barriers
    to addressing emotional and psycho-social
        needs, 263–64, 267
    to assessing mental health distress and
        suicidality, 67–69
cultural competency, and care in health and
        disease, 149–50
    ethical cultures, autonomy-based vs.
        family-centered, 150
cultural considerations, in cancer
    care, 76–77
cultural guidance, in caring for cancer
        patients in India, 475–76, 480–81
    implications for providing spiritual
        care, 479–80
    patient experiences, 478–79
    spiritual assessment, 479f
    spirituality in Indian context, 476–78
cultural guidance, in caring for cancer
        patients in Jamaica, 454, 465–67
    attitudes and beliefs regarding care, 463
    cultural factors modifying care, 454–63,
        456f, 457t, 458t, 462f
    diet, 462–63
    religious and spiritual factors modifying
        care, 464–65
    Spiritual Assessment Tool, 465, 466b
    spiritual care plan, 466b

cultural guidance, in caring for cancer patients in the Dominican Republic, 451–52
  cultural history and religious factors, 450–51
  economic factors, 449–50
  historical background, 446–47
  and practice of oncology, 447–48
  religion and spirituality, 448–49
cultural healing practices, and early cancer detection, 249, 255
  future research directions, 254–55
  help-seeking, impact on, 249–50
  help-seeking, influence of spirituality and religiosity on, 250–51
  sociocultural influences on cancer stage at diagnosis, 251–52
  traditional and complementary medicines, 252
  traditional and complementary medicines, and cancer outcomes, 254
  traditional and complementary medicines, disclosure of use, 253–54
  traditional and complementary medicines, reasons for use, 253
cultural influences
  and challenge of truth-telling, 45–47, 331–33
  on palliative care, 40–41
cultural influences, on advance care planning, 432–33
  advance directives, 437
  attitudes toward pain and illness, 435
  benefits of advance care planning, 433
  challenges in advance care planning, 433–34
  end-of-life medical care, 435
  ethnic aspects, 434–38
  euthanasia, 435
  hospice care, 436
  patient autonomy, 436
  sharing medical information, 437–38
cultural perspectives in cancer care, Middle Eastern, 357, 363
  communication practices, 362
  complementary and traditional medicine, 361–62
  culture, definition and purpose of, 357
  death and dying, taboos regarding, 363
  diagnosis and management, 359–62

  family values and dynamics, 358–59
  nondisclosure of diagnosis, 360
  and pain management, 362
  palliative care, 362–63
  religion and spiritual needs, 358
  screening and prevention, obstacles to, 358–59
  social views, 360
  spiritual perspectives, 360–61
  stigma and social values, 359
cultural-spiritual guidance for caregiving, Islam and, 339
  barriers to spiritual care provision in Iraq, 338
  benefits of spiritual care, 338
  cancer care in Iraq, 335–36
  case scenario, 333
  history and religious landscape of Iraq, 329
  Iraqi cultural attitudes toward illness and death, 329–30
  Iraqi families and kinship groups, 329
  Islamic medicine, tradition of, 330–31
  spiritual care in an Islamic context, 333–35
  truthful disclosure of cancer diagnosis, 331–33, 360–25
  values and beliefs regarding cancer patients, 336–38
cultural variations, on health and medicine, 302
culture
  and anticipation of death, 120
  and attempting cancer cures, 326
  definition and purpose of, 357
  definition of, 22, 117–18, 249, 295
  impact on help-seeking, 249–50
culture and beliefs, impact on cancer care, 367–68, 378
  acknowledgments and narratives, 378–81
  culture and traditions, 372–75
  patient experiences, 376–78
  spirituality, definitions and characteristics of, 371–72
  traditional beliefs and practices, 375–76
  in Uganda, 376t, 377t
culture and beliefs, impact on cancer care in Costa Rica
  beliefs about cancer, 354–55

culture and beliefs, impact on cancer care
in Costa Rica (cont.)
colonial times, 352
medical management, 354
myths about death and disease, 353
religion and spirituality, 353
witchdoctors and traditional healers, role
of, 352–53
culture and beliefs, impact on cancer care in
Iran, 215, 222–23
during course of disease, 217–18
in end-of-life care and death, 218–19
four stages of palliative care, 215–16
at onset of disease, 216–17
pain management, 217–18
prevention, screening, and early
diagnosis, 216
spiritual and religious beliefs, 221–22
traditional medicine, role of, 219–21
culture and beliefs, impact on care of brain-
tumor patients in Indonesia, 414, 419
beliefs of Indonesian brain-tumor
patients, 414–16
diagnosis, truthful disclosure of, 416–18
multidisciplinary management, challenges
of, 418–19
religion as coping mechanism, 418
culture and beliefs, influence on pain
management, 313–14
culture and faith, impact in cancer
care, 240
decision-making, and families, 243–45
family role in spiritual care, 241–42
filial piety, 241
providing diagnosis information, 242–43
spiritual care, 245–46
withholding diagnosis
information, 240–41
culture and spirituality interface, 22–23, 29
future research, 28–29
cure, patient expectations of, 48–49
customary heritage, contribution to
personalization of oncology, 422–
23, 429–30
medical psychology, role with
patients, 426–27
personalized medicine,
accomplishing, 423–24
spirituality and psychology, relationship
between, 427–28

death
Cosa Rican myths about, 353
cultural context and discussion of, 89–
91, 151
in Hinduism, 231–32, 237
in Iranian culture, 218–19
and Middle Eastern cultural perspectives
in cancer care, 363
perspectives on, 207–8
and sociocultural context of
discussion, 386–87
decision-making, and families in Chinese
culture, 243–45
decompensation phase, communication
in, 385
dependency phase, communication
in, 385–86
depression
assessment of, 79–81
definition of, 79
and loneliness among older adults, 101–4
management of, 81–82
nonpharmacological intervention, 81–82
pharmacological intervention, 81
and unmanaged psychological
disorders, 77
detection, and breast cancer survivorship in
Nigeria, 403–5
detection, cultural healing practices and early
cancer, 249, 255
future research directions, 254–55
help-seeking, impact on, 249–50
help-seeking, influence of spirituality and
religiosity on, 250–51
sociocultural influences on cancer stage at
diagnosis, 251–52
traditional and complementary
medicines, 252
traditional and complementary medicines,
and cancer outcomes, 254
traditional and complementary medicines,
disclosure of use, 253–54
traditional and complementary medicines,
reasons for use, 253
Devotions (Donne), 193–94
dharma, path of, 230
diagnosis
common reactions to cancer
diagnosis, 295
cultural considerations in early, 216

patient reaction to, 206
    sociocultural influences and cancer stage
        at, 251–52
    truthful disclosure in Indonesia, 416–18
    truthful disclosure of, 331–33, 360
    withholding information on, 240–41
diet, impact on cancer care in
        Jamaica, 462–63
dignity and hope, enhancing in palliative
        care, 132, 140
    concepts of dignity, 133
    during COVID-19 pandemic, 135, 137t
    dignity-conserving care, 133–39
    evaluating hope, 139–40
    fostering hope, 139–40, 141t
    Model of Dignity, 134f
    research on patients in Poland, 201
    toolkits for dignity, 135–39
    uncontrolled pain and symptoms,
        132–33
dignity therapy, 138–39, 201
distrust, and addressing psycho-social and
        emotional needs, 264
Dominican Republic
    Cultural Spiritual Guidance in Caring
        for Cancer Patients in the Dominican
        Republic, 446–53
    history and geography of, 446–47
    practice of oncology in, 447–48
Donne, John, 193–94
dyspnea
    as challenge for cancer patients, 34
    control in palliative care, 321

early cancer detection, and cultural healing
        practices, 249, 255
    future research directions, 254–55
    help-seeking, impact on, 249–50
    help-seeking, influence of spirituality and
        religiosity on, 250–51
    sociocultural influences on cancer stage at
        diagnosis, 251–52
    traditional and complementary
        medicines, 252
    traditional and complementary medicines,
        and cancer outcomes, 254
    traditional and complementary medicines,
        disclosure of use, 253–54
    traditional and complementary medicines,
        reasons for use, 253

economic factors, and caring for
        cancer patients in the Dominican
        Republic, 449–50
education, level of patient, 444
emotional and psychological aspects of
        cancer, 75–76
    adjustment disorders, 78
    assessment of anxiety and depression, 79–81
    cultural considerations, 76–77
    framework for clinical practice, 82
    management of anxiety and
        depression, 81–82
    psychological disorders among cancer
        patients, 78–79
    spiritual considerations, 76–77
    unmanaged psychological and psychiatric
        disorders, 77
emotional and psycho-social needs, barriers
        to addressing, 261–62, 269
    barriers for health care
        professionals, 264–67
    barriers originating from health
        system, 267–69
    barriers originating from patient and
        family, 262–64
    communication difficulties, 264
    lack of integrated model for care, 268–69
    stigmatization, fear of, 263–64
    unawareness and refusal, 262–63
emotional distress
    among challenges for cancer patients, 35
    influence of spirituality on, 180–81
emotional state, effect on acceptance of
        cancer, 391, 399
    hope and, 393–94
    and impact on illness experience, 392–94
emotional support, by nurses, 86–87
    attributes of, 91–93, 91t, 92f, 93b
    challenges in palliative care, 87–89
    cultural context, 89–91
    developing competency, 93–95
    spiritual distress, addressing, 92–93
emotional support, in palliative care, 325
empathy
    and emotional support by nurses, 93–95
    and physician-patient communication, 49
end-of-life care
    cultural preferences and aspects, 435
    in Iranian culture, 218–19
    for pediatric patients, 61

end-of-life care, impact of Latin American
cultural values, attitudes, and
preferences, 340–41, 344–46
caregiver's role, 345
decision-making processes, 344–45
integrating cultural values into care, 341–43
Latin American cultural context, 341
place of care and place of death, 345
spiritual care and relationships with
clinicians, 346
spirituality and religiosity, 343–44
end-of-life discussions
cultural influences on, 41
and team spiritual care, 18f
and traditional religious perspectives, 25
end-of-life spiritual care, a Jewish Israeli case
study, 275, 283–84
context for, 275–76
family member assessment, interventions,
outcomes, 283
family member spiritual-care visit, first, 280
family member spiritual-care visit,
second, 280–81
midrash, recitation of, 279–80
patient assessment, interventions,
outcomes, 281–83
patient spiritual-care visit, first, 276–78
patient spiritual-care visit, fourth, 279–80
patient spiritual-care visit, second, 278
patient spiritual-care visit, third, 278–79
scripture reading, 277–78
ethical cultures, autonomy-based *vs.* family-
centered, 150
euthanasia, cultural preferences and
aspects, 435
evaluation skills, education to further, 265
exercise, and holistic care, 38–39
existentialism and spirituality, in the healing
process, 285–86
accelerating access to care, 290–91
benefits of existential well-being, 287–88
capacity-building for spiritual care
providers, 291
and in terminal illness, 288–89

faith, role among palliative care patients in
coping with cancer, 205–6, 211–12
changes in religious habits and
practices, 209–10
coping methods, 210, 418
death, perspectives on, 207–8

Islam, principles of, 206
religious and cultural beliefs, impact of,
209, 211
spirituality, definition of, 207
types of coping, 208–9
faith and culture, impact in cancer care, 240
decision-making, and families, 243–45
family role in spiritual care, 241–42
filial piety, 241
providing diagnosis information, 242–43
spiritual care, 245–46
withholding diagnosis
information, 240–41
faith healing, spirituality and, 296–99
families
and barriers to addressing psycho-social
needs, 262–64
decision-making and, 243–45
family-centered ethical cultures,
150, 152–57
family values and dynamics, and Middle
Eastern perspectives in cancer
care, 358–59
the Filipino family and coping with
cancer, 152–57
the Indonesian family and truthful
disclosure of diagnosis, 417–18
and integrating cultural values into
care, 342–43
patient autonomy and, 122–23
psychosocial status of, 58–60
role in spiritual care, 241–42
See also pediatric cancer, providing
psychosocial-spiritual support in
fatigue
as challenge for cancer patients, 34
control in palliative care, 322
fear, manifestations of, 35
Feeling Good: The New Mood Therapy
(Burns), 192
FICA Spiritual Assessment Tool, 13t
filial piety
and Chinese culture, 241
and palliative care in Taiwan, 25
financial hardship, and psychosocial
status of pediatric patients and their
families, 59–60
France
Cancer Pain Care in French-speaking
African Countries and Access to
Analgesics, 309–18

Frankl, Viktor, 367, 394
Functional Assessment of Chronic Illness
    Therapy-Spiritual Scale, 164, 165*t*

gender-minority patients, psychosocial
    burden of cancer in, 107–8
    clinical care recommendations, 111
    disclosing sexual and gender-minority
        status, 110–11
    limited family and social support, 110
    specific cancer risks, incidence rates, and
        outcomes, 108
    understanding psychosocial
        burden, 109–11
global cancer burden, 148
grief
    coping with, 87–89
    manifestations of, 35
    rituals of, 86–87

healing process, existentialism and
    spirituality in the, 285–86
    accelerating access to care, 290–91
    benefits of existential well-being, 287–88
    capacity-building for spiritual care
        providers, 291
    and in terminal illness, 288–89
Healing Touch, and holistic care, 38
healthcare professionals
    attitudes and beliefs of, 264–65
    barriers to addressing psycho-social and
        emotional patient needs, 264–67
    inadequate support systems for, 267
    job description, lack of, 266
    need for cultural competence, 267
    and role of medical staff in spiritual care,
        199–200
    workload and lack of time, 266
healthcare professionals, psychosocial factors
    and quality of care, 65–66
    clinical implications and
        recommendations, 69–70
    mental health distress and suicidality,
        barriers to identifying, 66–69
healthcare team and culture, in Israeli cancer
    center, 117, 123–24
    clinical case 1: the ethical unit, 118–19
    clinical case 2: the value of life, 119–20
    culture, definition of, 117–18
    culture and anticipation of death, 120
    culture and the individual, 120–21

culture-based care, improving, 123
    demographics of Israel, 118
    Israel's Dying Patient Act 2006, 120
    Jewish law, 121
    patient autonomy and family
        consultation, 122–23
    rabbinical consultation, 121–22
health literacy, and approaching cancer
    patients, 444
health-related suffering, global burden
    of, 392*f*
health system, and barriers to addressing
    psycho-social and emotional patient
    needs, 14–18
help-seeking behavior
    influence of culture on, 249–50
    influence of spirituality and
        religiosity, 250–51
    sociocultural influences on cancer stage at
        diagnosis, 251–52
Herth Hope Index (HHI), 139–40
Hinduism
    basic tenets of, 229–30
    goals of human life, 231
    karma, principle of, 230, 233–34
    mind-body techniques, 235*f*, 235–36, 236*f*
    pain, suffering, and death in, 231–32
    path of nonattachment, 234–35
    and psychosocial-spiritual healing, 297
    role of rituals, 232–33
    spiritual concerns and healing in, 232–37
    traditional social system in, 232*t*
holistic care, 41–42
    components of care, 39–40
    cultural influences on palliative
        care, 40–41
    dyspnea, 34
    emotional distress, 35
    fatigue, 34
    fear, manifestations of, 35
    grief, manifestations of, 35
    interprofessional approach, 39–40
    nausea, 34
    nonpharmacological interventions, 37–39
    pain, occurrence in cancer, 34
    palliative *vs.* hospice care, 33–34
    social systems, 36
    spirituality, changes in, 35–36
    total pain model, 37*f*, 37
    unique challenges for cancer patients, 34–36
    workplace relationships, 36

hope
    and impact of emotional state on illness
        experience, 393–94
    preservation in patient
        communication, 47–52
    and role of faith in coping with cancer, 210
hope and dignity, enhancing in palliative
        care, 132, 140
    concepts of dignity, 133
    during COVID-19 pandemic, 135, 137t
    dignity-conserving care, 133–39
    evaluating hope, 139–40
    fostering hope, 139–40, 141t
    Model of Dignity, 134f
    research on patients in Poland, 201
    toolkits for dignity, 135–39
    uncontrolled pain and symptoms, 132–33
hospice care
    cultural preferences and aspects, 436
    finding meaning in, 151–52
    hospice movement in Poland, 197–98
    vs. palliative care, 33–34
Human Development Index (HDI),
        ratings from high to low-income
        countries, 368–71
human solidarity, in suffering and
        compassion, 193–94
hypnosis, and holistic care, 39

Ibn Al-Nafis, Islamic physician, 331
Ibn Sina, Islamic physician, 331
illness, perceptions of, 303–4
India
    culture and traditions, 374
    HDI rating, 60
    Indian Cultural-Spiritual Guidance in
        Caring for Cancer Patients, 475–83
    Sociocultural Context and Its Impact on
        Communication, 382–90
    Spiritual Healing in Cancer Care: A Hindu
        Perspective, 229–38
India, cultural and spiritual guidance in caring
        for cancer patients, 475–76, 480–81
    implications for providing spiritual
        care, 479–80
    patient experiences, 478–79
    spiritual assessment, 479f
    spirituality in Indian context, 476–78
indigenous populations, palliative care
        delivered to, 26–27

Indonesia
    Impact of Culture and Beliefs in
        Brain Tumor Patients' Care in
        Indonesia, 414–42
Indonesia, impact of culture and beliefs on
        brain-tumor patient care, 414, 419
    beliefs of Indonesian brain-tumor
        patients, 414–16
    diagnosis, truthful disclosure of, 416–18
    multidisciplinary management, challenges
        of, 418–19
    religion as coping mechanism, 418
interprofessional approach, and holistic
        care, 39–40
interventions, spiritual, 178–79
intervention skills, education to
        further, 265–66
intrinsic dignity, 133
Iran
    The Impact of Culture and Beliefs on
        Cancer Care, 215–28
Iranian medicine, role of traditional, 219–21
Iraq
    history and ethnic landscape of, 329
    history of, 329
    Islamic Cultural-Spiritual Guidance in
        Caring for Cancer Patients, 329
    major religious groups, 329
    See also Islam, cultural-spiritual guidance
        for caregiving
Ireland, HDI rating, 369–70
Islam
    major religious groups in Iraq, 329
    principles of, 206
    and psychosocial-spiritual healing, 297
    religious coping as adaptation
        tool, 398–99
Islam, cultural-spiritual guidance for
        caregiving, 339
    barriers to spiritual care provision in
        Iraq, 338
    benefits of spiritual care, 338
    cancer care in Iraq, 335–36
    case scenario, 333
    history and religious landscape
        of Iraq, 329
    Iraqi cultural attitudes toward illness and
        death, 329–30
    Iraqi families and kinship groups, 329
    Islamic medicine, tradition of, 330–31

spiritual care in an Islamic context, 333–35
truthful disclosure of cancer diagnosis,
    331–33, 360
values and beliefs regarding cancer
    patients, 336–38
isolation. *See* loneliness
Israel
    Differences in Attitudes toward Advanced
        Cancer Care Planning through the
        Scope of Culture, 432–40
    The Health-Care Team and Culture in an
        Israeli Cancer Center, 117–24
    A Jewish Israeli Case Study in End-of-Life
        Spiritual Care for a Cancer Patient, 275
    The Landscape of Loneliness: An
        Introspective Experience of Support and
        Depression in Older People Diagnosed
        with Cancer, 99–106
Israeli cancer center, healthcare team and
    culture in, 117, 123–24
    clinical case 1: the ethical unit, 118–19
    clinical case 2: the value of life, 119–20
    culture, definition of, 117–18
    culture and anticipation of death, 120
    culture and the individual, 120–21
    culture-based care, improving, 123
    demographics of Israel, 118
    Israel's Dying Patient Act 2006, 120
    Jewish law, 121
    patient autonomy and family
        consultation, 122–23
    rabbinical consultation, 121–22
Italy
    Enhancing Dignity and Hope in Caring
        for Cancer Patients through Palliative
        Care, 132–46
    Mindfulness and Compassion Practices for
        Cancer Patients: The Impact of Culture
        and Faith in Cancer Care, 125–31

Jamaica
    Jamaican Cultural and Spiritual Guidance
        in Caring for Cancer Patients, 454–74
    traditional treatments in, 454–61
Jamaica, cultural and spiritual guidance in
    caring for cancer patients, 454, 465–67
    attitudes and beliefs regarding care, 463
    cultural factors modifying care, 454–63,
        456f, 457t, 458t, 462f
    diet, 462–63

religious and spiritual factors modifying
    care, 464–65
Spiritual Assessment Tool, 465, 466b
spiritual care plan, 466b
Jewish Israeli case study, in end-of-life
    spiritual care, 275, 283–84
    context for, 275–76
    family member assessment, interventions,
        outcomes, 283
    family member spiritual-care visit, first, 280
    family member spiritual-care visit,
        second, 280–81
    midrash, recitation of, 279–80
    patient assessment, interventions,
        outcomes, 281–83
    patient spiritual-care visit, first, 276–78
    patient spiritual-care visit, fourth, 279–80
    patient spiritual-care visit, second, 278
    patient spiritual-care visit, third, 278–79
    scripture reading, 277–78
Job, compassion and biblical book of, 190–93
job description, lack of for healthcare
    professionals, 266

karma, principle of, 230, 233–34
Kenya
    HDI rating, 370
    Psychosocial-Spiritual Healing: An
        Impression of the Impact of Culture and
        Faith in Cancer Care in Africa., 295–300

Latin American cultural values, attitudes, and
    preferences, 346
    caregiver's role, 345
    decision-making processes, 344–45
    integrating cultural values into care, 341–43
    Latin American cultural context and
        palliative care, 341
    and palliative and end-of-life care, 340–
        41, 344–46
    place of care and place of death, 345
    spiritual care and relationships with
        clinicians, 346
    spirituality and religiosity, 343–44
loneliness, 99
    further research, 104
    older adults, impact of loneliness on health
        of, 101–4
    as public health crisis, 100
    vs. solitude, 100–1

Malaysia, HDI rating, 369
Man's Search for Meaning (Frankl), 367, 394
Maori culture and practices, 26–27
medical information, cultural patterns in
    sharing, 437–38
medical psychology
    role with oncology patients, 426–27
    spirituality and psychology, relationship
        between, 427–28
medical subculture, and challenge of truth-
    telling, 46–47
medicinal plants, and cancer care in Jamaica,
    455–61, 456f, 457t, 458t
mental health distress, associated
    sociodemographic and clinical
    factors, 65
mental health distress and suicidality,
    barriers to identifying, 66–69
    cultural barriers, 67–69
    psychological barriers, 66–67
    systemic barriers, 66
mental health distress and suicidality, clinical
    implications and recommendations for
    best practices, 69–70
Mexico
    Support and Palliative Care for Cancer
        Patients in Mexico, 319–28
Middle East Cancer Consortium, 187
    compassion, as a common
        language, 189–90
    compassion, examples of, 187–89
    and fulfilling a destiny, 195
    human solidarity in suffering and
        compassion, 193–94
    Job, compassion and biblical book
        of, 190–93
    lessons learned in suffering and
        compassion, 195–96
Middle Eastern cultural perspectives in
    cancer care, 357, 363
    communication practices, 362
    complementary and traditional
        medicine, 361–62
    culture, definition and purpose of, 357
    death and dying, taboos regarding, 363
    diagnosis and management, 359–62
    family values and dynamics, 358–59
    nondisclosure of diagnosis, 360
    and pain management, 362
    palliative care, 362–63

religion and spiritual needs, 358
screening and prevention, obstacles
    to, 358–59
social views, 360
spiritual perspectives, 360–61
stigma and social values, 359
midrash, recitation to patient, 279–80
mind-body techniques, and spiritual healing
    in Hinduism, 235f, 235–36
mindfulness and compassion practices for
    patients, 125–26, 129
    clinical practices and
        competencies, 128–29
    compassion-focused therapy (CFT), 126,
        127, 128–29
    transcultural and transreligious
        processes, 126–29
mindfulness-based interventions for
    pain, 38
Model of Dignity, 134f
moksha, goal of, 230
Montenegrin society, characteristics
    of, 424–26
    See also multiethnic societies,
        personalization of oncology in
Montenegro
    The Contribution of Spiritual, Religious,
        and Customary Heritage to the
        Personalization of Modern Oncology
        in Multiethnic Societies of Developing
        Countries, 422–30
Morocco
    Emotional State, Spirituality, and Religion's
        Effect on the Acceptance of Cancer,
        391–400
multidisciplinary management, and brain-
    tumor patients in Indonesia, 418–19
multiethnic societies, personalization of
    oncology in, 422–23, 429–30
    medical psychology, role with oncology
        patients, 426–27
    medical psychology, role with
        patients, 426–27
    personalized medicine,
        accomplishing, 423–24
    spirituality and psychology, relationship
        between, 427–28
multimodel interventions, 37–38
Murthy, Vivek, 100
music therapy, and holistic care, 38

Native American worldviews, medicine wheel and, 174
nausea
as challenge for patients, 34
control in palliative care, 322
New Zealand
Caring at the Culture and Spirituality Interface, 22–31
palliative care in, 26–27
Nigeria
Breast Cancer Survivorship in Nigeria, 401–13
HDI rating, 370–71
Nigeria, breast cancer survivorship in, 401–3, 409–10
detection and treatment, 403–5
experiences of survivorship, 406
narrative accounts of survivors, 403, 404f
support systems, 405–6
wider context of, 407–9
"No Man Is an Island" (Donne), 193–94
nonattachment, path of, 234–35
nonpharmacological interventions
anxiety and depression, 81–82
miracle drugs, 326
total pain model and, 37–39
nurses, emotional support and spiritual care by, 86–87
attributes of, 91–93, 91t, 92f, 93b
challenges in palliative care, 87–89
cultural context, 89–91
developing competency, 93–95
spiritual distress, addressing, 92–93
nurses, gender and culture as barriers to care, 216

older adults, impact of loneliness on health of, 101–4
Oman, Sultanate of
Healing the Psychological and Emotional Aspects of Cancer, 75–85
oncology
culturally competent care, 149–50
and finding meaning in cancer care, 149
history and practice in the Dominican Republic, 447–48
opioid consumption
in African countries, 310f, 311–13, 314, 315
attitudes and preferences in Latin America, 344

cultural messages regarding, 373
in Iraq, 336

pain
assessment and management in India, 478–79
control in palliative care, 321
in Hinduism, 231–32
nonpharmacological interventions, 37–39
prevalence in cancer, 34
total pain model, 37f, 37, 173, 174f
pain care, in French-speaking African countries, 309–11, 315–16
barriers to care, 311–15, 312t
and education and skills training in palliative care, 314–15
influence of beliefs and culture on, 313–14
main barriers to access, 311, 312t
opioid consumption, 310f, 311–13
opioid use, and training in palliative care, 314–15
opioid use, fear of, 314
opioid use, policies and regulations for, 315
pain management
attitudes and preferences in Latin America, 344
Filipino attitudes toward, 153–54
Iranian attitudes toward, 217–18
for Iraqi cancer patients, 217–18
and Middle Eastern cultural perspectives in cancer care, 362
"pain of the soul," and provision of spiritual care to patients and families, 86–87
palliative care
alleviating suffering in, 323–25
basic comfort, providing, 326–27
challenges to providing emotional support, 87–89
in China, 23–24
communication in, 323
cultural influences on, 40–41
emotional support by nurses, 93–95
emotional support in, 325
four stages of, 215–16
lack of education and skills training in, 314–15
and Middle Eastern cultural perspectives in cancer care, 362–63
in New Zealand, 26–27
for pediatric patients, 61

palliative care (*cont.*)
  pillars of, 319
  settings for, 205
  in Sub-Saharan Africa, 27–28
  in Taiwan, 24–25
  vs. hospice care, 33–34
palliative care, enhancing dignity and hope
    in, 132, 140
  concepts of dignity, 133
  during COVID-19 pandemic, 135, 137*t*
  dignity-conserving care, 133–39
  evaluating hope, 139–40
  fostering hope, 139–40, 141*t*
  Model of Dignity, 134*f*
  toolkits for dignity, 135–39
  uncontrolled pain and symptoms, 132–33
palliative care, impact of Latin American
    cultural values, attitudes, and
    preferences, 340–41, 344–46
  caregiver's role, 345
  decision-making processes, 344–45
  integrating cultural values into care, 341–43
  Latin American cultural context, 341
  place of care and place of death, 345
  spiritual care and relationships with
    clinicians, 346
  spirituality and religiosity, 343–44
palliative care, role of spirituality among
    patients in, 197, 201–2
  components of spirituality, 200
  and hospice movement in Poland, 197–98
  research on patients in Poland, 200–1
  role of chaplains, 198–99
  role of medical staff, 199–0
palliative care and support, in Mexico, 319
  alleviating suffering, 323–25
  basic comfort, 326–27
  communication, 323
  culture and attempting cancer cures, 326
  emotional support, 325
  pillars of palliative care, 319
  symptom control, 320–22
  symptom control, general principles
    of, 320
palliative care patients, role of faith in coping
    with cancer, 205–6, 211–12
  changes in religious habits and
    practices, 209–10
  coping, types of, 208–9, 418

  coping methods, 210, 418
  death, perspectives on, 207–8
  Islam, principles of, 206
  religious and cultural beliefs, impact of,
    209, 211
  spirituality, definition of, 207
Palliative Performance Scale (PPS), 3–4
pastoral care
  experiences in advanced cancer care, 166
  role of chaplains in spiritual care, 198–99
  as spiritual intervention, 178
patient autonomy, cultural preferences and
    aspects, 436
Patient Dignity Inventory, 138
Patient Dignity Question, 135–38
patients
  and barriers to addressing psycho-social
    needs, 262–64
  unique challenges for, 34–36
pediatric cancer, providing psychosocial-
    spiritual support in, 57, 61
  discussing diagnosis, 57–58
  end-of-life care and palliative care, 61
  psychosocial status of families, 58–60
  traditional attitudes, 60
personalization of oncology, in multiethnic
    societies, 422–23, 429–30
  medical psychology, role with
    patients, 426–27
  personalized medicine,
    accomplishing, 423–24
  spirituality and psychology, relationship
    between, 427–28
Philippine culture, religiosity and spirituality
    in, 150–52
Philippines
  Meaning-Making in Coping with
    Cancer, 148–58
physical distress, influence of spirituality
    on, 180
Plato, 100
Poland
  The Role of Spirituality among Palliative
    Care Patients in Poland, 197–203
Polish Association for Spiritual Care in
    Medicine, 200
Polish culture, religiosity and spirituality in,
    197, 200–1
prevention, cultural considerations in, 216

Primordial Energy of Activations and Transcendence (PEAT), 426–27
prognostic information
  compassionate truth-telling, 52–54, 331–33
  and physician-patient communication, 47–52
prostate cancer, impact of diet on, 462–63
Psalms, reading from, 277–78
psychological and emotional aspects of cancer, 75–76
  adjustment disorders, 78
  assessment of anxiety and depression, 79–81
  cultural considerations, 76–77
  framework for clinical practice, 82
  management of anxiety and depression, 81–82
  psychological disorders among cancer patients, 78–79
  spiritual considerations, 76–77
  unmanaged psychological and psychiatric disorders, 77
psychological and psychiatric disorders, consequences of unmanaged, 77
psychological assessment, 3–4
psychology and spirituality, relationship between, 427–28
psycho-oncology, mindfulness and compassion practices and, 125–26
psycho-social and emotional needs, barriers to addressing, 261–62, 269
  barriers for healthcare professionals, 264–67
  barriers originating from health system, 267–69
  barriers originating from patient and family, 262–64
  communication difficulties, 264
  lack of integrated model for care, 268–69
  stigmatization, fear of, 263–64
  unawareness and refusal, 262–63
psychosocial burden of cancer, in sexual and gender minority patients, 107–8
  clinical care recommendations, 111
  disclosing sexual and gender-minority status, 110–11
  limited family and social support, 110
  specific cancer risks, incidence rates, and outcomes, 108
  understanding psychosocial burden, 109–11

psychosocial factors, and quality of care, 65–66
  clinical implications and recommendations, 69–70
  mental health distress and suicidality, barriers to identifying, 66–69
psychosocial-spiritual healing, 295–96, 299
  cultural influences on care, 296
  spirituality and faith healing, 296–99
psychosocial-spiritual support, providing to children, 57, 61
  discussing diagnosis, 57–58
  end-of-life care and palliative care, 61
  psychosocial status of families, 58–60
  traditional attitudes, 60

Qanun (Canon), by Avicenna, 331
Qigong, and holistic care, 38
quality of care, psychosocial factors and, 65–66
  clinical implications and recommendations, 69–70
  mental health distress and suicidality, barriers to identifying, 66–69
quality of life, influence of spirituality on, 173, 180, 184
  assessment of spirituality, 175–78, 176t
  case study 1, 182
  case study 2, 182–83
  common terms and definitions, 174, 175t
  outcomes, 179–80
  physical distress, 180
  research considerations, 181
  social distress, 181
  spiritual interventions, 178–79, 179t
  total pain model, 173, 174f
Quran
  and effect of religion on acceptance of cancer, 397
  and religious coping as adaptation tool, 398
  and spiritual care in an Islamic context, 333–34

Al-Razi, famed Islamic physician, 331
Reiki, and holistic care, 38
religion, effect on acceptance of cancer, 391
  religious coping as adaptation tool, 397–99, 418

religion and spirituality
  and caring for cancer patients in the
    Dominican Republic, 448–49
  in Costa Rica, 353
  and Middle Eastern cultural perspectives
    in cancer care, 358
religiosity
  influence on help-seeking and treatment
    choices, 250–51
  and palliative care in Latin
    America, 343–44
  in Philippine culture, 150–52, 156
  in Poland, 197, 200–1
  religious coping as adaptation tool, 397–
    99, 418
  See also spirituality
religious beliefs, role in cancer
    management, 221–22
religious heritage, contribution to
    personalization of oncology, 422–
    23, 429–30
  medical psychology, role with
    patients, 426–27
  personalized medicine,
    accomplishing, 423–24
  spirituality and psychology, relationship
    between, 427–28
religious impacts, on advanced cancer care,
    163–64, 169–70
  Australian patients and caregivers,
    spiritual well-being and views, 164–67
  implications for care, 168–69
  importance of spirituality or
    religion, 164–65
  pastoral care, 166
  and religious affiliation, 165
  role of hospitals in supporting spiritual or
    religious requirements, 166–67
  spiritual requirements and
    concerns, 165–66
Republic, The (Plato), 100
resources and information, and approaching
    cancer patients, 444
rituals, and spiritual healing in
    Hinduism, 232–33
role, defining for healthcare
    professionals, 266

samsara, cycle of, 230f, 230
Saunders, Cecily, 386

school attendance, and pediatric cancer
    patients, 59
screening, cultural considerations in, 216
scripture reading, and end-of-life spiritual
    care, 277–78
sexual-minority patients, psychosocial
    burden of cancer in, 107–8
  clinical care recommendations, 111
  disclosing sexual and gender-minority
    status, 110–11
  limited family and social support, 110
  specific cancer risks, incidence rates, and
    outcomes, 108
  understanding psychosocial
    burden, 109–11
Singapore
  culture and traditions, 373
  HDI rating, 368–69
sleep disturbances, 34
social assessment, 3–4
social distress, influence of spirituality
    on, 181
social isolation. See loneliness
socialization, pediatric patients and their
    families, 59
social systems, 36
social values, and Middle Eastern
    perspectives in cancer care, 359
social views, and Middle Eastern perspectives
    in cancer care, 360
sociocultural context, and communication,
    382, 387
  ABCDE approach to exploring, 387
  death, discussion of, 386–87
  in decline and terminal phase, 386–87
  in decompensation phase, 385
  in dependency phase, 385–86
  diagnosis, disclosure of, 382–84
  family-centric communication, 384
sociocultural influences, and cancer stage at
    diagnosis, 251–52
solidarity, in suffering and
    compassion, 193–94
solitude vs. loneliness, 100–1
Spain
  Nurses Providing Emotional Support
    and Spiritual Care to Patients and
    Families, 86–98
Spanish society, religion and spirituality
    support in, 89–91

spiritual assessment, 3–4, 479f
spiritual assessment, methods and rationale
  for, 10–11, 18
  FICA Spiritual Assessment Tool, 13t
  health care providers, role of, 12–14,
    17, 18f
  methods for assessment, 12–14, 13t
  patient-initiated questions, 13–14
  patient interviews, 15–16
  patient interviews, timing and
    location of, 16
  referrals, 14
  vignette I, 11–12
  vignette I, analysis, 12–14
  vignette II, 14–15
  vignette II, analysis, 15–16
  vignette III, 16–17
  vignette III, analysis, 17
Spiritual Assessment Tool, and cancer care in
  Jamaica, 465, 466b
spiritual beliefs, role in cancer
  management, 221–22
spiritual care
  in an Islamic context, 333–35
  and assessment in whole-person care, 3–6
  barriers to provision in Iraq, 338
  and cancer patients in India, 479–80
  in Chinese culture, 245–46
  family role in, 241–42
  provision of, 76–77
  and relationships with clinicians, 346
  and whole-person approach to care, 1
spiritual care, by nurses, 86–87
  attributes of, 91–93, 91t, 92f, 93b
  challenges in palliative care, 87–89
  cultural context, 89–91
  developing competency, 93–95
  spiritual distress, addressing, 92–93
spiritual considerations, in cancer
  care, 76–77
spiritual distress
  addressing, 92–93
  manifestations of, 285–86
spiritual guidance, in caring for cancer
  patients in India, 475–76, 480–81
  implications for providing spiritual
    care, 479–80
  patient experiences, 478–79
  spiritual assessment, 479f
  spirituality in Indian context, 476–78

spiritual guidance, in caring for cancer
  patients in Jamaica, 454, 465–67
  attitudes and beliefs regarding care, 463
  cultural factors modifying care, 454–63,
    456f, 457t, 458t, 462f
  diet, 462–63
  religious and spiritual factors modifying
    care, 464–65
  Spiritual Assessment Tool, 465, 466b
  spiritual care plan, 466b
spiritual guidance, in caring for cancer patients
  in the Dominican Republic, 451–52
  cultural history and religious
    factors, 450–51
  economic factors, 449–50
  historical background, 446–47
  and practice of oncology, 447–48
  religion and spirituality, 448–49
spiritual guidance, in caring for cancer
  patients in Uganda, 441, 445
  approaches to cancer care, 442
  guidance on approaching cancer
    patients, 443–45
  and spiritual and cultural diversity, 441
  Ugandan context, 442–43
spiritual healing, Hindu perspective on,
  229, 237
  basic tenets of Hinduism, 229–30
  karma, principle of, 230, 233–34
  mind-body techniques, 235f, 235–36, 236f
  pain, suffering, and death, 231–32
  path of nonattachment, 234–35
  rituals, 232–33
  spiritual concerns and healing, 232–37
spiritual heritage, contribution to
  personalization of oncology, 422–
    23, 429–30
  medical psychology, role with
    patients, 426–27
  personalized medicine,
    accomplishing, 423–24
  spirituality and psychology, relationship
    between, 427–28
spiritual impacts, on advanced cancer care,
  163–64, 169–70
  Australian patients and caregivers,
    spiritual well-being and views, 164–67
  implications for care, 168–69
  importance of spirituality or
    religion, 164–65

spiritual impacts, on advanced
cancer care (*cont.*)
pastoral care, 166
and religious affiliation, 165
role of hospitals in supporting spiritual or
religious requirements, 166–67
spiritual requirements and
concerns, 165–66
spirituality
in an Indian context, 476–78
changes in, 35–36
components of, 200
definition of, 22–23, 76, 163, 207, 333
definitions and characteristics of, 371–72
and faith healing, 296–99
influence on help-seeking and treatment
choices, 250–51
and palliative care in Latin
America, 343–44
in Philippine culture, 150–52, 156
spirituality, and cancer care, 367–68, 378
acknowledgments and narratives, 378–81
culture and tradition, 372–75
definitions and characteristics of
spirituality, 371–72
other traditional beliefs and
practices, 375–76
patient experiences, 376–78
in Uganda, 376t, 377t
spirituality, effect on acceptance of cancer,
391, 399
impact of cancer on individual
spirituality, 396f
spiritual well-being before, during, and
after cancer, 394–96
spirituality, influence on quality of life, 173,
180, 184
assessment of spirituality, 175–78, 176t
case study 1, 182
case study 2, 182–83
common terms and definitions, 174, 175t
outcomes, 179–80
physical distress, 180
research considerations, 181
social distress, 181
spiritual interventions, 178–79, 179t
total pain model, 174f
spirituality, role among patients in palliative
care, 197, 201–2

components of spirituality, 200
and hospice movement in Poland, 197–98
research on patients in Poland, 200–1
role of chaplains, 198–99
role of medical staff, 199–0
spirituality and culture interface, 22–23, 29
future research, 28–29
spirituality and existentialism, in the healing
process, 285–86
accelerating access to care, 290–91
benefits of existential well-being, 287–88
capacity-building for spiritual care
providers, 291
and in terminal illness, 288–89
spirituality and psychology, relationship
between, 427–28
spirituality and religion
and caring for cancer patients in the
Dominican Republic, 448–49
in Costa Rica, 353
and Middle Eastern cultural perspectives
in cancer care, 358
spiritual well-being, before, during, and after
cancer, 394–96
stigmatization
and addressing emotional and psychosocial needs, 263–64
and Middle Eastern perspectives in cancer
care, 359
Sub-Saharan Africa
Caring at the Culture and Spirituality
Interface, 22–31
palliative care in, 27–28
sociocultural influences on cancer stage at
diagnosis, 251–52
suffering
alleviating in palliative care, 323–25
concept in Hinduism, 231–32
health-related suffering, global burden
of, 392f
suicidality, associated sociodemographic and
clinical factors, 65
suicide, moral views on, 67
Sultanate of Oman
Healing the Psychological and Emotional
Aspects of Cancer, 75–85
support systems
and breast cancer survivorship in
Nigeria, 405–6

inadequacy of for healthcare
   professionals, 267
survivorship, definition of, 402
   See also breast cancer survivorship, in
      Nigeria
symptom control, palliative care and, 320–22

Taiwan
   Caring at the Culture and Spirituality
      Interface, 22–31
   palliative care in, 24–25
terminal illness, existential healing in, 288–89
terminal phase, communication in, 386–87
Therapeutic Touch, and holistic care, 38
*Together: The Healing Power of Human
   Connection in a Sometimes Lonely World*
   (Murthy), 100
total pain model, 37*f*, 37
traditional treatments
   and cancer outcomes, 254
   disclosure of use, 253–54
   future research directions, 254–55
   guidance on approaching cancer
      patients, 445
   in Iran, 219–21
   in Jamaica, 454–61, 456*f*, 457*t*, 458*t*
   and Middle Eastern cultural perspectives
      in cancer care, 361–62
   miracle drugs, 326
   reasons for use, 253
   in Sub-Saharan Africa, 27–28
   in Uganda, 443
   use in low-to-middle-income
      countries, 252
treatment
   and breast cancer survivorship in
      Nigeria, 403–5
   influence of spirituality and religiosity on
      choices, 250–51
   and whole-person approach to care, 6–7
truth-telling, challenge of
   brain tumor diagnosis in
      Indonesia, 416–18
   compassionate truth-telling, 53*b*, 52–54
   cultural and historical backgrounds, 45–
      47, 331–33
   and medical subculture, 46–47
   preserving hope, possible ethical conflicts
      in, 47–52

Turkey
   Barriers to Addressing Emotional
      and Psycho-social Needs in Cancer
      Care, 261–74
   Cultural Challenges in Providing
      Psychosocial-Spiritual Support to
      Children with Cancer and Their
      Families, 57–64
   Psychosocial Aspects of Breast
      Cancer, 302–8
   The Role of Faith in Coping with Cancer
      among Palliative Care Patients in
      Turkey, 205–14
Turkish culture
   communication and psychosocial aspects
      of illness, 304–7
   and psychosocial aspects of illness, 303–4
Turkish society, religion and spirituality
   support in, 89–91

Uganda
   approaches to cancer care, 442
   Cultural Healing Practices and Influences
      on Early Cancer Detection and
      Treatment in Uganda, 249–59
   culture, spirituality, tradition, and cancer
      care in, 376*t*
   forms of advice and treatment in, 377*t*
   guidance on approaching cancer patients
      in, 443–45
   HDI rating, 370
   most common cancers in, 442
   spiritual and cultural diversity in, 441
   Spirituality, Culture, Traditions, and Other
      Beliefs Affecting Cancer Care, 367–81
   Ugandan Culture: Spiritual Guidance in
      Caring for Cancer Patients, 441–45
   use of traditional treatments in, 443
Unamuno, Miguel de, 195
United Kingdom
   Existentialism and Spirituality in the Healing
      Process of Cancer Patients, 285–94
   HDI rating, 369
United States
   The Challenge of Truth-Telling in Cancer
      Care", 45–56
   Existentialism and Spirituality in
      the Healing Process of Cancer
      Patients, 285–94

United States (*cont.*)
    Holistic Care of the Cancer Patient, 33–43
    The How and Especially *Why*
        Clinicians Should Do a Spiritual
        Assessment, 10–21
    The Influence of Spirituality on Quality of
        Life during Cancer, 173–86
    The Psychosocial Burden of Cancer
        in Sexual and Gender Minority
        Patients, 107–16
    Psychosocial Factors of Healthcare
        Professionals and Their Influence
        on Quality of Care for their Cancer
        Patient, 65–74
    The Soul of Health Care: Caring for the
        Whole Person, 1–9

vomiting, control in palliative care, 322

whole-person approach to care, 1–3, 8
    assessment, 3–6, 4*t*
    clinical example, 2–3, 6–7
    compassionate gaze, 7
    generalist specialist model, 1–2
    spiritual care, 1
    treatment plan, 6–7, 7*t*
witchdoctors and traditional healers, in
    Costa Rica, 352–53
workload, of healthcare professionals, 266
workplace relationships, 36
World Health Organization, on cancer pain
    relief, 368

yoga
    and holistic care, 38–39
    and spiritual healing in Hinduism, 235*f*,
    235–36